# Critical Care: The Essentials and More

# Critical Care:
# The Essentials and More

Editor: Anderson Murphy

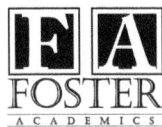

FA
FOSTER
ACADEMICS

www.fosteracademics.com

www.fosteracademics.com

FOSTER
ACADEMICS

Cataloging-in-Publication Data

Critical care : the essentials and more / edited by Anderson Murphy.
    p. cm.
Includes bibliographical references and index.
ISBN 978-1-63242-638-3
1. Critical care medicine. 2. Emergency medicine. 3. Intensive care units. I. Murphy, Anderson.
RC86.7 .C75 2019
616.025--dc23

Foster Academics,
118-35 Queens Blvd., Suite 400,
Forest Hills, NY 11375, USA

ISBN 978-1-63242-638-3 (Hardback)

# Contents

# Preface

Critical care medicine is the field of medicine that deals with life support for critically ill patients. Several hospitals have specifically designed intensive care areas for different specialties. Examples include the coronary intensive care unit (CICU) for heart disease and surgical intensive care unit (SICU) for surgeries. Some of the other types of intensive care units are neurological critical care unit, shock/trauma intensive-care unit (STICU), pediatric intensive care unit (PICU), neonatal intensive care unit (NICU), etc. The doctors who have specialized in the care and treatment of critically ill patients are known as intensivists. Most of the topics introduced in this book cover new techniques and the applications of critical care. It provides significant information of this discipline to help develop a good understanding of critical care and related fields. This book is a vital tool for all researching or studying critical care as it gives incredible insights into emerging trends and concepts.

The researches compiled throughout the book are authentic and of high quality, combining several disciplines and from very diverse regions from around the world. Drawing on the contributions of many researchers from diverse countries, the book's objective is to provide the readers with the latest achievements in the area of research. This book will surely be a source of knowledge to all interested and researching the field.

In the end, I would like to express my deep sense of gratitude to all the authors for meeting the set deadlines in completing and submitting their research chapters. I would also like to thank the publisher for the support offered to us throughout the course of the book. Finally, I extend my sincere thanks to my family for being a constant source of inspiration and encouragement.

**Editor**

# Glycocalyx and its involvement in clinical pathophysiologies

Akira Ushiyama[1], Hanae Kataoka[2] and Takehiko Iijima[2*] (iD)

## Abstract

Vascular hyperpermeability is a frequent intractable feature involved in a wide range of diseases in the intensive care unit. The glycocalyx (GCX) seemingly plays a key role to control vascular permeability. The GCX has attracted the attention of clinicians working on vascular permeability involving angiopathies, and several clinical approaches to examine the involvement of the GCX have been attempted. The GCX is a major constituent of the endothelial surface layer (ESL), which covers most of the surface of the endothelial cells and reduces the access of cellular and macromolecular components of the blood to the surface of the endothelium. It has become evident that this structure is not just a barrier for vascular permeability but contributes to various functions including signal sensing and transmission to the endothelium. Because GCX is a highly fragile and unstable layer, the image had been only obtained by conventional transmission electron microscopy. Recently, advanced microscopy techniques have enabled direct visualization of the GCX in vivo, most of which use fluorescent-labeled lectins that bind to specific disaccharide moieties of glycosaminoglycan (GAG) chains. Fluorescent-labeled solutes also enabled to demonstrate vascular leakage under the in vivo microscope. Thus, functional analysis of GCX is advancing. A biomarker of GCX degradation has been clinically applied as a marker of vascular damage caused by surgery. Fragments of the GCX, such as syndecan-1 and/or hyaluronan (HA), have been examined, and their validity is now being examined. It is expected that GCX fragments can be a reliable diagnostic or prognostic indicator in various pathological conditions. Since GCX degradation is strongly correlated with disease progression, pharmacological intervention to prevent GCX degradation has been widely considered. HA and other GAGs are candidates to repair GCX; further studies are needed to establish pharmacological intervention. Recent advancement of GCX research has demonstrated that vascular permeability is not regulated by simple Starling's law. Biological regulation of vascular permeability by GCX opens the way to develop medical intervention to control vascular permeability in critical care patients.

**Keywords:** Glycocalyx, Vascular permeability, Starling's law, Endothelial surface layer, Hyaluronan, Heparan sulfate, Syndecan-1, Sepsis, Lectin, Leukocyte

**Abbreviations:** ADHF, Acute decompensated heart failure; ANP, Atrial natriuretic hormone; BSA, Bovine serum albumin; ESL, Endothelial surface layer; FFP, Fresh frozen plasma; FITC, Fluorescein isothiocyanate; GAG, Glycosaminoglycan; GCX, Glycocalyx; HA, Hyaluronan; HS, Heparan sulfate; LPS, Lipopolysaccharide; PG, Proteoglycan; TEM, Transmission electron microscopy; TPLSM, Two-photon laser scanning microscope; VEGF, Vascular endothelial growth factor

* Correspondence: iijima@dent.showa-u.ac.jp
[2]Department of Perioperative Medicine, Division of Anesthesiology, Showa University, School of Dentistry, Tokyo, Japan
Full list of author information is available at the end of the article

## Background

More than 70 years ago, Danielli [1] and Chambers and Zweifach [2] introduced the concept of a thin non-cellular layer on the endothelial surface. This layer was thought to include absorbed plasma protein, although a direct demonstration of this layer was technically impossible at that time. About 20 years later, Copley [3] reported the endothelium–plasma interface and developed a concept in which the endothelial surface was covered by a thin molecular layer and an immobile sheet of plasma. The existence of the latter structure was identified when intravital microscopy was used to examine the hamster cheek pouch. In 1966, Luft used ruthenium red staining and electron microscopy to examine the endothelial surface [4]. Using this technique, Luft directly demonstrated the existence of an endocapillary layer that had evaded visualization using light or electron microscopy; this layer had a thickness in the range of 20 nm. Subsequent studies replicated these results and led to the concept that this layer was composed of proteoglycans (PGs) and glycosaminoglycans (GAGs) with a thickness of several tens of nanometers, as has been previously reviewed [5, 6]. Since the 1970s, the development of the intravital model for studying microcirculation has enabled several indirect and direct observations of the existence of an endothelial surface layer with a gel-like endothelial glycocalyx layer (GCX) located on the luminal surface of blood vessels [5].

## Biology of glycocalyx
### Structure of the endothelial GCX

The endothelial surface layer (ESL) is a multilayer structure that normally covers most of the surface of the endothelial cells and reduces the access of cellular and macromolecular components of the blood to the surface of the endothelium. The GCX, which is major constituent of the ESL, forms a luminal mesh that provides endothelial cells with a framework to bind plasma proteins and soluble GAGs. The GCX itself is inactive; however, once plasma constituents are bound with or immersed into the GCX, it forms the physiologically active ESL [7] (Fig. 1).

Glycoproteins and PGs form the bulk of the GCX [5, 8, 9]. PGs have a protein core to which are attached negatively charged GAG side chains. These PGs vary in the size of their core proteins, the number of GAG side chains, and their binding to the cell membrane (Table 1). The most common GAG (50–90 %) in the vascular system is heparan sulfate (HS) [10, 11], with the remainder composed of hyaluronic acid and chondroitin, dermatan, and keratan sulfates. HS is found on several core proteins including perlecan, glypican, and syndecans. Perlecan is a large HS proteoglycan found in the basement membrane. Glypicans are a family of cell surface HS proteoglycans having a glycosylphosphatidylinositol anchor [12, 13]. The syndecan family consists of transmembrane proteoglycans found in the GCX that are shed in a soluble form when the GCX becomes disordered. Each syndecan consists of an extracellular domain that contains GAG attachment sites, a single pass transmembrane domain, and a short cytoplasmic domain with phosphorylation sites. Other core proteins, such as versicans, decorins, biglycans, and mimecans, are chondroitin sulfate-bearing or dermatan sulfate-bearing proteoglycans [11, 14]. On the other, hyaluronic acid is a GAG that does not have the ability to bind to a protein core.

The composition and dimensions of the GCX fluctuate as it continuously replaces material sheared by flowing plasma [15], while throughout the vasculature, the thickness varies tenfold from several hundreds of nanometers to several micrometers [8]. The GCX forms a luminal mesh that provides endothelial cells with a framework to bind plasma proteins and soluble GAGs [16, 17].

## Physiological function of the ESL
### Vascular permeability barrier

The ESL and the GCX regulate vascular permeability [18]. The charged and complexed mesh structure of the GCX acts as a macromolecular sieve [16], repelling negatively charged molecules as well as white and red blood cells and platelets. For example, macromolecules larger than 70 kDa are known to be excluded from the GCX. Albumin is 67 kDa and has a net negative charge but binds tightly to the GCX [5] because of its

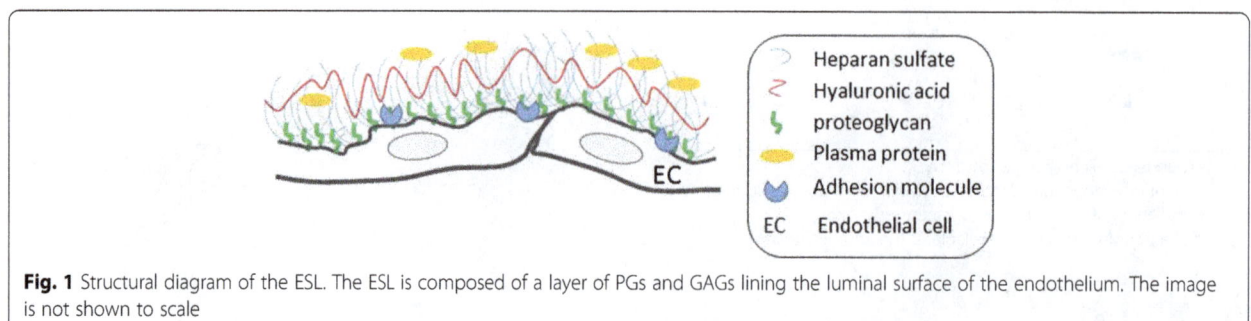

**Fig. 1** Structural diagram of the ESL. The ESL is composed of a layer of PGs and GAGs lining the luminal surface of the endothelium. The image is not shown to scale

**Table 1** Characterization of proteoglycan core proteins in glycocalyx

| Core protein | Core size (kDa) | Number of subtype | Structure characteristic | Linked GAG |
|---|---|---|---|---|
| Syndecan | 19–35 | 4 | Transmembrane protein | HS, CS |
| Glypican | 57–69 | 6 | GPI-anchored protein | HS, CS |
| Perlecan | 400 | 1 | Secreted | HS, CS |
| Versian | 370 | 1 | Secreted | CS, DS |
| Decorin | 40 | 1 | Secreted | CS, DS |
| Biglycan | 40 | 1 | Secreted | CS, DS |
| Minecan | 35 | 1 | Secreted | KS |

HS heparan sulfate, CS chondroitin sulfate, DS dermatian sulfate, KS keratan sulfate

amphoteric nature (it carries some positive charges along the protein chain). This binding reduces the hydraulic conductivity across the vascular barrier; therefore, some albumin leaks through the GCX [19]. Some pathophysiological statuses that are accompanied by the disruption of the GCX can lead to hyperpermeability.

### Mechanotransduction

The GCX also acts as a mechanotransducer, transmitting shear stress forces to endothelial cells thorough its intracellular protein domain [8, 18]. Conformational changes in the GCX, which can be induced by blood flow, trigger the release of nitric oxide, thereby contributing to the regulation of vasomotor tone and the peripheral distribution of oxygen. The GCX thus contributes to the maintenance of homeostasis in the peripheral tissues through this rheological mechanism [20].

### Vascular protection via the inhibition of coagulation and leukocyte adhesion

The GCX has been shown to be a significant binding site for blood proteins, such as antithrombin III, fibroblast growth factor, and extracellular superoxide dismutase. Based on these interactions, the most important physiological role of the endothelial GCX is vascular protection via the inhibition of coagulation and leucocyte adhesion [21, 22].

Cell adhesion molecules on the endothelium, such as integrins and immunoglobulins, are buried deep within the ESL. Under inflammatory conditions, the activation and/or externalization of proteases or glycosidases can lead to the degradation of the GCX through the digestion of PGs and/or GAGs. Shedding of the GCX may facilitate ligand-receptor interactions that promote the adhesion of leukocytes [23].

## Research methods

### Ultrastructure observation by electron microscopy

The first image of the endothelial GCX was obtained using conventional transmission electron microscopy (TEM), which revealed a small layer approximately 20 nm thick in capillaries [4]. Since then, several TEM approaches, along with various perfusates or fixatives, have demonstrated stained GCX structures with large variations in thickness [16, 24]. When fixation techniques were applied to stabilize and prevent the loss of negatively charged structures, such as lanthanum [25], evidence of a thick ESL (up to approximately 800 nm in width) was obtained [26, 27]. Lanthanum clearly stains the hair-like structure of GCX, which enables to measure the thickness of the GCX (Fig. 2). The differences in GCX thicknesses and structures can likely be attributed to the use of different TEM approaches and fixation methods (perfusion or immersion). The use of alcohol during specimen processing can led to the considerable collapse of the dehydrated gel-like state of the GCX and replacement with organic solvents. To avoid shrinkage by dehydration, Ebong et al. used rapid freeze technique to preserve the native state of the GCX structure, which preserves a high water content, with which thicknesses were quantified as 6 μm for rat fat pads and 11 μm for bovine aorta [28]. The thickness of GCX may be longer than ever expected. The measurement of thickness is also largely different between visualization techniques.

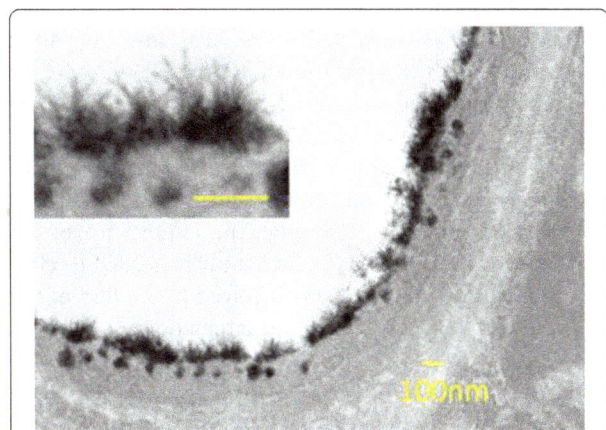

**Fig. 2** GCX layer visualized using transmission electron microscopy. Mice were fixed by perfusion with glutaraldehyde-lanthanum solution. The photos show a post-capillary venule under normal conditions. (The image was originally obtained by H. Kataoka)

## Visualization by intravital microscopy

Direct visualization of the GCX can be performed using several approaches, most of which use fluorescent-labeled lectins that bind to specific disaccharide moieties of GAG chains [29].

It has been examined a variety of fluorescent-labeled lectins for visualizing the ESL in vivo using fluorescence microscopy and shown that the specific binding of FITC (fluorescein isothiocyanate)-labeled WGA (wheat germ agglutinin) to the luminal surface of the vessel could be appropriately monitored in a mouse dorsal skinfold window [30, 31].

Recently, a novel technique that directly visualizes larger vessels using a two-photon laser scanning microscope (TPLSM) enabled a detailed description of the endothelial surface and the identification of the GCX [32, 33] because of its enhanced penetration depth, good resolution, and optical sectioning. It has been reported that thickness of the GCX of intact mouse carotid arteries was 4.5 μm by means of this technique [11].

## Functional analysis

### Leukocyte-endothelial interactions

Although the morphological profile of the GCX has begun to be elucidated, functional analyses are now needed to clarify the roles of the GCX. Receptors on the surface of the endothelium are assumed to hinder behind the GCX, and the degradation of the GCX exposes these receptors and triggers leukocyte-endothelial interactions. Lipopolysaccharide (LPS) may be a useful tool for triggering GCX degradation [34]. GCX degradation leads exteriorization of ICAM-1 (intercellular adhesion molecule 1) and/or VCAM-1 (vascular cell adhesion molecule 1) to the lumen of vasculature, which enhances leukocyte-endothelial interactions [35, 36]. The rolling leukocyte on the vessel wall is visualized in the septic model where the leukocyte is labeled with rhodamine 6G (Fig. 3a).

The heparanase-mediated mice also lose the ESL, which leads to the exposure of ICAM-1, VCAM-1 to circulating activated neutrophils, facilitating their adherence and extravasation [22, 37, 38]. Increases in the expressions of E-selectin, ICAM-1, and VCAM-1 have been reported in human microvascular endothelial cells [39, 40] and mice [41]. Although the importance of the GCX is being recognized, further study is needed to clarify the integrated mechanisms involved in the loss of the GCX and leukocyte-endothelium interactions.

### Vascular permeability

Another functional role of the GCX is as a barrier to vascular permeability. To observe changes in vascular permeability in vivo, a dye extraction method, such as the Evans blue method, has been used [42]. However, with the development of fluorescent imaging, the use of dextran

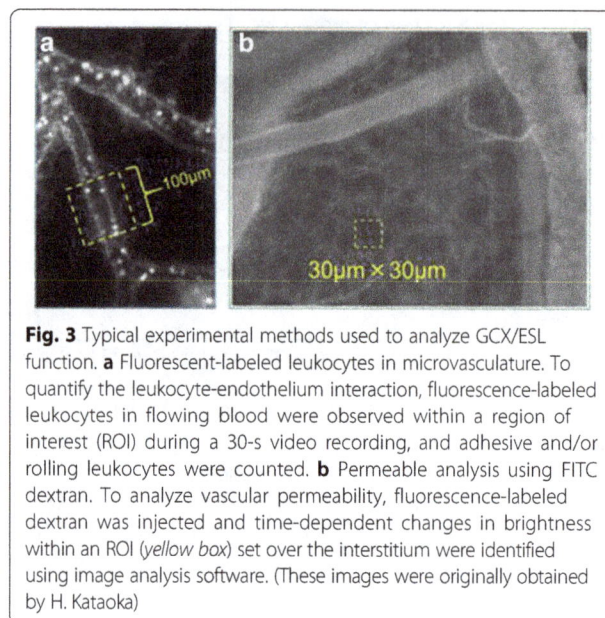

**Fig. 3** Typical experimental methods used to analyze GCX/ESL function. **a** Fluorescent-labeled leukocytes in microvasculature. To quantify the leukocyte-endothelium interaction, fluorescence-labeled leukocytes in flowing blood were observed within a region of interest (ROI) during a 30-s video recording, and adhesive and/or rolling leukocytes were counted. **b** Permeable analysis using FITC dextran. To analyze vascular permeability, fluorescence-labeled dextran was injected and time-dependent changes in brightness within an ROI (*yellow box*) set over the interstitium were identified using image analysis software. (These images were originally obtained by H. Kataoka)

covalently linked to a fluorophore has become the standard technique for qualifying and quantifying vascular permeability. In some studies, FITC-labeled bovine serum albumin (BSA; molecular weight, 66 kDa) has been used to determine the vascular permeability in rodent chamber models. As a substitute for BSA, dextran, a molecular weight of 70 kDa has also been used extensively, since it has a similar molecular weight. In a study performed by Alfieri [43], they used FITC albumin, and its leakage was quantified by using the alteration of fluorescence in the ROIs (region of interests) consisted of defined squares of 900 μm$^2$ (30 × 30 μm) located in three distinct interstitial areas. This technique can be applied to various weights of molecules. Kataoka and colleagues modified this method; FITC-labeled dextran (70 kDa) was injected intravenously in the mouse model, and the fluorescent intensity in ROIs (30 × 30 μm; Fig. 3b) using intravital microscopy was monitored. The data enabled the quantitative and continuous analysis of permeability under septic conditions (Kataoka et al., submitted).

## Pathophysiologies involving the GCX

### Revised Starling's law

### The GCX layer and its mechanism for controlling fluid movement

The GCX covers the luminal surface of the endothelium, which sieves molecules to the interstitium. The sub-GCX space in the intercellular cleft also forms a buffer space for molecules from the interstitium and intravascular spaces. This fragile and tiny structure acts as a barrier for the vessels. Studies on microvascular fluid exchange have attempted to estimate the accurate Pc (hydrostatic pressure) and π (osmotic pressure) and have revealed that the sub-GCX π is lower than the interstitial π. This means that the lower π space in the intercellular cleft insulates fluid movement along the osmotic gradient.

Based on these findings, Starling's law for fluid movement was revised [44, 45]. According to the revised Starling's principle, capillary hydrostatic pressure is the dominant factor in determining filtration and absorption (Fig. 4). Even at a low capillary pressure, absorption rarely occurs, and water movement is unidirectional. Under septic conditions, the profile for large pore filtration increases as the capillary pressure increases; this explains why fluid leakage is enhanced under septic conditions.

### Pathological alterations
#### GCX degradation and hyperpermeability
The GCX layer rarely allows water leakage through the ETC. However, once the GCX is disrupted, the permeability of the endothelial cells increases dramatically. Hyperpermeability induced by sepsis is a typical example in which GCX damage induces macromolecule leakage. However, the denudation of the vascular inner lumen itself cannot explain the leakage of water and other molecules, since endothelial cells bind tightly with neighboring cells via specific proteins, including cadherin and claudin [46, 47]. Therefore, the mechanism by which GCX degradation results in vascular hyperpermeability needs to be established. There are two pathways for the leakage of water and other molecules. The ETC has been suggested as one possible pathway and has been named the paracellular pathway [44]. This pathway requires the opening of intercellular keys, the proteins of which are known as tight junctions, adherent junctions, and gap junctions. This pathway seems to require intracellular signal conduction to loosen these junctions. A transcellular pathway has also been suggested. Vesicular transport to the interstitium has been confirmed during sepsis. The transcellular transport of macromolecules also results in interstitial edema.

#### GCX and vascular contraction
The GCX has been shown to sense blood flow and to regulate vascular tone via the production of NO (nitric oxide).

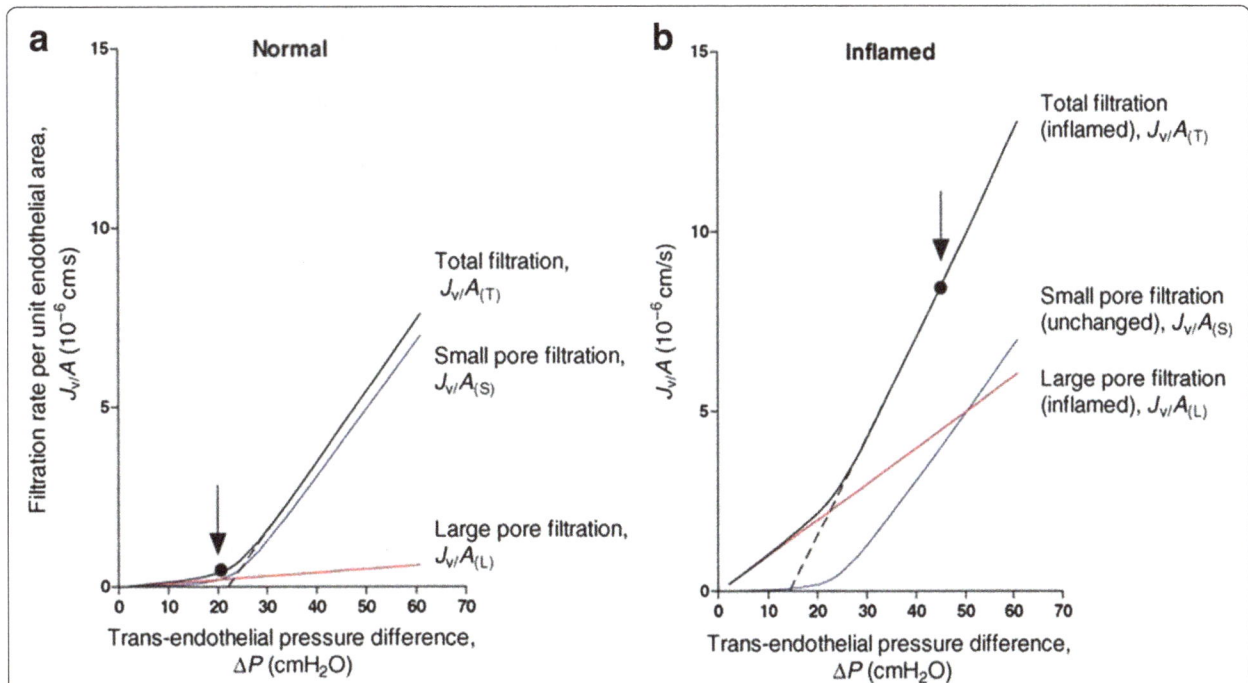

**Fig. 4** Steady-state fluid exchange simulated for a post-capillary venule, with the fluid-conducting pathways modeled as parallel small pore and large pore populations, under normal and inflamed conditions. **a** Basal low permeability state: 95 % of the hydraulic conductance is represented by small pores (radius = 4 nm; *blue curve*) and 5 % is represented by large pores (radius = 22.5 nm; *red curve*). The black solid curve shows the total fluid exchange (sum of the *red* and *blue* lines) at varying values of Pc. The vessel was perfused with Ringer solution containing serum albumin ($\Pi p$ = 25 cmH$_2$O). Pi was assumed to be constant, and the aquaporin pathway was negligible (≤10 % of total conductance). **b** Steady-state fluid exchange under increased permeability conditions in the same vessel as that shown in **a**. The *red curve* represents the flow through the large pore system after inflammation had increased the number of large pores by tenfold. The small pore population remained unchanged. The *dashed lines* represent extrapolations of the linear parts of the steady-state summed relations to the pressure axis, where their intersection gives the value of the effective COP opposing fluid filtration (reduced during inflammation). The *vertical arrows* show the typical microvascular pressures under the basal condition (A) and during mild inflammation (**b**). The increase in pressure contributed to the dramatic 17-fold increase in the filtration rate (cited from Levick JR, Michel CC. Cardiovasc Res. 2010;87(2):198–210.)

Yen et al. demonstrated that the denudation of the GCX by heparinase III reduced NO production; thus, the GCX has a physiological role in mechanosensing [48, 49], which may have an important role in the development of angiopathies and arteriosclerosis. According to the proposed hypothesis, GAGs holds negatively charged HS and consists of the structured water area. This area excludes the blood stream and protects the endothelial surface from being damaged. Positively charged cells or substances streaming in a column of negative charges create an electromagnetic field, resulting in the production of NO [50]. NO physiologically dilates vessels; if the dilation is sustained pathologically, NO further triggers free radicals and disrupts the ESL [51]. This disruption was suggested to trigger cholesterol accumulation, resulting in arteriosclerosis. Since the GCX is an insulator, this hypothesis is convincing. Further study may unveil the mechanism responsible for vascular aging, which would promote additional investigations of the GCX.

## Clinical implications
### Clinical monitoring of the GCX
Angiopathy is a frequent pathological feature involved in a wide range of diseases. The GCX has attracted the attention of clinicians working on angiopathies, and several clinical approaches to examining the involvement of the GCX have been attempted. A biomarker of GCX degradation has been clinically applied as a marker of

vascular damage caused by surgery. Fragments of the GCX, such as syndecan-1 and/or hyaluronan (HA), have been examined, and their validity is now being examined. Various clinical studies have also been reported.

The GCX is assumed to act as a size barrier for albumin filtration. Thus, GCX fragments could be a biomarker of renal disease [52]. Plasma HA is increased in patients with chronic kidney disease [53], kidney failure, hemodialysis, or peritoneal dialysis [54]. Whether this change should be interpreted as indicating degradation or increased turnover remains uncertain. However, a high concentration of HA seems to be a predictor of survival [55]. Acute decompensated heart failure (ADHF) is closely associated with AKI (acute kidney injury) [56]. Syndecan-1 has been assumed to be a predictor of death from ADHF [56], and syndecan-1 was selected as a significant predictor (odds ratio, 1.461; 95 % confidence interval, 1.256–1.677). In addition, biomarkers of the GCX are also being considered as possible indicators of the prognosis and diagnosis of various other diseases. Positive associations with these biomarkers have already been demonstrated for diabetes mellitus [57], cardiac surgery [58], Alzheimer disease [59], hematological disease [60, 61], and Crohn's disease [62] (Table 2). Thus, damage to the GCX, as reflected by the plasma syndecan-1 concentration, is attracting attention in critical care fields. Even transfusions could potentially damage the GCX. Larsen demonstrated that the expression of syndecan-1 increased 24 h after red blood

**Table 2** Clinical assessments of GCX damage

Fragment detection

| Authors | Subjects | Substances | Results |
|---|---|---|---|
| Ostrowski [65] | Trauma | Soluble VEGF receptor 1 | Positive correlation with injury severity |
| Padberg [53] | CKD | Syn-1, HA, sFlt-1, sVCAM-1, vWF, angiopoietin-2 | Syn-1, HA increased in parallel with CKD stage |
| Larsen [60] | RBC transfusion | Syn-1, sICAM-1, sVE-cadherin, hyaluronan | Slight increase in syn-1 at 24 h after transfusion |
| Larsen [61] | Myeloid leukemia | Syn-1, sICAM-1, sVE-cadherin, hyaluronan | High syn-1 was associated with bleeding, impaired platelet function |
| Neves [56] | Acute decompensated heart failure | Syn-1 | Syn-1 was high in AKI |
| Cekic [62] | Crohn's disease | Syn-1 | Disease activity was correlated with syn-1 |
| Page [63] (review) | Infectious disease | Ang-1,-2, vWF, thrombomodulin, sE-selectin, sICAM-1, sVCAM-1 | A biomarker with consistent clinical utility was not identified |

Intravital microscopy

| Authors | Subjects | Results |
|---|---|---|
| Nussbaum [57] | Children, diabetes mellitus type 1 | GCX thickness was inversely correlated with glucose |
| Koning [68] | Cardiac surgery | Pulsatile and non-pulsatile reduced perfusion density zone |
| Broekhuizen [67] | Diabetes mellitus type 2 | Sulodexide increased GCX thickness |

*syn-1* syndecan-1, *HA* hyaluronan, *sFlt-1* soluble fms-like tyrosine kinase-1, *sVCAM-1* soluble vascular adhesion molecule-1, *vWF* von-Willebrand factor, *sVE-cadherin* soluble vascular endothelial cadherin

cell or platelet transfusion in patients with hematological disease [60]. This data suggests that the detection of GCX fragments may indicate physiological turnover of the GCX. Finally, Page et al. reviewed the clinical utility of various endothelial biomarkers for infectious disease [63] and concluded that so far, none of the examined biomarkers are clinically useful as a reliable diagnostic or prognostic indicator in sepsis.

The GCX covers various receptors on the endothelial surface. Vascular endothelial growth factor (VEGF) is an important regulator of angiogenesis as well as permeability and vasodilation. This factor binds two types of receptors: VEGFR1 and VEGFR2. The binding of these receptors is regulated by soluble Fms-like tyrosine kinase receptor (sFlt-1). Reportedly, elevations in sFlt-1 are closely correlated with the APACHE II (Acute Physiology and Chronic Health Evaluation II) score, and the sFlt-1 level might be useful as a predictor of survival [64]. This receptor fragment on the endothelial surface is conceivably induced by GCX degradation. Actually, a close association has been shown between an elevation in syndecan-1 and the sVEGFR1 level ($r = 0.76$, $P < 0.001$) [65]. The appearance of this receptor fragment in the blood may reflect the extent of GCX degradation.

The diameters of peripheral vessels can be measured microscopically. The GCX layer covers the luminal surface, and red blood cells cannot pass through this layer. Consequently, visualization of the red blood cell stream

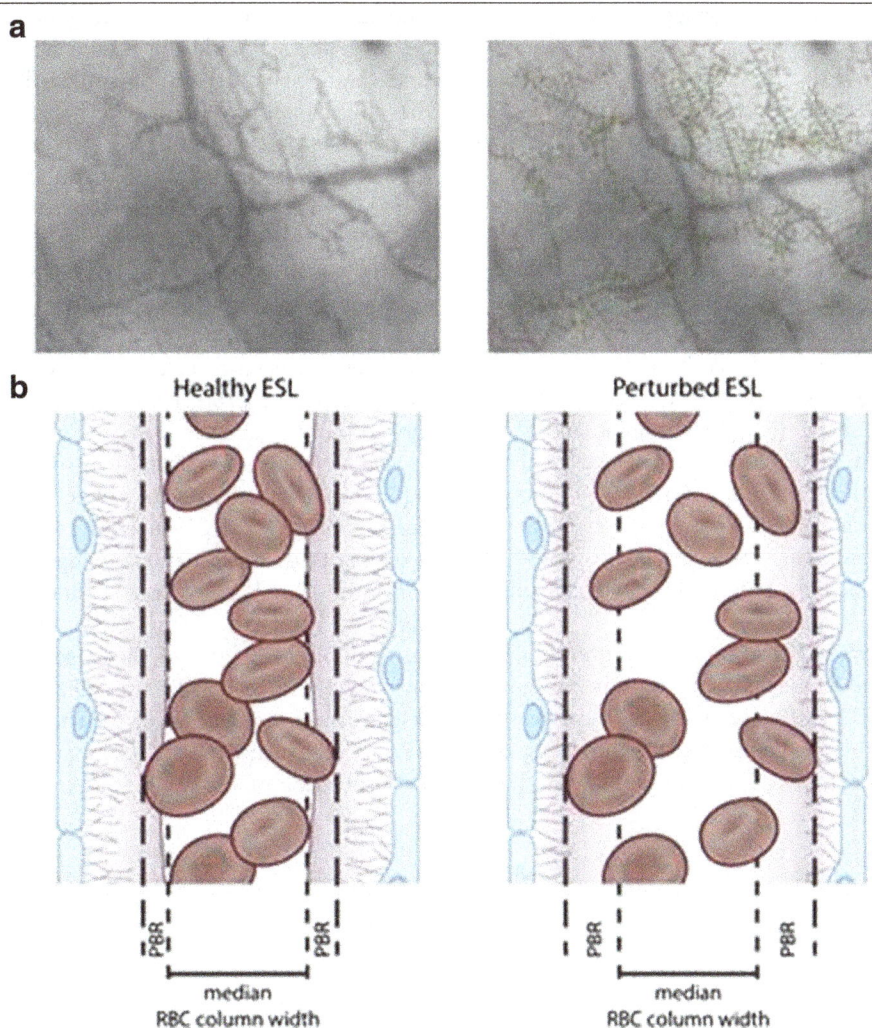

**Fig. 5** Sidestream dark field (SDF) imaging for measuring the perfused boundary region (PBR) in the sublingual capillary bed. **a** Recording of the sublingual capillary bed captured using an SDF camera (*left*). The capillaries are automatically recognized and analyzed after various quality checks (*right*). Based on the shift in the red blood cell (RBC) column width over time, the PBR can be calculated. **b** Model of a blood vessel showing the PBR under healthy conditions (*left*). The EG prevents the RBC from approaching the endothelial cell; thus, the PBR is relatively small. Under disease conditions (*right*) or after enzymatic breakdown of the EG in an animal model, the damaged EG allows the RBCs to approach the endothelium more often. This results in a higher variation in RBC column width, which is reflected as a high PBR. ESL, endothelial surface layer (cited from Dane MJ, van den Berg BM, et al. Am J Physiol Renal Physiol. 2015,308(9):F956–F966)

can be used to demarcate the GCX layer. Several clinical studies have been reported, and changes in the GCX layer have been confirmed using this technique [66]. Sidestream dark field imaging is a unique measurement for assessing damage to the GCX in situ. This measurement observes superficial vessels (sublingual vessels) and the red blood cell stream simultaneously (Fig. 5). An exclusion space exists between the vessel wall surface and the red blood cell stream. The width of this space corresponds to the thickness of the GCX or ESL. This system can be used to estimate GCX damage in patients. Several clinical reports have already been published, and significant illness-induced changes in GCX thickness have been reported [67]. Patients who have undergone cardiopulmonary bypass (CPB) have a thinner GCX in sublingual vessels, suggesting that CPB might damage the GCX [58, 68].

*Pharmacological preservation and intervention*
Since GCX degradation is strongly correlated with disease progression, pharmacological intervention to prevent GCX degradation has been widely considered (Table 3). Hyperpermeability and thrombotic activation may be targets of such interventions. HA is expected to help repair damaged GCX [69]. Sulodexide is a highly purified mixture of GAGs composed of low molecular weight heparin (80 %) and dermatan sulfate (20 %). Sulodexide has been used to treat patients with type 2 diabetes mellitus, and a restoration of the GCX thickness was shown [67]. Antithrombin and hydrocortisone have been reported to prevent the ischemia-induced release of HA and syndecan-1 [70, 71]. Immobilizing multi-arm heparin has also been used in an animal model to prevent thrombin formation and to protect the ESL during the induction of ischemic reperfusion injury (IRI) [72].

Hydroxyethyl starch has been reported to prevent capillary leakage [73], and its mechanism is assumed to have a plugging effect on ESL pores caused by GCX degradation [74, 75]. Whether the mechanism involves plugging or a specific interaction with the GCX remains uncertain [76].

Hydrocortisone is expected to reduce GCX damage [70]; this result has been obtained in an animal model, which also exhibited a reduction in sydecan-1 release, and tissue edema. Further experiments have shown that this mechanism involves the prevention of IRI-induced platelet adhesion [77, 78]. Sevoflurane also has a protective effect on the GCX by preventing IRI-induced leukocyte and platelet adhesion [79, 80].

Atrial natriuretic hormone (ANP) is assumed to cause the GCX shedding. ANP is excreted from the atrium and plays a role in regulating the intravascular volume. Physiological levels of this peptide have been shown to result in the GCX shedding and the promotion of vascular leakage [81]. Hypervolemia itself triggers ANP excretion. Since hypervolemia is harmful to thin layers, such as in the lung or other organs, excessive water should be drained. ANP may act to open water channels to the interstitium, resulting in the efflux of water [82]. Whether ANP is a regulator of the strength of the GCX seal or the disruption of the GCX is uncertain. In this context, matrix metalloprotease has been experimentally shown to reduce GCX damage. This pathway has also attracted attention in terms of protecting the GCX.

Although pharmacological intervention to GCX is widely challenged, the physiological synthesis and turnover has not been elucidated. There may be a key point to preserve and protect GCX from various kind of injury. Albumin has been shown to reduce GCX shedding caused by cold ischemia [83]. Also fresh frozen plasma (FFP) has been shown to protect vascular endothelial permeability [84]. GCX layer is coated by albumin and proteins; thus, these natural components may not only constitute the barrier against flowing substances but may nourish GCX. Schött et al. hypothesize that FFP may inhibit or neutralize sheddases (a diverse group of proteases) and/or that FFP mobilizes intracellular stores of preformed syndecans [85]. Further research to elucidate natural turn-over of GCX may disclose the theoretical protection of GCX.

**Table 3** Pharmacological intervention for GCX protection

| Authors | Study subjects | Substances | Insults | Results |
|---|---|---|---|---|
| Broekhuizen [67] | Patients | Sulodexide | Diabetes mellitus type 2 | GCX thickness increased |
| Gao [71] | Rats | Hydrocortisone | Pancreatitis | Improved intestinal perfusion Attenuation of Syn-1 and HA release |
| Nordling [72] | Endothelial cells | Immobilized heparin conjugate | IRI | Attenuation of thrombotic disorder |
| Strunden [75] | Isolated mouse lung | HES | Heparinase | HES attenuated interstitial edema, increased pulmonary arterial pressure |
| Chappell [70] | Isolated guinea pig heart | Corticosteroid | IRI | Increase in Syn-1 and reduction in HS |
| Chappell [79] | Isolated guinea pig heart | Sevoflurane | IRI | Increase in Syn-1 and reduction in HS |

*IRI* ischemia reperfusion injury

## Conclusions

The GCX is an extracellular matrix that covers the luminal surface of the vascular system. This structure is not just a barrier for vascular permeability but contributes to various functions including signal sensing and transmission to the endothelium. Thus, pathological changes to this structure are involved in the development of various diseases. Further research on the GCX is expected to provide useful information for the regulation of vascular-related pathophysiologies.

**Acknowledgements**
Not applicable.

**Funding**
We use no specific funding for writing this review.

**Authors' contributions**
TI conceived, planned, and organized the manuscript. AU drafted the "Biology of glycocalyx" section, HK drafted the "Research methods" section, and TI drafted the "Pathophysiologies involving the GCX" section. All authors critically revised the manuscript for important intellectual content. All authors read and approved the final manuscript.

**Competing interests**
The authors declare that they have no competing interests.

**Author details**
[1]Department of Environmental Health, National Institute of Public Health, Saitama, Japan. [2]Department of Perioperative Medicine, Division of Anesthesiology, Showa University, School of Dentistry, Tokyo, Japan.

## References

1.  Danielli J. Capillary permeability and oedema in the perfused frog. J Physiol. 1940;98:109–29.
2.  Chambers R, Zweifach B. Intercellular cement and capillary permeability. Physiol Rev. 1947;27:436–63.
3.  Copley A. Hemorheological aspects of the endothelium-plasma interface. Microvasc Res. 1974;8:192–212.
4.  Luft JH. Fine structures of capillary and endocapillary layer as revealed by ruthenium red. Fed Proc. 1966;25(6):1773–83.
5.  Pries AR, Secomb TW, Gaehtgens P. The endothelial surface layer. Pflugers Arch. 2000;440:653–66.
6.  Weinbaum S, Tarbell JM, Damiano ER. The structure and function of the endothelial glycocalyx layer. Annu Rev Biomed Eng. 2007;9:121–67.
7.  Jacob M, Bruegger D, Rehm M, Stoeckelhuber M, Welsch U, Conzen P, Becker BF. The endothelial glycocalyx affords compatibility of Starling's principle and high cardiac interstitial albumin levels. Cardiovasc Res. 2007;73:575–86.
8.  Becker BF, Chappell D, Bruegger D, Annecke T, Jacob M. Therapeutic strategies targeting the endothelial glycocalyx: acute deficits, but great potential. Cardiovasc Res. 2010;87:300–10.
9.  Alphonsus CS, Rodseth RN. The endothelial glycocalyx: a review of the vascular barrier. Anaesthesia. 2014;69:777–84.
10. Ihrcke NS, Wrenshall LE, Lindman BJ, Platt JL. Role of heparan sulfate in immune system-blood vessel interactions. Immunol Today. 1993;14:500–5.
11. Reitsma S, Slaaf DW, Vink H, van Zandvoort MA, oude Egbrink MG. The endothelial glycocalyx: composition, functions, and visualization. Pflugers Arch. 2007;454:345–59.
12. Fransson L-Å, Belting M, Cheng F, Jönsson M, Mani K, Sandgren S. Novel aspects of glypican glycobiology. Cell Mol Life Sci CMLS. 2004;61:1016–24.
13. Iozzo RV, Cohen IR, Grässel S, Murdoch AD. The biology of perlecan: the multifaceted heparan sulphate proteoglycan of basement membranes and pericellular matrices. Biochem J. 1994;302:625.
14. Iozzo RV. Matrix proteoglycans: from molecular design to cellular function. Annu Rev Biochem. 1998;67:609–52.
15. Lipowsky HH. Microvascular rheology and hemodynamics. Microcirculation. 2005;12:5–15.
16. van den Berg BM, Nieuwdorp M, Stroes ES, Vink H. Glycocalyx and endothelial (dys) function: from mice to men. Pharmacol Rep. 2006;58(Suppl):75–80.
17. Gouverneur M, Berg B, Nieuwdorp M, Stroes E, Vink H. Vasculoprotective properties of the endothelial glycocalyx: effects of fluid shear stress. J Intern Med. 2006;259:393–400.
18. Curry FE, Adamson RH. Endothelial glycocalyx: permeability barrier and mechanosensor. Ann Biomed Eng. 2012;40:828–39.
19. Levick J. Capillary filtration-absorption balance reconsidered in light of dynamic extravascular factors. Exp Physiol. 1991;76:825–57.
20. Tarbell JM, Pahakis M. Mechanotransduction and the glycocalyx. J Intern Med. 2006;259:339–50.
21. Lipowsky HH. The endothelial glycocalyx as a barrier to leukocyte adhesion and its mediation by extracellular proteases. Ann Biomed Eng. 2012;40:840–8.
22. Mulivor AW, Lipowsky HH. Role of glycocalyx in leukocyte-endothelial cell adhesion. Am J Physiol Heart Circ Physiol. 2002;283:H1282–91.
23. Shuvaev VV, Tliba S, Nakada M, Albelda SM, Muzykantov VR. Platelet-endothelial cell adhesion molecule-1-directed endothelial targeting of superoxide dismutase alleviates oxidative stress caused by either extracellular or intracellular superoxide. J Pharmacol Exp Ther. 2007;323:450–7.
24. van den Berg B, Vink H. Glycocalyx perturbation: cause or consequence of damage to the vasculature? Am J Physiol Heart Circ Physiol. 2006;290:H2174–5.
25. Chappell D, Jacob M, Paul O, Rehm M, Welsch U, Stoeckelhuber M, Conzen P, Becker BF. The glycocalyx of the human umbilical vein endothelial cell: an impressive structure ex vivo but not in culture. Circ Res. 2009;104:1313–7.
26. van den Berg BM, Spaan JA, Vink H. Impaired glycocalyx barrier properties contribute to enhanced intimal low-density lipoprotein accumulation at the carotid artery bifurcation in mice. Pflugers Arch. 2009;457:1199–206.
27. van den Berg BM, Vink H, Spaan JA. The endothelial glycocalyx protects against myocardial edema. Circ Res. 2003;92:592–4.
28. Ebong EE, Macaluso FP, Spray DC, Tarbell JM. Imaging the endothelial glycocalyx in vitro by rapid freezing/freeze substitution transmission electron microscopy. Arterioscler Thromb Vasc Biol. 2011;31:1908–15.
29. Salmon AH, Ferguson JK, Burford JL, Gevorgyan H, Nakano D, Harper SJ, Bates DO, Peti-Peterdi J. Loss of the endothelial glycocalyx links albuminuria and vascular dysfunction. J Am Soc Nephrol. 2012;23:1339–50.
30. Ushiyama A, Yamada S, Ohkubo C. Microcirculatory parameters measured in subcutaneous tissue of the mouse using a novel dorsal skinfold chamber. Microvasc Res. 2004;68:147–52.
31. Kataoka H, Ushiyama A, Kawakami H, Akimoto Y, Matsubara S, Iijima T. Fluorescent imaging of endothelial glycocalyx layer with wheat germ agglutinin using intravital microscopy. Microsc Res Tech. 2016;79:31–7.
32. Megens RT, oude Egbrink MG, Merkx M, Slaaf DW, van Zandvoort MA. Two-photon microscopy on vital carotid arteries: imaging the relationship between collagen and inflammatory cells in atherosclerotic plaques. J Biomed Opt. 2008;13:044022.
33. Megens RT, Reitsma S, Prinzen L, oude Egbrink MG, Engels W, Leenders PJ, Brunenberg EJ, Reesink KD, Janssen BJ, ter Haar Romeny BM, et al. In vivo high-resolution structural imaging of large arteries in small rodents using two-photon laser scanning microscopy. J Biomed Opt. 2010;15:011108.
34. Marechal X, Favory R, Joulin O, Montaigne D, Hassoun S, Decoster B, Zerimech F, Neviere R. Endothelial glycocalyx damage during endotoxemia coincides with microcirculatory dysfunction and vascular oxidative stress. Shock. 2008;29:572–6.

35. Yang Y, Schmidt EP. The endothelial glycocalyx: an important regulator of the pulmonary vascular barrier. Tissue Barriers. 2013;1, e23494.

36. Schmidt EP, Yang Y, Janssen WJ, Gandjeva A, Perez MJ, Barthel L, Zemans RL, Bowman JC, Koyanagi DE, Yunt ZX. The pulmonary endothelial glycocalyx regulates neutrophil adhesion and lung injury during experimental sepsis. Nat Med. 2012;18:1217–23.

37. Bashandy GM. Implications of recent accumulating knowledge about endothelial glycocalyx on anesthetic management. J Anesth. 2015;29:269–78.

38. Reitsma S, oude Egbrink MG, Vink H, van den Berg BM, Passos VL, Engels W, Slaaf DW, van Zandvoort MA. Endothelial glycocalyx structure in the intact carotid artery: a two-photon laser scanning microscopy study. J Vasc Res. 2011;48:297–306.

39. Myers CL, Wertheimer SJ, Schembri-King J, Parks T, Wallace RW. Induction of ICAM-1 by TNF-alpha, IL-1 beta, and LPS in human endothelial cells after downregulation of PKC. Am J Phys Cell Phys. 1992;263:C767–72.

40. Haraldsen G, Kvale D, Lien B, Farstad IN, Brandtzaeg P. Cytokine-regulated expression of E-selectin, intercellular adhesion molecule-1 (ICAM-1), and vascular cell adhesion molecule-1 (VCAM-1) in human microvascular endothelial cells. J Immunol. 1996;156:2558–65.

41. Henninger DD, Panes J, Eppihimer M, Russell J, Gerritsen M, Anderson DC, Granger DN. Cytokine-induced VCAM-1 and ICAM-1 expression in different organs of the mouse. J Immunol. 1997;158:1825–32.

42. Udaka K, Takeuchi Y, Movat HZ. Simple method for quantitation of enhanced vascular permeability. Exp Biol Med. 1970;133:1384–7.

43. Alfieri A, Watson JJ, Kammerer RA, Tasab M, Progias P, Reeves K, Brown NJ, Brookes ZL. Angiopoietin-1 variant reduces LPS-induced microvascular dysfunction in a murine model of sepsis. Crit Care. 2012;16:R182.

44. Levick JR, Michel CC. Microvascular fluid exchange and the revised Starling principle. Cardiovasc Res. 2010;87:198–210.

45. Woodcock TE, Woodcock TM. Revised Starling equation and the glycocalyx model of transvascular fluid exchange: an improved paradigm for prescribing intravenous fluid therapy. Br J Anaesth. 2012;108:384–94.

46. Mehta D, Ravindran K, Kuebler WM. Novel regulators of endothelial barrier function. Am J Physiol Lung Cell Mol Physiol. 2014;307:L924–35.

47. Marsolais D, Rosen H. Chemical modulators of sphingosine-1-phosphate receptors as barrier-oriented therapeutic molecules. Nat Rev Drug Discov. 2009;8:297–307.

48. Yen W, Cai B, Yang J, Zhang L, Zeng M, Tarbell JM, Fu BM. Endothelial surface glycocalyx can regulate flow-induced nitric oxide production in microvessels in vivo. PLoS One. 2015;10, e0117133.

49. Tarbell JM, Simon SI, Curry FR. Mechanosensing at the vascular interface. Annu Rev Biomed Eng. 2014;16:505–32.

50. Seneff S, Davidson RM, Lauritzen A, Samsel A, Wainwright G. A novel hypothesis for atherosclerosis as a cholesterol sulfate deficiency syndrome. Theor Biol Med Model. 2015;12:9.

51. Dull RO, Dinavahi R, Schwartz L, Humphries DE, Berry D, Sasisekharan R, Garcia JG. Lung endothelial heparan sulfates mediate cationic peptide-induced barrier dysfunction: a new role for the glycocalyx. Am J Physiol Lung Cell Mol Physiol. 2003;285:L986–95.

52. Dane MJ, van den Berg BM, Lee DH, Boels MG, Tiemeier GL, Avramut MC, van Zonneveld AJ, van der Vlag J, Vink H, Rabelink TJ. A microscopic view on the renal endothelial glycocalyx. Am J Physiol Renal Physiol. 2015;308: F956–66.

53. Padberg JS, Wiesinger A, di Marco GS, Reuter S, Grabner A, Kentrup D, Lukasz A, Oberleithner H, Pavenstadt H, Brand M, Kumpers P. Damage of the endothelial glycocalyx in chronic kidney disease. Atherosclerosis. 2014;234:335–43.

54. Vlahu CA, Krediet RT. Can plasma hyaluronan and hyaluronidase be used as markers of the endothelial glycocalyx state in patients with kidney disease? Adv Perit Dial. 2015;31:3–6.

55. Stenvinkel P, Heimburger O, Wang T, Lindholm B, Bergstrom J, Elinder CG. High serum hyaluronan indicates poor survival in renal replacement therapy. Am J Kidney Dis. 1999;34:1083–8.

56. Neves FM, Meneses GC, Sousa NE, Menezes RR, Parahyba MC, Martins AM, Liborio AB. Syndecan-1 in acute decompensated heart failure—association with renal function and mortality. Circ J. 2015;79:1511–9.

57. Nussbaum C, Cavalcanti Fernandes Heringa A, Mormanova Z, Puchwein-Schwepcke AF, Bechtold-Dalla Pozza S, Genzel-Boroviczeny O. Early microvascular changes with loss of the glycocalyx in children with type 1 diabetes. J Pediatr. 2014;164:584–9. e1.

58. Bruegger D, Brettner F, Rossberg I, Nussbaum C, Kowalski C, Januszewska K, Becker BF, Chappell D. Acute degradation of the endothelial glycocalyx in infants undergoing cardiac surgical procedures. Ann Thorac Surg. 2015;99:926–31.

59. Nagga K, Hansson O, van Westen D, Minthon L, Wennstrom M. Increased levels of hyaluronic acid in cerebrospinal fluid in patients with vascular dementia. J Alzheimers Dis. 2014;42:1435–41.

60. Larsen AM, Leinoe EB, Johansson PI, Birgens H, Ostrowski SR. Haemostatic function and biomarkers of endothelial damage before and after RBC transfusion in patients with haematologic disease. Vox Sang. 2015;109:52–61.

61. Larsen AM, Leinøe EB, Johansson PI, Larsen R, Wantzin P, Birgens H, Ostrowski SR. Haemostatic function and biomarkers of endothelial damage before and after platelet transfusion in patients with acute myeloid leukaemia. Transfus Med. 2015;25(3):174–83.

62. Cekic C, Kirci A, Vatansever S, Aslan F, Yilmaz HE, Alper E, Arabul M, Saritas Yuksel E, Unsal B. Serum syndecan-1 levels and its relationship to disease activity in patients with Crohn's disease. Gastroenterol Res Pract. 2015;2015:850351.

63. Page AV, Liles WC. Biomarkers of endothelial activation/dysfunction in infectious diseases. Virulence. 2013;4:507–16.

64. van der Flier M, van Leeuwen HJ, van Kessel KP, Kimpen JL, Hoepelman AI, Geelen SP. Plasma vascular endothelial growth factor in severe sepsis. Shock. 2005;23:35–8.

65. Ostrowski SR, Sorensen AM, Windelov NA, Perner A, Welling KL, Wanscher M, Larsen CF, Johansson PI. High levels of soluble VEGF receptor 1 early after trauma are associated with shock, sympathoadrenal activation, glycocalyx degradation and inflammation in severely injured patients: a prospective study. Scand J Trauma Resusc Emerg Med. 2012;20:27.

66. Goedhart PT, Khalilzada M, Bezemer R, Merza J, Ince C. Sidestream dark field (SDF) imaging: a novel stroboscopic LED ring-based imaging modality for clinical assessment of the microcirculation. Opt Express. 2007;15:15101–14.

67. Broekhuizen LN, Lemkes BA, Mooij HL, Meuwese MC, Verberne H, Holleman F, Schlingemann RO, Nieuwdorp M, Stroes ES, Vink H. Effect of sulodexide on endothelial glycocalyx and vascular permeability in patients with type 2 diabetes mellitus. Diabetologia. 2010;53:2646–55.

68. Koning NJ, Vonk AB, Vink H, Boer C. Side-by-side alterations in glycocalyx thickness and perfused microvascular density during acute microcirculatory alterations in cardiac surgery. Microcirculation. 2016;23:69–74.

69. Wheeler-Jones CP, Farrar CE, Pitsillides AA. Targeting hyaluronan of the endothelial glycocalyx for therapeutic intervention. Curr Opin Investig Drugs. 2010;11:997–1006.

70. Chappell D, Jacob M, Hofmann-Kiefer K, Bruegger D, Rehm M, Conzen P, Welsch U, Becker BF. Hydrocortisone preserves the vascular barrier by protecting the endothelial glycocalyx. Anesthesiology. 2007;107:776–84.

71. Gao SL, Zhang Y, Zhang SY, Liang ZY, Yu WQ, Liang TB. The hydrocortisone protection of glycocalyx on the intestinal capillary endothelium during severe acute pancreatitis. Shock. 2015;43:512–7.

72. Nordling S, Hong J, Fromell K, Edin F, Brannstrom J, Larsson R, Nilsson B, Magnusson PU. Vascular repair utilising immobilised heparin conjugate for protection against early activation of inflammation and coagulation. Thromb Haemost. 2015;113:1312–22.

73. Huang CC, Kao KC, Hsu KH, Ko HW, Li LF, Hsieh MJ, Tsai YH. Effects of hydroxyethyl starch resuscitation on extravascular lung water and pulmonary permeability in sepsis-related acute respiratory distress syndrome. Crit Care Med. 2009;37:1948–55.

74. Vincent JL. Plugging the leaks? New insights into synthetic colloids. Crit Care Med. 1991;19:316–8.

75. Strunden MS, Bornscheuer A, Schuster A, Kiefmann R, Goetz AE, Heckel K. Glycocalyx degradation causes microvascular perfusion failure in the ex vivo perfused mouse lung: hydroxyethyl starch 130/0.4 pretreatment attenuates this response. Shock. 2012;38:559–66.

76. Tatara T, Itani M, Sugi T, Fujita K. Physical plugging does not account for attenuation of capillary leakage by hydroxyethyl starch 130/0.4: a synthetic gel layer model. J Biomed Mater Res B Appl Biomater. 2013;101:85–90.

77. Chappell D, Brettner F, Doerfler N, Jacob M, Rehm M, Bruegger D, Conzen P, Jacob B, Becker BF. Protection of glycocalyx decreases platelet adhesion after ischaemia/reperfusion: an animal study. Eur J Anaesthesiol. 2014;31:474–81.

78. Chappell D, Dorfler N, Jacob M, Rehm M, Welsch U, Conzen P, Becker BF. Glycocalyx protection reduces leukocyte adhesion after ischemia/reperfusion. Shock. 2010;34:133–9.

79. Chappell D, Heindl B, Jacob M, Annecke T, Chen C, Rehm M, Conzen P, Becker BF. Sevoflurane reduces leukocyte and platelet adhesion after ischemia-reperfusion by protecting the endothelial glycocalyx. Anesthesiology. 2011;115:483–91.

80. Annecke T, Rehm M, Bruegger D, Kubitz JC, Kemming GI, Stoeckelhuber M, Becker BF, Conzen PF. Ischemia-reperfusion-induced unmeasured anion generation and glycocalyx shedding: sevoflurane versus propofol anesthesia. J Invest Surg. 2012;25:162–8.

81. Bruegger D, Jacob M, Rehm M, Loetsch M, Welsch U, Conzen P, Becker BF. Atrial natriuretic peptide induces shedding of endothelial glycocalyx in coronary vascular bed of guinea pig hearts. Am J Physiol Heart Circ Physiol. 2005;289:H1993–9.

82. Chappell D, Bruegger D, Potzel J, Jacob M, Brettner F, Vogeser M, Conzen P, Becker BF, Rehm M. Hypervolemia increases release of atrial natriuretic peptide and shedding of the endothelial glycocalyx. Crit Care. 2014;18:538.

83. Jacob M, Paul O, Mehringer L, Chappell D, Rehm M, Welsch U, Kaczmarek I, Conzen P, Becker BF. Albumin augmentation improves condition of guinea pig hearts after 4 hr of cold ischemia. Transplantation. 2009;87:956–65.

84. Pati S, Matijevic N, Doursout MF, Ko T, Cao Y, Deng X, Kozar RA, Hartwell E, Conyers J, Holcomb JB. Protective effects of fresh frozen plasma on vascular endothelial permeability, coagulation, and resuscitation after hemorrhagic shock are time dependent and diminish between days 0 and 5 after thaw. J Trauma. 2010;69 Suppl 1:S55–63.

85. Schott U, Solomon C, Fries D, Bentzer P. The endothelial glycocalyx and its disruption, protection and regeneration: a narrative review. Scand J Trauma Resusc Emerg Med. 2016;24:48.

# 2

# AN69ST membranes adsorb nafamostat mesylate and affect the management of anticoagulant therapy

Takahiro Hirayama[1,2]* (iD), Nobuyuki Nosaka[3,5], Yasumasa Okawa[4], Soichiro Ushio[4], Yoshihisa Kitamura[4], Toshiaki Sendo[4], Toyomu Ugawa[2] and Atsunori Nakao[2]

## Abstract

**Background:** In Japan, nafamostat mesylate (NM) is frequently used as an anticoagulant during continuous renal replacement therapy (CRRT). The dialyzer membrane AN69ST has been reported to adsorb NM and affect the management of anticoagulant therapy. However, the adsorbed amount has not yet been quantitatively assessed. Therefore, in this study, we evaluated the pre- and post-hemofilter prolongation of the activated clotting time (ACT) in patients with AN69ST and PS membranes. We also measured the adsorption of NM in three types of CRRT membranes using an experimental model.

**Methods:** In a study of patients who underwent CRRT using AN69ST or PS membranes in 2015 at the Advanced Emergency and Critical Care Center, Okayama University Hospital, pre- and post-hemofilter ACT measurements were extracted retrospectively, and the difference was calculated. In addition, AN69ST (sepXiris100), PS (HEMOFEEL SHG-1.0), and PMMA membranes (HEMOFEEL CH-1.0N) were used in an in vitro model of a dialysis circuit, and the concentrations of NM were measured in pre- and post-hemofilter membranes and filtrates.

**Results:** The ACT difference was significantly lower in the group using AN69ST membranes ($p < 0.01$). In the in vitro model ($n = 4$) with adsorption and filtration, the post-hemofilter and filtrate concentrations of NM in AN69ST membranes were significantly lower than those in the PS and PMMA membranes ($p < 0.01$). The NM adsorption clearance of the AN69ST membrane was significantly higher than that of the PS and PMMA membranes.

**Conclusions:** The AN69ST membrane had higher NM adsorption than the PS and PMMA membranes. This may have resulted in the lower ACT difference in patients undergoing CRRT using the AN69ST membrane than in patients undergoing CRRT using PS or PMMA membranes.

**Keywords:** AN69ST, Nafamostat mesylate, Continuous renal replacement therapy, Adsorption, Anticoagulant therapy

* Correspondence: ce-hirayama@cc.okayama-u.ac.jp
[1]Department of Clinical Engineering, Okayama University Hospital, 2-5-1 Shikata-cho, Kita-ku, Okayama city 700-8558, Japan
[2]Department of Emergency and Critical Care Medicine, Okayama University Graduate School of Medicine, Dentistry and Pharmaceutical Sciences, Okayama University Hospital, 2-5-1 Shikata-cho, Kita-ku, Okayama city 700-8558, Japan
Full list of author information is available at the end of the article

## Background

Continuous renal replacement therapy (CRRT) has a milder impact on hemodynamics than intermittent hemodialysis therapy and enables strict management of the body fluid balance, acid-base equilibrium, electrolytes, and plasma osmotic pressure. Accordingly, CRRT has been widely used in the treatment of acute renal injury [1]. However, CRRT requires long-term anticoagulation management [2]. In Japan, nafamostat mesylate (NM) is used in most patients receiving CRRT because it does not affect the patient's coagulability in vivo [3]. NM is a serine protease inhibitor with a molecular weight of 539 Da that exerts non-antithrombin III-mediated anticoagulant effects by strongly inhibiting activated coagulation factors, such as factor IIa (thrombin), factor Xa, and factor XIIa. In addition, NM also has an inhibitory effect on platelet coagulability. In the blood, NM is rapidly degraded by carboxylesterase; as a result, its active half-life in the blood ($\beta$-phase) is 23.1 min. NM can also be eliminated through dialysis. Therefore, NM exerts anticoagulant effects only in extracorporeal circulation circuits, whereas in vivo, NM is quickly inactivated, enabling safe management of coagulation [4].

The AN69ST membrane is currently attracting attention in the field of intensive care because of its ability to adsorb cytokines, making it potentially beneficial in the treatment of patients with septic shock [5, 6]. The AN69ST membrane was developed based on the AN69 membrane, which was released in the market in France in 1969. Because the AN69 membrane has a strong negative charge, it poses problems such as induction of bradykinin production [7] and adsorption of pharmacological agents such as NM [8]. Therefore, with the AN69ST membrane, surface treatment has been performed to neutralize the negative charge at the surface of the membrane. Additionally, reduction of bradykinin production has been achieved by reducing the zeta potential at the point of contact between the blood and the surface of the membrane to a level that is lower than that found in the AN69 membrane [9]. However, few studies have examined the adsorption of drugs by the AN69ST membrane, and no previous studies have quantitatively assessed the amount of adsorption.

Therefore, in this study, the pre- and post-hemofilter difference in the activated clotting time (ACT) in patients using the AN69ST membrane was calculated, and the values were compared with those in patients who used PS membranes. In addition, the amounts of NM adsorbed on AN69ST, PS, and PMMA membranes were quantitatively measured and compared in an in vitro model, and the capacity of the AN69ST membrane to adsorb NM was evaluated.

## Methods

### Measurement of the ACT and calculation of its difference

This study was performed in patients who were hospitalized at the Advanced Emergency and Critical Care Center, Okayama University Hospital in 2015, and who were receiving CRRT with AN69ST or PS membranes. In addition, we extracted data for patients whose respective pre- and post-hemofilter ACT was measured simultaneously after initiation of CRRT, and we calculated the ACT difference (ACT difference [s] = ACT post-hemofilter – ACT pre-hemofilter). For the measurement of the ACT, we used a Hemochron Response device (Heiwa Bussan, Co. Ltd., Tokyo, Japan) and Hemochron ACT tubes (Celite ACT; FTCA510; Heiwa Bussan, Co. Ltd.; Fig. 1). This study was approved by the Ethics Committee of Okayama University Hospital (approval no. Ken1610-510).

### In vitro model of a dialysis circuit and measurement of NM levels

The following hemofilters were used ($n = 4$ each): AN69ST membrane (sepXiris100; Baxter Co. Ltd., Tokyo, Japan), PS membrane (Hemofeel SHG1.0; Toray Medical Co., Ltd., Tokyo, Japan), and PMMA membrane

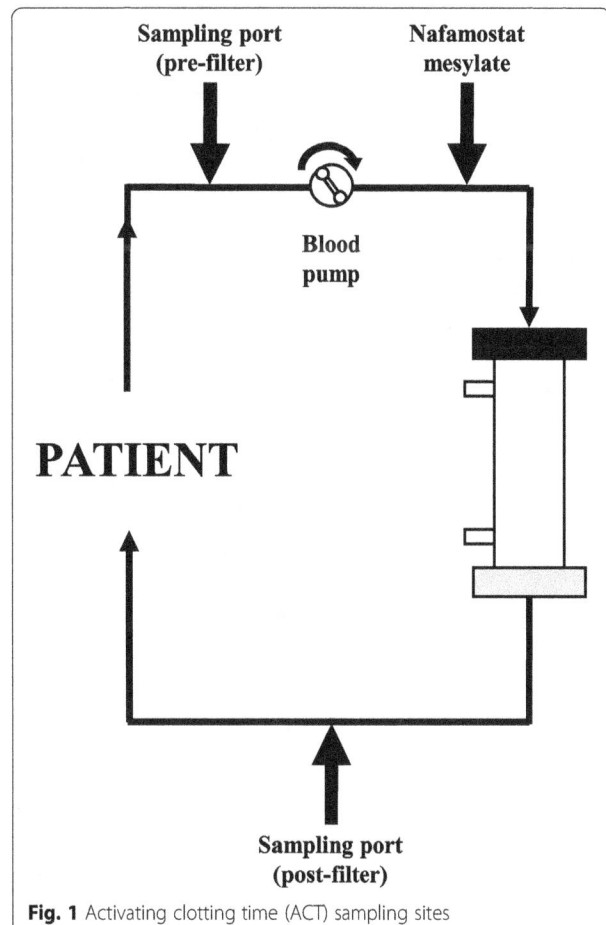

**Fig. 1** Activating clotting time (ACT) sampling sites

(Hemofeel CH1.0N; Toray Medical Co., Ltd.; Table 1). The device used in this study was a JUN-505 (Junken Medical, Co., Ltd., Tokyo, Japan). Only normal saline solution was used as the filling solution to eliminate the influence of other substances. In the clinical setting, heparin coating was performed by adding heparin sodium to the filling solution; however, because the presence or absence of heparin has been reported to not result in any differences in the amount of adsorption of high-mobility group box-1 [10], heparin priming was not performed in our study.

To calculate the NM clearance, pre- and post-hemofilter samples and filtrates were collected under the following conditions: blood pump, 80 mL/min; filtrate pump, 1000 mL/h; NM, 100 mg/h (Fig. 2). Although pre-hemofilter samples were collected from the site before administering NM in the clinical setting to observe excess or shortage of anticoagulant, we collected pre-hemofilter samples from the site after administering NM in an in vitro setting to quantify NM adsorption by each membrane. To normalize the sample concentrations, the timing of blood sampling was aligned with that of the time elapsed since the activation of the pump. The timing for sampling was considered as the time when the NM had fully reached the sampling port, which was determined based on measurement of the priming volume of the blood circuit.

The NM used in this study was nafamostat mesylate (MEEK; Meiji Seika Pharma Co. Ltd, Tokyo, Japan), and the normal saline solution used in this study was Terumo (Terumo Corp., Tokyo, Japan). Nafamostat mesylate (Wako Pure Chemical Industries, Ltd., Tokyo, Japan) was used as the standard substance, and ethyl p-hydroxybenzoate (Wako Pure Chemical Industries, Ltd) was used as the internal standard substance.

NM was quantified by high-performance liquid chromatography (HPLC). Measurement devices from Shimadzu Emit Co., Ltd. were used (pump: LC-20AT; ultraviolet/visible detector: SPD-20A; column oven: CTO-20AC; degasser: DGU-20A5R). The HPLC conditions were as follows: flow rate, 1.0 mL/min; wavelength, 260 nm; injection volume, 100 μL; C18-Supersphar column (4 μm, 125 mm × 4 mm); and column temperature, 40 °C. The mobile phase consisted of 0.1 M acetic acid (sodium 1-heptanesulfonate 6.07 g/L):acetonitrile (70:30). An isocratic analysis was performed.

Various equations were used for calculation of NM clearance (Table 2). In addition, for the AN69ST, PS, and PMMA membranes, the sieving coefficient (SC) was 1.0.

## Statistical analysis

All data are expressed as the mean ± standard deviation (SD) and were compared using chi-squared tests, Mann-Whitney $U$ tests, or one-way analysis of variance followed by Tukey's post-test where appropriate. $p < 0.05$ was considered significant. All statistical calculations were performed using GraphPad Prism 6.0 (GraphPad Software, San Diego, CA, USA).

## Results

### The difference in ACT was significantly lower with the AN69ST membrane

There were 122 and 37 ACT measurements in 19 AN69ST-treated patients and 11 PS-treated patients, respectively. Table 3 shows the characteristics of the patients participating in this study. The proportion of sepsis patients was significantly higher in the AN69ST group. Figure 3a shows the pre- and post-filter average ACT in each membrane. Compared with the PS group, the AN69ST group had higher and lower pre- and post-filter ACT values, respectively ($p < 0.01$). Figure 3b shows the pre- and post-filter ACT difference in the AN69ST and PS membrane groups. The ACT difference was significantly lower in the AN69ST membrane group ($p < 0.01$). The amounts of NM used with the AN69ST and PS membranes were 16.8 ± 7.1 and 17.7 ± 8.4 mg/h, respectively, and this difference was not significant.

### NM adsorption was significantly higher with the AN69ST membrane

Figure 4 shows the NM concentrations in pre- and post-hemofilter samples and in filtrate samples when both the blood pump and filtrate pump were activated. The concentrations of NM in the filtrate and post-hemofilter samples were significantly lower in the circuit using the AN69ST membrane than in circuits using the two other membranes ($p < 0.05$; Fig. 4). Finally, we calculated the clearance of NM with each type of hemofilter (Fig. 5). The highest clearance of NM was found when the AN69ST membrane was used ($p < 0.01$); in comparison with the findings obtained with the other membranes,

**Table 1** Characteristics of the three hemofilters

| Dialysis membrane | Material | Structure | Surface area (m$^2$) | Inner diameter (μm) | Wall thickness (μm) | Priming volume (mL) |
|---|---|---|---|---|---|---|
| sepXiris100 | Polyacrylonitrile (surface treated) | Symmetric | 1.0 | 240 | 50 | 69 |
| Hemofeel SHG-1.0 | Polysulfone | Asymmetric | 1.0 | 200 | 40 | 67 |
| Hemofeel CH-1.0N | Polymethylmethacrylate | Symmetric | 1.0 | 200 | 30 | 58 |

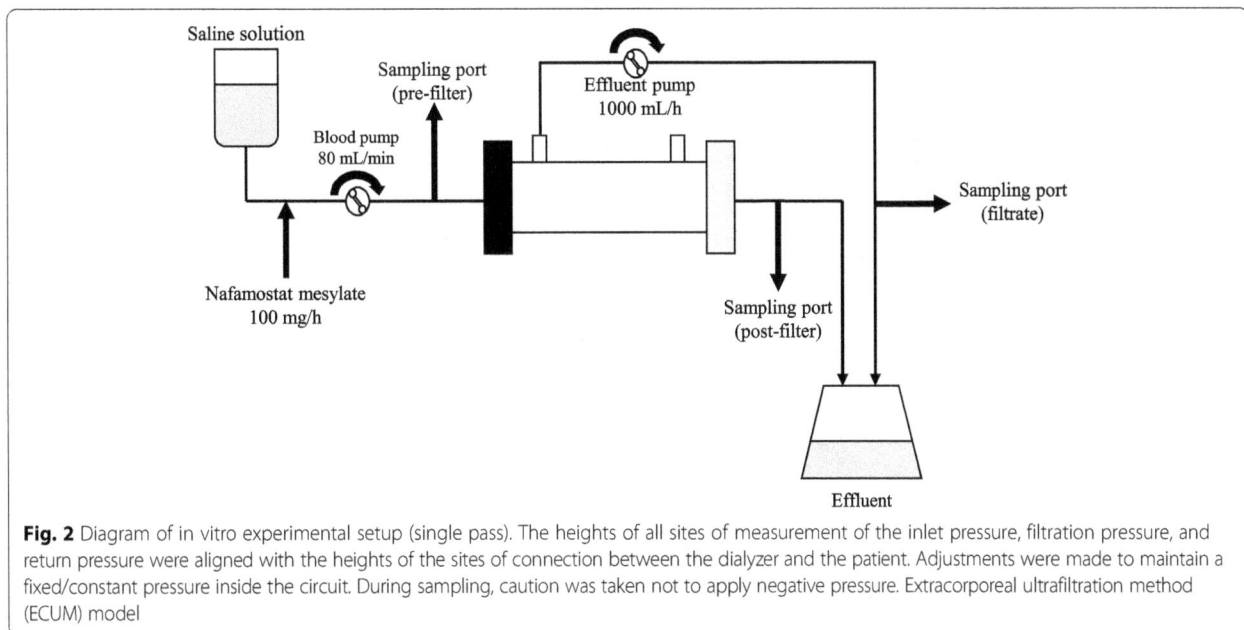

**Fig. 2** Diagram of in vitro experimental setup (single pass). The heights of all sites of measurement of the inlet pressure, filtration pressure, and return pressure were aligned with the heights of the sites of connection between the dialyzer and the patient. Adjustments were made to maintain a fixed/constant pressure inside the circuit. During sampling, caution was taken not to apply negative pressure. Extracorporeal ultrafiltration method (ECUM) model

the adsorption clearance ($CL_{ad}$) accounted for a significantly larger proportion, whereas the filtration clearance ($CL_f$) did not contribute substantially ($p < 0.01$). Comparable $CL_f$ values were found with the PS and PMMA membranes, whereas the $CL_{ad}$ tended to be higher with the PMMA membrane.

## Discussion

AN69 membranes are copolymers of acrylonitrile and sodium methallyl sulfonate and are characterized by their strong negative charge. As a result, positively charged cytokines and NM are adsorbed into the hemofilter through ion binding. For generation of AN69ST membranes, AN69 membranes were subjected to surface treatment with biocompatible polyethyleneimine, resulting in a weaker negative charge [11]. In the clinical setting, heparin priming is generally performed, where the membrane surface is coated with heparin [12]; thus, the negative charge is attenuated by addition of positive charges to the membrane. However, because some negative charges still remain, NM is adsorbed.

The basic principles of substance removal by hemofilters involve the following three elements: dialysis

(diffusion), filtration (convection), and adsorption. Given that there is no NM adsorption, diffusion would be the main removal mechanism because NM is small with a molecular weight of 539 Da. Diffusion is correlated with the ratio between the blood pump flow rate (QB) and dialysate pump flow rate (QD). In this study, however, we found a significantly smaller ACT difference between pre- and post-AN69ST hemofilter application, despite the significantly lower QD, indicating low diffusion capability. This finding suggested that NM was removed by adsorption to the AN69ST membrane.

**Table 3** Patient summary

| Dialysis membrane | AN69ST | PS | P value |
|---|---|---|---|
| Age (years) | 69.8 ± 11.4 | 67.4 ± 19.6 | N.S. |
| Sex (male:female) | 13:6 | 6:5 | N.S. |
| Body weight | 58.2 ± 14.6 | 62.3 ± 16.9 | N.S. |
| SOFA | 11.1 ± 4.0 | 9.5 ± 4.4 | N.S. |
| APACHE II | 27.6 ± 10.0 | 26.9 ± 10.4 | N.S. |
| Mortality | 6/19 (32%) | 3/11 (27%) | N.S. |
| Sepsis | 13/19 (68%) | 3/11 (27%) | 0.03 |
| QB (mL/min) | 95.9 ± 8.9 | 95.1 ± 15.4 | N.S. |
| QD (mL/h) | 934.8 ± 329.6 | 1422.4 ± 602.5 | <0.01 |
| QS (mL/h) | 517.7 ± 152.5 | 602.6 ± 312.8 | N.S. |
| QF (mL/h) | 1471.7 ± 414.7 | 1852.4 ± 662.2 | <0.01 |

Data are the mean and standard deviation or number. For intergroup testing, the Mann-Whitney $U$ test or the $\chi^2$ test was performed at suitable locations. *AN69ST* polyacrylonitrile (surface treated), *PS* polysulfone, *N.S.* not significant, *SOFA* Sequential Organ Failure Assessment, *APACHE II* Acute Physiology and Chronic Health Evaluation II score, *QB* blood pump flow rate, *QD* dialysate pump flow rate, *QF* filtration pump flow rate, *QS* substitution fluid pump flow rate

**Table 2** Clearance formulas

| | |
|---|---|
| Solution clearance (mL/min) | $CL_s = (CB_i - CB_o)/CB_i \times (QB - QF) + QF$ |
| Filtrate clearance (mL/min) | $CL_f = CF/CB_i \times QF$ |
| Adsorption clearance (mL/min) | $CL_{ad} = CL_s - CL_f$ |
| Sieving coefficient | $SC = 2CF/(C_{Bi} + C_{Bo})$ |

$C_{Bi}$ inlet (pre-hemofilter) solute concentration, $C_{Bo}$ outlet (post-hemofilter) solute concentration, *CF* filtrate solute concentration, *QB* blood flow, *QF* filtration flow

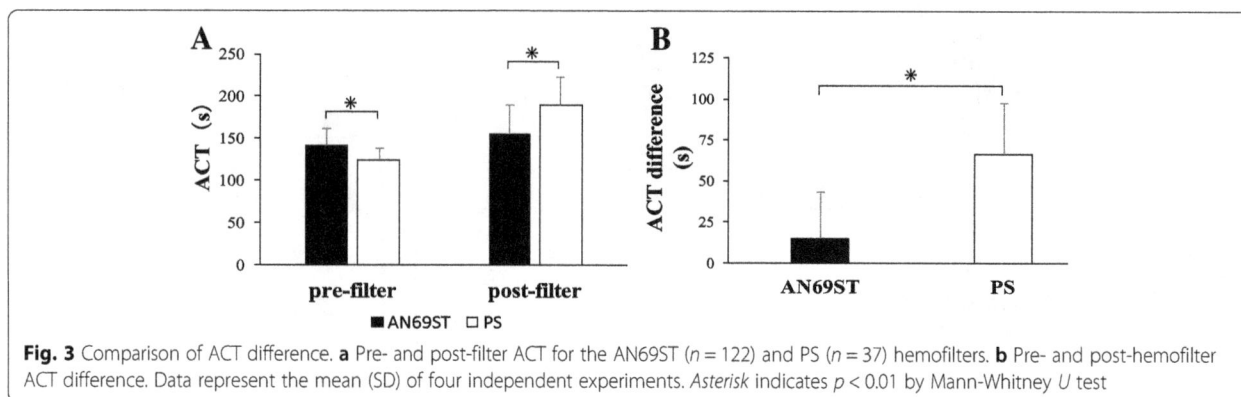

**Fig. 3** Comparison of ACT difference. **a** Pre- and post-filter ACT for the AN69ST ($n = 122$) and PS ($n = 37$) hemofilters. **b** Pre- and post-hemofilter ACT difference. Data represent the mean (SD) of four independent experiments. *Asterisk* indicates $p < 0.01$ by Mann-Whitney $U$ test

The substance removal capability of each hemofilter can be calculated using the clearance equation. In the model that we used in our experiment, the dialysate was not used to eliminate the effects of solutes other than NM. Therefore, the elimination of NM was examined as a phenomenon that was due to filtration and adsorption. $CL_{ad}$ is defined by the structure and charge of the membrane; the interactions among the charge, half-life, and size of the target substance; and the blood pump flow rate QB. Accordingly, the value of QB is considered to be the maximum value for $CL_{ad}$ [13]. Our experiment was performed with a QB of 80 mL/min; therefore, the maximum value of $CL_{ad}$ was 80 mL/min. In our experimental results, the $CL_{ad}$ of the AN69ST membrane reached a level equivalent to the theoretical maximum value, showing the strength of the membrane's adsorptive power with regard to NM. $CL_f$ represents the product of the filtration pump flow rate (QF) and the sieving coefficient (SC), and the SC is the percentage of solutes that pass through the pores of the hemofilter as a result of the filtration of substances. The three types of hemofilters that we used in our study had a maximal SC value of nearly 1.0 for NM (539.58 Da); therefore, $CL_f = QF \times 1.0$, and theoretically, the maximum value of $CL_f$ was equal to the QF value [14, 15]. The experiments conducted in our study were performed with a

QF of 1000 mL/h, i.e., 17 mL/min. The $CL_f$ of the AN69ST membrane was extremely low because most of the NM was lost through adsorption ($CL_f = 0.3$ mL/min). Additionally, for both the PS and PMMA membranes, the $CL_f$ reached the theoretical maximum value, showing that these membranes had high filtration capacity in the filtration of NM. The PMMA membrane had a neutral to weakly negative charge and had the ability to adsorb substances in the pores inside the membrane. As a result, the $CL_{ad}$ of the PMMA membrane tended to be higher than that of the PS membrane.

There are some limitations in this study. First, the patient sample size was small. The proportions of men differed greatly; however, there were no significant differences between groups, possibly because of the small sample size. Second, the proportion of patients with sepsis was significantly higher in the AN69ST group. Sepsis-associated factors may have affected the NM adsorption ability of the AN69ST filter. Third, further studies are necessary to determine how the adsorption capacity of the circuit model used in our study may change over time. Additionally, only NM was measured in this study. Accordingly, measurements were performed using normal saline solution as the filling solution. In the clinical setting, various substances and drugs in the blood are also believed to be adsorbed.

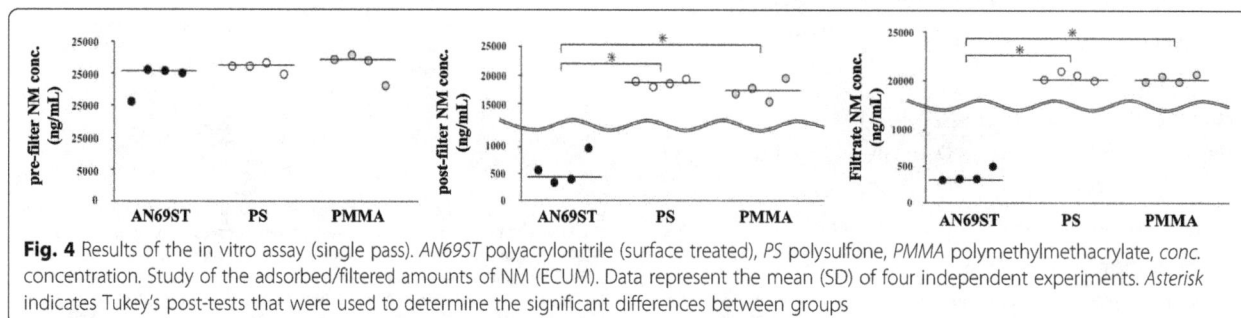

**Fig. 4** Results of the in vitro assay (single pass). *AN69ST* polyacrylonitrile (surface treated), *PS* polysulfone, *PMMA* polymethylmethacrylate, *conc.* concentration. Study of the adsorbed/filtered amounts of NM (ECUM). Data represent the mean (SD) of four independent experiments. *Asterisk* indicates Tukey's post-tests that were used to determine the significant differences between groups

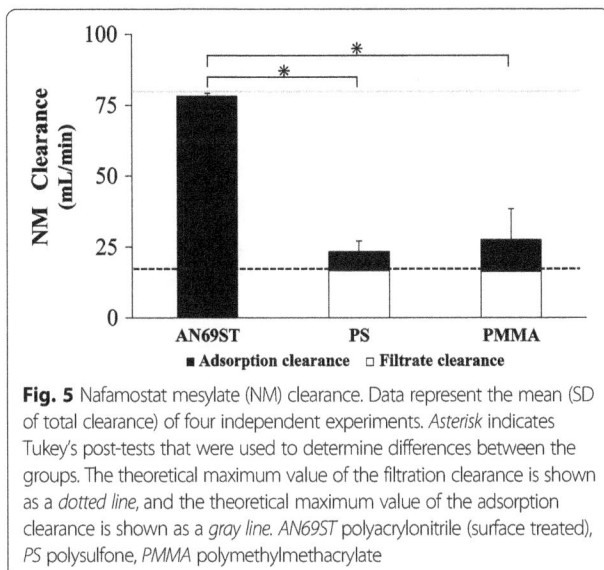

**Fig. 5** Nafamostat mesylate (NM) clearance. Data represent the mean (SD of total clearance) of four independent experiments. *Asterisk* indicates Tukey's post-tests that were used to determine differences between the groups. The theoretical maximum value of the filtration clearance is shown as a *dotted line*, and the theoretical maximum value of the adsorption clearance is shown as a *gray line*. *AN69ST* polyacrylonitrile (surface treated), *PS* polysulfone, *PMMA* polymethylmethacrylate

Therefore, NM concentrations may need to be measured from samples collected from dialysis circuits attached to actual patients.

## Conclusions

In summary, a comparison of pre- and post-hemofilter findings revealed that in dialysis patients, the ACT difference was significantly lower with the AN69ST membrane than with the PS membrane. Moreover, our study showed that this was due to the high NM adsorption capacity of the AN69ST membrane. We suggest that in dialysis circuits using AN69ST membranes, administration of additional post-hemofilter doses of NM may be useful for the management of anticoagulant therapy.

## Abbreviations
ACT: Activated clotting time; AN69: Polyacrylonitrile; AN69ST: Polyacrylonitrile (surface treated); $CL_{ad}$: Adsorption clearance; $CL_f$: Filtration clearance; CRRT: Continuous renal replacement therapy; ECUM: Extracorporeal ultrafiltration method; NM: Nafamostat mesylate; PMMA: Polymethylmethacrylate; PS: Polysulfone; QB: Blood pump flow rate; QD: Dialysate pump flow rate; QF: Filtration pump flow rate; QS: Substitution fluid pump flow rate; SC: Sieving coefficient; SDs: Standard deviations

## Acknowledgements
We would like to thank Mr. Satoru Ezumi at the Department of Pharmacy, Okayama University Hospital; Dr. Tetsuya Yumoto at the Department of Emergency and Critical Care Medicine, Okayama University Graduate School of Medicine, Dentistry and Pharmaceutical Sciences; and Mr. Jun-ichi Ono at the Kawasaki University of Medical Welfare for substantial contributions to data management.

## Funding
This study was supported by the Department of Traumatology and Emergency Intensive Care Medicine, Okayama University Graduate School of Medicine, Dentistry and Pharmaceutical Sciences and the Department of Pharmacy, Okayama University Hospital.

## Authors' contributions
TH designed the study protocols, acquired the data, and performed the statistical analysis. NN helped with the statistical analysis and completed the manuscript for publication. YO and SU helped with acquiring data and advised the study methodology. YK, TS, TU, and AN supervised the interpretation of the results and writing of the reports. All authors have read and approved the final version of the manuscript.

## Competing interests
The authors declare that they have no competing interests.

## Author details
[1]Department of Clinical Engineering, Okayama University Hospital, 2-5-1 Shikata-cho, Kita-ku, Okayama city 700-8558, Japan. [2]Department of Emergency and Critical Care Medicine, Okayama University Graduate School of Medicine, Dentistry and Pharmaceutical Sciences, Okayama University Hospital, 2-5-1 Shikata-cho, Kita-ku, Okayama city 700-8558, Japan. [3]Department of Pediatrics, Okayama University Hospital, 2-5-1 Shikata-cho, Kita-ku, Okayama city 700-8558, Japan. [4]Department of Pharmacy, Okayama University Hospital, 2-5-1 Shikata-cho, Kita-ku, Okayama city 700-8558, Japan. [5]Department of Pediatrics, Division of Infectious Diseases and Immunology, Cedars-Sinai Medical Center, 8700 Beverly Blvd., Los Angeles, CA 90048, USA.

## References
1. Forni LG, Hilton PJ. Continuous hemofiltration in the treatment of acute renal failure. N Engl J Med. 1997;336:1303–9.
2. Morabito S, Guzzo I, Solazzo A, Muzi L, Luciani R, Pierucci A. Continuous renal replacement therapies: anticoagulation in the critically ill at high risk of bleeding. J Nephrol. 2003;16:566–71.
3. Ohtake Y, Hirasawa H, Sugai T, Oda S, Shiga H, Matsuda K, et al. Nafamostat mesylate as anticoagulant in continuous hemofiltration and continuous hemodiafiltration. Contrib Nephrol. 1991;93:215–7.
4. Akizawa T, Koshikawa S, Ota K, Kazama M, Mimura N, Hirasawa Y. Nafamostat mesilate: a regional anticoagulant for hemodialysis in patients at high risk for bleeding. Nephron. 1993;64:376–81.
5. Shiga H, Hirasawa H. Continuous hemodiafiltration with a cytokine-adsorbing hemofilter in patients with septic shock: a preliminary report. Blood Purif. 2014;38:211–8.
6. Hattori N, Oda S. Cytokine-adsorbing hemofilter: old but new modality for septic acute kidney injury. Renal Replace Ther. 2016;41:2.
7. Renaux J, Thomas M, Crost T, Loughraieb N, Vantard G. Activation of the kallikrein-kinin system in hemodialysis: role of membrane electronegativity, blood dilution, and pH. Kidney Int. 1999;55:1097–103.
8. Inagaki O, Nishian Y, Iwaki R, Nakagawa K, Takamitsu Y, Fujita Y. Adsorption of nafamostat mesilate by hemodialysis membranes. Artif Organs. 1992;16: 553–8.
9. Désormeaux A, Moreau ME, Lepage Y, Chanard J, Adam A. The effect of electronegativity and angiotensin-converting enzyme inhibition on the kinin-forming capacity of polyacrylonitrile dialysis membranes. Biomaterials. 2008;29:1139–46.
10. Nishida O, Yumoto M, Moriyama K, Shimomura Y, Miyasho T, Yamada S. Possible adsorption mechanism of high mobility group box 1 protein on polyacrylonitrile (AN69ST) membrane filter. Crit Care. 2012;16:135–6.

11. Jacques C, Sylvie L, Randoux C, Rieu P. New insights in dialysis membrane biocompatibility: relevance of adsorption properties and heparin binding. Nephrol Dial Transplant. 2003;18:252–7.

12. Chanard J, Lavaud S, Paris B, Toure F, Rieu P, Renaux JL, et al. Assessment of heparin binding to the AN69 ST hemodialysis membrane: I. Preclinical studies. ASAIO J. 2005;51:342–7.

13. Nishida O. A reconsideration of effective mediator removal based on hemofiltration principles—taking the HMGB1, notable alarmin, removal by hemofiltration for instance. J Jpn Soc Blood Purif Crit Care. 2011;2:52–60 [in Japanese].

14. Moriyama K, Soejima Y. Continuous hemodiafiltration using PMMA membrane: clinical efficacy and its mechanisms. Contrib Nephrol. 1999;125: 222–32.

15. Yumoto M, Nishida O. In vitro evaluation of high mobility group box 1 protein removal with various membranes for continuous hemofiltration. Ther Apher Dial. 2011;15:385–93.

# 3

# Psychological rumination and recovery from work in intensive care professionals: associations with stress, burnout, depression and health

Tushna Vandevala[1*], Louisa Pavey[1], Olga Chelidoni[2], Nai-Feng Chang[1], Ben Creagh-Brown[3,4] and Anna Cox[2]

## Abstract

**Background:** The work demands of critical care can be a major cause of stress in intensive care unit (ICU) professionals and lead to poor health outcomes. In the process of recovery from work, psychological rumination is considered to be an important mediating variable in the relationship between work demands and health outcomes. This study aimed to extend our knowledge of the process by which ICU stressors and differing rumination styles are associated with burnout, depression and risk of psychiatric morbidity among ICU professionals.

**Methods:** Ninety-six healthcare professionals (58 doctors and 38 nurses) who work in ICUs in the UK completed a questionnaire on ICU-related stressors, burnout, work-related rumination, depression and risk of psychiatric morbidity.

**Results:** Significant associations between ICU stressors, affective rumination, burnout, depression and risk of psychiatric morbidity were found. Longer working hours were also related to increased ICU stressors. Affective rumination (but not problem-solving pondering or distraction detachment) mediated the relationship between ICU stressors, burnout, depression and risk of psychiatric morbidity, such that increased ICU stressors, and greater affective rumination, were associated with greater burnout, depression and risk of psychiatric morbidity. No moderating effects were observed.

**Conclusions:** Longer working hours were associated with increased ICU stressors, and increased ICU stressors conferred greater burnout, depression and risk of psychiatric morbidity via increased affective rumination. The importance of screening healthcare practitioners within intensive care for depression, burnout and psychiatric morbidity has been highlighted. Future research should evaluate psychological interventions which target rumination style and could be made available to those at highest risk. The efficacy and cost effectiveness of delivering these interventions should also be considered.

**Keywords:** Intensive care, Critical care, Stress, Burnout, Health, Rumination

* Correspondence: t.vandrevala@kingston.ac.uk
[1]School of Social and Behavioural Sciences, Criminology and Sociology, Faculty of Arts & Social Sciences, Kingston University, Penrhyn Road, Kingston, Surrey KT1 2EE, UK
Full list of author information is available at the end of the article

## Background

Majority of admissions into ICU are unplanned emergencies where ICU professionals are often required to rapidly attend to complex situations of uncertain outcomes. Several international studies have found that professionals working in ICU experience high levels of stress, moral distress, burnout, anxiety, depression and posttraumatic stress disorder [1–10]. Environmental factors (e.g. heavy workload, long working hours), patient factors (e.g. critical illness or end of life, witnessing pain and suffering from futile treatments) and ethical issues relating to communication lead to ICU professionals experiencing moral distress, burnout, ill health and staff turnover [2, 7, 11–15]. Uncertainty and responsibilities associated with end-of-life (EOL) decisions are associated with an increased burden [16]. A recent systematic review found that working in an intensive care setting correlated with substantial risks of emotional distress [8, 17].

Work recovery or unwinding from work is a process that facilitates psychological and physical restoration, and the impairment of recovery from work stress may result in poor health [18]. The recovery process is largely influenced by the extent to which individuals disengage (or disconnect) from their work demands and related thoughts [19]. Rumination can be defined as "passively and repetitively focusing on one's symptoms of distress and the circumstances surrounding these symptoms" ([20], p. 855). Ruminative response to stress has been identified as contributing to the development and maintenance of depression [21], impaired somatic and mental health [22] and increase in work-related fatigue [23]. Evidence suggests the importance of rumination as a mediator [24, 25], while other studies have failed to find a mediation effect of work-related rumination [19]. Rumination per se may not be associated with impaired health, but the emotional component of rumination may evoke negative effects of other stressors [26].

Previous research has shown clear associations between stress, burnout and poor psychological health and has found these symptoms to be highly prevalent in ICU healthcare professionals. In this study, we aimed to confirm these associations and to investigate the potential mediating process of rumination style. We predicted that the association between work stressors, burnout, depression and risk of psychiatric morbidity would be mediated by rumination.

This study's objectives were

(1) To determine the association between ICU stressors, burnout, depression and risk of psychiatric morbidity
(2) To determine the mediating effects of the three types of work-related rumination (affective rumination, problem-solving pondering and distraction detachment) on the relationship between ICU stressors

and each of the outcome variables (burnout, depression and risk of psychiatric morbidity)
(3) To determine the impact of occupational role (doctors vs. nurses), working hours (more than 40 h per week vs. 40 h per week or less) and gender (male vs. female) on rumination (affective rumination, problem-solving pondering, distraction detachment), ICU stressors, burnout, depression and risk of psychiatric morbidity

## Methods

### Design

A cross-sectional design was used.

### Participants

The sample consisted of 96 professionals working in ICU (46 males and 50 females; 58 doctors and 38 nurses) in three different hospitals in the UK. The majority of the doctors and nurses were aged between 31 and 50 years and married. The sample had a range of years of experience in intensive care ranging from 0–5 years to more than 20 years. Fifty-four participants (56.3%) worked a 40-h week or less, while 41 participants (42.7%) worked more than 40 h per week (one missing data for work hours). For full participant statistics, see Table 1.

### Materials

The *General Health Questionnaire* (GHQ-12) developed by Goldberg was used to assess the risk of psychiatric morbidity. The GHQ-12 is a 12-item, self-administered questionnaire designed to detect risk for non-psychotic psychiatric morbidity in non-clinical adult populations [27]. It measures psychiatric symptoms such as depression, sleep

**Table 1** Participants demographic characteristics (N = 96)

| Variable | | Doctors | Nurses | Overall |
|---|---|---|---|---|
| Gender | Male | 40 (69%) | 6 (15.8%) | 46 (47.9%) |
| | Female | 18 (31%) | 32 (84.2%) | 50 (52.1%) |
| Age (years) | 18–30 | 4 (6.9%) | 13 (34.2%) | 17 (17.7%) |
| | 31–50 | 48 (82.8%) | 24 (63.2%) | 72 (75%) |
| | 51–65 | 6 (10.3%) | 1 (2.6%) | 7 (7.3%) |
| Marital status | Single | 4 (6.9%) | 8 (21.1%) | 12 (12.%) |
| | Married | 44 (75.9%) | 20 (52.6%) | 64 (66.7%) |
| | In a relationship | 9 (15.5%) | 7 (18.4%) | 16 (16.7%) |
| | Divorced | 1 (1.7%) | 3 (7.9%) | 4 (4.2%) |
| Experience in ICU | 0–5 years | 15 (25.9%) | 20 (52.6%) | 35 (36.5%) |
| | 6–10 years | 17 (29.3%) | 10 (26.3%) | 27 (28.1%) |
| | 11–20 years | 15 (25.9%) | 5 (13.2%) | 20 (20.8%) |
| | >20 years | 11 (19%) | 3 (7.9%) | 14 (14.6%) |
| Work hours | ≤40 h/week | 23 (39.7%) | 31 (81.6%) | 54 (56.3%) |
| | >40 h/week | 34 (58.6%) | 7 (18.4%) | 41 (42.7%) |

disorders and loss of self-confidence. Responses were coded as 0 (e.g. better or same as usual) or 1 (e.g. less than usual, much less than usual) and summed to give an overall score ranging from 0 to 12, as recommended by the authors. In the present study, the tool demonstrated satisfactory reliability, Cronbach's $\alpha$ = .81.

The *Oldenburg Burnout Inventory* (OLBI) developed by Demerouti et al. [28] is a well-validated psychometric tool that assesses burnout syndrome and contains two subscales of exhaustion and disengagement. Exhaustion subscale refers to emotions of emptiness, the need to take time off from work and physical symptoms of exhaustion. Disengagement subscale refers to negative and cynical views towards work [28]. The items for each subscale were summed to give an overall score ranging from 0 to 32, Cronbach's $\alpha$ = .69 (disengagement) and $\alpha$ = .73 (emotional exhaustion).

The *Inventory of Depressive Symptomatology, Self-Reported* (IDS-SR) developed by Rush et al. is a 30-item self-reported scale which measures depressive signs and symptoms [29]. This inventory is useful in evaluating the severity of depression, and the cut-off score in detecting endogenous depression suggested by Rush et al. [30] is adopted in the specific study. Items were summed to give a total score ranging from 0 to 90, with satisfactory reliability, Cronbach's $\alpha$ = .86.

The *ICU-related stressors questionnaire* developed by Coomber et al. [2] was used to identify the frequency and the stress severity of ICU-specific factors. Participants were asked to indicate how often they deal with (0 = never, 1 = occasionally, 2 = often) and how stressful they perceive (0 = not at all, 1 = slightly, 2 = moderately, 3 = very, 4 = extremely) 30 ICU-specific situations, such as bed allocation, dealing with death, treatment withdrawal and effects of stress/hours on personal/family life were included. An overall score was calculated by multiplying the frequency and stress ratings for each stressor and summing the totals, giving an ICU stressor score ranging from 0 to 240, Cronbach's $\alpha$ = .84.

The *Work-Related Rumination Questionnaire* (WRRQ) developed by Cropley et al. [26] explores the unwinding process of switching off from work and evaluates one's tendencies and directions to ruminative thinking. It consists of three subscales: (1) affective rumination refers to the state of fatigue and distress that participants experience when they think of issues related to work; (2) problem-solving pondering focuses on the logic and cognitive way of organising work issues; and (3) distraction detachments focuses on the unwinding process that takes place after the individual has left the work environment. Items were summed to give a total score of 24 for each subscale (affective rumination: Cronbach's $\alpha$ = .83; problem-solving pondering: Cronbach's $\alpha$ = .43; distraction detachment: Cronbach's $\alpha$ = .76).

**General personal information** Participants were asked general personal information such as age, gender, marital status, specialty and years of experience within ICU. Participants were asked how many hours per week they work at the indicated job (less than 40 per week, 40 per week, more than 40 per week) and how often do they face EOL decision-making procedures (once every week, twice a week, more than twice a week, once a day, more than once a day).

### Procedure

The permission of heads of the ICU departments in hospitals within four National Health Service (NHS) Trusts in the South of England was sought before an invitation letter was sent to their staff. The information sheet and invitation letter was sent to all prospective participants inviting them to complete an online questionnaire. A researcher also visited the hospitals to increase response rate and administered paper versions of the questionnaires. The online questionnaire was also made openly available to doctors who were registered with https://www.doctors.net.uk (an online database of over 220,000 doctors in the UK). Web-based questionnaires which are open to all users make calculation of a response rate more difficult, and in this instance, it was not possible. There were no differences in demographic characteristics between participants recruited online and in person. Ethical review and governance permissions were sought and received from the Faculty of Arts and Human Sciences, University of Surrey Ethics Committee (1003-PSY-14), the Faculty of Arts and Social Sciences, Kingston University Ethics Committee (1314/5/3) and the Research and Development Department of the participating NHS Trust in the South of England.

### Statistical analysis

Bivariate correlations were conducted to determine the associations between ICU stressors, burnout, depression and risk of psychiatric morbidity. Regression, mediation and moderation analyses were then conducted using the PROCESS software [31] to test the indirect effect of ICU stressors on each of the outcome variables via the types of work-related rumination. To determine the impact of occupational role, working hours and gender on rumination, ICU stressors, burnout, depression and risk for psychiatric morbidity, $t$ tests were conducted with the Bonferroni correction for multiple comparisons.

### Results

#### Sample characteristics

The means and standard deviations for each of the measured variables by occupational role, working hours and gender are shown in Table 2. After applying cut-off scores for risk of psychiatric morbidity and depression, 32.3% of

**Table 2** Differences in ICU stressors and burnout between gender, occupation type and working hours

|  | Overall mean (SD) | Doctors' mean (SD) | Nurses' mean (SD) | Males | Females | ≤40 h per week | >40 h per week |
|---|---|---|---|---|---|---|---|
| ICU stressors | 49.5 (26.09) | 45.50 (24.63) | 55.84 (27.43) | 46.38 (28.37) | 52.55 (23.67) | 39.71 (15.69) | 53.83 (27.64) |
| Burnout: emotional exhaustion | 20.12 (3.09) | 19.91 (3.14) | 20.45 (3.04) | 19.48 (3.49) | 20.72 (2.57) | 19.71 (3.01) | 20.46 (3.35) |
| Burnout: disengagement | 17.65 (3.1) | 17.60 (3.01) | 17.71 (3.28) | 17.67 (2.95) | 17.62 (3.26) | 16.90 (2.76) | 18.07 (3.42) |

the sample was at risk of psychiatric morbidity and 18.8% were at risk of depression.

### The effects of ICU stressors on burnout, depression and risk of psychiatric morbidity

Correlation analyses indicated that ICU stressors were significantly associated with burnout (emotional exhaustion, $r(96) = .43$, $p < .001$ and disengagement, $r(96) = .42$, $p < .001$). Logistic regression analysis indicated that ICU stressors were a significant predictor of depression, $\beta = .04$, $p = .002$, but were not associated with the risk of psychiatric morbidity, $\beta = .01$, $p = .353$.

### The effects of gender, occupational role and working hours

Independent sample $t$ tests were conducted to assess any differences in ICU stressors and burnout (emotional exhaustion and disengagement) between gender (males vs. females), occupation (doctors vs. nurses) and working hours (40 h per week or less vs. more than 40 h per week). There was a significant difference in burnout according to gender (emotional exhaustion), $t(94) = -2.00$, $p = .049$, with female ICU workers showing greater emotional exhaustion than male ICU workers. There were no other significant gender differences, and no significant differences between nurses and doctors for any of the other variables (the means and standard deviations are displayed in Table 2). There was a significant difference between those working 40 h per week or less and those working more than 40 h in ICU stressors, $t(68) = -2.63$, $p = 0.011$, with those working more than 40 h reporting greater ICU stressors than those working 40 h per week or less (means and standard deviations are displayed in Table 2). Part-time workers ($N = 28$) were excluded from this analysis due to the qualitatively different nature of the work and stress they encounter.

Chi square analyses were conducted to determine the differences in the risk of psychiatric morbidity and depression between gender (males vs. females), occupation (doctors vs. nurses) and working hours (40 h per week or less vs. more than 40 h per week). There was a significant association between gender and risk of psychiatric morbidity, with females displaying a greater incidence of being at risk of psychiatric morbidity than males, $X^2(1) = 8.97$, $p = .003$. There was also a significant association between occupational role and risk of psychiatric morbidity,

with nurses displaying a greater incidence of being at risk of psychiatric morbidity than doctors, $X^2(1) = 4.46$, $p = .035$. There was no significant association between working hours and risk of psychiatric morbidity, and no significant associations between gender, occupation, working hours and depression.

### The mediating and moderating role of rumination styles

Four mediation analyses were conducted to determine the mediating effects of the work-related rumination (affective rumination, problem-solving pondering and distraction detachment) on the relationship between ICU stressors and each of the four outcome variables. The full correlation matrix is displayed in Table 3. Linear regression was used for the two continuous outcome variables (emotional exhaustion and disengagement, see Table 4), and logistic regression for the two binary variables (depression and risk of psychiatric morbidity, see Table 5).

Results showed significant effects of ICU stressors on affective rumination ($\beta = .47$, $t = 4.74$, $p < .001$) and distraction detachment ($\beta = .31$, $t = 2.85$, $p = .005$), but not on problem-solving pondering ($\beta = .17$, $t = 1.60$, $p = .113$).

When ICU stressors and the three mediating variables were added to each regression model simultaneously, affective rumination was the only variable to significantly predict emotional exhaustion ($\beta = .53$, $t = 4.50$, $p < .001$), disengagement ($\beta = .45$, $t = 3.49$, $p < .001$), depression ($\beta = .44$, $z = 3.14$, $p = .002$) and risk of psychiatric morbidity ($\beta = .21$, $z = 2.37$, $p = .018$). The effect of ICU stressor on each of the outcome variables diminished when rumination styles were added to the analysis (see Tables 4 and 5).

Inspection of the indirect effects revealed a significant effect of ICU stressors on emotional exhaustion via

**Table 3** Bivariate correlations for continuous predictor, mediating and outcome variables ($N = 96$)

|  | 2 | 3 | 4 | 5 | 6 |
|---|---|---|---|---|---|
| 1. ICU stressors | .47** | .17 | .31** | .43** | .42** |
| 2. Affective rumination | – | .45** | .50** | .58** | .40** |
| 3. Problem-solving pondering |  | – | .35** | .21* | .02 |
| 4. Distraction detachment |  |  | – | .36** | .08 |
| 5. Emotional exhaustion |  |  |  | – | .62** |
| 6. Disengagement |  |  |  |  | – |

*$p < .05$; **$p < .01$

**Table 4** Linear regression models examining the effect of ICU stressors on burnout (emotional exhaustion and disengagement), mediated by rumination style (affective rumination, problem-solving pondering and distraction detachment)

|  | Emotional exhaustion | | Disengagement | |
| --- | --- | --- | --- | --- |
|  | β | t | β | t |
| Step 1 | | | | |
| ICU stressors | 0.43 | 4.26** | 0.42 | 4.16* |
| $R^2$ | .43** | | .42** | |
| Step 2 | | | | |
| ICU stressors | 0.17 | 1.73 | 0.26 | 2.41* |
| Affective rumination | 0.53 | 4.50** | 0.45 | 3.49** |
| Problem-solving pondering | −0.05 | −0.52 | −0.13 | −1.24 |
| Distraction detachment | 0.06 | 0.57 | −0.09 | −0.81 |
| $R^2$ | .64** | | .54** | |

*$p < .05$; **$p < .01$

affective rumination (95% CI [0.01, 0.06]) but not via problem-solving pondering (95% CI [−0.01, 0.01]) or distraction detachment (95% CI [−0.01, 0.01]). There was also a significant effect of ICU stressors on disengagement via affective rumination (CI 0.01, 0.06) but not via problem-solving pondering (CI −0.01, 0.001) or distraction detachment (CI −0.001, 0.01). The same result was found for depression: there was a significant indirect effect found between ICU stressors and depression via affective rumination (95% CI [0.01, 0.07]) but not via problem-solving pondering (95% CI [−0.01, 0.02]) or distraction detachment (95% CI [−0.03, 0.02]). Although there was no significant direct effect of ICU stressors on risk of psychiatric morbidity, there was a significant indirect effect of ICU stressors on risk of psychiatric morbidity via affective rumination (95% CI [0.01, 0.03]) but not via problem-solving pondering (95% CI [−0.01, 0.01]) or distraction detachment (95% CI

[−0.01, 0.02]). Path models with standardised beta weights are shown in Fig. 1.

Overall, the results suggest that affective rumination, but not problem-solving pondering or distraction detachment, significantly mediated the effect of ICU stressor on each of the outcome variables (burnout, depression and risk of psychiatric morbidity). Moderation analysis revealed no significant moderation effects of rumination style on the association between ICU stressors and the four outcome variables.

## Discussion

The findings from the current study indicated that staff working in an ICU can experience significant stress and this was negatively associated with health and wellbeing: 32% of the sample were categorised as being at risk of psychiatric morbidity and 18% as being at risk of depression. These findings are comparable with empirical evidence that between 20 and 30% of ICU professionals are at risk of psychiatric morbidity [1, 2] and 10–25% express depressive symptoms [2, 32]. Prevalence estimates for common mental disorder from population studies range from 14 to 31%, with the prevalence of psychiatric morbidity in health professionals approximately 30% [33]. Participants who worked more than 40 h per week reported experiencing higher levels of ICU stressors, and ICU stressors were associated with higher incidences of burnout and depression. The current study did not account for shift patterns and night working but showed evidence that working in excess of 40 h may leave little time for actual recovery from work. It is possible that those working weekends or shift pattern may experience increased fatigue, irritability, decreased work efficiency and reduced mental agility [34].

The mediation analysis from the current study showed that ICU stressors per se may not lead to negative health outcomes and highlighted the importance of rumination

**Table 5** Logistic regression models examining the effect of ICU stressors on depression and risk of psychiatric morbidity, mediated by rumination style (affective rumination, problem-solving pondering and distraction detachment)

|  | Depression | | | Risk of psychiatric morbidity | | |
| --- | --- | --- | --- | --- | --- | --- |
|  | β | Wald | Odds ratio | β | t | Odds ratio |
| Step 1 | | | | | | |
| ICU stressors | 0.35 | 8.41** | 1.04 | 0.01 | 0.86 | 1.00 |
| Nagelkerke $R^2$ | .17** | | | .02 | | |
| Step 2 | | | | | | |
| ICU stressors | 0.02 | 2.40 | 1.02 | −0.01 | 0.44 | .99 |
| Affective rumination | 0.34 | 10.78** | 1.40 | 0.21 | 5.60* | 1.23 |
| Problem-solving pondering | −0.14 | 0.09 | .87 | −0.03 | 0.13 | .97 |
| Distraction detachment | −0.09 | 0.09 | .14 | 0.07 | 0.57 | 1.07 |
| Nagelkerke $R^2$ | .37** | | | .18* | | |

*$p < .05$; **$p < .01$

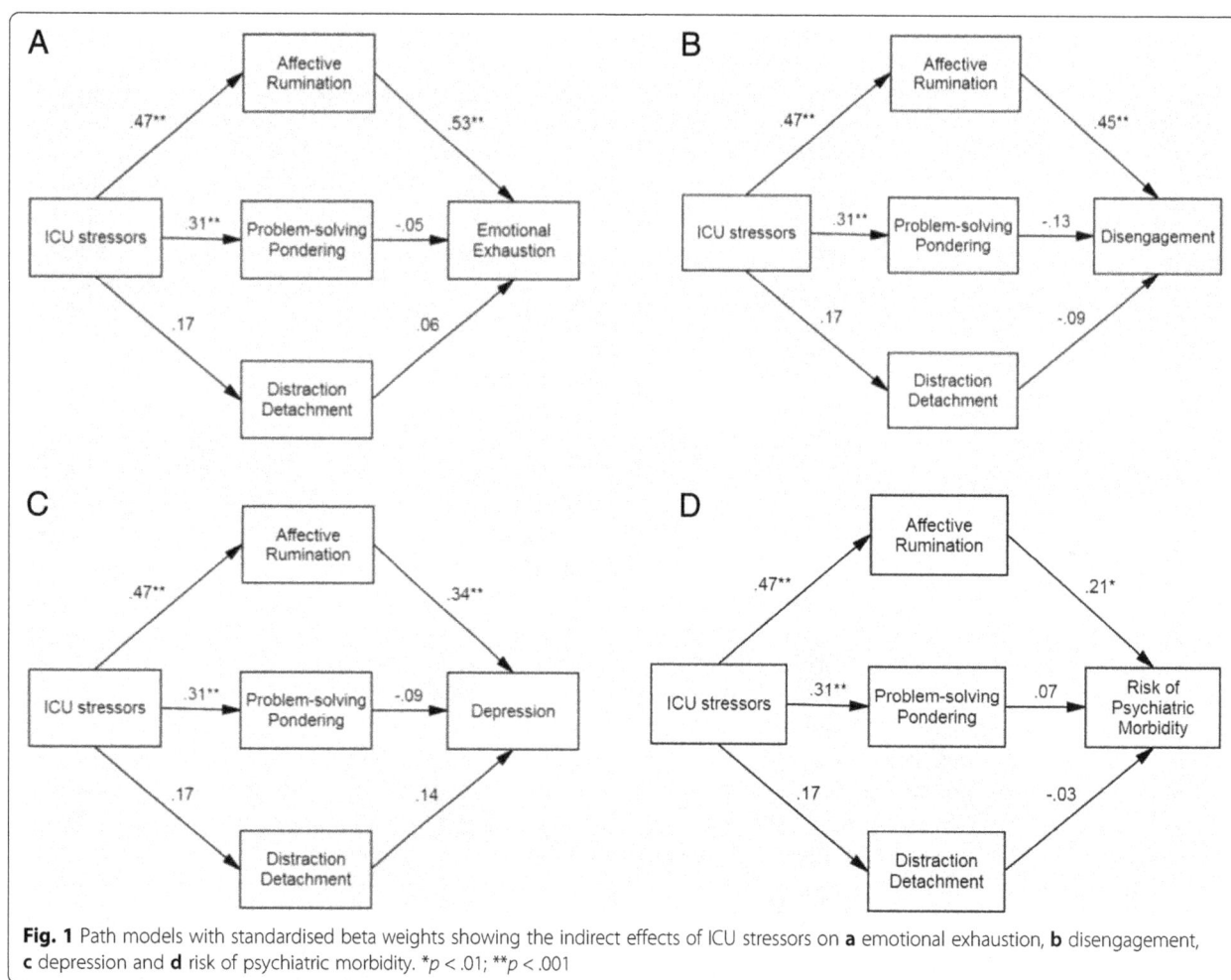

**Fig. 1** Path models with standardised beta weights showing the indirect effects of ICU stressors on **a** emotional exhaustion, **b** disengagement, **c** depression and **d** risk of psychiatric morbidity. $*p < .01$; $**p < .001$

style. Our findings corroborate and build on previous research suggesting that rumination is an important link between stress at work and negative health outcomes [24]. Our study reports that there were significant indirect effects of ICU stressors on burnout, depression and risk of psychiatric morbidity via affective rumination, but not via problem-solving pondering or distraction detachment. The results suggest that affective rumination style may hinder the process of recovery from work, leading to negative psychological health outcomes. Even though the maladaptive nature of rumination has been previously stressed, it remains a debate whether there are some adaptive aspects to it. Previous research has suggested that problem-solving pondering expresses a creative aspect of rumination that enables the individual to engage with the task and gain an enjoyable experience [19]. Unlike affective rumination, problem-solving pondering may offer benefit to the individual [35].

Our findings also suggest that distraction detachment rumination does not mediate the relationship between ICU stressors and ill health. Studies have found that psychological detachment or mentally distancing oneself

from work has positive impacts on mood and low fatigue; however, high time pressure and high workload can make it difficult to psychologically detach from work [36]. Psychological detachment acts as a potential buffer of the negative impacts of job stressors on strain reaction [37], while other studies have found that psychological detachment does not mediate the relationship between job demands and cognitive failures [38]. In the current study, the impact of individual ICU stressors on rumination styles, and the impact of work–home conflict or family–work conflict (family or home responsibilities interfering with work) on rumination styles, was not investigated.

There are some limitations that need to be considered. Data collection was restricted to four intensive care units in the South of England and an online survey to doctors, which limits the generalizability of the findings. It is possible that the self-selecting nature of the sample may have resulted in those experiencing high levels of stress and burnout not participating in the study. Even though the study took into account the different dimensions of rumination, the frequency and duration of the ruminating thought was not explored. Further to this, relatively low reliability indicators for the WRRQ were obtained in this sample, particularly for the problem-solving pondering subscale. Although the three subscales of this questionnaire have shown good reliability and clear factor loadings in the previous studies, the scale is relatively new and has not yet been widely used, particularly in more diverse samples. Further research is needed to determine whether modifications of this questionnaire are needed, as the low inter-item reliability of this subscale may have contributed to null mediation findings for this subscale in the current study. Finally, our study included a specific sample of healthcare professionals working in ICU; it would be interesting to replicate our findings in other healthcare professionals facing a high workload and high emotional demands.

## Conclusions

This study demonstrates the potential value for screening healthcare practitioners within intensive care in order to provide targeted interventions. Affective rumination can act as a precursor to developing psychological problems, such as depression and anxiety and long-term health consequences, including cardiovascular disease and other chronic conditions [39]. Screening and identifying those with an affective rumination style and those working in excess of 40 h per week may protect healthcare practitioners from burnout, depression and psychiatric morbidity.

Intervention programmes to reduce burnout found that person-directed interventions, such as cognitive behavioural therapy (CBT) and relaxation exercises, led to a significant reduction in burnout, in comparison with organisational-directed interventions [40]. These person-directed interventions can effectively reduce negative rumination styles, such as affective rumination, and encourage recovery from work [41]. There may be a potential to further develop mindfulness meditation for ICU professionals with affective rumination styles to prevent stress, which could enable them to pay attention in the present moment, rather than react later with negative feeling [17]. The quality of care for ICU patients and their relatives may be compromised through long-term absenteeism or skill drain if healthcare professionals leave their jobs prematurely to preserve their health, ultimately leading to economic burdens [17].

### Acknowledgements
We are grateful to all participants and their managers for giving their time so generously.

### Funding
This research did not receive any specific grant from funding agencies in the public, commercial or not-for-profit sectors.

### Authors' contributions
TV and AC designed the study contributed to the interpretation of results and drafted the manuscript. LP substantially contributed to the data analysis and interpretation of results and helped draft the manuscript. LC and OC collected the data. B C-B contributed to the design of the study, access to participants and drafting of the manuscript. All authors have read and approved the final manuscript.

### Competing interests
The authors declare that they have no competing interests.

### Author details
[1]School of Social and Behavioural Sciences, Criminology and Sociology, Faculty of Arts & Social Sciences, Kingston University, Penrhyn Road, Kingston, Surrey KT1 2EE, UK. [2]School of Health Sciences, Faculty of Health and Medical Sciences, University of Surrey, Guildford, Surrey GU2 7XH, UK. [3]Intensive Care Unit, Royal Surrey County Hospital, Egerton Road, Guildford, Surrey GU2 7XX, UK. [4]Surrey Perioperative Anaesthesia Critical Care Collaborative Research Group (SPACeR), Department of Clinical and Experimental Medicine, Faculty of Health and Medical Sciences, University of Surrey, Guildford GU2 7XH, UK.

### References
1. Asai M, Morita T, Akechi T, Sugawara Y, Fukimori M, Nakano T, et al. Burnout and psychiatric morbidity among physicians engaged in end-of-life care for cancer patients: a cross-sectional nationwide survey in Japan. Psychooncology. 2007;16:421–8.
2. Coomber S, Todd C, Park G, Baxter P, Firth-Cozens J, Shore S. Stress in UK intensive care unit doctors. Br J Anaesth. 2002;89:873–81.
3. Curtis JR, Vincent JL. Ethics and end-of-life care for adults in intensive care unit. Lancet. 2010;376:1347–57.
4. Day T. Review: symptoms of posttraumatic stress disorder, anxiety and depression among Czech critical care and general surgical and medical ward nurses. J Res Nurs. 2015;20:310–1.
5. Dodek PM, Wong H, Norena M, Ayas N, Reynolds SC, Keenan SP, et al. Moral distress in intensive care unit professionals is associated with profession, age and years of experience. J Crit Care. 2016;31:178–82.
6. De Villers MJ, DeVon HA. Moral distress and avoidance behaviour in nurses working in critical care and noncritical care units. Nurs Ethics. 2013;20:589–603.
7. Reader TW, Cuthbertson BH, Decruyenaere J. Burnout in the ICU: potential consequences for staff and patient well-being. J Intensive Care Med. 2007. doi:10.1007/s00134-007-0908-4.
8. Rushton CH, Batcheller J, Schroeder K, Donohue P. Burnout and resilience among nurses practicing in high-intensity settings. Am J Crit Care. 2015;24:412–20.
9. Ulrich CM, Taylor C, Soeken K, O'Donnell P, Farrar A, Danis M, et al. Everyday ethics: ethical issues and stress in nursing practice. J Adv Nurs. 2010;66:2510–9.
10. Janda R, Jandova E. Symptoms of posttraumatic stress disorder, anxiety and depression among Czech critical care and general surgical and medical ward nurses. J Res Nurs. 2015;20:298–309.
11. Escriba-Aguir V, Martin-Baena D, Perez-Hoyos S. Psychosocial work environment and burnout among emergency medical and nursing staff. Int Arch Occup Environ Health. 2006;80:127–33.
12. Escriba-Aguir V, Perez-Hoyos S. Psychological well-being and psychosocial work environment characteristics among emergency medical and nursing staff. Stress Health. 2007;23:153–60.
13. Ozden D, Karagozogly S, Yildirim G. Intensive care nurses' perception of futility: job satisfaction and burnout dimensions. Nurs Ethics. 2013;20:436–47.
14. Teixeira C, Ribeiro O, Fonseca AM, Carvalho AS. Ethical decision making in intensive care units: a burnout risk factor? Results from a multicentre study conducted with physicians and nurses. J Med Ethics. 2014;40:97–103.
15. van Dam K, Meewis M, van der Heijden BI. Securing intensive care: towards a better understanding of intensive care nurses' perceived work pressure and turnover intention. J Adv Nurs. 2012;69:31–40.

16. Konstantara E, Vandrevala T, Cox A, Creagh-Brown BC, Ogden J. Balancing professional tension and deciding upon the status of death: making end-of-life decisions in intensive care units. Health Psychol Open. 2016;3:1–9.

17. van Mol MMC, Kompanje EJO, Benoit DD, Bakker J, Nijkamp MD. The prevalence of compassion fatigue and burnout among healthcare professionals in intensive care units: a systematic review. PLoS One. 2015;10:e0136955.

18. Zijlstra FRH, Sonnentag S. After work is done: psychological perspectives on recovery from work. Eur J Work Organ Psy. 2006;15:129–38.

19. Cropley M, Dijk D-J, Stanley N. Job strain, work rumination and sleep in school teachers. Eur J Work Organ Psy. 2006;15:181–96.

20. Nolen-Hoeksema S, McBride A, Larson J. Rumination and psychological distress among bereaved partners. J Pers Soc Psychol. 1997;72:855–62.

21. Watkins ER. Constructive and unconstructive repetitive thought. Psychol Bull. 2008;134:163–206.

22. Sansone RA, Sansone LA. Antidepressant adherence: are patients taking their medications? Innov Clin Neurosci. 2012;9:41–6.

23. Querstret D, Cropley M. Exploring the relationship between work-related rumination, sleep quality and work-related fatigue. J Occup Health Psychol. 2012;17:341–53.

24. Berset M, Semmer NK, Elfering A, Jacobshagen N, Meier LL. Does stress at work make you gain weight? A two year longitudinal study. Scand J Work Environ Health. 2011;37:45–53.

25. Zawadzki MJ, Graham JE, Gerin W. Rumination and anxiety mediate the effect of loneliness on depressed mood and sleep quality in college students. Health Psychol. 2013;32:212–22.

26. Cropley M, Michalianou G, Pravettoni G, Millward LJ. The relation of post-work ruminative thinking with eating behaviour. Stress Health. 2012;28:23–30.

27. Goldberg DP, Hillier VF. A scaled version of the Psychological Wellbeing Questionnaire. Psychol Med. 1978;9:139–45.

28. Demerouti E, Bakker AB, Nachreiner F, Ebbinghaus M. From mental strain to burnout. Eur J Work Organ Psy. 2002;11:423–41.

29. Rush AJ, Giles DE, Schlesser MA, Fulton CL, Weissenburger J, Burns C. The inventory for depressive symptomatology (IDS): preliminary findings. Psychiatry Res. 1986;18:65–87.

30. Rush AJ, Hiser W, Giles DE. A comparison of self-reported versus clinical rated symptoms of depression. J Clin Psychiatry. 1987;48960:246–8.

31. Hayes AF, Preacher KJ. Conditional process modeling: using structural equation modeling to examine contingent causal processes. In: Hancock GR, Mueller RO, editors. Structural equation modeling: a second course. 2nd ed. Charlotte: Information Age Publishing Inc; 2013. p. 219–66.

32. Embriaco N, Hraiech S, Azoulay E, Baumstarck-Barrau K, Forel J-M, Kentish-Barnes N, Pochard F, Loundou A, Roch A, Papazian L. Symptoms of depression in ICU physicians. Ann Intensive Care. 2012;2:34–42.

33. Goodwin N, Sonola L, Thiel V, Kodner D. Co-ordinated care for people with complex chronic conditions: key lessons and markers for success. In: The King's Fund. 2013. https://pdfs.semanticscholar.org/2ad6/035496f6d09d1573a976500de43506fa9f6d.pdf. Accessed 5 Dec 2016.

34. Bajraktarov S, Novotni A, Manuseva N, Richter K. Main effects of sleep disorders related to shift work—opportunities for preventive programs. EPMA J. 2011;2:365–70.

35. Cropley M, Zijlstra FRH. Work and rumination. In: Langan-Fox J, Cooper CL, editors. Handbook of stress in the occupations. UK: Edward Elgar Publishing Ltd; 2011. p. 487–503.

36. Sonnentag S, Bayer UV. Switching off mentally: predictors and consequences of psychological detachment from work during off-job time. J Occup Health Psychol. 2005;10:393–414.

37. Sonnentag S, Kuttler I, Fritz C. Job stressors, emotional exhaustion, and need for recovery: a multi-source study on the benefits of psychological detachment. J Vocat Behav. 2010;76:355–65.

38. Safstrom M, Hartig T. Psychological detachment in the relationship between job stressors and strain. Behav Sci. 2013;3(3):418–33.

39. Brosschot JF, Gerin W, Thayer JF. The perseverative cognition hypothesis: a review of worry, prolonged stress-related physiological activation, and health. J Psychosom Res. 2006;60:113–24.

40. Awa WL, Plaumann M, Walter U. Burnout prevention: a review of intervention programs. Patient Educ Couns. 2010;78:184–90.

41. Querstret D, Cropley M. Assessing treatments used to reduce rumination and/or worry: a systematic review. Clin Psychol Rev. 2013;33:996–1009.

4

# The relationship between cerebral regional oxygen saturation during extracorporeal cardiopulmonary resuscitation and the neurological outcome in a retrospective analysis of 16 cases

Naoki Ehara[1], Tomoya Hirose[2*], Tadahiko Shiozaki[2], Akinori Wakai[1], Tetsuro Nishimura[1], Nobuto Mori[2], Mitsuo Ohnishi[2], Daikai Sadamitsu[1] and Takeshi Shimazu[2]

## Abstract

**Background:** In recent years, the measurement of cerebral regional oxygen saturation ($rSO_2$) during resuscitation has attracted attention. The objective of this study was to clarify the relationship between the serial changes in the cerebral $rSO_2$ values during extracorporeal cardiopulmonary resuscitation (ECPR) and the neurological outcome.

**Methods:** We measured the serial changes in the cerebral $rSO_2$ values of patients with out-of-hospital cardiac arrest before and after ECPR in Osaka National Hospital.

**Results:** From January 2013 through March 2015, the serial changes in the cerebral $rSO_2$ values were evaluated in 16 patients. Their outcomes, as measured by the Glasgow Outcome Scale (GOS) score at discharge, included good recovery (GR) ($n = 4$), vegetative state (VS) ($n = 2$), and death (D) ($n = 10$). In the poor neurological group (VS and D: $n = 12$; age, $52.8 \pm 4.0$ years), the cerebral $rSO_2$ values showed a significant increase during ECPR (5 min before ECPR: $52.0 \pm 1.8\%$; 2 min before ECPR: $56.1 \pm 2.3\%$; 2 min after ECPR: $63.5 \pm 2.2\%$; 5 min after ECPR: $66.4 \pm 2.2\%$; 10 min after ECPR: $67.6 \pm 2.3\%$ [$P < 0.01$]). In contrast, in the good neurological group (GR: $n = 4$; age, $53.8 \pm 6.9$ years), the cerebral $rSO_2$ values did not increase to a significant extent during ECPR (5 min before ECPR: $61.9 \pm 3.1\%$; 2 min before ECPR: $57.1 \pm 4.0\%$; 2 min after ECPR: $59.6 \pm 3.8\%$; 5 min after ECPR: $61.0 \pm 3.7\%$; 10 min after ECPR: $62.0 \pm 3.8\%$ [$P = 0.88$]). Our study suggested that the patients whose cerebral $rSO_2$ values showed no significant improvement after ECPR might have had a good neurological prognosis.

**Conclusions:** The serial changes in the cerebral $rSO_2$ values during ECPR may predict a patient's neurological outcome. The further evaluation of the validity of $rSO_2$ monitoring during ECPR may lead to a new resuscitation strategy.

**Keywords:** Cerebral regional oxygen saturation, Extracorporeal cardiopulmonary resuscitation, Neurological outcome, Out-of-hospital cardiac arrest, Near-infrared spectroscopy

* Correspondence: htomoya1979@hp-emerg.med.osaka-u.ac.jp
[2]Department of Traumatology and Acute Critical Medicine, Osaka University Graduate School of Medicine, 2-15 Yamadaoka, Suita, Osaka 565-0871, Japan
Full list of author information is available at the end of the article

## Background

Sudden cardiac arrest is one of the most important causes of death and an important public health problem in the industrialised world [1]. However, survival from out-of-hospital cardiac arrest (OHCA) is still low [2], and to improve it, we think that a new resuscitation strategy is needed.

In recent years, the measurement of cerebral regional oxygen saturation ($rSO_2$) by near-infrared spectroscopy (NIRS) during resuscitation has attracted attention. We have already reported the serial changes in the cerebral $rSO_2$ values during resuscitation in patients with OHCA [3]. Chest compression alone could not increase the cerebral $rSO_2$ value, which was found to gradually increase with a return of spontaneous circulation (ROSC). The cerebral $rSO_2$ value also increased promptly after the initiation of extracorporeal cardiopulmonary resuscitation (ECPR) [4]. However, we could not predict the neurological outcome by evaluating the cerebral $rSO_2$ value in patients with OHCA in 2010 [4].

It is challenging to predict the neurological outcome following OHCA. Although some researchers have reported that the cerebral $rSO_2$ value at hospital arrival can predict the neurological outcome in patients with OHCA [5–7], we thought that this conclusion was incorrect. Because the $rSO_2$ values always change depending on the patient's situation at the time when the cerebral $rSO_2$ is measured [4, 8], we hypothesise that the serial change in the $rSO_2$ values is important rather than a single measured value.

By chance, we detected a difference in the way the values of cerebral $rSO_2$ in patients with OHCA changed before and after the application of ECPR. Thus, the objective of this study was to clarify the relationship between the serial changes in the cerebral $rSO_2$ value during ECPR and the neurological outcome.

## Methods

### Study design and data collection

This retrospective study was approved by the Ethics Committee of National Hospital Organization Osaka National Hospital (Osaka, Japan). The subjects were all cardiopulmonary arrest (CPA) patients who were transferred to National Hospital Organization Osaka National Hospital by emergency life-saving technicians (ELTs). At the emergency department, a sensor was attached to the patient's forehead to continuously monitor the cerebral $rSO_2$ value during resuscitation. ELTs and medical staff performed cardiopulmonary resuscitation according to the recommendations of the Japan Resuscitation Council Guidelines 2010, which were based on the American Heart Association and the International Liaison Committee on Resuscitation guidelines [9]. The medical staff could see the $rSO_2$ values during resuscitation, and the values were automatically recorded. However, they did not change the treatment according to the cerebral $rSO_2$ data. We retrospectively collected and analysed data from the CPA patients undergoing ECPR.

The variables that were analysed included the age, sex, initial rhythm, whether the OHCA was witnessed, and whether a bystander performed cardiopulmonary resuscitation (CPR). We evaluated the patient's cerebral $rSO_2$ values at 5 and 2 min before the application of ECPR and at 2, 5, and 10 min after the application of ECPR. The neurological prognosis was evaluated according to the Glasgow Outcome Scale (GOS) score. The normal range of cerebral $rSO_2$ was determined from 15 healthy adult volunteers whose values were measured on room air.

### The NIRS-based $rSO_2$ monitoring system

An $rSO_2$ monitor (TOS-OR; TOSTEC Co., Tokyo, Japan) was used to measure the cerebral $rSO_2$ value. The monitor measures the oxygen saturation based on the Beer-Lambert law, using three different wavelengths of near-infrared LED light, which have specific absorbance in oxyhaemoglobin and deoxyhaemoglobin. The lights pass through the skin to a depth of approximately 3 cm, and the reflected lights are sensed by a photodiode. The reflected lights mainly represent the haemoglobin information in the cerebral cortex. The system can measure $rSO_2$ data every second without the need for pulsation. It is therefore possible to continuously monitor the $rSO_2$ values of CPA patients.

### Data analysis

Two $rSO_2$ values (on the left side and right side) were acquired continuously. The average of these two values was then calculated. If the value of one of the two values appeared to be in error, then the other value was used for the data analysis. Finally, graphs were drawn of the serial changes in the cerebral $rSO_2$ values.

### Statistical analysis

All of the data are represented as the mean ± standard deviation (SD). The Wilcoxon rank sum test was used to compare the differences between the two groups at each measurement point. A one-way repeated-measures analysis of variance (ANOVA) was used to evaluate the differences among the measured points. $P$ values of $<0.05$ were considered to indicate statistical significance. All of the statistical analyses were performed using the JMP Pro 11 for Windows software program (SAS Institute Inc., Cary, NC, USA).

## Results

### Normal range of cerebral $rSO_2$

The normal range of cerebral $rSO_2$ in the healthy adult volunteers ($n = 15$; age, $43.2 \pm 8.9$ years; 10 men and 5 women) was $71.2 \pm 3.9\%$ (on room air).

## Patient characteristics

From January 2013 through March 2015, the serial changes in the cerebral $rSO_2$ values of 16 patients were evaluated. Their outcomes, as measured by the GOS score at discharge, included a good recovery (GR) ($n$ = 4), vegetative state (VS) ($n$ = 2), and death (D) ($n$ = 10). The time from the onset of cardiac arrest to the initiation of ECPR did not differ to a statistically significant extent between the poor neurological group (VS and D: $64.6 \pm 22.6$ min) and the good neurological group (GR: $49.5 \pm 5.7$ min) ($P$ = 0.11). The characteristics of the patients with OHCA are shown in Table 1.

## The relationship between the cerebral $rSO_2$ values during ECPR and the neurological outcome

The serial changes in the cerebral $rSO_2$ values during ECPR for each patient are shown in Fig. 1. The serial changes in the mean cerebral $rSO_2$ value during ECPR in the good and poor neurological outcome groups are shown in Fig. 2. The only significant difference in the cerebral $rSO_2$ values of the two groups was observed at 5 min before ECPR ($P < 0.05$) (2 min before ECPR: $P$ = 0.95; 2 min after ECPR: $P$ = 0.36; 5 min after ECPR: $P$ = 0.20; and 10 min after ECPR: $P$ = 0.21). In the poor neurological group (VS and D: $n$ = 12; age, $52.8 \pm 4.0$ years), the cerebral $rSO_2$ values increased significantly during ECPR (5 min before ECPR: $52.0 \pm 1.8\%$; 2 min before ECPR: $56.1 \pm 2.3\%$; 2 min after ECPR: $63.5 \pm 2.2\%$; 5 min after ECPR: $66.4 \pm 2.2\%$; and 10 min after

**Table 1** The characteristics of the patients with out-of-hospital cardiac arrest

| | Good neurological outcome group (GR) | Poor neurological outcome group (VS and D) |
|---|---|---|
| Number | 4 | 12 |
| Age (±SD) (years) | 53.8 ± 6.9 | 52.9 ± 4.0 |
| Male (%) | 4 (100%) | 10 (83.3%) |
| Initial rhythm | | |
| VF (%) | 4 (100%) | 6 (50.0%) |
| PEA (%) | 0 | 4 (33.3%) |
| Asystole (%) | 0 | 2 (16.7%) |
| Witnessed | | |
| Yes (%) | 4 (100%) | 11 (91.7%) |
| No (%) | 0 | 1 (8.3%) |
| Bystander CPR | | |
| Yes (%) | 4 (100%) | 10 (83.3%) |
| No (%) | 0 | 2 (16.7%) |
| The time from the onset of cardiac arrest to the initiation of ECPR (min) | 49.5 ± 5.7 | 64.6 ± 22.6 |

*CPR* cardiopulmonary resuscitation, *D* death, *GR* good recovery, *PEA* pulseless electrical activity, *VF* ventricular fibrillation, *VS* vegetative state

ECPR: $67.6 \pm 2.3\%$ [$P < 0.01$]) (Figs. 1a and 2). In contrast, in the good neurological group (GR: $n$ = 4; age, $53.8 \pm 6.9$ years), the cerebral $rSO_2$ values did not increase to a statistically significant extent during ECPR (5 min before ECPR: $61.9 \pm 3.1\%$; 2 min before ECPR: $57.1 \pm 4.0\%$; 2 min after ECPR: $59.6 \pm 3.8\%$; 5 min after ECPR: $61.0 \pm 3.7\%$; and 10 min after ECPR: $62.0 \pm 3.8\%$ [$P$ = 0.88]) (Figs. 1b and 2).

## Discussion

Recently, a systematic review and meta-analysis reported by Sanfilippo et al. [10] showed that higher initial and average cerebral $rSO_2$ values were both associated with a greater chance of achieving an ROSC in patients with cardiac arrest; however, they could not show a relationship between the cerebral $rSO_2$ value and the neurological outcome of patients resuscitated from cardiac arrest. Both Ito et al. [5] and Storm et al. [11] revealed significantly higher cerebral $rSO_2$ values on hospital arrival in patients with a good neurological outcome, but the cerebral $rSO_2$ values of the good and poor outcome groups varied widely and there was a large amount of overlap. We hypothesised that a single measurement of cerebral value might not be important because the $rSO_2$ values always change depending on the patient's situation at the time of the $rSO_2$ measurement [4, 8]. Therefore, we think that the value of NIRS should be assessed by trend value, not by absolute value.

Counterintuitively, the results of this study suggested that the patients whose cerebral $rSO_2$ values did not show a significant improvement after ECPR might have had a good neurological prognosis (Figs. 1b and 2). We thought that, in the good neurological group, the brain blood flow was recovered by ECPR, the oxygen was delivered to brain tissue, and the brain tissue might start to consume oxygen. These events continuously change. So, we believe that the most important factor when evaluating the cerebral $rSO_2$ value during resuscitation to predict the neurological outcome is serial change in the cerebral $rSO_2$ values. Two reports have shown a significant increase in the cerebral $rSO_2$ value after the application of ECPR in patients with OHCA; however, all of the reported patients had a poor neurological outcome or died [4, 12]. One report showed that the tissue oxygen index decreased in a patient with a favourable neurological outcome ($n$ = 1) but that it did not change in patients with unfavourable neurological outcome ($n$ = 14) [13]. These reports also failed to show a relationship between the cerebral $rSO_2$ value during ECPR and the neurological outcome.

We hypothesised that the cerebral $rSO_2$ values of the patients in the good neurological outcome group did not change before or after ECPR because their brain tissue might have been consuming oxygen; therefore, we began

**a**

rSO$_2$ (%)

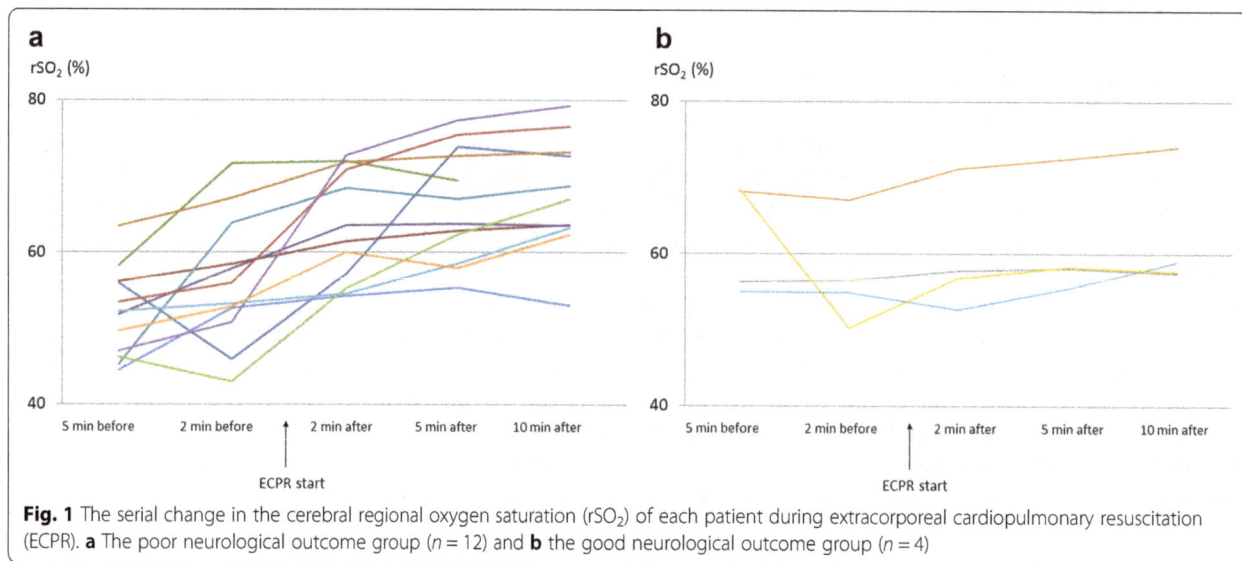

**b**

rSO$_2$ (%)

**Fig. 1** The serial change in the cerebral regional oxygen saturation (rSO$_2$) of each patient during extracorporeal cardiopulmonary resuscitation (ECPR). **a** The poor neurological outcome group (n = 12) and **b** the good neurological outcome group (n = 4)

to evaluate the cerebral rSO$_2$ value during intensive care unit (ICU) treatment after the ROSC. In Fig. 3, we show one patient with an ROSC who displayed a decreasing cerebral rSO$_2$ value but who experienced a GR. When we started to perform cerebral rSO$_2$ measurement in this patient, his cerebral rSO$_2$ value was 66%, and it gradually dropped to 57% after 12 min. His neurological outcome was good. We think that the ROSC led to the recovery of the cerebral blood flow, and because in patients with a good neurological outcome oxygen consumption might increase, as a result, his cerebral rSO$_2$ value decreased. Our study investigates the serial changes in the cerebral rSO$_2$ value during ICU after an ROSC treatment is currently ongoing. In the future, additional studies should be performed to investigate the relationship between the

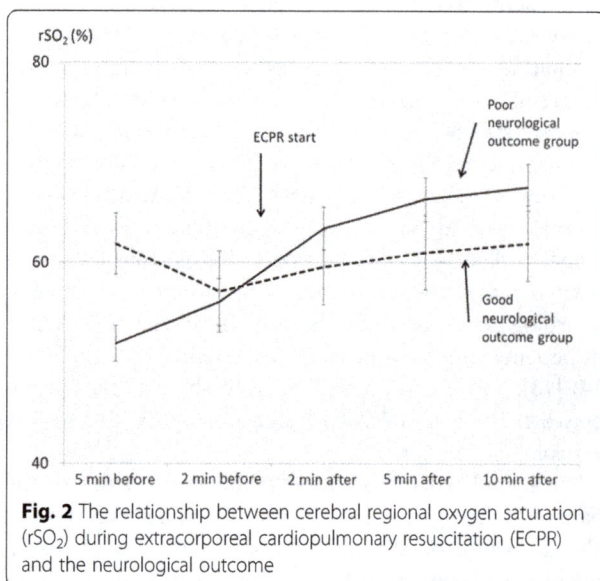

**Fig. 2** The relationship between cerebral regional oxygen saturation (rSO$_2$) during extracorporeal cardiopulmonary resuscitation (ECPR) and the neurological outcome

serial changes in the cerebral rSO$_2$ value after an ROSC and the neurological outcome.

A recent review on ECPR revealed that the outcome of ECPR in patients with in-hospital cardiac arrest was satisfactory, with good survival rates and good neurological outcome [14]. However, it is more challenging to achieve satisfactory ECPR results in OHCA patients, and a good outcome can only be obtained in 15–20% of the patients, provided that the time from cardiac arrest to the initiation of ECPR is shorter than 60 min. Our results may be useful for helping to establish a new ECPR strategy for cardiac arrest patients. If we can predict the neurological outcome during ECPR, we might be able to develop innovative methods to further improve the neurological outcome of these patients.

The present study is associated with some limitations. Firstly, the present study is a single-centre, retrospective study with a small population. There was no ECPR protocol and the application of ECPR depended on the physician's decision. Furthermore, it was not possible to evaluate the cerebral rSO$_2$ value in all of the patients who underwent ECPR during this study period. The number of CPA cases was 420 during the study period. Second, only the patients whose cerebral rSO$_2$ values were recorded during resuscitation were included in the present study. So, we could not evaluate the relationship between the cerebral rSO$_2$ values and the cardiac index, the timing of ROSC and blood pressure. In this study, all patients did not get ROSC during the evaluation of the cerebral rSO$_2$. Third, we did not evaluate the relationship between the cerebral rSO$_2$ values and the blood sample parameters such as the SaO$_2$, PaO$_2$, PaCO$_2$, haematocrit, and lactate values. Fourth, we could not evaluate brain function such as electroencephalogram. Moreover, we did not evaluate the cerebral rSO$_2$ values in the pre-hospital setting.

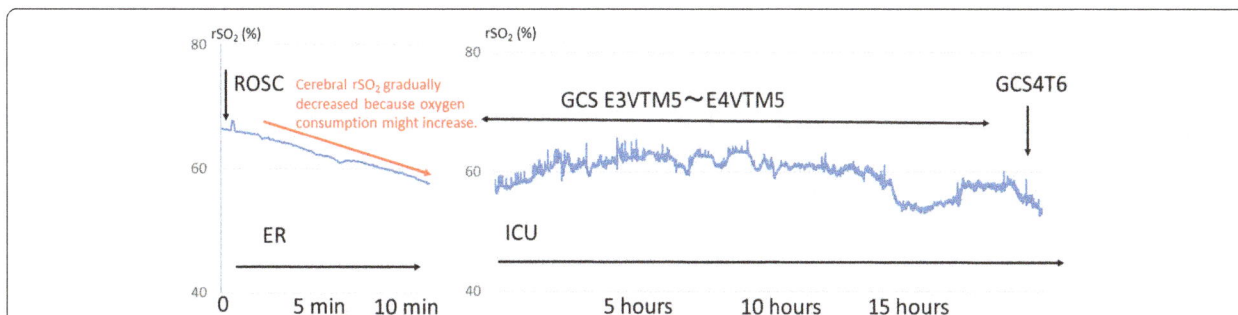

**Fig. 3** The serial change in the cerebral regional oxygen saturation of a 74-year-old male patient during ICU treatment after the ROSC. When we started cerebral rSO$_2$ measurement in this patient, the cerebral rSO$_2$ value was 66%; it gradually fell to 57% after 12 min. His neurological outcome was good. We think that the ROSC led to the recovery of the cerebral blood flow, and because the oxygen consumption of patients with a good neurological outcome might increase, the cerebral rSO$_2$ value can be expected to decrease. *ER* emergency room, *GCS* Glasgow Coma Scale, *ICU* intensive care unit, *ROSC* return of spontaneous circulation, *rSO$_2$* regional saturation of oxygen

Recently, we developed a portable rSO$_2$ monitor (HAND ai TOS®; TOSTEC Co.), which is $170 \times 100 \times 50$ mm in size and 600 g in weight and which is small enough to carry in the pre-hospital settings. Thus, we can now measure the pre-hospital rSO$_2$ values [8]. There is a need for a prospective multi-centre study that includes measurements from the pre-hospital setting.

## Conclusions

The cerebral rSO$_2$ value during ECPR may predict the neurological outcome. The further evaluation of the validity of cerebral rSO$_2$ monitoring during ECPR may lead to a new resuscitation strategy.

### Acknowledgements
We gratefully acknowledge the devoted cooperation of the medical staff in the Traumatology and Critical Care Medical Center, National Hospital Organization Osaka National Hospital.

### Funding
This work was supported by Grants-in-Aid for Scientific Research from the Ministry of Education, Culture, Sports, Science, and Technology in Japan (no. 15H05007).

### Authors' contributions
NE, TH, TS, and MO designed the study. NE, AW, TN, and DS collected and generated the data. NE, TH, TS, AW, TN, NM, and MO analysed the data. NE and TH wrote the first draft. TS, NM, MO, DS, and TS helped to draft the manuscript. All of the authors read and approved the final manuscript.

### Competing interests
The authors declare that they have no competing interests.

### Author details
[1]Traumatology and Critical Care Medical Center, National Hospital Organization Osaka National Hospital, 2-1-14 Hoenzaka Chuo-ku, Osaka, Osaka 540-0006, Japan. [2]Department of Traumatology and Acute Critical Medicine, Osaka University Graduate School of Medicine, 2-15 Yamadaoka, Suita, Osaka 565-0871, Japan.

### References
1. Kitamura T, Iwami T, Kawamura T, Nitta M, Nagao K, Nonogi H, et al. Nationwide improvements in survival from out-of-hospital cardiac arrest in Japan. Circulation. 2012;126:2834–43.
2. Berdowski J, Berg RA, Tijssen JG, Koster RW. Global incidences of out-of-hospital cardiac arrest and survival rates: systematic review of 67 prospective studies. Resuscitation. 2010;81:1479–87.
3. Nakahori Y, Shimizu K, Shiozaki T, Ogura H, Tasaki O, Kuwagata Y, et al. The change of cerebral rSO$_2$ during cardiopulmonary resuscitation. Crit Care Med. 2008;36:A152.
4. Nakahori Y, Hirose T, Shiozaki T, Ogawa Y, Ohnishi M, Fujimi S, et al. Serial changes in values of cerebral regional saturation of oxygen (rSO$_2$) during resuscitation in patients with out-of-hospital cardiac arrest. Nihon Kyukyu Igakukai Zasshi. 2013;24:774–80 (Abstract in English).
5. Ito N, Nishiyama K, Callaway CW, Orita T, Hayashida K, Arimoto H, et al. Noninvasive regional cerebral oxygen saturation for neurological prognostication of patients with out-of-hospital cardiac arrest: a prospective multicenter observational study. Resuscitation. 2014;85:778–84.
6. Hayashida K, Nishiyama K, Suzuki M, Abe T, Orita T, Ito N, et al. Estimated cerebral oxyhemoglobin as a useful indicator of neuroprotection in patients with post-cardiac arrest syndrome: a prospective, multicenter observational study. Crit Care. 2014;18:500.
7. Nishiyama K, Ito N, Orita T, Hayashida K, Arimoto H, Beppu S, et al. Regional cerebral oxygen saturation monitoring for predicting interventional outcomes in patients following out-of-hospital cardiac arrest of presumed cardiac cause: a prospective, observational, multicentre study. Resuscitation. 2015;96:135–41.
8. Tajima G, Shiozaki T, Izumino H, Yamano S, Hirao T, Inokuma T, et al. Portable system for monitoring of regional cerebral oxygen saturation during prehospital cardiopulmonary resuscitation: a pilot study. Acute Med Surg. 2015;2:48–52.
9. Hazinski MF, Nolan JP, Billi JE, Böttiger BW, Bossaert L, de Caen AR, et al. Part 1: Executive summary: 2010 International Consensus on Cardiopulmonary Resuscitation and Emergency Cardiovascular Care Science with Treatment Recommendations. Circulation. 2010;122:S250–75.
10. Sanfilippo F, Serena G, Corredor C, Benedetto U, Maybauer M, Al-Subaie N, et al. Cerebral oximetry and return of spontaneous circulation after cardiac arrest: a systematic review and meta-analysis. Resuscitation. 2015;94:67–72.
11. Storm C, Leithner C, Krannich A, Wutzler A, Ploner CJ, Trenkmann L, et al. Regional cerebral oxygen saturation after cardiac arrest in 60 patients—a prospective outcome study. Resuscitation. 2014;85:1037–41.

12. Taccone FS, Fagnoul D, Rondelet B, Vincent JL, de Backer D. Cerebral oximetry during extracorporeal cardiopulmonary resuscitation. Crit Care. 2013;17:409.

13. Yagi T, Nagao K, Sakatani K, Kawamorita T, Soga T, Kikushima K, et al. Changes of cerebral oxygen metabolism and hemodynamics during ECPR with hypothermia measured by near-infrared spectroscopy: a pilot study. Adv Exp Med Biol. 2013;789:121–8.

14. Fagnoul D, Combes A, De Backer D. Extracorporeal cardiopulmonary resuscitation. Curr Opin Crit Care. 2014;20:259–65.

# 5

# Acetylcholinesterase and butyrylcholinesterase in cardiosurgical patients with postoperative delirium

Mira John[1]*, E. Wesley Ely[2,3], Dorothee Halfkann[1], Julika Schoen[1], Beate Sedemund-Adib[1], Stefan Klotz[4], Finn Radtke[5], Sebastian Stehr[1] and Michael Hueppe[1]

## Abstract

**Background:** Patients in intensive care units (ICU) are often diagnosed with postoperative delirium; the duration of which has a relevant negative impact on various clinical outcomes. Recent research found a potentially important role of acetylcholinesterase (AChE) and butyrylcholinesterase (BChE) in delirium of critically ill patients on non-surgical ICU or in non-cardiac-surgery patients. We tested the hypothesis that AChE and BChE have an impact on patients after cardiac surgery with postoperative delirium.

**Methods:** After obtaining approval from the local ethics committee, this mechanistic study gathered data of all 217 patients included in a randomized controlled trial testing non-pharmacological modifications of care in the cardiac surgical ICU to reduce delirium.
Delirium was assessed with the Confusion Assessment Method for the Intensive Care Unit (*CAM-ICU*) and the Nursing Delirium Screening Scale (*Nu-DESC*) twice a day for the first 3 days after surgery. Further outcome variables were somatic laboratory parameters and variables regarding surgery, anesthesia, and postsurgical recovery. 10 μl venous or arterial blood was drawn and AChE and BChE were determined with *ChE check mobile* from Securetec.

**Results:** Of 217 patients, 60 (27.6%) developed postsurgical delirium (POD). Patients with POD were older ($p = 0.005$), had anemia ($p = 0.01$), and worse kidney function ($p = 0.006$). Furthermore, these patients had lower intraoperative cerebral saturation (NIRS) ($p < 0.001$) and higher intraoperative need of catecholamines ($p = 0.03$). Delirious patients showed more inflammatory response ($p < 0.001$). AChE and BChE values were mainly inside the norm. Patients with values outside the norm did not have POD more often than others. Regarding AChE and BChE patients did not differ in having delirium or not ($p > 0.10$).

**Conclusions:** Postoperative measurement of AChE and BChE did not discern between patients with and without POD. The effect of the cardiac surgical procedure on AChE and BChE remains unclear. Further studies with patients in cardiac surgery are needed to evaluate a possible combination of delirium and the cholinergic transmitter system. There might be possible interactions with AChE/BChE and blood products and the use of cardiopulmonary bypass, which should be investigated more intensively.

**Keywords:** Delirium, Cardiac surgery, Intensive care unit, Acetylcholinesterase, Butyrylcholinesterase, CAM-ICU, Nu-DESC

* Correspondence: mira.john@uksh.de
[1]Clinic for Anaesthesiology and Intensive-Care Medicine, UKSH Campus Luebeck, Ratzeburger Allee 160, 23538 Luebeck, Germany
Full list of author information is available at the end of the article

# Background

The definition of delirium according to DSM-5 criteria includes a transient and serious disturbance in attention and cognition and the development over a short period of time. The symptoms tend to fluctuate during the day and cannot be explained by a pre-existing neurocognitive disorder [1].

Delirium is a complex symptom which is very common in operative and non-operative disciplines in the course of hospital stay. The incidence is especially high among patients undergoing heart surgery [2]. The incidence in this patient population has been described to be from 30 up to 80% [2–4].

The duration of delirium has a relevant negative impact on various clinical outcomes. Patients stay longer on the ICU, they suffer from more complications, are immobilized for a longer period of time, have a higher 6-months-mortality, and have long-term cognitive impairment [3–8].

The causes for delirium are numerous. Intoxication, drugs, alcohol, hypoglycaemia, hypoxia, or anemia might lead to cognitive dysfunction. The pre-, intra-, and postoperative status of patients might also trigger symptoms of delirium. Especially, a pre-existing dementia, fluid loss, abnormal electrolyte concentrations, use of benzodiazepines, and hypotension belong to those trigger factors. Especially older patients tend to develop delirium more often. This might be a result of hearing impairment, changes of the environment, and a limited bladder- and bowl function; in particular, during stay in hospital [9].

Other hypotheses assume an influence of infection and stress (also postoperative stress) with a higher level of cytokines (IL-1, IL-6) and a higher level of cortisol inside the cerebrospinal fluid [10, 11].

In addition, neuronal metabolism and changes in transmitter interaction have been implicated to play a central role in delirium (e.g., acetylcholine and dopamine) [12, 13]. Previous studies show that patients with preoperative lower levels of cholinesterase are postoperatively more often diagnosed with delirium [14]. Those patients might have a higher function of serum-cholinesterase. Additionally, pilot studies show that the use of indirect parasympathomimetics (e.g., physostigmine) may reduce the severity of delirium [15–17]. Worek et al. found a procedure which provides a simple method for sensitive and precise determination of AChE in whole blood samples [18].

Due to recent studies that found a potentially important mechanistic role of acetylcholinesterase (AChE) and butyrylcholinesterase (BChE) in delirium of critically ill patients on non-surgical ICU or in non-cardiac surgery patients, the main focus of this paper was to examine AChE and BChE in patients after cardiac surgery and their association with postoperative delirium [12, 14, 16, 19].

# Methods

## Study design

We designed a mechanistic study of data from all patients included in a randomized controlled trial. The two investigators were blinded against each other. The study was conducted after the positive vote of the local ethics committee and was registered in the German Register for Clinical Trials (German Clinical Trials Register: DRKS00006217). All patients gave informed consent to take part in this study.

## Patient population

Patients were enrolled from June 1st, 2014 until December 20th, 2014. All patients had an elective cardiosurgical procedure with a postoperative stay on the ICU.

Inclusion criteria: minimum age of 18 years, men and women were equally considered, command of the German language.

Exclusion criteria: missing consent, preoperative diagnosis of delirium (with *CAM-ICU*), psychiatric pre-diagnosis of schizophrenia, preoperative indications for cognitive dysfunction (*abbreviated mental test* < 7 points), *RASS-Score* < −2 for the current test, and neurological complications (e.g., media infarction).

## Independent variable

The intervention itself was the study's independent variable and the assignment to control- or intervention group. Patients in the intervention group received special exercises for orientation: standardized acoustic, visual, olfactory, and tactile stimulation (see Table 1). The intervention was performed twice a day for the first 3 days after surgery.

## Dependent variable

### Delirium

Occurrence of postsurgical delirium (POD) was the dependent variable (i.e., the primary outcome variable), as measured using a combination of the Confusion Assessment Method for the Intensive Care Unit (CAM-ICU) [20] and the Nursing Delirium Screening Scale (Nu-DESC) [21, 22] twice a day for the first 3 days after surgery (morning and late afternoon). Both screening tools were tested for ICU patients and show high sensitivity and specificity.

CAM-ICU was performed identically each time and inspired by the CAM-ICU worksheet. All four features were conducted (acute onset or fluctuating course, inattention, altered level of consciousness, disorganized thinking); the inattention was tested via the letters in the word ANANASBAUM, explained once at the beginning and in case of patients failing to squeeze on the letter "A" and when the patients squeezed on any letter other than "A" errors were counted.

**Table 1** Exercises for orientation

| Stimulation | Contents | Summary |
|---|---|---|
| Acoustic/visual stimulation | Time of year, date, time of day, weather, place, reason for stay, day of surgery/duration of stay<br>News of the day (newspaper article with picture) | Summary with pictures of temporal and local orientation |
| Olfactory stimulation | Lemon<br>Peppermint<br>Orange | Summary with plants suitable to the smelling and view at the items of tactile stimulation |
| Tactile stimulation | Screw<br>Cotton pad<br>Sandpaper | |

Annotation: acoustic stimulation contained questions for the time of year, the date and time of day as well as the weather, place, reason, and duration of stay. Patients were corrected in case of false answer or supported in case of correct answers. The information was summarized by the investigator and was enhanced with suitable pictures. Afterwards patients got to read out a newspaper article. In the olfactory stimulation, patients got to smell three different smellings (lemon, peppermint, and orange).
The answers were corrected or supported and summarized with special pictures. The tactile stimulation in the end included a screw, cotton pad, and a sandpaper. The answers were corrected or supported, and patients could have a look at the items they felt before

Patients with a Richmond Agitation Sedation Scale (RASS) $\leq -2$ were excluded for the current testing. A positive delirium diagnoses was given if patients got a positive result in CAM-ICU and/or Nu-DESC at least once within the 3 days of measurement.

### Cognitive dysfunction

For recognition of cognitive dysfunction, the abbreviated mental test (AMT) was performed once a day (in the evening) for the first 3 days after surgery. Especially for cardiosurgical patients the AMT is a very useful tool in detection for cognitive function.

### Anxiety and pain

According to the current DAS-Guidelines (Guideline for **D**elirium management, **A**nalgesia, **S**edative medication on the ICU), patients were interviewed for anxiety and pain also twice a day for the first 3 days after surgery. It was assessed with the numeric rating scale (NRS; score: 0 = no pain–10 = maximum pain). Pain was separated into resting pain and pain on movement.

### Somatic laboratory parameters

Blood was drawn from each patient twice a day after each testing. All patients had a central venous catheter or an arterial catheter where 10 µl venous or arterial blood was taken out and used for determination of AChE and BChE. The measurement was performed immediately with *ChE check mobile* from Securetec [18]. The reference range is for AChE: 26.7–50.9 U/gHb and for BChE 2300–7000 U/L.

Furthermore, postoperative leukocytes, C-reactive protein (CRP), creatine kinase (CK), heart-enzymes (CK-MB), and creatinine were tested once every day in the normal laboratory control.

### Preoperative variables

Patients were evaluated for psychological and cognitive function. After a written consent, patients received a 12-sided questionnaire with special questions about personal, the Hospital Anxiety and Depression Scale in a German version (HADS-D), the Pain Sensitivity Questionnaire (PSQ), and finally questions for life quality (SF-12). Questions about the person itself contained information about age, gender, education, previous surgery, regular use of nicotine and alcohol, other illnesses, and use of drugs.

Preoperative assessment of CRP, leukocytes, hemoglobin, and creatinine was performed.

### Variables of surgery and anesthesia

From the anesthesia report duration of surgery, method of narcosis and its duration as well as intraoperative cerebral saturation (near infra-red spectrometry, NIRS), lactate, hemoglobin, and the used drugs were noticed. Furthermore, transfusion of blood products, the use of catecholamines, and any complications were written down.

### Postoperative variables

Especially important was the duration of mechanical ventilation and the time of stay on the ICU and in hospital in total. The need of blood transfusion, given psychiatric drugs, and any other medication was collected. Furthermore, any complication in recovery time was noticed.

### Study protocol

All elective cardiosurgical patients were assessed for eligibility. In case of meeting the inclusion criteria, a written consent from patients were evaluated and randomized. The randomization was performed by the project leader (M.H.) who was not involved in the delirium assessment and the implementation of the intervention. The program BiAS was used for randomization.

All patients were postoperatively admitted to the ICU mechanically ventilated and hemodynamic supported. As soon as patients met the extubation criteria and were extubated, both investigators visited the patients separately (blinded by each other) twice a day (in the morning and in the late afternoon) for the first 3 days after surgery. The intervention, delirium assessment, and the postoperative evaluation were performed each time of measurement.

## Statistical analysis

Statistical analysis was performed by chi-square tests, $t$ tests, and analysis of variance using SPSS 22. $P$ values lower 0.05 were considered statistically significant.

## Results
### Sample of analysis

332 patients were assessed for eligibility. All those patients had an elective cardiosurgical procedure. Eighty-one patients had to be excluded due to declining participation ($n = 47$), missing inclusion criteria ($n = 20$), or others ($n = 14$). In total, 251 patients were randomized and allocated to intervention ($n = 129$) or control group ($n = 122$). Due to canceled surgery ($n = 3$) or later decline of participation ($n = 6$), preoperative tests that revealed exclusion criteria ($n = 3$), postoperative decease of patients ($n = 3$), diagnosed media infarction ($n = 10$), or others ($n = 9$), a total number of 217 patients were included in the analysis (see Fig. 1). Within this mechanistic study in up to six patients few data was missing.

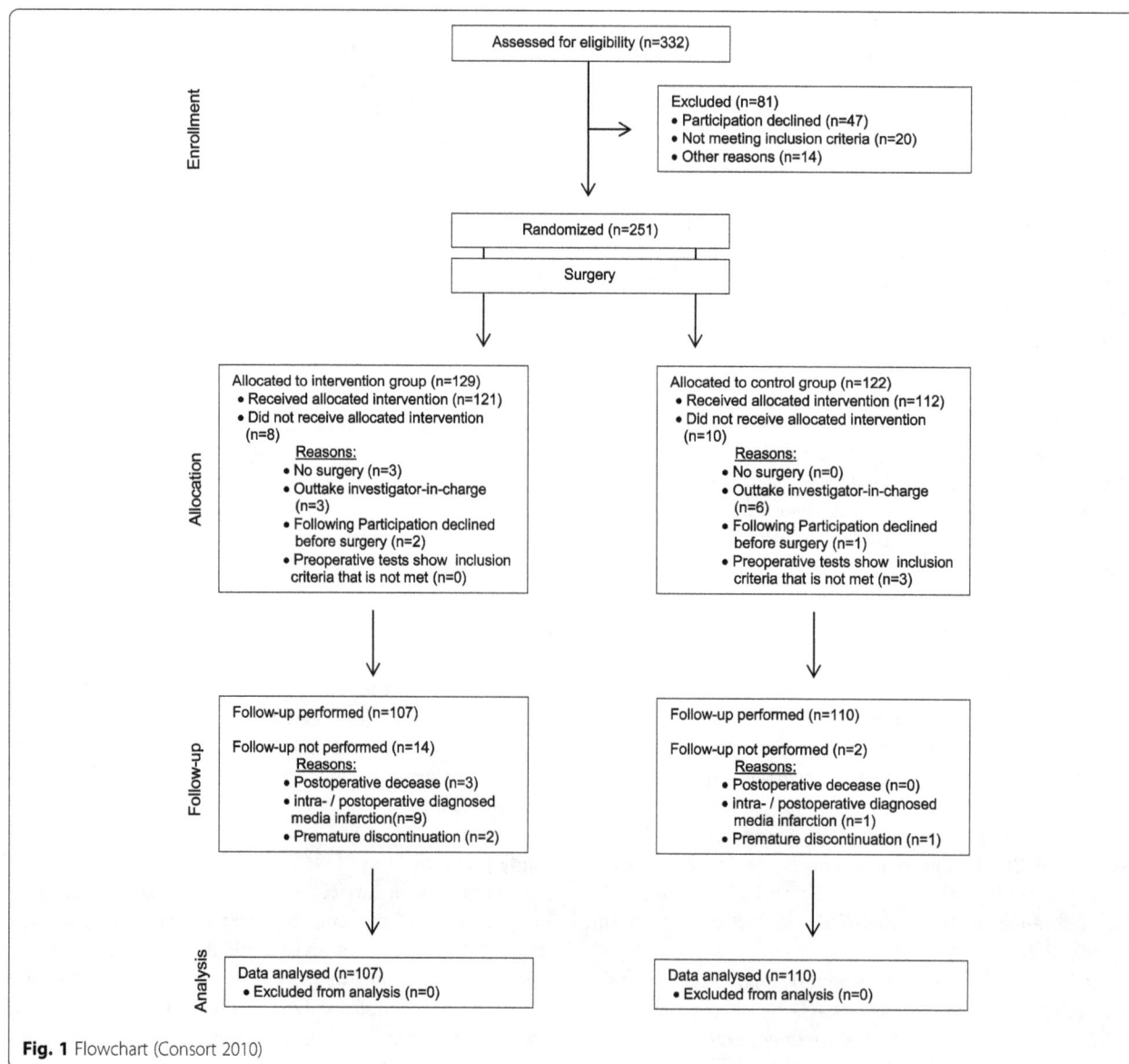

**Fig. 1** Flowchart (Consort 2010)

## Description of sample of analysis

Most participants were male gender (71.4%), had a lower education and any previous surgeries. Patients were classified as ASA-PS III in 92.6% (patients with illnesses with marked impairment). All patients received a balanced anesthesia with propofol, sufentanil, remifentanil and sevoflurane. Most patients had coronary surgery (40.6%). The mean duration of the anesthetic procedure was 5.5 h, surgery lasted about 4.75 h. Cardiac bypass time was 2 h in average. Patients were sedated and ventilated for about 3.5 h in postoperative ICU care. All patients got opiates for analgesia. In case they developed delirium, they got lorazepam or haloperidol. If they could not be extubated early, they had a combined sedation with dexmedetomidine or propofol and opiates. In case the weaning lasted more than a week, propofol was replaced by midazolam. On average, patients were discharged to a normal ward after 2.1 days and left the hospital after 12.6 days. Table 2 gives an overview of sample of analysis description.

## Incidence of delirium

Of 217 patients, 60 (27.6%) developed postoperative delirium according to the results of CAM-ICU and Nu-DESC combined together. Considering just the results from CAM-ICU, only 26 patients had a positive result (12.0%). There were no differences in transient and continuously delirious patients. Most patients developed their delirium on the second day after surgery.

## Differences between patients with and without postoperative delirium

### Preoperative variables

Patients who developed postoperative delirium were older ($p = 0.005$). They did not differ in their education. Values of hemoglobin were already preoperatively lower in patients developing delirium afterwards ($p = 0.01$). Furthermore, those patients had worse kidney function ($p = 0.006$). We did not see a difference in preoperatively recognized higher inflammatory response regarding the delirium diagnosis. Patients with delirium did not have a higher ASA-PS-Score preoperatively than patients without delirium.

### Intraoperative variables

If patients had a lower intraoperative cerebral saturation they developed delirium postoperatively more often ($p = 0.001$). Additionally, those patients had a higher need of noradrenaline ($p = 0.03$) during surgery. The duration of anesthesia, surgery or time of bypass was not longer in patients with postoperative delirium ($p > 0.05$). Furthermore, there was no relation in occurrence of complications (heart arrhythmia and intubation problems) and a higher rate of delirium afterwards.

**Table 2** Description of sample of analysis

| Characteristic | Total sample ($n = 217$) |
|---|---|
| Age (years) [M (SD)] | 65.4 (12.3) |
| Sex [$n$ (%)] | |
|   Male | 155 (71.4) |
|   Female | 62 (28.6) |
| Education [$n$ (%)] | |
|   No graduation | 7 (3.2) |
|   Low graduation | 89 (41.0) |
|   Middle graduation | 52 (24.0) |
|   Polytechnic secondary school | 28 (12.9) |
|   Higher graduation | 21 (9.7) |
|   A-level | 20 (9.2) |
| ASA-PS [$n$ (%)] | |
|   2 | 2 (0.9) |
|   3 | 201 (92.6) |
|   4 | 14 (6.5) |
|   LV-EF in % [M (SD)] | 57.9 (13.4) |
| Anesthesia [$n$ (%)] | |
|   Balanced | 217 (100.0) |
|   Pulmonary artery catheter | 59 (28.5) |
|   NIRS | 217 (100.0) |
|   TEE | 169 (81.6) |
|   BIS | 217 (100.0) |
| Operative procedure [$n$ (%)] | |
|   Coronary surgery | 88 (40.6) |
|   Valve surgery (even multiple valves) | 46 (21.2) |
|   Coronary and valve surgery | 22 (10.1) |
|   Aorta ascendens replacement | 2 (0.9) |
|   Valve surgery + aorta ascendens replacement | 12 (5.5) |
|   Other combinations | 35 (16.1) |
|   Other surgery | 12 (5.5) |
| Intraoperative variables [M (SD)] | |
|   Duration of anesthesia (min) | 329.2 (81.1) |
|   Duration of surgery (min) | 258.5 (79.1) |
|   Time of bypass (min) | 123.2 (58.9) |
|   Duration of mechanical ventilation after surgery (min) [M (SD)] | 334.5 (658.3) |
|   Duration of stay on the ICU (days) [M (SD)] | 2.1 (2.8) |
|   Duration of stay in hospital (days) [M (SD)] | 12.6 (6.2) |

Abbreviation: *M* mean, *SD* standard deviation, *n* number of patients, *%* percent, *min* minutes. *ASA* risk score American Society of Anesthesiologists, *LVEF* left ventricular ejection fraction, *NIRS* near infrared spectrometry, *TEE* transesophageal echocardiography, *BIS* bispectral index)

### Postoperative variables

Patients with POD had a longer duration of ventilation after surgery ($p = 0.004$) and increased length of ICU as well as in hospital stay (both $p = 0.01$). Neurological complications during hospital stay were seen more often in patients with delirium ($p = 0.001$). Anemia was also more often present in patients with POD than without ($p = 0.01$). Other complications were recorded more often in delirium patients, but without reaching the level of significance.

Patients with delirium did show lower value of hemoglobin ($p = 0.002$), higher inflammatory response (CRP: $p = 0.01$), higher rate of heart enzymes (CK: $p = 0.03$; CK-MB: $p = 0.04$), and worse kidney function (creatinine: $p = 0.001$). Leukocytes did not differ in patients with or without delirium.

Leukocytes and heart enzymes declined during the 3 days of measurement. CRP reached its maximum on the third day after surgery. Hemoglobin and creatinine remained stable. Table 3 shows values in detail.

**Table 3** Pre-, intra-, and postoperative variables

| Variables | Delirum | n | M | SD | p value |
|---|---|---|---|---|---|
| Preoperative variables | | | | | |
| Age | No | 157 | 64.0 | 12.8 | *0.005* |
| | Yes | 60 | 69.2 | 10.1 | |
| Hemoglobin (g/dl) | No | 157 | 13.6 | 1.8 | *0.01* |
| | Yes | 60 | 13.0 | 1.8 | |
| Creatinine (µmol/l) | No | 155 | 93.3 | 39.5 | *0.006* |
| | Yes | 59 | 116.4 | 81.4 | |
| Intraoperative variables | | | | | |
| Duration of anesthesia (min) | No | 157 | 323.3 | 77.3 | 0.08 |
| | Yes | 60 | 344.7 | 89.1 | |
| Duration of surgery (min) | No | 151 | 252.4 | 74.3 | 0.07 |
| | Yes | 60 | 274.0 | 88.7 | |
| Time of bypass (min) | No | 152 | 119.9 | 57.2 | 0.35 |
| | Yes | 60 | 128.3 | 63.6 | |
| NIRS (low) | No | 157 | 69.5 | 8.2 | *0.001* |
| | Yes | 60 | 65.4 | 7.6 | |
| Nor-adrenaline | No | 157 | 2.9 | 2.8 | *0.03* |
| | Yes | 60 | 3.8 | 2.4 | |
| Postoperative variables | | | | | |
| Mechanical ventilation (min) | No | 157 | 254.4 | 178.8 | *0.004* |
| | Yes | 60 | 544.1 | 1200.2 | |
| Stay on the ICU (days) | No | 157 | 1.9 | 2.5 | *0.01* |
| | Yes | 60 | 2.9 | 3.4 | |
| Stay in hospital (days) | No | 157 | 11.9 | 5.3 | *0.01* |
| | Yes | 60 | 14.3 | 8.0 | |

Abbreviation: *M* mean, *SD* standard deviation, *n* number of patients, *min* minutes
$p < 0.05$ is statistically significant

### AChE and BChE

AChE increased within the first 3 days after surgery ($p = 0.02$), BChE decreased ($p < 0.001$) (Table 4). Patients with and without delirium did not differ (Figs. 2 and 3).

Just a few values were outside the normal range; however, those patients did not develop delirium more often than others. Additionally, AChE and BChE levels were not affected by the study intervention.

### Cognitive function

Patients with postoperative delirium did not have a worse AMT preoperatively in comparison to patients without delirium. Patients reached a worse result in AMT during an episode of postoperative delirium ($p < 0.001$).

### Anxiety and pain

Patients with and without delirium did not differ in having resting pain and pain under movement. Patients showed significantly more anxiety when they developed delirium ($p = 0.001$).

## Discussion
### Summary of key findings

The focus of this analysis was a comparison of patients with and without delirium after cardiac surgery.

Within this patient population, the incidence of postoperative delirium was 27.6%. Secondary outcome variables showed that patients with delirium were older, had anemia, a worse kidney function, a lower cerebral saturation during surgery, and a higher need of noradrenaline. Furthermore, those patients had a higher inflammatory response.

The main result was that AChE and BChE values were mainly inside the norm and did not differ in patients having postoperative delirium or not.

Due to recent studies which supposed an important role of AChE and BChE in delirium of critically ill patients this study focused on AChE and BChE in patients after cardiac surgery and its impact on postoperative delirium. Results of this study did not show a difference in AChE and BChE of patients suffering from delirium than those who did not.

### Strengths and limitations

This analysis was designed as a mechanistic study from all patients included in a randomized controlled trial. The investigators were blinded against each other. Those two facts show the quality and strength of this study. Additionally, patients were visited twice a day which takes the cycling of delirious symptoms into account. Furthermore, most patients undergoing heart surgery participated and responded very well. The dependent variable (the occurrence of postoperative delirium) was assessed with CAM-ICU and Nu-DESC. Both screening

**Table 4** AChE and BChE values (in detail)

| Variable | Day | Delirium | | No delirium | | Analysis of variance | | | | | |
| --- | --- | --- | --- | --- | --- | --- | --- | --- | --- | --- | --- |
| | | | | | | Group | | Time | | G × T | |
| | | M | SD | M | SD | F | p | F | p | F | p |
| AChE | 1 | 47.2 | 5.8 | 45.8 | 6.2 | 2.2 | 0.14 | 4.3 | 0.02 | 0.2 | 0.78 |
| | 2 | 47.7 | 5.4 | 46.0 | 5.9 | | | | | | |
| | 3 | 47.9 | 4.8 | 46.4 | 6.3 | | | | | | |
| BChE | 1 | 2613.8 | 639.5 | 2710.2 | 632.2 | 0.7 | 0.41 | 62.7 | <0.001 | 0.5 | 0.58 |
| | 2 | 2399.8 | 574.6 | 2446.3 | 534.0 | | | | | | |
| | 3 | 2291.7 | 548.0 | 2394.2 | 522.4 | | | | | | |

Abbreviation: *M* mean, SD standard deviation, *p* p - value, *G × T* group × time

tools are characterized by its good test quality criteria (sensitivity and specificity) and the easy use for critically ill patients on the ICU. Additionally, testing was performed by a qualified investigator who was independent of the work on the ICU. As shown in the section of results, this study could reproduce previous findings in delirious patients. The differences in patients with and without delirium are plausibly significant. As well as other studies have already shown patients with delirium were older, had more often anemia, were mechanically ventilated longer, had longer ICU and hospital stays; furthermore, as previously shown, those patients had a higher rate of cognitive dysfunction. These facts indicate the strength and validity of this analysis.

Limitations of this study might be the short duration of 3 days measurement, no preoperative values of AChE and BChE as well as no long-term follow-up was performed. Blood was taken from each patient; in case the analysis could not be performed immediately, the sample

was cooled down in a refrigerator. Maybe values of AChE and BChE changed in combination with lower temperatures. During analysis, the blood needed to be mixed with a substance in the cap; maybe there is a difference in strength of shaking and final discrepancies of the mixed samples. Furthermore, it was only one measurement performed with each sample, so no control values could be achieved.

In addition, not all patients got a measurement due to technical problems (long wait for material) and removed central line catheters which implicated missing values afterwards.

Previous studies assumed an interaction of delirium and the immune and cholinergic systems [12] and identified plasma cholinesterase activity as a useful biomarker to identify patients with a higher risk for postoperative delirium [14]. As shown in this study AChE increased within the first 3 days after surgery and BChE decreased. We do know from previous studies that serum cholinesterase

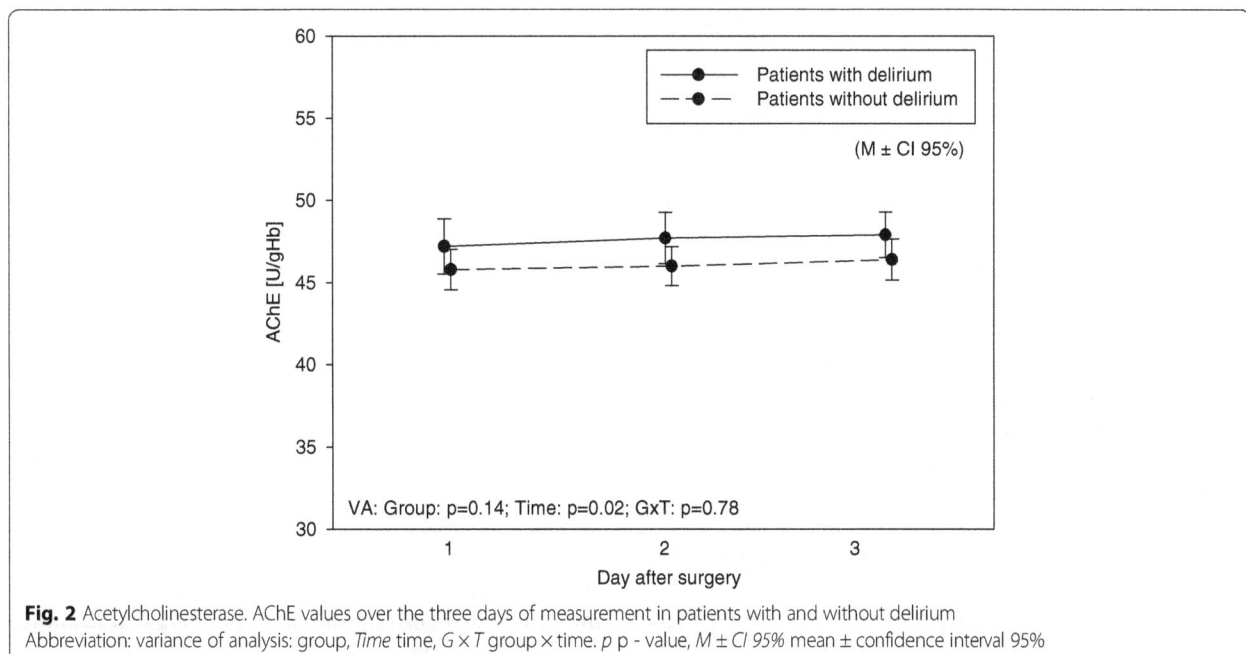

**Fig. 2** Acetylcholinesterase. AChE values over the three days of measurement in patients with and without delirium
Abbreviation: variance of analysis: group, *Time* time, *G × T* group × time. *p* p - value, *M ± CI 95%* mean ± confidence interval 95%

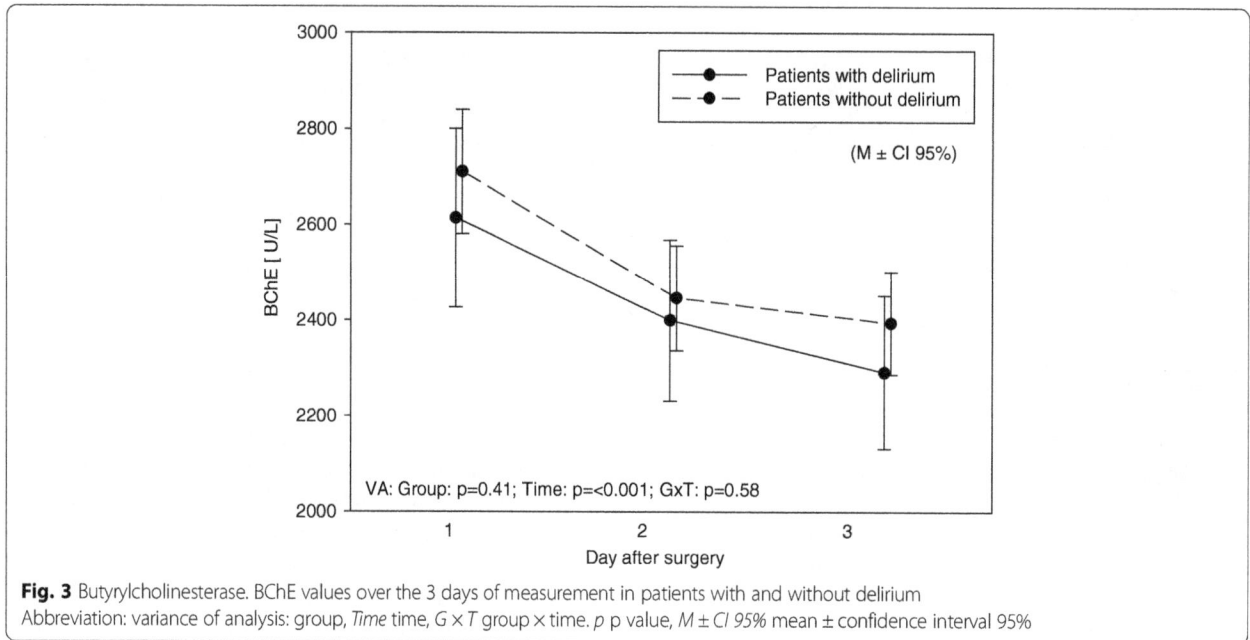

**Fig. 3** Butyrylcholinesterase. BChE values over the 3 days of measurement in patients with and without delirium
Abbreviation: variance of analysis: group, *Time* time, *G × T* group × time. *p* p value, *M ± CI 95%* mean ± confidence interval 95%

(BChE) is the major enzyme hydrolysing AChE in the blood. The role of this enzyme during inflammation has not been fully understood yet. However, studies show that the reduction of BChE activity could early indicate the onset on the systemic inflammatory response. Therefore, BChE could decline due to the inflammatory response in the neurosystem after surgery.

Studies with an interventional approach using cholinesterase inhibitors such as physostigmine were performed. Dawson et al. proposed the use in anticholinergic delirium that did not respond to non-pharmacological delirium management [16]. In contrast, Jackson et al. assumed that simple enhancement of cholinergic neurotransmission may not be sufficient enough to treat delirium [23]. Most studies which were previously performed did not include patients undergoing cardiac surgery. There are various studies with patients in general surgery or on the internal ICU.

Potentially, there is an interaction of AChE and BChE and the use of a cardiopulmonary bypass. A different medication is used for those patients as well. Furthermore, patients after cardiac surgery are critically ill and do need transfusion of blood products. Until now no studies were performed which evaluated AChE and BChE and possible interactions of blood products. A recent study with patients undergoing venoarterial ECMO therapy after cardiac surgery however revealed BChE as a strong predictor of all-cause and cardiovascular mortality [19].

Another fact to mention is the different concentration of AChE at the perisynaptic space and the blood. Although previous studies show that the blood concentration is strongly related to the rate of delirium

and a method for testing was developed, the pathophysiology is not clearly understood yet.

The latest systematic review about published RCTs evaluated the use of acetylcholinesterase inhibitors for delirium treatment. No efficacy for the prevention or management of delirium could be found [17].

Incidence of delirium measured with CAM-ICU was much lower than with Nu-DESC. Possible reasons might be more subjective evaluation of patients with Nu-DESC. Patients just need two points out of ten to be marked positive for delirium; that means already two items can be judged as low remarkable. Patients after cardiac surgery might easily be scored with positive items due to long duration of surgery. In general, those patients are more often very critically ill which also supports this statement. Another aspect might however also be that delirium assessment with Nu-DESC might identify patients in a prodromal stage of delirium. Furthermore, both methods have a different approach. Nu-DESC is a test with external assessment, *CAM-ICU* needs a reaction and interaction of the patient [21, 24].

**Conclusions**

In conclusion, we could reproduce results regarding delirium as previously shown. Delirium is a serious complex of various symptoms, which need to be recognized early to initiate a correct and effective treatment. In this analysis, no difference of AChE and BChE in cardiosurgical patients with or without postoperative delirium could be found.

Further studies are needed to evaluate a possible connection of delirium and the cholinergic transmitter system. Studies which investigate the pathophysiology of the cholinergic system are essential. Furthermore, a possible association of cardiosurgical patients on the ICU and the cholinergic transmitter system should be examined. Studies measuring acetylcholinesterase and butyrylcholinesterase in surgical patients should include preoperative values and need to be continued during surgery and postoperatively (probably over more than three days after surgery). Not to mention the fact that the use of anticholinergic medication should be handled with care. Furthermore, the measurement should be performed more than twice a day and probably even at night. Due to the fact that mostly patients after cardiac surgery develop delirium, and due to the negative impact on clinical outcomes, more studies with this patient population should be conducted in the future.

## Abbreviations

AChE: Acetylcholinesterase; AMT: Abbreviated mental test; ASA-PS: American Society of Anesthesiologists–Physical Status; BChE: Butyrylcholinesterase; BIS: Bispectral index; CAM-ICU: Confusion Assessment Method for the Intensive Care Unit; CI: Confidence interval; CK: Creatine kinase; CK-MB: Creatine kinase, myocardial subtype; CRP: C-reactive protein; DSM-5: Diagnostic and Statistical Manual of Mental Disorders, Fifth Edition; ECMO: Extra-corporal-membrane-oxygenation; HADS-D: Hospital Anxiety and Depression Scale—German version; ICU: Intensive care unit; IL-1/IL-6: Interleukin-1/-6; LVEF: Left ventricular ejection fraction; M: Mean; NIRS: Near-infrared spectroscopy; NRS: Numeric rating scale; Nu-DESC: Nursing Delirium Screening Scale; p: p value; POD: Postoperative delirium; PSQ: Pain Sensitivity Questionnaire; RASS-Score: Richmond Agitation Sedation Score; RCT: Randomized controlled trial; SD: Standard deviation; SF-12: Questionnaire for Quality of life; TEE: Transesophageal echocardiography

## Acknowledgements

We would like to thank all participants in this study for their support during the whole research. We are grateful to all doctors and nurses on the ICU, the intermediate care ward, and the ward for cardiosurgical patients. We would like to thank Securetec and Koehler Chemie for providing a device for measuring acetylcholinesterase and butyrylcholinesterase.

## Funding

Not applicable.

## Authors' contributions

MJ designed the study, performed the data collection, analysis, and interpretation and was the major contributor in writing this manuscript. WE supported the work with his expertise and helped write this manuscript. DH performed the data collection of the dependent variable. JS, BSA, FR, and SS supported the work with their expertise. SK enabled the patient enrolment. MH was the project leader. All authors read and approved the final manuscript. All authors read and approved the final manuscript.

## Competing interests

MJ's traveling costs for the HAI in Berlin 2016 were paid by Koehler Chemie. The other authors declare that they have no competing interests.

## Author details

[1]Clinic for Anaesthesiology and Intensive-Care Medicine, UKSH Campus Luebeck, Ratzeburger Allee 160, 23538 Luebeck, Germany. [2]Pulmonary and Critical Care Medicine, Vanderbilt University, Nashville, Tennessee, USA. [3]Geriatric Research Education Clinical Center (GRECC) of the Tennessee Valley Veterans Administration, Nashville, Tennessee, USA. [4]Department of Cardiac and Thoracic Vascular Surgery, UKSH Campus Luebeck, Luebeck, Germany. [5]Clinic for Anaesthesiology and Operative Intensive-Care Medicine, Charité University Hospital Berlin, Berlin, Germany.

## References

1. The dsm-5 criteria, level of arousal and delirium diagnosis. Inclusiveness is safer. BMC Med. 2014;12:141.
2. Klugkist M, Sedemund-Adib B, Schmidtke C, Schmucker P, Sievers HH, Huppe M. Confusion assessment method for the intensive care unit (cam-icu): diagnosis of postoperative delirium in cardiac surgery. Anaesthesist. 2008;57:464–74.
3. Ely EW, Shintani A, Truman B, Speroff T, Gordon SM, Harrell Jr FE, Inouye SK, Bernard GR, Dittus RS. Delirium as a predictor of mortality in mechanically ventilated patients in the intensive care unit. JAMA. 2004;291:1753–62.
4. Ouimet S, Kavanagh BP, Gottfried SB, Skrobik Y. Incidence, risk factors and consequences of icu delirium. Intensive Care Med. 2007;33:66–73.
5. Jackson JC, Gordon SM, Hart RP, Hopkins RO, Ely EW. The association between delirium and cognitive decline: a review of the empirical literature. Neuropsychol Rev. 2004;14:87–98.
6. Thomason JW, Shintani A, Peterson JF, Pun BT, Jackson JC, Ely EW. Intensive care unit delirium is an independent predictor of longer hospital stay: a prospective analysis of 261 non-ventilated patients. Crit Care. 2005;9:R375–81.
7. Milbrandt EB, Deppen S, Harrison PL, Shintani AK, Speroff T, Stiles RA, Truman B, Bernard GR, Dittus RS, Ely EW. Costs associated with delirium in mechanically ventilated patients. Crit Care Med. 2004;32:955–62.
8. Wacker P, Nunes PV, Cabrita H, Forlenza OV. Post-operative delirium is associated with poor cognitive outcome and dementia. Dement Geriatr Cogn Disord. 2006;21:221–7.
9. McNicoll L, Pisani MA, Zhang Y, Ely EW, Siegel MD, Inouye SK. Delirium in the intensive care unit: occurrence and clinical course in older patients. J Am Geriatr Soc. 2003;51:591–8.
10. Cerejeira J, Lagarto L, Mukaetova-Ladinska EB. The immunology of delirium. Neuroimmunomodulation. 2014;21:72–8.
11. Pearson A, de Vries A, Middleton SD, Gillies F, White TO, Armstrong IR, Andrew R, Seckl JR, MacLullich AM. Cerebrospinal fluid cortisol levels are higher in patients with delirium versus controls. BMC Res Notes. 2010;3:33.
12. Cerejeira J, Nogueira V, Luis P, Vaz-Serra A, Mukaetova-Ladinska EB. The cholinergic system and inflammation: common pathways in delirium pathophysiology. J Am Geriatr Soc. 2012;60:669–75.
13. Trzepacz PT. Update on the neuropathogenesis of delirium. Dement Geriatr Cogn Disord. 1999;10:330–4.
14. Cerejeira J, Batista P, Nogueira V, Firmino H, Vaz-Serra A, Mukaetova-Ladinska EB. Low preoperative plasma cholinesterase activity as a risk marker of postoperative delirium in elderly patients. Age Ageing. 2011;40:621–6.
15. Zujalovic B, Barth E. Delirium accompanied by cholinergic deficiency and organ failure in a 73-year-old critically ill patient: physostigmine as a therapeutic option. Case Rep Crit Care. 2015;2015:793015.
16. Dawson AH, Buckley NA. Pharmacological management of anticholinergic delirium-theory, evidence and practice. Br J Clin Pharmacol. 2016;81:516–24.
17. Tampi RR, Tampi DJ, Ghori AK. Acetylcholinesterase inhibitors for delirium in older adults. Am J Alzheimers Dis Other Demen. 2016;31:305–10.
18. Worek F, Mast U, Kiderlen D, Diepold C, Eyer P. Improved determination of acetylcholinesterase activity in human whole blood. Clin Chim Acta. 1999; 288:73–90.
19. Distelmaier K, Winter M-P, Rützler K, Heinz G, Lang IM, Maurer G, Koinig H, Steinlechner B, Niessner A, Goliasch G. Serum butyrylcholinesterase predicts survival after extracorporeal membrane oxygenation after cardiovascular surgery. Crit Care. 2014;18:R24.
20. Ely EW, Inouye SK, Bernard GR, Gordon S, Francis J, May L, Truman B, Speroff T, Gautam S, Margolin R, Hart RP, Dittus R. Delirium in mechanically ventilated patients: validity and reliability of the confusion assessment method for the intensive care unit (cam-icu). JAMA. 2001;286:2703–10.

21. Lutz A, Radtke FM, Franck M, Seeling M, Gaudreau JD, Kleinwachter R, Kork F, Zieb A, Heymann A. Spies CD: [the nursing delirium screening scale (nu-desc)]. AINS. 2008;43:98–102.

22. Gaudreau JD, Gagnon P, Harel F, Tremblay A, Roy MA. Fast, systematic, and continuous delirium assessment in hospitalized patients: the nursing delirium screening scale. J Pain Symptom Manage. 2005;29:368–75.

23. Jackson TA, Moorey HC, Sheehan B, Maclullich AM, Gladman JR, Lord JM. Acetylcholinesterase activity measurement and clinical features of delirium. Dement Geriatr Cogn Disord. 2016;43:29–37.

24. Radtke FM, Gaudreau JD, Spies C. Diagnosing delirium. JAMA. 2010;304: 2125. author reply 2126-2127.

# 6

# Initial central venous pressure could be a prognostic marker for hemodynamic improvement of polymyxin B direct hemoperfusion

Hiroyuki Yamada[1,2]*, Tatsuo Tsukamoto[1], Hiromichi Narumiya[2,3], Kazumasa Oda[3], Satoshi Higaki[3], Ryoji Iizuka[3], Motoko Yanagita[1] and Masako Deguchi[2]

## Abstract

**Background:** Direct hemoperfusion with polymyxin B-immobilized fiber column (PMX-DHP) could improve the hemodynamic status of septic shock patients. As PMX-DHP is an invasive and costly procedure, it is desirable to estimate the therapeutic effect before performing the therapy. However, it is still unclear when this therapy should be started and what type of sepsis it should be employed for. In this study, we retrospectively examined the clinical effect of patients treated with PMX-DHP by using central venous pressure (CVP).

**Methods:** Seventy patients who received PMX-DHP for septic shock during the study period were recruited and divided into a low CVP group ($n = 33$, CVP < 12 mmHg) and a high CVP group ($n = 37$, CVP≧12 mmHg). The primary endpoint was vasopressor dependency index at 24 hours after starting PMX-DHP, and the secondary endpoint was the 28-day survival rate. Additionally, we performed a multivariate linear regression analysis on the difference in the vasopressor dependency index.

**Results:** The vasopressor dependency index significantly improved at 24 h in the low CVP group (0.33 to 0.16 mmHg$^{-1}$; $p < 0.01$) but not in the high CVP group (0.43 to 0.34 mmHg$^{-1}$; $p = 0.41$), and there was a significant difference between the two groups in the index at 24 h ($p = 0.02$). The 28-day survival rate was higher in the low CVP group (79 vs. 43 %; $p < 0.01$). Multivariate linear regression analysis showed that CVP ($p = 0.04$) was independently associated with the difference in the vasopressor dependency index.

**Conclusions:** Our study indicates that the clinical effect of PMX-DHP for septic shock patients with higher CVP (≧12 mmHg) might be limited and that the initial CVP when performing PMX-DHP could function as an independent prognostic marker for the hemodynamic improvement.

**Keywords:** Polymyxin B, Hemoperfusion, Septic shock, Central venous pressure, PMX-DHP

* Correspondence: hyamada@kuhp.kyoto-u.ac.jp
[1]Department of Nephrology, Graduate School of Medicine, Kyoto University, 54 Shogoin-Kawahara-cho, Sakyo-ku, Kyoto 606-8507, Japan
[2]Department of Metabolism, Nephrology and Rheumatology, Japanese Red Cross Kyoto Daini Hospital, 355-5 Haruobi, Kamigyo-ku, Kyoto 602-8026, Japan
Full list of author information is available at the end of the article

## Background

Both the 2008 and 2012 Surviving Sepsis Campaign Guidelines (SSCG) recommend the rapid infusion of intravenous fluids until a central venous pressure (CVP) of 8–12 mmHg is achieved during initial resuscitation [1, 2]. However, many studies show that excess fluid accumulation is associated with adverse outcomes in critically ill patients [3–5]. In particular, positive fluid balance seems to be harmful for patients whose comorbid burden includes chronic heart failure and/or chronic kidney disease [6, 7]. In order to avoid excess volume expansion in those patients, it is important to carefully monitor intravascular volume by the following parameters: CVP, stroke volume variance, or extravascular lung water.

Direct hemoperfusion with a polymyxin B-immobilized fiber column (PMX-DHP), which can effectively adsorb bacterial endotoxin and lead to an earlier recovery from shock state, was first reported in 1994, and it has been used for the treatment of septic shock in many countries [8–11]. Although many clinical reports, including two randomized control trials, have shown the clinical effect of adapting PMX-DHP for septic shock patients, there is no clear consensus about the effect of the hemoperfusion [9–12]. As PMX-DHP is an invasive and costly procedure, it is desirable to accurately estimate the therapeutic effect before performing the therapy [11]. However, it is still unclear when this therapy should be started and what type of sepsis it should be employed for.

The utility of CVP as a marker of intravascular volume has been questioned for many years [13, 14]. However, we consider that CVP is one of the most widely used hemodynamic parameters because of the promptness of the measurement and the ability to perform it in any hospital facility. Actually, many clinical studies also demonstrated that high CVP was associated with positive fluid balance [1, 5, 15].

In this study, in order to clarify the application of PMX-DHP for septic shock patients, we retrospectively examined the hemodynamic improvement and the mortality of patients treated with PMX-DHP by using CVP values. Moreover, we investigated whether the CVP values at the start of PMX-DHP could function as an independent prognostic factor for the hemodynamic improvement of the hemoperfusion.

## Methods

### Patients

We conducted a retrospective cohort study among all consecutive patients who received PMX-DHP for septic shock between May 2008 and April 2013 in the intensive care unit (ICU), high care unit (HCU), and cardiovascular care unit (CCU) at the Japanese Red Cross Kyoto Daini Hospital and the Kyoto University Hospital in Japan. After initial resuscitation to achieve the early goal directed therapy (EGDT), PMX-DHP was applied along the Japanese health insurance system, as follows [1]: septic shock patients who require vasopressor support because of endotoxin or gram-negative bacteria. The following patients were excluded: (1) those who were under 18 years old, (2) those who were admitted to the ICU, HCU, or CCU for reasons other than sepsis, (3) those who were not given vasopressors when starting PMX-DHP, and (4) those in whose medical records CVP was not sufficiently recorded.

The Ethics Committee of Kyoto University Graduate School and Faculty of Medicine approved the protocol (E2153). This study was retrospective and used only a data bank while employing the highest privacy policy standards. Therefore, the requirement of informed consent was waived.

### Procedures

Vascular access was placed at the femoral or the internal jugular vein. PMX-DHP with PMX-20R (Toray Industries, Tokyo, Japan) was performed for at least 120 min per session once or twice per patient per day for 2 days. The blood flow volume was 80–120 mL/min. The duration of hemoperfusion was decided by the attending physician. The therapy was terminated when the attending physician deemed it appropriate to conclude PMX-DHP for any reason. The anticoagulant used in PMX-DHP was nafamostat mesilate, low molecular weight heparin, or unfractionated heparin. All other cardiovascular management, including cardiac output management, setting of blood pressure goals, and fluid and inotropic therapy, were performed on the basis of SSCG recommendations by the attending physician.

### Definitions and classification

In this study, we classified the patients into two groups: patients with CVP values greater than or equal to ($\geq$) 12 mmHg when starting PMX-DHP were placed in the high CVP group, while the remaining patients whose CVP values were less than ($<$) 12 mmHg were placed in the low CVP group. CVP was measured using the standard method when starting PMX-DHP and expressed as mmHg, as described previously [16, 17]. This classification is also based on the SSCG recommendations, which suggest that in mechanical ventilation patients, a higher target CVP of 12 mmHg should be achieved [2].

### Data collection

We employed three parameters in order to compare hemodynamic status among the patients in this study: mean arterial pressure (MAP), inotropic score, and vasopressor dependency index, as described in the preceding studies [9, 18]. Namely, the inotropic score was calculated as follows:

$$(\text{dopamine dose } [\mu g/kg/\min])$$
$$\times\ 1\ +\ (\text{dobutamine } [\mu g/kg/\min])$$
$$\times\ 1\ +\ (\text{epinephrine dose } [\mu g/kg/\min])$$
$$\times\ 100\ +\ (\textit{n}\text{orepinephrine dose } [\mu g/kg/\min])$$
$$\times\ 100\ +\ (\text{phenylephrine dose } [\mu g/kg/\min])\ \times\ 100$$

And, vasopressor dependency index was calculated as the inotropic score/MAP. The parameters were calculated before the first PMX-DHP, immediately thereafter and 24 h after the first PMX-DHP.

Relevant clinical background, medical history, and clinical data of all patients were collected at appropriate times during the treatment for sepsis. Basic cardiopulmonary data and laboratory data obtained at the time of starting PMX-DHP were considered baseline values. These included age, sex, body mass index, systolic blood pressure, diastolic blood pressure, dopamine infusion rate, noradrenaline infusion rate, inotropic score, vasopressor dependency index, heart rate, central venous pressure, cardiac output, cardiac index, body temperature, arterial pH, lactate, arterial oxygen tension ($PaO_2$)/fractional inspired oxygen ($FiO_2$) ratio (P/F ratio), positive end-expiratory pressure (PEEP), renal replacement therapy, surgery, hemoglobin, platelet count, C-reactive protein (CRP), total bilirubin, total protein, Acute Physiologic and Chronic Health Evaluation II (APACHE II) score, Sequential Organ Failure Assessment (SOFA) score, time from admission to care units until starting PMX-DHP, duration of PMX-DHP, total fluid dosage from ICU admission until starting PMX-DHP, site of infection, and microorganism types. Cardiac output and cardiac index were measured by an arterial catheter attached to the Flotrac$^{\text{TM}}$ pulse counter device (Vigileo$^{\text{TM}}$, Edwards Lifesciences, Irvine, CA, USA) or a pulmonary artery catheter attached to Vigilance$^{\text{TM}}$ monitor (Vigileo$^{\text{TM}}$, Edwards Lifesciences, Irvine, CA, USA).

## Study outcomes

The primary outcome was vasopressor dependency index at 24 h after starting PMX-DHP. The secondary outcome was the 28-day survival rate.

## Statistical analysis

Statistical analysis was performed using JMP for Macintosh version 10.0.2 software (SAS Institute, Tokyo, Japan). Categorical variables are expressed as the number of patients (%) and were analyzed by using the $\chi^2$ test or Fisher's exact test. Continuous variables are expressed as means and 95 % confidence intervals (CIs). Comparison of continuous variables between the two groups was conducted with the $t$ test

or the Mann-Whitney $U$ test, according to the distribution of the variables. Evaluation of significance between groups over time points was done by repeated measure ANOVA. As post hoc analysis, the three pair-wise comparisons of the hemodynamic status within a single group among different time points were made using Bonferroni adjustment. Therefore, $p$ values less than 0.016 were considered significant only in this comparison. In the other comparisons, statistical significance was defined as $p$ values <0.05. Kaplan-Meier curves were constructed for the comparison of the survival rate in the two groups and were tested for difference using the log-rank test.

To ensure the assumption that the CVP at the beginning of PMX-DHP could be an independently prognostic factor for the hemodynamic improvement of the hemoperfusion, we performed a multivariate linear regression analysis that focused on the difference in the vasopressor dependency index before PMX-DHP and 24 h after hemoperfusion. The relationships between the parameter and continuous variables were examined using Pearson's correlation coefficient, and categorical variables were examined using Spearman's R test. All variables with $p$ values <0.20 in the univariate analysis were included in the multivariate analysis. To ensure that the assumptions for regression analysis were not violated, an analysis of residuals was carried out. Moreover, we performed multivariate Cox regression analysis to assess the covariates that were associated with time to mortality.

## Results
### Patient characteristics

Although 112 patients received PMX-DHP for septic shock during the study period, 70 patients met the inclusion criteria, while 42 patients were excluded for a variety of reasons (age, 2; reasons for admission to ICU, 13; vasopressors not used, 9; no record of CVP, 18). Of these 70 patients, the initial CVP of 33 patients when receiving PMX-DHP was <12 mmHg, and the initial CVP of the other 37 patients was ≥12 mmHg, as shown in Fig. 1. The baseline characteristics of the study population are described in Table 1. Although the SOFA score, in particular SOFA liver and SOFA hematological, was significantly higher in the high CVP group than in the low CVP group, the APACHE II score was not significantly different between the two groups. Arterial pH was also significantly lower in the high CVP group. There were no significant differences in the other parameters except CVP. Although cardiac pump dysfunction could have a serious influence on CVP value, there was not a significant difference between the two groups in cardiac output and cardiac index before starting PMX-DHP.

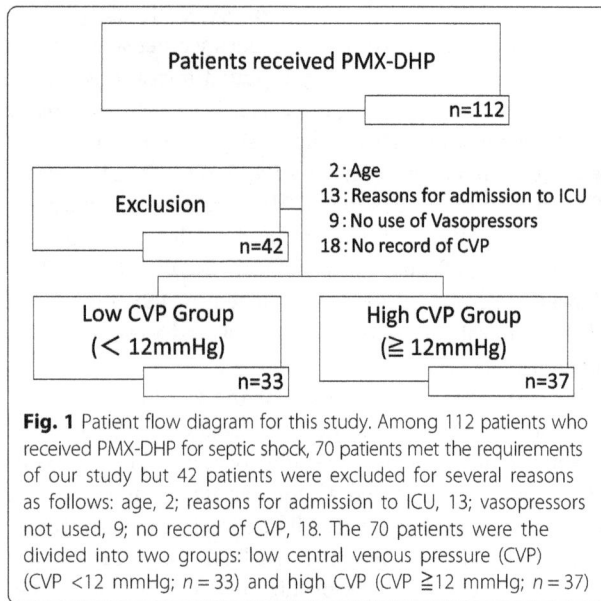

**Fig. 1** Patient flow diagram for this study. Among 112 patients who received PMX-DHP for septic shock, 70 patients met the requirements of our study but 42 patients were excluded for several reasons as follows: age, 2; reasons for admission to ICU, 13; vasopressors not used, 9; no record of CVP, 18. The 70 patients were the divided into two groups: low central venous pressure (CVP) (CVP <12 mmHg; $n = 33$) and high CVP (CVP $\geqq$12 mmHg; $n = 37$)

Table 2 shows the site of infection and microorganism types in both groups. There were also no significant differences between them.

### Primary outcome
Repeated measures ANOVA for the vasopressor dependency index revealed that the index in the low CVP group improved more significantly than in the high CVP group (for each $p < 0.01$) (Fig. 2). As for post hoc analysis, the vasopressor dependency index decreased significantly at 24 h (0.16 mmHg$^{-1}$; 95 % CI, 0.05–0.28; $p < 0.01$) but not after PMX-DHP (0.24 mmHg$^{-1}$; 95 % CI, 0.15–0.34; $p = 0.14$) in the low CVP group whereas the decrease was observed neither after PMX-DHP (0.39 mmHg$^{-1}$; 95 % CI, 0.30–0.49; $p = 1.00$) nor at 24 h (0.34 mmHg$^{-1}$; 95 % CI, 0.25–0.44; $p = 0.41$) in the high CVP group. Additionally, we could observe a significant difference in the index at 24 h between the two groups ($p < 0.05$) (Fig. 3). Thus, PMX-DHP appeared to be more effective for the hemodynamic status in the low CVP group than in the high CVP group.

### Secondary outcome
The survival rates of both groups after 28 days were analyzed by the Kaplan-Meier method (Fig. 3). The survival rate was significantly higher in the low CVP group than in the high CVP group ($p < 0.01$), as determined by log-rank test.

### Regression analysis
Correlation analyses were performed to identify factors associated with the difference in the vasopressor dependency index before and 24 h after PMX-DHP (Additional file 1: Table S1). In the univariate regression analysis, age statistically significantly correlated with the difference ($p = 0.03$). Subsequent multivariate linear regression confirmed CVP ($p = 0.04$) and age ($p = 0.03$) as independent prognosis factors regarding the hemodynamic improvement of PMX-DHP (Table 3). This also indicates that the higher the CVP at the start of hemoperfusion is, the less it improves the hemodynamic state.

### Discussion
In this study, we observed the association between CVP and the hemodynamic improvement with PMX-DHP. Our results yielded two interesting findings. First, the hemodynamic status of patients with higher CVP did not improve significantly by PMX-DHP. In other words, our retrospective results did not support the guideline's recommendations, which suggested that septic shock patients with mechanical ventilation should achieve a higher target of CVP 12 to 15 mmHg$^2$. Second, the initial CVP when performing PMX-DHP could function as an independent prognostic factor for the hemodynamic improvement of the therapy. To the best of our knowledge, this is the first study that investigated this particular association and prognosis.

Although CVP is one of the most popular hemodynamic parameters, we cannot deny that CVP values may not reflect intravascular volume accurately. In fact, recent reviews reported that the CVP value is mainly determined by two factors: cardiac pump function and venous return function [17, 19, 20]. In terms of cardiac function, a high CVP indicates a decrease in contractility, diastolic dysfunction, valvular disease, and cardiomyopathy in these patients, although in our study, there was not a significant difference in cardiac output and cardiac index [19, 20]. On the other hand, venous return is determined by the gradient between CVP and the mean circulatory filling pressure (MCFP), as shown in the formula below:

$$\text{venous return} = (\text{MCFP} - \text{CVP})/\text{venous resistance}$$

[19] MCFP is the pressure in the vasculature when the heart is stopped (zero flow) and the pressures in all segments of the circulatory system have equalized [21, 22]. Thus, an increase in CVP values leads to the decrease in venous return [19–22]. Because PMX-DHP does not directly affect these pressures and cardiac function, it is difficult for the hemoperfusion to improve the hemodynamic status for septic shock patients with high CVP.

Actually, in this study, we observed that the patients in the high CVP group suffered from hemodynamic impairment due to high CVP. The proportion of patients who received renal replacement therapy was non-significantly larger in the high CVP group, which suggests that many

**Table 1** Baseline characteristics of the patients

| | Low CVP group $n = 33$ Median (95 % CI) | High CVP group $n = 37$ Median (95 % CI) | p value |
|---|---|---|---|
| Age, year | 72 (68–76) | 67 (64–71) | 0.07 |
| Male, n(%) | 20 (61) | 26 (70) | 0.46 |
| Body mass index, kg/m$^2$ | 22 (20–23) | 23 (21–24) | 0.37 |
| Systolic blood pressure, mmHg | 99 (90–106) | 92 (84–99) | 0.22 |
| Diastolic blood pressure, mmHg | 50 (47–53) | 48 (44–51) | 0.30 |
| Mean blood pressure, mmHg | 66 (62–70) | 62 (59–66) | 0.17 |
| Dopamine infusion rate, µg/kg/min | 5.0 (3.5–6.6) | 5.8 (4.4–7.3) | 0.45 |
| Noradrenaline infusion rate, µg/kg/min | 0.12 (0.09–0.16) | 0.16 (0.12–0.20) | 0.20 |
| Inotropic score | 20 (15–25) | 25 (21–30) | 0.14 |
| Vasopressor dependency index, mmHg$^{-1}$ | 0.33 (0.23–0.45) | 0.43 (0.34–0.53) | 0.15 |
| Heart rate, bpm | 109 (103–116) | 115 (109–121) | 0.18 |
| CVP, mmHg | 8 (7–9) | 15(14–16) | <0.01 |
| Cardiac output, L/min | 4.6 (3.3–5.8) | 5.7 (4.6–5.7) | 0.18 |
| Cardiac index, L/min/m$^2$ | 2.8 (2.3–3.4) | 3.3 (2.8–3.7) | 0.23 |
| Body temperture, °C | 36.8 (36.4–37.2) | 36.8 (36.4–37.2) | 0.92 |
| Arterial pH | 7.36 (7.32–7.41) | 7.27 (7.23–7.31) | <0.01 |
| Lactate, mmol/L | 3.9 (2.6–5.3) | 4.0 (2.9–5.2) | 0.94 |
| P/F ratio | 220 (181–258) | 168 (131–206) | 0.06 |
| PEEP, cmH$_2$O | 8 (6–10) | 9 (7–11) | 0.32 |
| Renal replacement therapy, n(%) | 13 (39) | 23 (62) | 0.06 |
| Surgery, n(%) | 21 (64) | 17 (46) | 0.16 |
| Hemoglobin, g/dL | 10.4 (9.7–11.1) | 10.3 (9.6–11.0) | 0.78 |
| Platelet count, ×10$^9$/L | 111 (87–134) | 81 (59–104) | 0.08 |
| CRP, mg/dL | 17.7 (11.4–24.0) | 17.6 (11.6–23.5) | 0.97 |
| Total Bilirubin, mg/dL | 1.7 (0.2–3.1) | 3.6 (2.2–5.0) | 0.06 |
| Total Protein, mg/dL | 4.9 (4.5–5.3) | 4.6 (4.2–4.9) | 0.17 |
| APACHE II score | 26 (25–28) | 28 (26–30) | 0.23 |
| SOFA score | 12 (11–13) | 14 (13–15) | 0.01 |
| SOFA cardiovascular | 3.5 (3.3–3.7) | 3.7 (3.5–3.9) | 0.29 |
| SOFA renal | 1.9 (1.4–2.4) | 2.3 (1.8–2.8) | 0.22 |
| SOFA hematological | 1.6 (1.2–2.0) | 2.1 (1.8–2.5) | 0.05 |
| SOFA respiratory | 2.4 (1.9–2.8) | 2.8 (2.4–3.2) | 0.15 |
| SOFA liver | 0.8 (0.4–1.2) | 1.4 (1.0–1.7) | 0.04 |
| SOFA central nerve system | 2.0 (1.6–2.5) | 2.0 (1.5–2.4) | 0.83 |
| Time from ICU admission until starting PMX-DHP, min | 441 (98–802) | 829 (498–1159) | 0.11 |
| PMX-DHP duration, min | 354 (249–458) | 366 (263–469) | 0.97 |
| Total fluid dosage from ICU admission until starting PMX-DHP, ml | 2970 (1200–4760) | 3212 (1223–5203) | 0.86 |

*APACHE* Acute Physiologic and Chronic Health Evaluation, *CRP* c-reactive protein, *CVP* central venous pressure, *ICU* intensive care unit, *PEEP* positive end-expiratory pressure, *P/F ratio* arterial oxygen tension/fractional inspired oxygen ratio *PMX-DHP* direct hemoperfusion with polymyxin B-immobilized fiber column, *SOFA* Sequential Organ Failure Assessment

of the attending physicians might think the intravascular volume in the high CVP group patients is too large. Additionally, the P/F ratio and PEEP were also non-significantly lower in the high CVP group, which indicated that some of the patients had a high intrathoracic pressure. Hence, we consider that high CVP group patients did not have adequate venous return because excess fluid therapy or high intrathoracic pressure reduces the

**Table 2** Isolated microorganisms by treatment group

|  | Low CVP group $n = 33$ | High CVP group $n = 37$ |
|---|---|---|
| Site of infection |  |  |
| Abdomen | 13 | 15 |
| Lung | 6 | 13 |
| Urinary tract | 7 | 2 |
| Skin | 2 | 1 |
| Blood stream | 0 | 1 |
| Others | 5 | 5 |
| Microorganism type |  |  |
| Escherichia coli | 7 | 5 |
| Staphylococcus species | 2 | 5 |
| Streptococcus species | 1 | 4 |
| Enterococcus species | 1 | 2 |
| Pseudomonas species | 1 | 2 |
| Bacteroides species | 1 | 1 |
| Klebsiella species | 2 | 0 |
| Serratia species | 1 | 1 |
| Acinetobacter species | 1 | 0 |
| Citrobacter species | 0 | 1 |
| Clostridium species | 1 | 0 |
| Morallexa species | 0 | 1 |
| Stenotrophomonas species | 0 | 1 |

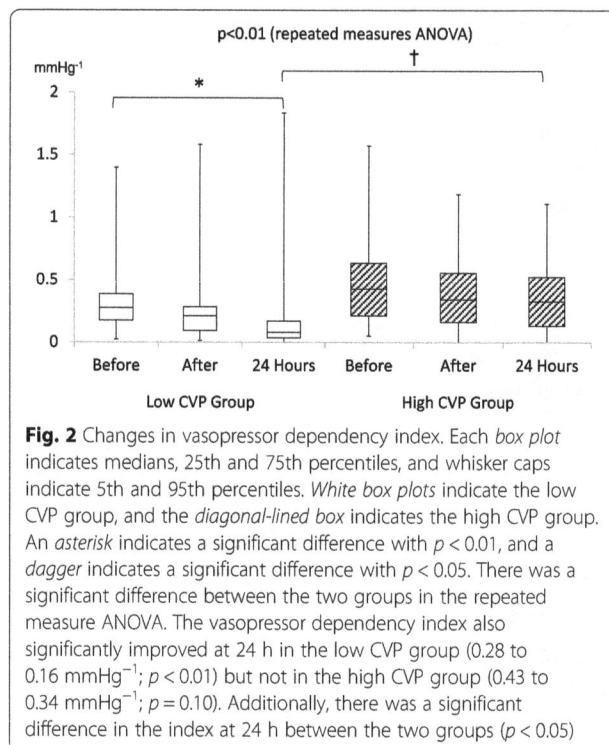

**Fig. 2** Changes in vasopressor dependency index. Each *box plot* indicates medians, 25th and 75th percentiles, and whisker caps indicate 5th and 95th percentiles. *White box plots* indicate the low CVP group, and the *diagonal-lined box* indicates the high CVP group. An *asterisk* indicates a significant difference with $p < 0.01$, and a *dagger* indicates a significant difference with $p < 0.05$. There was a significant difference between the two groups in the repeated measure ANOVA. The vasopressor dependency index also significantly improved at 24 h in the low CVP group (0.28 to 0.16 mmHg$^{-1}$; $p < 0.01$) but not in the high CVP group (0.43 to 0.34 mmHg$^{-1}$; $p = 0.10$). Additionally, there was a significant difference in the index at 24 h between the two groups ($p < 0.05$)

gradient between MCFP and CVP. On the other hand, the significant improvement in the low CVP group could be because they genuinely received the clinical effect of PMX-DHP. Generally, PMX-DHP can reduce plasma cytokine levels by absorbing endotoxin, immune cells, and anandamide [23–25]. These physiological and pathological responses could be equivalent in both groups in our study. However, the harmful effect of high CVP at the start of PMX-DHP differentiated the clinical effect of both groups. In other words, fluid toxicity or increase in intrathoracic pressure might be deleterious beyond the beneficial effect of PMX-DHP in patients with high CVP in our study.

Previous studies have reported that early initiation of PMX-DHP reduced the catecholamine requirement and that early improvement in inotropic score and vasopressor dependency index after PMX-DHP might be a prognostic factor [18, 23, 26]. In our study, the patients in the low CVP group who received PMX-DHP earlier also tended to show a decrease in their vasopressor dependency index. Meanwhile, in terms of the time between ICU admission and starting PMX-DHP, there was neither a statistical difference between the two groups nor a significant association with hemodynamic improvement in our study. However, because the sample size of our study was not large

enough to demonstrate the association, our results should be viewed with this limitation in mind. In addition, although we performed PMX-DHP for around 6 h in both groups, a recent study has indicated that a longer duration of PMX-DHP therapy can be expected to improve the hemodynamics and pulmonary oxygenation capacity of patients with severe sepsis/septic shock [27]. Thus, longer operation of PMX-DHP might contribute to improve the outcome of patients with low CVP.

Other limitations of our study need to be acknowledged. First, we could not show the data on intrinsic PEEP, so-

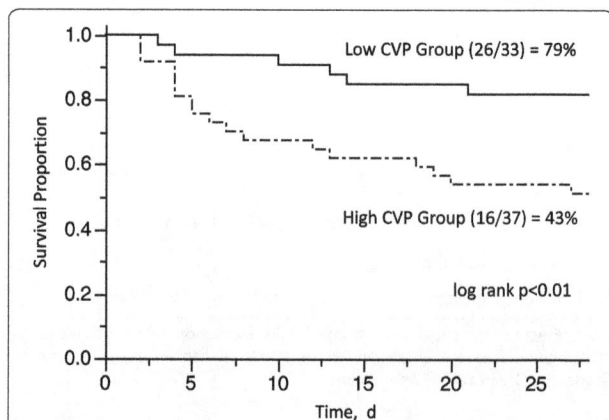

**Fig. 3** Survival rate of each group by Kaplan-Meier analysis. Although patients in both groups were similarly treated with PMX-DHP, patients in the low CVP group showed a better survival rate in this study

**Table 3** Results of multivariate regression analysis for the difference in the vasopressor dependency index between before and 24 h after PMX-DHP

| Selected variables | Regression coefficient (β) | 95 % CI | Partial correlations | p value | $r^2$ |
|---|---|---|---|---|---|
| Age | −0.2972 | −0.0168 – −0.0009 | −0.0089 | 0.03 | 0.180 |
| CVP | −0.3155 | −0.0348 – −0.0007 | −0.0178 | 0.04 | |
| SOFA | 0.1530 | −0.0166 – 0.0497 | 0.0165 | 0.32 | |
| Arterial pH | −0.2871 | −1.2656 – −0.0171 | −0.6242 | 0.06 | |

*CVP* central venous pressure, *PMX-DHP* direct hemoperfusion with polymyxin B-immobilized fiber column, *SOFA* Sequential Organ Failure Assessment

called auto-PEEP, which might have a direct influence on the CVP values in the high CVP group. However, we consider that it may not fundamentally change our conclusion. Auto-PEEP-induced hypotension is not a result of hyper-inflammatory response to sepsis, but it is rather a patient-ventilator interaction. Thus, it is obvious that PMX-DHP is less effective for the high CVP patients with auto-PEEP-induced hypotension. Additionally, this clinical study is not for acute exacerbation of chronic obstructive pulmonary disease, bronchial asthma, or acute respiratory distress syndrome, and it only evaluated patients with septic shock. Thus, we consider that there were not a large proportion of the study patients with auto-PEEP in our study. Second, the previous studies reported that high CVP was associated with a poor prognosis [28, 29]. Indeed, high CVP might have a negative influence on the cardiac function during the treatment in patients with high CVP group, although cardiac output and index were not significantly different in both groups at the beginning of the hemoperfusion [29]. Therefore, regardless of the effect of PMX-DHP, there may be a possibility of observing the clinical course of patients with a poor prognosis. Third, this study was not a randomized controlled trial, and we cannot rule out the possibility of selection bias, especially referral bias and Neyman bias. Fourth, perhaps we could not extract the patients whose conditions changed rapidly or whose case was extremely severe because our study patients had enough time to receive the hemoperfusion. Fifth, vasopressors were regulated by local physicians, depending on the patient's condition. Therefore, the protocol for titrating the vasopressors was different among the attending physicians. Further study is required to clarify these unsolved issues.

## Conclusions

Our study indicated that the effect of PMX-DHP for septic shock patients with higher CVP (≥12 mmHg) may be limited and that the initial CVP in performing PMX-DHP could be an independent prognostic marker for hemodynamic improvement. Further study is required to clarify the mechanisms of PMX-DHP that affect sepsis treatment.

**Abbreviations**
APACHE: Acute Physiologic and Chronic Health Evaluation; CCU: Cardiovascular care unit; CRP: C-reactive protein; CVP: Central venous pressure; EGDT: Early goal directed therapy; ER: Emergency room; HCU: High care unit; ICU: Intensive care unit; MAP: Mean arterial pressure; MCFP: Mean circulatory filling pressure; P/F ratio: Arterial oxygen tension/fractional inspired oxygen ratio; PEEP: Positive end-expiratory pressure; PMX-DHP: Direct hemoperfusion with polymyxin B-immobilized fiber column; SOFA: Sequential Organ Failure Assessment; SSCG: Surviving Sepsis Campaign Guidelines

**Acknowledgements**
We thank Juan Alejandro Oliva Trejo (Medical Innovation Center, TMK project, Graduate School of Medicine, Kyoto University) for serving as an advisor and the medical staff of the intensive care unit, high care unit, and cardiac care unit of both the Japanese Red Cross Kyoto Daini Hospital and Kyoto University Hospital.

**Funding**
None of the authors received any funding for this study.

**Authors' contributions**
HY designed the study protocols, acquired the data, performed the statistical analysis, and completed the manuscript for publication. TT revised the manuscript and approved it for publication. HN and KO helped with the data analysis. SH, RI, MY, and MD supervised the interpretation of the results and writing of the reports. All authors have read and approved the final version of the manuscript.

**Competing interests**
The authors declare that they have no competing interests.

**Previous presentations**
This study was presented in part at the 10th International Society for Apheresis Congress May 15, 2015, Cancun, Mexico, and at the 26th Annual Meeting of the Japan Society for Blood Purification in Critical Care October 9, 2015, Tokyo, Japan.

**Author details**

[1]Department of Nephrology, Graduate School of Medicine, Kyoto University, 54 Shogoin-Kawahara-cho, Sakyo-ku, Kyoto 606-8507, Japan. [2]Department of Metabolism, Nephrology and Rheumatology, Japanese Red Cross Kyoto Daini Hospital, 355-5 Haruobi, Kamigyo-ku, Kyoto 602-8026, Japan. [3]Department of Emergency, Japanese Red Cross Kyoto Daini Hospital, 355-5 Haruobi, Kamigyo-ku, Kyoto 602-8026, Japan.

## References

1. Rivers E, Nguyen B, Havstad S, et al. Early goal-directed therapy in the treatment of severe sepsis and septic shock. N Engl J Med. 2001;345(19):1368–77.

2. Dellinger RP, Levy MM, Rhodes A, et al. Surviving sepsis campaign. Crit Care Med. 2013;41(2):580–637.

3. Wiedemann HP, Wheeler AP, Bernard GR, et al. Comparison of two fluid-management strategies in acute lung injury. N Engl J Med. 2006;354(24):2564–75.

4. Bouchard J, Soroko SB, Chertow GM, et al. Fluid accumulation, survival and recovery of kidney function in critically ill patients with acute kidney injury. Kidney Int. 2009;76(4):422–7.

5. Boyd JH, Forbes J, Nakada T-a, Walley KR, Russell JA. Fluid resuscitation in septic shock: a positive fluid balance and elevated central venous pressure are associated with increased mortality*. Crit Care Med. 2011;39(2):259–65.

6. Yancy CW, Jessup M, Bozkurt B, et al. 2013 ACCF/AHA guideline for the management of heart failure: a report of the American College of Cardiology Foundation/American Heart Association Task Force on Practice Guidelines. J Am Coll Cardiol. 2013;62(16):e147–239.

7. Tsai YC, Tsai JC, Chen SC, et al. Association of fluid overload with kidney disease progression in advanced CKD: a prospective cohort study. Am J Kidney Dis. 2014;63(1):68–75.

8. Shoji H. Extracorporeal endotoxin removal for the treatment of sepsis: endotoxin adsorption cartridge (toraymyxin). Ther Apher Dial. 2003;7(1):108–14.

9. Cruz DN, Antonelli M, Fumagalli R, et al. Early use of polymyxin B hemoperfusion in abdominal septic shock: the EUPHAS randomized controlled trial. JAMA. 2009;301(23):2445–52.

10. Berto P, Ronco C, Cruz D, Melotti RM, Antonelli M. Cost-effectiveness analysis of polymyxin-B immobilized fiber column and conventional medical therapy in the management of abdominal septic shock in Italy. Blood Purif. 2011;32(4):331–40.

11. Cruz DN, Perazella MA, Bellomo R, et al. Effectiveness of polymyxin B-immobilized fiber column in sepsis: a systematic review. Crit Care. 2007;11(2):R47.

12. Payen DM, Guilhot J, Launey Y, et al. Early use of polymyxin B hemoperfusion in patients with septic shock due to peritonitis: a multicenter randomized control trial. Intensive Care Med. 2015;41(6):975–84.

13. Hoffman MJ, Greenfield LJ, Sugerman HJ, Tatum JL. Unsuspected right ventricular dysfunction in shock and sepsis. Ann Surg. 1983;198(3):307–19.

14. Marik PE, Cavallazzi R. Does the central venous pressure predict fluid responsiveness? An updated meta-analysis and a plea for some common sense*. Crit Care Med. 2013;41(7):1774–81.

15. Van Biesen W, Yegenaga I, Vanholder R, et al. Relationship between fluid status and its management on acute renal failure (ARF) in intensive care unit (ICU) patients with sepsis: a prospective analysis. J Nephrol. 2005;18(1):54–60.

16. Magder S. Central venous pressure: a useful but not so simple measurement. Crit Care Med. 2006;34(8):2224–7.

17. Magder S, Bafaqeeh F. The clinical role of central venous pressure measurements. J Intensive Care Med. 2007;22(1):44–51.

18. Kobayashi A, Iwasaki Y, Kimura Y, Kawagoe Y, Ujike Y. Early recovery in hemodynamics after direct hemoperfusion with polymyxin B-immobilized fibers may predict mortality rate in patients with septic shock. J Anesth. 2010;24(5):709–15.

19. Gelman S. Venous function and central venous pressure: a physiologic story. Anesthesiology. 2008;108(4):735–48.

20. Magder S. Bench-to-bedside review: an approach to hemodynamic monitoring—Guyton at the bedside. Crit Care. 2012;16(5):236.

21. Marik PE. Iatrogenic salt water drowning and the hazards of a high central venous pressure. Ann Intensive Care. 2014;4:21.

22. Henderson WR, Griesdale DE, Walley KR, Sheel AW. Clinical review: Guyton—the role of mean circulatory filling pressure and right atrial pressure in controlling cardiac output. Crit Care. 2010;14(6):1.

23. Ikeda T, Ikeda K, Nagura M, et al. Clinical evaluation of PMX-DHP for hypercytokinemia caused by septic multiple organ failure. Ther Apher Dial. 2004;8(4):293–8.

24. Nishibori M, Takahashi HK, Katayama H, et al. Specific removal of monocytes from peripheral blood of septic patients by polymyxin B-immobilized filter column. Acta Med Okayama. 2009;63(1):65–9.

25. Kohro S, Imaizumi H, Yamakage M, et al. Anandamide absorption by direct hemoperfusion with polymyxin B-immobilized fiber improves the prognosis and organ failure assessment score in patients with sepsis. J Anesth. 2006;20(1):11–6.

26. Takeyama N, Noguchi H, Hirakawa A, et al. Time to initiation of treatment with polymyxin B cartridge hemoperfusion in septic shock patients. Blood Purif. 2012;33(4):252–6.

27. Yamashita C, Hara Y, Kuriyama N, Nakamura T, Nishida O. Clinical effects of a longer duration of polymyxin B-immobilized fiber column direct hemoperfusion therapy for severe sepsis and septic shock. Ther Apher Dial. 2015;19(4):316–23.

28. Wang XT, Yao B, Liu DW, Zhang HM. Central venous pressure dropped early is associated with organ function and prognosis in septic shock patients: a retrospective observational study. Shock. 2015;44(5):426–30.

29. Damman K, van Deursen VM, Navis G, Voors AA, van Veldhuisen DJ, Hillege HL. Increased central venous pressure is associated with impaired renal function and mortality in a broad spectrum of patients with cardiovascular disease. J Am Coll Cardiol. 2009;53(7):582–8.

# 7

# Interruption of enteral nutrition in the intensive care unit: a single-center survey

Midori Uozumi[1], Masamitsu Sanui[2]* iD, Tetsuya Komuro[2], Yusuke Iizuka[2], Tadashi Kamio[2], Hiroshi Koyama[2], Hideyuki Mouri[2], Tomoyuki Masuyama[2], Kazuyuki Ono[1] and Alan Kawarai Lefor[3]

## Abstract

**Background:** Interruption of enteral nutrition (EN) in the intensive care unit (ICU) occurs frequently for various reasons including feeding intolerance and the conduct of diagnostic and therapeutic procedures. However, few studies have investigated the details of EN interruption practices including reasons for and duration of interruptions. There is no standard protocol to minimize EN interruptions.

**Methods:** This is a retrospective review of 100 patients in the ICU staying more than 72 h and receiving EN in a 12-bed, medical/surgical ICU in a tertiary care center in 2013. Data collected include total time designated for EN; the number of EN interruption episodes; reason for each interruption categorized as diagnostic study, therapeutic intervention, or gastrointestinal (GI) event, and their individual subcategories; duration of each interruption; and the presence of written orders for interruptions.

**Results:** One hundred patients staying in the ICU for at least 72 h and receiving EN were included. There were 567 episodes of EN interruption over a median ICU length of stay of 17.1 (interquartile range 8.0–22.0) days. There were a median of three EN interruption episodes per patient. EN interruption was performed for undetermined reasons (166 episodes, 29%), airway manipulation (103 episodes, 18%), GI events (78 episodes, 14%), and intermittent dialysis (71 episodes, 13%). Median duration of EN interruption in all patients was 5.5 (3.0–10.0) h. The cumulative interruption time corresponds to 19% of the total time designated for EN. Duration of EN interruption varied according to reason, including airway manipulation (9.0 [5.0–21.0] h), tracheostomy (9.5 [7.5–14.0] h), and GI events (6.5 [3.0–14.0] h). The average calorie deficits due to interruptions were 11.5% of daily target calories. Only 60 episodes (12%) had clear written orders for interruption.

**Conclusions:** Based on this single-center retrospective chart review, interruption of EN in the ICU is frequent, reasons for and duration of interruption varied, and airway procedures are associated with a relatively longer duration of interruption. Documentation and orders were frequently missing. These results warrant development of a protocol for EN interruption.

**Keywords:** Interruption of enteral nutrition, Diagnostic procedures, Therapeutic interventions, Nutritional protocol, Energy deficit

\* Correspondence: msanui@mac.com
[2]Department of Anesthesiology and Critical Care Medicine, Division of Critical Care Medicine, Jichi Medical University Saitama Medical Center, 1-847 Amanumacho, Omiya-ku, Saitama-shi, Saitama 330-8503, Japan
Full list of author information is available at the end of the article

## Background

In the intensive care unit (ICU), the interruption of enteral nutrition (EN) occurs frequently for various reasons including feeding intolerance, and the conduct of diagnostic and therapeutic procedures [1–3]. However, guidelines for administration of EN to critically ill patients [4–6] only indicate that "efforts should be taken to reduce EN interruptions due to diagnostic and therapeutic procedures" [5, 7], without offering specific protocols for minimizing EN interruptions [6].

In fact, there are several existing studies on the effect of EN interruption [2, 3, 8], suggesting that EN interruption is common in the ICU. However, one study did not evaluate the interruptions associated with diagnostic procedures [3], and another study failed to assess the duration of the interruptions [8]. No studies have apparently investigated the effectiveness of EN interruption protocols in the literature.

To establish effective interruption protocols in the future, obtaining accurate information regarding the current status of EN interruptions is an important initial step. Therefore, we conducted a single-center retrospective observational study to evaluate the frequency, duration, and reasons for EN interruptions, and the presence of written orders for interruption.

## Methods

This study was approved by the Institutional Research Ethics Review Committee, and consent for research participation was waived due to the retrospective study design. The study was performed in a 12-bed combined surgical and medical ICU at the Jichi Medical University Saitama Medical Center, Saitama, Japan. Patients aged 18 years or older who stayed in the ICU for 72 h or longer and who commenced EN from January 1 to December 31, 2013, were included. Data collection was terminated when a study patient was discharged from the ICU or placed on either an oral diet or intermittent EN. All data were retrospectively retrieved from hospital electronic medical records (COSMOS®, IBM, Tokyo, Japan) and the electronic ICU chart system (PIMS®, Phillips, Tokyo, Japan).

As an institutional practice at the time of study initiation, the initiation of EN within 48 h of ICU admission was encouraged unless contraindicated [5]. In patients for whom EN was indicated, incremental continuous feeding was initiated at 20 kcal/h for the energy and protein target, calculated as 25 kcal multiplied by ideal body weight and 1.2–1.5 g/ideal body weight. Every morning, a daily goal for energy and protein administration was determined at the physician's discretion and documented in the electronic chart. If a patient was considered stable enough to tolerate a full diet, the rate of continuous feeding was increased by 20 kcal/h every 4 h. Measurement of gastric residual volume was not routinely performed but was performed if events such as gastric discomfort or fullness, obvious regurgitation and active vomiting occurred. In those cases, metoclopramide and erythromycin were used to promote gastric motility with transient interruption of the EN at the discretion of the physician. However, definitive protocols regarding interruption of EN did not exist except that an effort was made to achieve the daily goal by increasing the rate of administration after restarting EN. Once a patient was stabilized with a daily nutritional target achieved by continuous administration of EN at a rate of 60–80 kcal/h, intermittent administration or daytime continuous administration (e.g., 7 am–7 pm) was allowed at the physician's discretion.

Data collected include the total administration time of EN (from start to end), the number of EN interruption episodes, the proportion of daily target calorie administration missed due to interruptions, the reasons for EN interruption (e.g., diagnostic testing, therapeutic interventions, and gastrointestinal (GI) events), duration of each interruption, time interval from the beginning of the interruption to beginning of the procedure, time interval from the end of the procedure to resumption of EN, the presence or absence of physician orders for EN interruption and its resumption, and the presence or absence of an endotracheal tube.

Reasons for interruption were categorized as follows: "undetermined" for patients where a clear reason for interruption could not be identified; "GI event" for abdominal pain, significant gastric residual volume, vomiting, diarrhea, or gastrointestinal bleeding; "airway manipulation" for intubation, cricothyroidotomy, tracheotomy tube replacement, successful tracheal extubation, or extubation attempt for situations where weaning of the ventilator was attempted but patients did not pass the spontaneous breathing trial, and for cases where the clinical load did not allow the extubation of those patients; "T-piece trial" for liberation from the ventilator using a weaning protocol; "tracheostomy" for tracheostomies performed either in the ICU or the operating room; "ICU diagnostic and therapeutic procedures" for bronchoscopy, transesophageal echocardiography, or placement or removal of central venous lines, extracorporeal membrane oxygenation, or other devices and endoscopy; "Procedures outside of the ICU" for radiological diagnostic procedures or interventions performed outside of the ICU; "Intermittent dialysis" for intermittent dialysis performed in either a dialysis suite or ICU; and "daytime only administration" for cases where EN was administered during the daytime only for the purpose of preventing airway trouble during the night.

The proportion of calorie deficits in daily caloric goals due to the interruption (%) was calculated as daily calorie deficits due to the interruption divided by the daily caloric goal. Daily calorie deficits (kcal) due to interruptions were calculated by subtracting the actual energy administered from a daily caloric goal determined at the physician's discretion, both of which were retrieved from the ICU electronic medical record.

For data presentation, categorical variables are expressed as numbers (%), and continuous variables are expressed as mean ± standard deviation or median with interquartile range (IQR), as appropriate.

## Results

Patient demographics are shown in Table 1. Between January 1 and December 31, 2013, a total of 100 patients stayed in the ICU for at least 72 h and received EN. Patient age was 66.7 ± 14.4 years, and 63 (63%) patients were men. Acute Physiology and Chronic Health Evaluation II score was 21.8 ± 6.8. A total of 95 (95%) patients were endotracheally intubated at the time of study inclusion, ICU stay was 17.1 (8.0–22.0) days, and in-hospital mortality was 19%. There were 567 episodes of EN interruptions, including 515 episodes in intubated patients (90%). The number of EN interruptions per patient was 3.0 (1.0–5.3) (Table 1).

The most common reason for EN interruption was undetermined (166 episodes, 29%), followed by airway

**Table 1** Baseline characteristics of study patients (N = 100)

| Characteristic | Value |
|---|---|
| Age, mean (SD) | 66.7 (14.4) |
| Male gender, N (%) | 63 (63.0) |
| APACHE II score, mean (SD) | 21.8 (6.8) |
| Intubated (endotracheal) patients at time of study inclusion, N (%) | 95 (95.0) |
| ICU length of stay, median (IQR) (days) | 17.1 (8.0–22.0) |
| Diagnosis, N | |
|   Cardiovascular surgery | 57 |
|   Surgical | 6 |
|   Neurosurgical | 2 |
|   Medical | 35 |
| Total episodes of EN interruption, N | 567 |
|   Episodes in endotracheally intubated patients, N (%) | 515 (90.8) |
| Number of EN interruptions per patient, median (IQR) | 3.0 (1.0–5.3) |
| Caloric deficit of daily caloric goal due to EN interruptions, % | 11.5 |
| EN interruption orders documented, % | 12.0 |
| EN resumption orders documented, % | 8.0 |
| Number of patients with a feeding tube placed post-pyloric region | 11 |
| Number of patients given prokinetic agents | 34 |

*APACHE II* Acute Physiology and Chronic Health Evaluation II, *SD* standard deviation, *IQR* interquartile range, *EN* Enteral nutrition, *ICU* Intensive Care Unit

manipulation (103 episodes, 18%), GI events (78 episodes, 14%), intermittent dialysis (71 episodes, 13%), and ICU diagnostic and therapeutic procedures (61 episodes, 11%) (Fig. 1).

Median values and IQR of duration of EN interruption by category are shown in Table 2. The median duration of EN interruption in all patients was 5.5 (3.0–10.0) h. The proportion of EN interruption duration to total EN administration was 19% (data not shown). Events with relatively long total EN interruption include surgery, airway manipulation, and daytime-only administration. Events with a large variation in interruption duration were GI events, airway manipulation, and undetermined. Events with a relatively short total EN interruption duration include ICU diagnostic and therapeutic procedures, T-piece trials, and physical therapy.

The time intervals between EN interruption and procedure start are shown in Table 3. The time interval from EN interruption until the event (procedure, etc.) start was 1.2 (0.3–3.7) h. Relatively long intervals between EN interruption and procedure start were documented for tracheostomy (5.8 [4.0–9.3]). The time from the end of an event until EN restart was 1.8 (0.8–4.2) h (Table 4). In a majority of the reasons for EN interruption, a substantial delay for restart of EN was documented. After tracheostomy, 3.2 (1.0–3.6) h were consumed until EN restart. Also, not significantly long but substantial delays were detected for intermittent dialysis, procedures outside of the ICU, and ICU procedures. Relatively large variations were found for most reasons of EN interruption including intervals from EN interruption to procedure start and the interval from procedure end until EN restart.

Average calorie deficits in daily caloric goal due to interruptions were 11.5% (Table 1). EN interruption orders were clearly documented for only 12% of the total interruption episodes, and the EN resume orders were present in 8% (Table 1).

## Discussion

This retrospective observational study in a single-center mixed ICU demonstrates that EN interruption is frequent, relatively long, and associated with substantial calorie deficits for various reasons. Airway procedures are associated with relatively longer durations of interruption compared to other reasons. Documentation and orders are frequently missing.

Previous studies [2, 8, 9] have reported GI dysfunction and interruptions due to therapeutic procedures to be the most common reasons for EN interruption. Although the current study observed similar trends, previous studies did not categorize the procedure details [2, 8, 9], and invasive procedures were excluded [3]. To our knowledge, this is the first study to evaluate the relationship between the reasons for and duration of EN interruption.

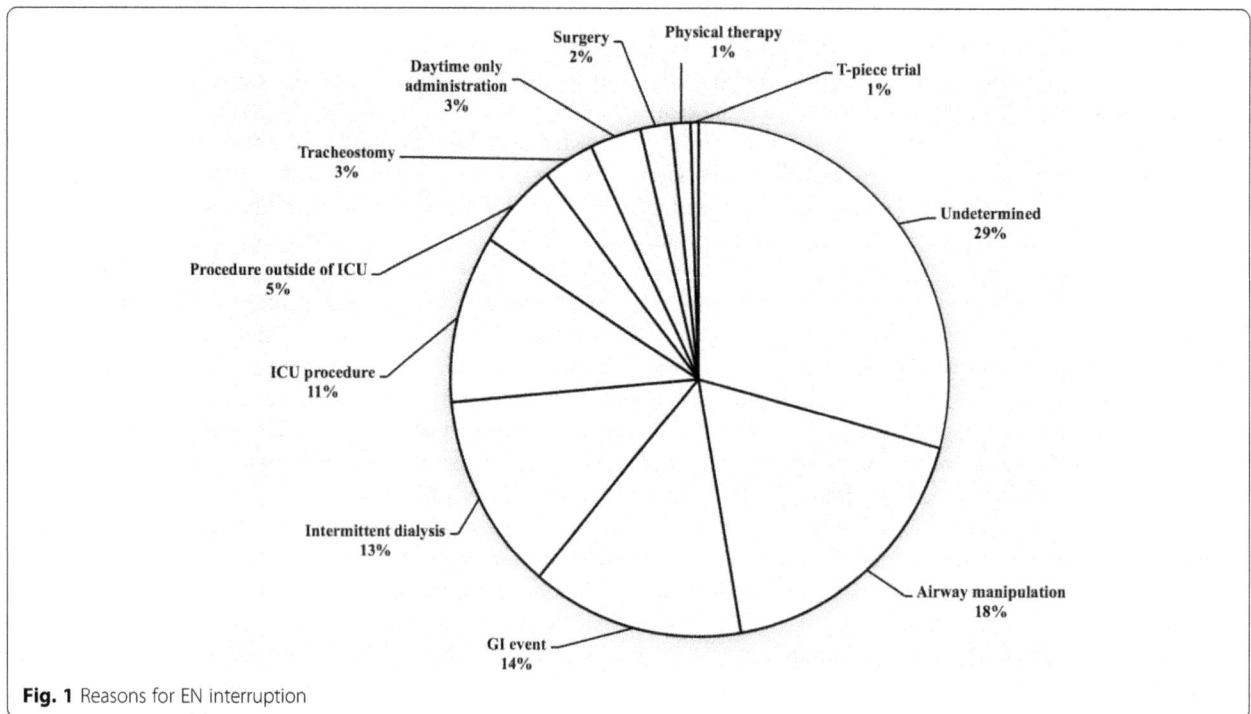

**Fig. 1** Reasons for EN interruption

To achieve the goal of minimizing calorie deficits while preventing EN-associated complications, nutritional protocols should focus on minimizing the interruption of nutrition along with enhancing administration. To establish an efficient interruption protocol, it is essential to evaluate the duration of the interruption for each procedure since different procedures have different safety margins for the duration of the interruption. Each interruption can be divided into several components. Whether the time of EN interruption before or after the procedure has a greater impact on nutritional deficits is a valid question since the

cause for delay and the longest part of the interruption duration differs among procedures. McClave et al. investigated the durations and reasons for interruption of EN in a medical ICU [2], showing the proportion of interruption in the total duration of EN administration for an individual reason, but did not present the actual length of time for the interruption [2]. Passier et al. described the duration of interruptions, partitioning into two durations before and after the procedures, but the numbers presented in the study were only the average durations among all patients and were not individualized according

**Table 2** Duration of enteral nutrition interruption per episode

| Reason for enteral nutrition interruption[a] | Time, median (IQR), h |
|---|---|
| Total | 5.5 (3.0–10.0) |
| Gastrointestinal event | 6.5 (3.0–14.0) |
| Airway manipulation | 9.0 (5.0–21.0) |
| T-piece trial | 3.0 (2.5–4.5) |
| Tracheostomy | 9.5 (7.5–14.0) |
| Surgery | 29.6 (11.0–34.3) |
| Intermittent dialysis | 6.0 (5.0–8.0) |
| Procedure outside of ICU | 4.0 (3.0–6.0) |
| ICU procedure | 4.0 (2.0–5.5) |
| Physical therapy | 1.0 (1.0–2.5) |
| Daytime only administration | 10.0 (9.0–10.5) |
| Undetermined | 4.0 (2.5–6.0) |

[a]Detailed explanation of each category are documented in the text
*IQR* interquartile range

**Table 3** Interval between enteral nutrition interruption and start of procedure

| Reasons for enteral nutrition interruption[a] | Time, median (IQR), hours |
|---|---|
| Total | 1.2 (0.3–3.7) |
| Airway manipulation[b] | 3.9 (1.8–5.8) |
| T-piece trial | 2.3 (2.0–2.3) |
| Tracheostomy | 5.8 (4.0–9.3) |
| Surgery | 6.2 (0.5–9.8) |
| Intermittent dialysis | 0.3 (0.0–0.6) |
| Procedure outside of ICU | 0.6 (0.3–0.7) |
| ICU procedure | 1.3 (0.5–2.5) |
| Physical therapy | 0.0 (0.0–0.5) |

[a]Detailed explanation of each category is documented in the text
[b]Patients in whom the ventilator weaning and tracheal extubation attempt failed, or patients where clinical load did not allow extubation were not included in this category
*IQR* interquartile range, *ICU* intensive care unit

**Table 4** Interval from end of procedure to restarting enteral nutrition

| Reasons for enteral nutrition interruption[a] | Time, median (IQR), h |
|---|---|
| Total | 1.8 (0.8–4.2) |
| Airway manipulation[b] | 7.7 (3.0–21.8) |
| T-piece trial | 0.3 (0.2–0.3) |
| Tracheostomy | 3.2 (1.0–3.6) |
| Surgery | 7.0 (1.7–16.8) |
| Intermittent dialysis | 1.0 (0.3–1.8) |
| Procedure outside of ICU | 1.2 (0.5–2.3) |
| ICU procedure | 1.5 (0.7–3.0) |
| Physical therapy | 0.6 (0.3–2.0) |

[a]Detailed explanation of each category are documented in the text
[b]Patients in whom ventilator weaning and tracheal extubation attempt failed, or patients where clinical load did not allow extubation were not included in this category
*IQR* interquartile range, *ICU* intensive care unit

to the reasons for interruption [3]. Adam et al. investigated interruptions and their reasons and energy deficits in five ICUs in the UK [8], but a thorough description of the interruption reasons was not performed in this study. In contrast with these studies, we describe the duration of the interruption for each reason, and the duration of interruptions for the procedure and from the time of the procedure to restart for each reason.

The duration of EN interruption related to either patient GI symptoms or respiratory and airway manipulations was long, and large variations found. Large variations were observed for interruptions for diagnostic tests or therapeutic interventions, both in the time from EN interruption until treatment start and the time from treatment end until EN restart. Reasons for the long, varying durations of these interruptions may be due to a lack of a clear interruption protocol, leading to a long unnecessary interruption, and a delay in early restart after a procedure. External factors including excess clinical load in the ICU and other departments involved in patient care may affect the timing of diagnostic and therapeutic procedures. Extended duration until EN restart after procedures may be due to insufficient staff awareness of the calorie deficit caused by the interruption, which might worsen patient outcomes [1]. Intervals between EN interruption and tracheostomy (5.8 [4.0–9.3] h) could be shortened in at least half of the patients, if the general consensus of a 6-h interruption before the procedure is followed. Substantial delay until restart of EN could also be improved for tracheostomy (3.2 [1.0–3.6] h), intermittent dialysis (1.0 [0.3–1.8] h), procedures outside of the ICU (1.2 [0.5–2.3] h), and ICU procedures (1.5 [0.7–3.0] h).

In this study, the average nutritional deficit due to EN interruption for the daily caloric goal was 11.5%. Adam et al. [8] reported an average deficit in prescribed

calories of 24% in five facilities studied, while other studies have reported calorie deficits of 13–40% [9–11]. The results of the current study are better than those in previous reports, probably due to efforts to supplement substantial calorie deficits, not by reducing the duration of the interruption but by increasing the rate of administration after restarting EN. However, depending on an increased rate of administration is a potential source of GI complications of EN. In one ICU with an EN administration protocol, calorie administration was closer to prescribed targets compared to ICUs without a protocol [8]. Although details of this protocol are unknown, EN administration protocols may affect the resulting calorie deficit.

In the current study, the most common reason for EN interruption was "undetermined." Clear orders for EN interruption and resumption were not documented in most cases. Insufficient nutrition in critically ill patients is related to increased mortality rates [1]. Many institutions adopt an efficient EN protocol for achieving calorie targets and reducing interruption by EN intolerance. However, a practical protocol for reducing interruption time due to the procedures has not yet been made available [12]. Busy ICU staff may fail to pay sufficient attention to nutritional deficits due to interruptions but would become more cautious of the interruption if a clear interruption protocol existed.

The current study has several limitations. First, a single-center design may hamper generalizability of the results. Nutritional policies and practices in an individual ICU vary and change over time. These findings may not be applicable in a substantial number of ICUs. However, it is noteworthy that even in a closed ICU as in the study institution, the absence of an interruption protocol and documentation may result in calorie deficits. These data may be of value in institutions considering implementation of a protocol, especially in open ICUs. Second, due to the retrospective study design, various errors could be possibly included. However, data from an electronic chart system, as in the current study, could allow more accurate documentation of the initiation and cessation of EN and amounts given than by a manual system.

## Conclusions

This retrospective single-center study evaluated details regarding interruption of enteral feeding administration and shows that durations of interruption were long for a variety of reasons. In addition, the most frequent reasons for interruption were undetermined, and documentation and orders were frequently missing. These findings may be of use in institutions considering the development and verification of an interruption minimizing protocol.

## Abbreviations
EN: Enteral nutrition; GI: Gastrointestinal; ICU: Intensive care unit; IQR: Interquartile range

## Acknowledgements
The authors thank Kentaro Koguchi, graduate student Department of Chemical Engineering, graduate school of Tokyo Institute of Technology.

## Funding
The authors declare that they have no funding for this study.

## Authors' contributions
UM designed the study, analyzed the data, and drafted the manuscript. MS was involved in the conception and design of the study, and critical revision of the manuscript. AKL and KO were involved in critical revision of the manuscript. YI, TKo, TKa, HK, HM, and TM contributed to the protocol development of the study, and collection and interpretation of patient data. All authors have read and approved the final manuscript.

## Competing interests
The authors declare that they have no competing interest.

## Author details
[1]Emergency and Critical Care Medicine, Dokkyo Medical University, Mibumachi, Shimotsuga-gun, Tochigi, Japan. [2]Department of Anesthesiology and Critical Care Medicine, Division of Critical Care Medicine, Jichi Medical University Saitama Medical Center, 1-847 Amanumacho, Omiya-ku, Saitama-shi, Saitama 330-8503, Japan. [3]Department of Surgery, Jichi Medical University, 3311-1 Yakushiji, Shimotsuke-shi, Tochigi 329-0498, Japan.

## References
1. Alberda C, Gramlich L, Jones N, et al. The relationship between nutritional intake and clinical outcomes in critically ill patients: results of an international multicenter observational study. Intensive Care Med. 2009;35: 1728–37.
2. McClave SA, MD, sexton LK. RPh et al. Enteral tube feeding in the intensive care unit: factors impeding adequate delivery. Crit Care Med 1999;27(7): 1252-1256.
3. Passier RH, et al. Periprocedural cessation of nutrition in the intensive care unit: opportunities for improvement. Intensive Care Med. 2013;39:1221–6.
4. Doig GS, Simpson F, Finfer S, et al. Nutrition guidelines investigators of the ANZICS clinical trials group: effect of evidence-based feeding guidelines on mortality of critically ill adults: a cluster randomized controlled trial. JAMA. 2008;300:2731–41.
5. Taylor BE, McClave SA, Martindale RG, et al. Guidelines for the provision and assessment of nutrition support therapy in the adult critically ill patient: Society of Critical Care Medicine (SCCM) and American Society for Parenteral and Enteral Nutrition (a.S.P.E.N.). Crit Care Med. 2016;44:390–438.
6. Kreymann KG, Berger MM, Deutz NEP, et al. ESPEN guidelines on enteral nutrition: intensive care. Clin Nutr. 2006;25:210–23.
7. Singer P, Anbar R, Cohen J, et al. The tight calorie control study (TICACOS): a prospective, randomized, controlled pilot study of nutritional support in critically ill patients. Intensive Care Med. 2011;37:601–9.
8. Adam S, Batson S. A study of problems associated with the delivery of enteral feed in critically ill patients in five ICUs in the UK. Intensive Care Med. 1997;23:261–6.
9. Cahill NE, Dhaliwal R, Day AG, et al. Nutrition therapy in the critical care setting: what is "best achievable" practice? An international multicenter observational study. Crit Care Med. 2010;38:395–401.
10. Koruda MJ, Guenter P, Rombeau JL, et al. Enteral nutrition in the critically ill. Crit Care Clin. 1987;3:133–53.
11. Heyland DK, Cook DJ, Guyatt GH. Does the formulation of enteral feeding products influence infectious morbidity and mortality rates in the critically ill patient? A critical review of the evidence. Crit Care Med. 1994;22:1192–202.
12. Higashibeppu N, Sanui M, et al. Current nutritional therapy in Japanese intensive care units: what did we learn from the international nutritional survey? J Jpn Soc Intensive Care Med. 2014:243–52.

# 8

# Predictors of intracranial hemorrhage in adult patients on extracorporeal membrane oxygenation

Alexander Fletcher Sandersjöö[1,2*], Jiri Bartek Jr.[1,2,3], Eric Peter Thelin[2,4], Anders Eriksson[5], Adrian Elmi-Terander[1], Mikael Broman[5,6] and Bo-Michael Bellander[1,2]

## Abstract

**Background:** Intracranial hemorrhage (ICH) is a recognized complication of adults treated with extracorporeal membrane oxygenation (ECMO) and is associated with increased morbidity and mortality. However, the predictors of ICH in this patient category are poorly understood. The purpose of this study was to identify predictors of ICH in ECMO-treated adult patients.

**Methods:** We conducted a retrospective review of adult patients (≥18 years) treated with ECMO at the Karolinska University Hospital (Stockholm, Sweden) between September 2005 and June 2016, excluding patients with ICH upon admission or those who were treated with ECMO for less than 12 h. In a comparative analysis, the primary end-points were the difference in baseline characteristics and predictors of hemorrhage occurrence (ICH vs. non-ICH cohorts). The secondary end-point was difference in mortality between groups. Paired testing and uni- and multivariate regression models were applied.

**Results:** Two hundred and fifty-three patients were included, of which 54 (21%) experienced an ICH during ECMO treatment. The mortality for patients with ICH was 81% at 1 month and 85% at 6 months, respectively, compared to 28 and 33% in patients who did not develop ICH. When comparing ICH vs. non-ICH cohorts, pre-admission antithrombotic therapy ($p = 0.018$), high pre-cannulation Sepsis-related Organ Failure Assessment (SOFA) coagulation score ($p = 0.015$), low platelet count ($p < 0.001$), and spontaneous extracranial hemorrhage ($p = 0.045$) were predictors of ICH. In a multivariate regression model predicting ICH, pre-admission antithrombotic therapy and low platelet count demonstrated independent risk association. When comparing the temporal trajectories for coagulation variables in the days leading up to the detection of an ICH, plasma antithrombin significantly increased per patient over time ($p = 0.014$). No other temporal trajectories were found.

**Conclusions:** ICH in adult ECMO patients is associated with a high mortality rate and independently associated with pre-admission antithrombotic therapy and low platelet count, thus highlighting important areas of potential treatment strategies to prevent ICH development.

**Keywords:** Intracranial hemorrhage, Extracorporeal membrane oxygenation, Adults, Predictors, Risk factors

* Correspondence: alexander.fletcher-sandersjoo@stud.ki.se
[1]Department of Neurosurgery, Karolinska University Hospital, Stockholm, Sweden
[2]Department of Clinical Neuroscience, Karolinska Institutet, Stockholm, Sweden
Full list of author information is available at the end of the article

## Background

Extracorporeal membrane oxygenation (ECMO) for respiratory and circulatory support—frequently used in pediatric intensive care [1]—is increasingly being employed in adults [2–4]. In addition to the critical condition of the patients treated, there is significant morbidity associated with the ECMO treatment itself [5]. A frequent complication is bleeding, a result of the systemic effects of cardiopulmonary bypass, causing platelet dysfunction, platelet consumption, and hemodilution of clotting factors, in combination with the anticoagulation and antiplatelet therapy administered to reduce the risk of circuit clotting [6]. In all probabilities, intracranial hemorrhage is the most devastating bleeding complication that can occur (ICH) [7] and has previously been associated with increased mortality in adults receiving ECMO treatment [8–10]. Despite this, the predictors of ICH in adult patients treated with ECMO are poorly understood.

So far, studies investigating the predictors of ICH in ECMO patients have focused on the pediatric population [11, 12] with only three studies looking into possible predictors in adults. In these studies, female sex, thrombocytopenia, use of heparin, dialysis, creatinine >2,6 mg/dl (230 μmol/L), duration of ECMO treatment, increased activated clotting time (ACT), spontaneous extracranial hemorrhage, renal failure upon intensive care unit (ICU) admission as well as rapid $PaO_2$ increase and $PaCO_2$ decrease upon ECMO initiation have been identified as predictors of ICH [13–15]. Generally, these studies have been constrained by the limited number of patients included, making statistical modeling difficult. In addition, only one of them included patients treated with both venoarterial (VA) and venovenous (VV) ECMO.

In this largest retrospective observational cohort study to date, we explored possible predictors of ICH in ECMO-treated adult patients.

## Methods

### Patients

All adult patients (≥18 years) treated with VA or VV ECMO at the Karolinska University Hospital, Stockholm, Sweden, between September 2005 and June 2016 were eligible for inclusion. Patients with intracranial hemorrhage upon admission were excluded. To reduce the influence of precipitating events, patients were required to have been on ECMO support for at least 12 h prior to decannulation or the development of an ICH. Medical records, including clinical notes, laboratory analysis, monitoring reports, and brain imaging data were collected from patient charts. The outcome variable was the presence of an ICH on a computed tomography (CT) scan.

## Variables

### Pre-cannulation data

Medical history and clinical charts were retrospectively reviewed, and the following pre-cannulation data were collected: age, sex, comorbidities (including a calculation of the Charlson comorbidity index [16]), Sepsis-related Organ Failure Assessment (sometimes referred to as Sequential Organ Failure Assessment) (SOFA) scores [17], and an arterial blood gas analysis within 2 h before cannulation. Ongoing antithrombotic therapy prior to admission (defined in our study as both antiplatelet and anticoagulation therapy), as well as cardiopulmonary resuscitation at any point during hospitalization were also noted.

### ECMO data

ECMO data included the indication for ECMO treatment, the ECMO mode employed (VA or VV ECMO), and whether conversion (shifting from one mode to the other) was necessary. Common complications that occurred during the ECMO treatment were also registered, including septic shock, dialysis, spontaneous extracranial hemorrhage, and administered blood products post-cannulation (plasma, platelets, and erythrocyte concentrate). We also noted the lowest recorded value during the ECMO treatment for platelet count, fibrinogen concentration, $P_vCO_2$ and axillary body temperature, as well as the highest recorded value for antithrombin concentration, international normalized ratio (INR), venous lactate concentration, venous pH, $P_vO_2$, and mean arterial blood pressure (MAP). By registering the highest/lowest values, as opposed to medians or means, we were able to catch temporary critical levels that could precipitate ICH development, for example, unexpected increases in MAP or acute decreases in platelet count. For patients that developed an ICH, variables were only recorded until the detection of the ICH, which in turn was determined according to the time the CT scan was performed. Registered follow-up data were 1-month and 6-month mortality. In addition, for patients with ICH, we registered hemorrhage location, hemorrhage volume (calculated by multiplying the hemorrhage length × width × height and dividing by two), and Fisher scale [18]. We also registered the daily mean platelet count, antithrombin concentration, fibrinogen concentration, INR and activated partial thromboplastin time (APTT) on the day the ICH was diagnosed as well as in the 4 days preceding diagnosis—an arbitrary time frame we believe would incorporate any clinically important information.

### Patient management during ECMO

Patients with potentially reversible acute respiratory and/or cardiac failure were considered for ECMO treatment. In acute respiratory failure, a ratio of arterial oxygen partial pressure to fraction of inspired oxygen ($P_aO_2/F_iO_2$ ratio) <80 mmHg ($FiO_2$ 1.0) was required. Other criteria included peak inspiratory pressure >35 $cmH_2O$ (pressure control), prolonged refractory hypercarbia with acidosis (pH < 7.10), and Murray score >3 [19]. In acute cardiac failure, the following criteria increased the chance of acceptance for ECMO treatment: central venous oxygen saturation ($S_{cv}O_2$) <55%, cardiac index <2 L/min m$^2$ [20], acidaemia, lactatemia, or vasoactive-inotropic score >45–50 µg/kg min$^{-1}$ [21].

Anticoagulation was achieved by a continuous intravenous infusion of unfractionated heparin (UFH) targeting an APTT of 60–80 s, which was assessed three times daily. Hourly monitoring using arterial and/or venous blood gas analysis was performed (Radiometer, Copenhagen, Denmark), including a separate assessment for activated clotting time (ACT) (Hemochron Mini II, Helena Laboratories, Beaumont, TX, USA, or Hemochron Junior, Scandinavian Medical Partner, Gothenburg, Sweden) with a treatment target of 180–220 s. After arrival at our ICU, a tracheostomy was performed within 2 to 3 days, after which the patients' sedation was reduced with the goal of keeping the patient awake with analgosedation. The bedside nurse and the physician in charge of the patient continuously monitored the central nervous system through serial neurological examinations. This included calculation of the Glasgow Coma Scale [22], response to verbal directives or pain, brainstem reflexes, eye opening, and pupil examination. When an unexpected neurological event occurred (e.g., seizures, mydriasis, anisocoria, delirium, confusion, motor function deficits, or failure to wake up following withdrawal of sedation), a cerebral CT scan was performed. Additional cerebral CT scans were also performed whenever the patient was referred for a thoracic or abdominal CT scan, even without any apparent clinical indication. A description of the ECMO pumps, oxygenators, ventilators, cannulas and patients monitoring systems used is included in Additional file 1.

### Statistical analysis

For descriptive purposes, continuous data are presented as medians (interquartile range) and categorical data as numbers (proportion). Mann-Whitney $U$ test and chi-square test were used to compare continuous and categorical variables, respectively. A univariate regression analysis was then used to correlate factors indicating a significant trend ($p < 0.1$) between ICH and non-ICH cohorts ("lrm" function in R, "rms"-package) [23]. In the univariate model, unimputed data were used. Nagelkerke's pseudo-$R^2$ was used to illustrate the pseudo explained variance, where "0" does not explain and "1" fully explains the model. A multivariate model, bias-adjusted for multiple parameters, was performed to determine independent risk factors for ICH. In order to detect significant temporal trajectories in the

coagulation variables of patients that developed an ICH, a paired $t$ test was used. Moreover, a student's $t$ test was used to detect any statistically significant change in the coagulation variables between the day of ICH diagnosis vs. 4 days prior. The statistical significance level was set to $p < 0.05$. The statistical program R was used, utilizing the interface R-studio Version 1.0.136 [23].

### Results

During the study period, 311 adults were admitted for ECMO treatment. Of these, 24 were excluded from our study due to <12 h of ECMO treatment, four were excluded due to the presence of an ICH upon admission and 30 were excluded because their ECMO treatment was partially conducted at a different hospital. Two hundred and fifty-three patients were included in the study, 161 of whom were treated with VV ECMO and 92 treated with VA ECMO, while 42 required conversion at least once. Pulmonary indications were by far the most common reason for ECMO treatment ($n = 224$, 89%). The majority of patients (98.4%) received intravenous heparin infusion to prevent clotting. The patients that did not receive heparin infusion did so because they had ongoing bleeding complications.

### ICH events and patient outcome

Fifty-four patients (21%) developed an ICH during their ECMO treatment. Forty-one of these were intracerebral hemorrhages (76%), 12 were subarachnoid hemorrhages (22%), and one was a subdural hemorrhage (2%). The median hematoma volume for the intracerebral hemorrhages was 22.8 mL, and the median Fisher scale for the subarachnoid hemorrhages was grade 2 (Table 1). The median time to ICH development from ECMO initiation was 7 days (4.0–14.5) (Table 4). Compared to non-ICH cohorts, ICH development was strongly associated with increased 1-month mortality (81 vs. 28%, $p < 0.001$, pseudo-$R^2 = 0.258$) and 6-month mortality (85 vs. 33%, $p < 0.001$, pseudo-$R^2 = 0.248$). There was no significant difference in ICH occurrence between VV and VA ECMO patients (19 and 27%, respectively, $p = 0.283$).

**Table 1** ICH characteristics

| Variables | ICH cohort ($n = 54$) |
| --- | --- |
| Intracerebral hemorrhage | 41 (76%) |
| Hematoma volume (mL)[a] | 22.8 (6.24–56.7) |
| Subdural hemorrhage | 1 (2%) |
| Hematoma volume (mL)[a] | 25.0 (range N/A) |
| Subarachnoid hemorrhage | 12 (22%) |
| Fisher grade | 2 (2–4) |

Values are expressed as median (interquartile range) or numbers (proportion)
*Abbreviation: ICH* intracranial hemorrhage
[a]Calculated by multiplying the length × width × height of the hemorrhage and dividing by two

### Predictors of ICH

When comparing ICH with non-ICH cohorts, increased risk of ICH was associated with the following: pre-admission antithrombotic therapy ($p = 0.018$), high pre-cannulation SOFA coagulation score ($p = 0.015$) (Table 2), low platelet count ($p < 0.001$) (Table 3), spontaneous extracranial hemorrhage ($p = 0.045$), amount of administered platelets ($p = 0.004$), and amount of administered erythrocyte concentrate ($p = 0.014$) (Table 4).

### Independent predictors of ICH

In the regression analysis, we included variables with $p < 0.1$. The pre-cannulation SOFA coagulation score was not included because the data was missing in 50% of patients (the parameter was not registered at our center prior to 2012), which would require a high degree of imputation and weaken any conclusions. The SOFA coagulation score is determined by the platelet count,

where a lower platelet count yields a higher score [17]. As expected, a strong co-variance between the pre-cannulation SOFA coagulation score and low platelet count (pseudo-$R^2 = 0.156$, data not shown) was also found, further supporting the removal of this variable from the regression analysis. Furthermore, due to a high degree of treatment intensity bias, we also disregarded the variables concerning administered blood products in the regression analysis. The univariate regression analysis confirmed pre-admission antithrombotic therapy ($p = 0.014$), low platelet count ($p < 0.001$), and spontaneous extracranial hemorrhage ($p = 0.031$) as predictors of ICH. It also recognized septic shock ($p = 0.043$) and dialysis ($p = 0.020$) as predictors. In the multivariate analysis, pre-admission antithrombotic therapy ($p = 0.011$, $R^2 = 0.037$) and low platelet count ($p = 0.035$, $R^2 = 0.074$) demonstrated independent risk association (Table 5).

**Table 2** ICH vs. non-ICH cohorts: demographics, pre-admission morbidity, pre-cannulation SOFA score, ECMO mode, and indication

| Variable | ICH cohort ($n = 54$) | Non-ICH cohort ($n = 199$) | $p$ value |
|---|---|---|---|
| Demographics | | | |
| Age (years) | 51.5 (40–61) | 50 (32–60) | 0.158 |
| Male sex | 35 (65%) | 127 (64%) | 1.000 |
| Pre-admission morbidity | | | |
| Hypertension | 9 (17%) | 36 (18%) | 0.967 |
| Insulin-dependent diabetes mellitus | 5 (9%) | 22 (11%) | 0.896 |
| Chronic renal disease | 2 (4%) | 1 (1%) | 0.116 |
| Antithrombotic therapy | 7 (13%) | 7 (4%) | *0.018* |
| Charlson comorbidity index | 0 (0–1) | 0 (0–1) | 0.373 |
| Pre-cannulation SOFA score | | | |
| Total | 14 (10.8–16) (26 missing, 48%) | 13 (10–15) (106 missing, 53%) | 0.443 |
| Respiration | 4 (4–4) (25 missing, 46%) | 4 (4–4) (95 missing, 48%) | 0.340 |
| Coagulation | 2 (0–3) (26 missing, 48%) | 1 (0–2) (100 missing, 50%) | *0.015* |
| Liver | 1 (0–2) (26 missing, 48%) | 1 (0–2) (102 missing, 51%) | 0.960 |
| Cardiovascular | 4 (3–4) (25 missing, 46%) | 4 (3–4) (95 missing, 48%) | 0.742 |
| Neurological | 1 (0–2) (25 missing, 46%) | 1 (0–2) (98 missing, 49%) | 0.726 |
| Renal | 1.5 (1–4) (26 missing, 48%) | 1 (0–4) (101 missing, 51%) | 0.606 |
| ECMO Indication | | | |
| Pulmonary | 48 (89%) | 176 (88%) | |
| Cardiac | 2 (4%) | 17 (9%) | |
| ECPR | 4 (7%) | 6 (3%) | |
| ECMO mode | | | |
| Venovenous | 31 (57%) | 130 (65%) | 0.361 |
| Venoarterial | 23 (43%) | 69 (35%) | 0.361 |

Values are expressed as median (interquartile range) or numbers (proportion)
Italicized text in the $p$ value column indicates a statistically significant correlation ($p < 0.05$)
Pulmonary indications included pneumonia ($n = 102$), sepsis ($n = 78$), respiratory failure ($n = 18$), ARDS ($n = 17$), trauma ($n = 6$), and drowning ($n = 3$). Cardiac indications included cardiogenic shock ($n = 18$) and pulmonary embolism ($n = 1$)
*Abbreviations: SOFA* Sepsis-related Organ Failure Assessment (also known as Severity Organ Failure Assessment), *ECMO* extracorporeal membrane oxygenation, *ICH* intracranial hemorrhage, *ECPR* extracorporeal cardiopulmonary resuscitation

**Table 3** ICH vs. non-ICH cohorts: laboratory variables

| Variable | ICH cohort (n = 54) | Non-ICH cohort (n = 199) | p value |
|---|---|---|---|
| Lab biochemistry | | | |
| Platelet count[a] ($\times 10^9$/mL) | 31 (17–46) | 48 (27–84) | *<0.001* |
| INR[b] | 1.5 (1.2–1.8) | 1.4 (1.2–1.6) | 0.147 |
| Antithrombin[b] (kIU/L) | 0.90 (0.78–1.06) | 0.93 (0.82–1.09) | 0.542 |
| Fibrinogen[a] (g/L) | 2.8 (1.5–4.3) | 2.7 (1.6–3.8) | 0.814 |
| v-Lactate[b] (mmol/L) | 4.7 (3.0–9.7) (4 missing, 7%) | 3.7 (2.7–7.7) (22 missing, 11%) | 0.174 |
| Blood gas analysis | | | |
| Arterial[c] | | | |
| a-pH | 7.26 (7.18–7.33) (16 missing, 30%) | 7.25 (7.16–7.34) (51 missing, 26%) | 0.703 |
| $P_aCO_2$ (kPa) | 6.90 (6.10–7.65) (17 missing, 31%) | 7.27 (6.00–9.90) (50 missing, 25%) | 0.481 |
| $P_aO_2$ (kPa) | 7.39 (6.36–8.81) (16 missing, 30%) | 7.34 (6.17–9.00) (50 missing, 25%) | 0.661 |
| Venous | | | |
| v-pH[a] | 7.22 (7.17–7.26) (4 missing, 7%) | 7.23 (7.17–7.28) (22 missing, 11%) | 0.184 |
| $P_vCO_2$ (kPa)[b] | 7.80 (7.38–8.95) (4 missing, 7%) | 8.04 (7.25–9.00) (22 missing, 11%) | 0.890 |
| $P_vO_2$ (kPa)[a] | 4.30 (3.73–4.80) (4 missing, 7%) | 4.46 (4.00–5.00) (22 missing, 11%) | 0.105 |

Values are expressed as median (interquartile range) or numbers (proportion)
Italicized text in the *p* value column indicates a statistically significant correlation (*p* < 0.05)
*Abbreviations: ICH* intracranial hemorrhage, *INR* international normalized ratio
[a]Lowest value during ECMO support and before ICH diagnosis (if applicable)
[b]Highest value during ECMO support and before ICH diagnosis (if applicable)
[c]Registered within 2 h before cannulation

**Table 4** ICH vs. non-ICH cohorts: clinical variables

| Variable | ICH cohort (n = 54) | Non-ICH cohort (n = 199) | p value |
|---|---|---|---|
| Administered blood products[a] | | | |
| Plasma (mL) | 2804 (1434–5674) (3 missing, 6%) | 1873 (690–4887) (22 missing, 11%) | 0.061 |
| Platelets (mL) | 1239 (275–3265) (3 missing, 6%) | 370 (0–2072) (22 missing, 11%) | *0.004* |
| Erythrocyte concentrate (mL) | 3576 (2155–6848) (3 missing, 6%) | 2471 (1027–6531) (22 missing, 11%) | *0.014* |
| Mean arterial pressure[b] (mmHg) | 99 (89–113) (1 missing, 2%) | 100 (92–109) (16 missing, 8%) | 0.791 |
| Axillary temperature <36 °C[a] | 12 (23%) (1 missing, 2%) | 53 (29%) (16 missing, 8%) | 0.463 |
| Spontaneous extracranial hemorrhage[a] | 32 (59%) | 85 (43%) | *0.045* |
| CPR[c] | 11 (20%) | 34 (17%) | 0.719 |
| Septic shock[a] | 24 (44%) | 59 (30%) | 0.059 |
| Dialysis[a] | 52 (96%) | 171 (86%) | 0.063 |
| Converted | 12 (22%) | 30 (15%) | 0.296 |
| ECMO days at ICH diagnosis | 7 (4.0–14.5) | – | – |
| Days on ECMO | 12 (5–19) | 7 (4.0–15) | 0.057 |
| 1-month mortality | 44 (81%) | 52 (28%) (13 missing, 7%) | *<0.001* |
| 6-month mortality | 46 (85%) | 61 (33%) (13 missing, 7%) | *<0.001* |

Values are expressed as median (interquartile range) or numbers (proportion)
Italicized text in the *p* value column indicates a statistically significant correlation (*p* < 0.05)
*Abbreviations: ICH* intracranial hemorrhage, *CPR* cardiopulmonary resuscitation, *ECMO* extracorporeal membrane oxygenation
[a]During ECMO support and before ICH diagnosis (if applicable)
[b]Highest value during ECMO support and before ICH diagnosis (if applicable)
[c]During hospitalization and before ICH diagnosis (if applicable)

**Table 5** ICH risk factors: uni- and multivariate analysis

| Variable | Univariate p value | Nagelkerke's pseudo $R^2$ | Multivariate p value |
|---|---|---|---|
| Pre-admission antithrombotic therapy | 0.014 | 0.036 | 0.011 |
| Platelet count | <0.001 | 0.074 | 0.035 |
| Septic shock | 0.043 | 0.025 | 0.280 |
| Dialysis | 0.020 | 0.033 | 0.215 |
| Spontaneous extracranial hemorrhage | 0.031 | 0.028 | 0.221 |

Italicized text in the p value column indicates a statistically significant correlation (p < 0.05)
*Abbreviations: ICH* intracranial hemorrhage, *ECMO* extracorporeal membrane oxygenation

### Coagulation trajectories prior to ICH

APTT, platelet count, INR, antithrombin, and fibrinogen concentration during the 4 days preceding the diagnosis of an ICH as well as on the day of ICH diagnosis were assessed. Figure 1 displays the daily means for each patient, and Table 6 demonstrates the combined mean values on the day of ICH diagnosis and 4 days prior to this. The results show that, on both an individual and group level, the APTT consistently stayed within the therapeutic range and there was no significant change in APTT preceding ICH diagnosis ($t$ test $p = 0.289$, paired $t$ test $p = 0.254$, Fig. 1, Table 6). In the paired $t$ test, the only parameter that significantly changed per patient over time preceding ICH diagnosis was antithrombin (increasing levels) ($p = 0.014$). Apart from this, no other significant temporal trajectories

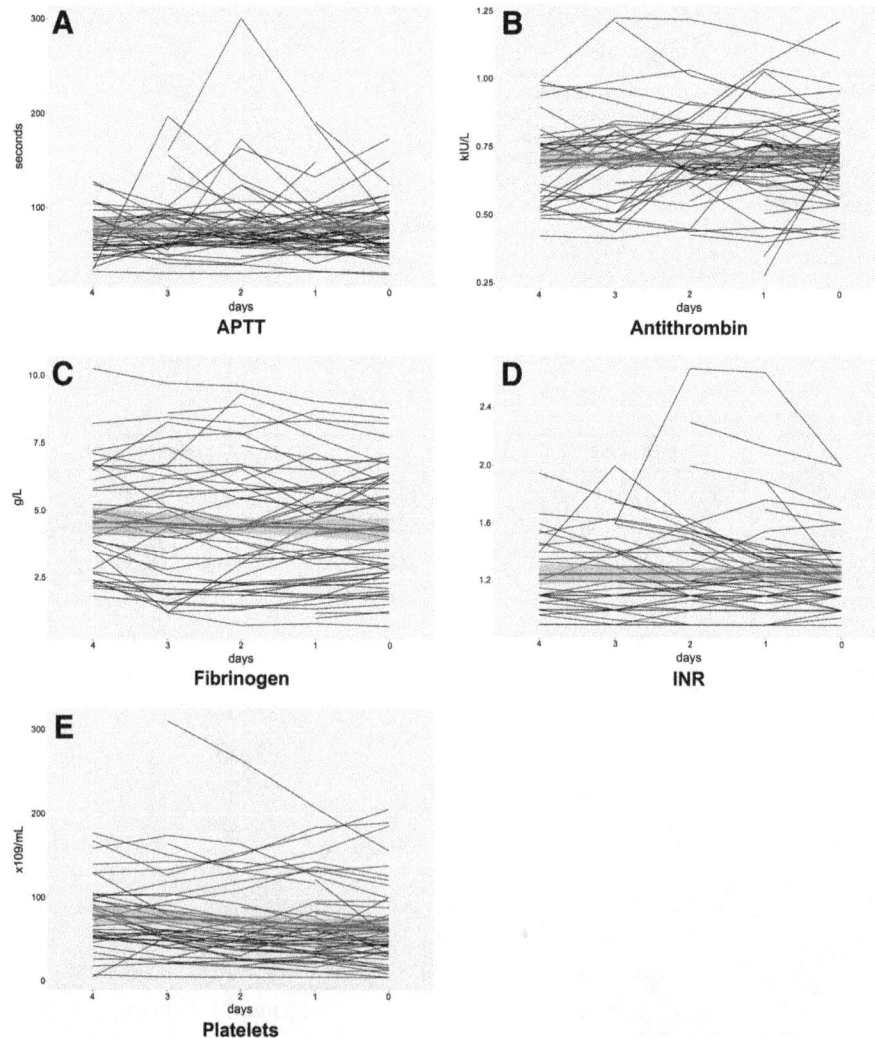

**Fig. 1** ICH cohort: temporal trajectories for coagulation variables prior to ICH diagnosis. Calculated using the daily means in the 4 days preceding the diagnosis of an ICH as well as on the day of ICH diagnosis. The *horizontal axis* indicates the amount of days prior to detection of an ICH, where "0" is the same day that the ICH was later detected. The *horizontal blue lines* represent the combined daily mean values for all patients, and the *gray area* represents the corresponding 95% confidence interval. *APTT* activated partial thromboplastin time, *INR* international normalized ratio

**Table 6** ICH cohort: coagulation variables on the day of ICH diagnosis and 4 days prior

| Variable | 4 days prior to ICH diagnosis | Day of ICH diagnosis | t test p value | Paired t test p value |
|---|---|---|---|---|
| APTT (s) | 69 (57–89) | 78 (60–95) | 0.289 | 0.254 |
| Platelet count (×10$^9$/mL) | 76 (52–99) | 54 (35–77) | 0.156 | 0.263 |
| Antithrombin (kIU/L) | 0.70 (0.56–0.76) | 0.71 (0.63–0.80) | 0.374 | *0.014* |
| Fibrinogen (g/L) | 4.50 (2.80–6.13) | 4.40 (2.70–6.00) | 0.467 | 0.496 |
| INR | 1.13 (1.05–1.40) | 1.20 (1.10–1.30) | 0.816 | 0.054 |

Values are expressed as medians (interquartile range)
Italicized text in the p value column indicates a statistically significant correlation ($p < 0.05$)
*Abbreviations: APTT* activated partial thromboplastin time, *INR* international normalized ratio

were found and no significant difference on group level could be detected.

## Discussion

In this observational cohort study, we sought to identify predictors of ICH in adult patients receiving ECMO treatment. Out of 253 patients, 54 (21%) developed an ICH. In patients that developed an ICH, the mortality was 81% at 1 month and 85% at 6 months, compared to 28 and 33%, respectively, in patients without an ICH. We identified (i) pre-admission antithrombotic therapy, (ii) high pre-cannulation SOFA coagulation score, (iii) low platelet count, (iv) septic shock, (v) dialysis, (vi) spontaneous extracranial hemorrhage, (vii) administered platelets, and (viii) administered erythrocyte concentrate as predictors of ICH development. Of these, pre-admission antithrombotic therapy and low platelet count were independent risk factors. Notably, this is the first time that pre-admission antithrombotic therapy, high pre-cannulation SOFA coagulation score, and septic shock have been identified as predictors of ICH. In addition, when comparing the temporal trajectories for coagulation variables in the days leading up to the detection of an ICH, there was a significant per patient increase in antithrombin concentration over time, while the means remained largely unchanged. To the best of our knowledge, this is the largest study of ICH predictors in adult patients on ECMO and contributes new findings that are important for patient management and future study design.

We included both VA and VV ECMO patients in our study, contrary to one of the previous studies that excluded VA patients on the basis of an increased risk of systemic thromboembolism from thrombus formation within the ECMO unit [15]. However, this complication is infrequent [24] due to the heparin infusion regimen as well as the bedside staffs' continuous attentive observation of the ECMO circuit for signs of clotting. Moreover, to the best of our knowledge, a comparison between VA and VV ECMO of the frequency of systemic thromboembolism has not been studied in the adult population and is thus only theoretical, further supporting the inclusion of both patient categories in the analysis.

Twenty-one percent of our patients experienced an ICH during ECMO treatment. This is in the upper range of the 7–19% previously reported in similar studies [13–15]. However, in a number of cases, the ICHs we identified were diagnosed using CT scans performed in the absence of neurological symptoms (i.e., a cerebral CT scan that was performed at the same time as a CT scan of the thorax or abdomen). A previous study, conducted at our center, on adult and pediatric ECMO patients treated between 1994 and 2004 found that 24% of those with an intracranial pathology (defined as ICH, cerebral infarction, or general edema) presented with no clinical neurological signs before performing the diagnostic CT, further suggesting that low utilization of neuroimaging contributed to underreporting of ICH [25]. It is possible, therefore, that our CT examination policy was a contributing factor to the high diagnostic rate of ICH in our cohort. However, in previous studies, the routine for performing cerebral CT scans in the absence of neurological symptoms is poorly described, making comparison difficult. With respect to outcome, we found that the 1-month mortality rate for patients who experienced an ICH was 81%, compared to 28% in non-ICH patients, which is in accordance with current literature [8, 13–15]. Consequently, ICH was associated with a considerable risk for mortality in this ECMO population, with a somewhat higher incidence of ICH occurrence compared to previous studies.

Pulmonary indications were the most common reasons for ECMO treatment in this cohort (n = 224, 89%). Previously, other groups have tried to establish if the indication for ECMO was associated with a higher risk of ICH [13, 14] but were limited by few data points in several of the subgroups, making statistical analysis unreliable. Moreover, while we determined indications for ECMO treatment by denoting the most severely affected organ system, patients usually presented with failure of multiple organ systems, further confounding this parameter. Thus, we chose not to include this variable in further analysis.

Prior to our study, pre-admission antithrombotic therapy as a predictor of ICH had not been assessed in ECMO-treated adults [7, 13–15]. We identified the parameter as an independent predictor of ICH, with 50% of patients with pre-admission antithrombotic therapy who were admitted for ECMO treatment developing an ICH. In theory, long-term antithrombotic therapy could have rendered these patients hemostatically difficult to control using the heparin infusion regimen. Alternatively, there could be a prolonged drug effect at play that is difficult to take into account. However, we have not found any studies to guide us in this area. A limitation to the variable was that we did not differentiate between different forms of antithrombotics. This could be important as they have different mechanisms of action, although differentiating and subgrouping the antithrombotics would yield extremely small subgroups and make statistical modeling difficult. For descriptive purposes, a compilation of the different forms of pre-admission antithrombotic therapy is included in Additional file 2: Table S1. Our results imply that patients with pre-admission antithrombotic therapy were at increased risk of developing an ICH during ECMO treatment, but its specific role in different subgroups needs to be further evaluated.

We further identified low platelet count, amount of administered platelets, and high pre-cannulation SOFA coagulation score as predictors of ICH. Low platelet count, determined by the lowest platelet count recorded during the ECMO treatment, was identified as an independent predictor. Previously, Kasirajan et al. reported that thrombocytopenia was an independent predictor of ICH [13] but the results have not been confirmed by others, possibly due to a high platelet count and/or due to the low incidence of ICH in the patient cohorts in similar studies [14, 15]. The impact of high pre-cannulation SOFA coagulation score has been assessed once before, albeit not as a continuous variable, when Luyt et al. distinguished patients with a SOFA coagulation score >2, compared to those with a score ≤2, at ECMO initiation. However, in their cohort of 12 patients with an ICH, only one met these criteria [15]. The total amount of administered platelets was another predictor of ICH in our study and has been identified as such previously [14]. However, since patients are administered platelet transfusions to combat their low platelet count, thus introducing a potent treatment bias, this parameter can just as easily be interpreted as an identification of patients with thrombocytopenia rather than acting a risk factor on its own. Although this remains unknown, no prospective study has been designed to address the issue. Clinically, if there were no signs of bleeding, we used platelet counts $<25-30 \times 10^9$/mL as the arbitrary threshold for platelet transfusion. Lastly, in the temporal trajectories of patients with ICH, there was no significant change in platelet levels in the days leading up to the detection of an ICH. This can be attributed to the fact that not all bleedings were detected following the development of a neurological symptom(s), which makes it

more difficult to determine the exact time of ictus. In addition, the values were achieved by calculating the daily average of each patients' platelet count, which meant that momentary decreases, which could have led to hemorrhaging, did not show if the rest of the platelet counts that day were normal. Hence, low platelet count, both pre-cannulation and during ECMO treatment, was a predictor of ICH.

Spontaneous extracranial hemorrhage as a significant predictor of ICH in adult patients treated with ECMO has only been assessed once previously, with significant results [14]. This can be attributed to the loss of platelets and coagulation factors that occur following major bleeding, or to the fact that patients who are hemostatically unstable are more likely to bleed. The most common bleeding sites in our study were pulmonary, cannula insertion sites, gastrointestinal tract, abdominal cavity, and thoracic cavity. The amount of administered erythrocyte concentrate was also identified as a predictor of ICH. However, since patients are administered erythrocyte concentrate transfusions following major bleeding, this parameter is probably an identification of the patients with extracranial hemorrhage rather than a risk factor on its own, even if this remains unknown as no prospective study addressing this exists. Hence, spontaneous extracranial hemorrhage is associated with an increased risk for ICH but the precise mechanism behind it needs to be further assessed.

The risk of ICH was higher in patients who required dialysis, which is in accordance with previous studies; Kasirajan et al. showed that dialysis and hypercreatininemia predicted ICH development [13], and Luyt et al. showed a correlation between renal failure at ICU admission and increased risk of ICH [15]. However, the precise mechanism of action needs to be further assessed. Evidence is also warranted to determine if the increased risk of ICH is a result of the dialysis treatment or the conditions that require dialysis. Overhydration was the main indication for dialysis at our ECMO center, with acute kidney injury as the second most common indication, and the number of patients who received dialysis was high in both ICH and non-ICH cohorts (96 and 86%, respectively).

Finally, antithrombin significantly increased over time in patients who developed an ICH, with INR increase showing a trend towards significance. However, as shown in Fig. 1b, most ICH patients had antithrombin values within the reference range, making it difficult to draw conclusions based on the temporal trajectories alone. One could hypothesize that the significant temporal trajectory found was due to a general improvement of hemostatically unstable patients' coagulation ability over time. Alternatively, it could be attributed to the fact that patients were, in some cases, administered antithrombin to combat heparin resistance, facilitate heparin effect, or reduce fibrin deposition in the ECMO circuit. However, the exact role of this correlation remains to be determined. Moreover, there was no significant change in APTT (Table 6), indicating that this per patient trajectory probably played a minor role in the development of ICH. The results also showed that the average patient had an APTT within the therapeutic range (Fig. 1a, Table 6). In the clinical setting, APTT is used to guide the heparin infusion regimen. This therefore suggests that the bleedings were not caused by heparin treatment errors (i.e., overdose). However, there are some solitary outliers in Fig. 1a, which could be the result of incorrect heparin administration or repetitive contamination when conducting the laboratory measurements of APTT. APTT was not included in the paired testing between ICH and non-ICH cohorts due to the risk of bias, as APPT is controlled by the amount of administered heparin and, accordingly, a non-therapeutic APPT also results in the physician adjusting the heparin infusion. To conclude, antithrombin significantly increased over time in patients who developed an ICH, but the clinical significance behind this is debatable. In addition, due to the lack of significant change in APTT in the days leading up to ICH diagnosis, coupled with the fact that the average patients' APTT was within the therapeutic range, we concluded that the ICHs were not the result of incorrect heparin administration.

## Clinical implications and future research

Although this is a retrospective study, with its inherent limitations, our research highlights the importance of closely monitoring predictors of ICH. While we acknowledge that ECMO is a last resort treatment that is considered only after great scrutiny, it is important to identify the ICH predictors that can be targeted with interventions or where earlier weaning from ECMO could be attempted. Low platelet count can be combated by decreasing the threshold for platelet transfusion; this must however be balanced against the risk for thrombosis. Also, considering the fact that a number of patients developed ICH despite a normal mean platelet count, as is highlighted in Fig. 1e, one should consider the value of performing "thrombocyte function tests" (i.e., multiplate) on this patient group on a regular basis, as platelet dysfunction can lead to the development of ICH even in the absence of thrombocytopenia [26]. Pre-admission antithrombotic therapy, high pre-cannulation SOFA coagulation score, septic shock, dialysis, and spontaneous extracranial hemorrhage may help to identify the patients prone to ICH where more rigorous neurological checks and earlier weaning from ECMO could be attempted. Considering the high mortality associated with an ICH in patients on ECMO, prospective studies evaluating risk factors for ICH in this patient group are warranted, as well as studies on management and predictors of outcome after the occurrence of an ICH.

## Conclusions

ICH is a frequent complication in adult patients treated with ECMO and associated with increased mortality. We identified pre-admission antithrombotic therapy, low platelet count, high pre-cannulation SOFA coagulation score, spontaneous extracranial hemorrhage, dialysis, and septic shock as predictors of ICH during ECMO treatment, with pre-admission antithrombotic therapy and low platelet count identified as independent risk factors. In the clinical setting, risk factor identification may help initiate steps to lower the risk of ICH in patients undergoing ECMO treatment. Prospective trials are warranted to identify additional risk factors and their mechanisms of action.

## Additional files

> **Additional file 1:** ECMO circuit. A description of the ECMO pumps, oxygenators, ventilators, cannulas and patients monitoring system used for the patients included in the study. (DOCX 84 kb)
>
> **Additional file 2: Table S1.** A compilation of the different forms of pre-admission antithrombotic therapy in ICH vs. non-ICH cohorts. (DOCX 48 kb)

### Abbreviations

ACT: Activated clotting time; APTT: Activated partial thromboplastin time; CT: Computed tomography; ECMO: Extracorporeal membrane oxygenation; ECPR: Extracorporeal cardiopulmonary resuscitation; FiO$_2$: Fraction of inspired oxygen; Fr.: French; ICH: Intracranial hemorrhage; ICU: Intensive care unit; INR: International normalized ratio; MAP: Mean arterial blood pressure; P$_a$O$_2$: Arterial partial pressure of oxygen; P$_v$CO$_2$: Venous partial pressure of carbon dioxide; P$_v$O$_2$: Venous partial pressure of oxygen; S$_{cv}$O$_2$: Central venous oxygen saturation; SOFA: Sepsis-related organ failure assessment; UFH: Unfractionated heparin; VA ECMO: Venoarterial extracorporeal membrane oxygenation; VV ECMO: Venovenous extracorporeal membrane oxygenation

### Acknowledgements
Not applicable.

### Funding
Eric Peter Thelin is funded by Swedish Society of Medicine (Grant No. SLS-587221). The funders had no role in the design of the study or preparation of the manuscript.

### Authors' contributions
AFS, JB, ET, AE, AET, and BB contributed to the study design. AFS and JB contributed to the data collection. ET contributed to the statistical analysis. AFS, JB, ET, MB, and BB contributed to the data interpretation. AFS, JB, and ET contributed to the draft of the manuscript. BB contributed to the study supervision. All authors contributed to the revision and approval of the manuscript.

### Competing interests
The authors declare that they have no competing interests.

**Author details**

[1]Department of Neurosurgery, Karolinska University Hospital, Stockholm, Sweden.
[2]Department of Clinical Neuroscience, Karolinska Institutet, Stockholm, Sweden.
[3]Department of Neurosurgery, Copenhagen University Hospital Rigshospitalet,
Copenhagen, Denmark. [4]Division of Neurosurgery, Department of Clinical
Neurosciences, Cambridge Biomedical Campus, University of Cambridge,
Cambridge, UK. [5]ECMO Center Karolinska, Department of Pediatric Perioperative
Medicine and Intensive Care, Karolinska University Hospital, Stockholm, Sweden.
[6]Department of Physiology and Pharmacology, Karolinska Institutet, Stockholm,
Sweden.

**References**

1.  Shanley CJ, Hirschl RB, Schumacher RE, Overbeck MC, Delosh TN, Chapman RA, et al. Extracorporeal life support for neonatal respiratory failure; a 20-year experience. Ann Surg. 1994;220:269–82.
2.  Gerke AK, Tang F, Cavanaugh JE, Doerschug KC, Polgreen PM. Increased trend in extracorporeal membrane oxygenation use by adults in the United States since 2007. BMC Res Notes. 2015;8:686.
3.  McCarthy FH, McDermott KM, Kini V, Gutsche JT, Wald JW, Xie D, et al. Trends in U.S. extracorporeal membrane oxygenation use and outcomes: 2002–2012. Semin Thorac Cardiovasc Surg. 2015;27:81–8.
4.  Sauer CM, Yuh DD, Bonde P. Extracorporeal membrane oxygenation use has increased by 433% in adults in the United States from 2006 to 2011. ASAIO J. 2015;61:31–6.
5.  Aubron C, Cheng AC, Pilcher D, Leong T, Magrin G, Cooper DJ, et al. Factors associated with outcomes of patients on extracorporeal membrane oxygenation support: a 5-year cohort study. Crit Care. 2013;17:R73.
6.  Hampton CR, Verrier ED. Systemic consequences of ventricular assist devices: alterations of coagulation, immune function, inflammation, and the neuroendocrine system. Artif Organs. 2002;26:902–8.
7.  Aubron C, DePuydt J, Belon F, Bailey M, Schmidt M, Sheldrake J, et al. Predictive factors of bleeding events in adults undergoing extracorporeal membrane oxygenation. Ann Intensive Care. 2016;6:97.
8.  Nasr DM, Rabinstein AA. Neurologic complications of extracorporeal membrane oxygenation. J Clin Neurol. 2015;11:383–9.
9.  Risnes I, Wagner K, Nome T, Sundet K, Jensen J, Hynås IA, et al. Cerebral outcome in adult patients treated with extracorporeal membrane oxygenation. Ann Thorac Surg. 2006;81:1401–7.
10. Mateen FJ, Muralidharan R, Shinohara R, Parisi J, Schears G, Wijdicks E. Neurological injury in adults treated with extracorporeal membrane oxygenation. Arch Neurol. 2011;68:1543–9.
11. Hardart GE, Fackler JC. Predictors of intracranial hemorrhage during neonatal extracorporeal membrane oxygenation. J Pediatr. 1999;134:156–9.
12. Doymaz S, Zinger M, Sweberg T. Risk factors associated with intracranial hemorrhage in neonates with persistent pulmonary hypertension on ECMO. J Intensive Care. 2015;3:6.
13. Kasirajan V, Smedira NG, Mccarthy JF, Casselman F, Boparai N, McCarthy PM. Risk factors for intracranial hemorrhage in adults on extracorporeal membrane oxygenation. Eur J Cardiothoracic Surg. 1999;15:508–14.
14. Omar HR, Mirsaeidi M, Mangar D, Camporesi EM. Duration of ECMO is an independent predictor of intracranial hemorrhage occurring during ECMO support. ASAIO J. 2016;62:634–6.
15. Luyt C-E, Bréchot N, Demondion P, Jovanovic T, Hékimian G, Lebreton G, et al. Brain injury during venovenous extracorporeal membrane oxygenation. Intensive Care Med. 2016;42:897–907.
16. Charlson ME, Pompei P, Ales KL, MacKenzie CR. A new method of classifying prognostic comorbidity in longitudinal studies: development and validation. J Chronic Dis. 1987;40:373–83.
17. Vincent JL, Moreno R, Takala J, Willatts S, De Mendonça A, Bruining H, et al. The SOFA (Sepsis-related Organ Failure Assessment) score to describe organ dysfunction/failure. On behalf of the Working Group on Sepsis-Related Problems of the European Society of Intensive Care Medicine. Intensive Care Med. 1996;22:707–10.
18. Fisher CM, Kistler JP, Davis JM. Relation of cerebral vasospasm to subarachnoid hemorrhage visualized by computerized tomographic scanning. Neurosurgery. 1980;6:1–9.
19. Murray JF, Matthay MA, Luce JM, Flick MR. An expanded definition of the adult respiratory distress syndrome. Pulm Perspect. 1988;138:720–3.
20. Tibby SM, Murdoch IA. Monitoring cardiac function in intensive care. Arch Dis Child. 2003;88:46–52.
21. Gaies MG, Gurney JG, Yen AH, Napoli ML, Gajarski RJ, Ohye RG, et al. Vasoactive-inotropic score as a predictor of morbidity and mortality in infants after cardiopulmonary bypass. Pediatr Crit Care Med. 2010;11:234–8.
22. Teasdale G, Jennett B. Assesment of coma and impaired consciousness. Lancet. 1974;304:81–4.
23. R Development Core Team. A language and environment for statistical computing. Vienna: R Foundation for Statistical Computing; 2011.
24. Makdisi G, Wang I. Extra corporeal membrane oxygenation (ECMO) review of a lifesaving technology. J Thorac Dis. 2015;7:E166–76.
25. Lidegran MK, Mosskin M, Ringertz HG, Frenckner BP, Lindén VB. Cranial CT for diagnosis of intracranial complications in adult and pediatric patients during ECMO: clinical benefits in diagnosis and treatment. Acad Radiol. 2007;14:62–71.
26. Nekludov M, Bellander BM, Blomback M, Wallen HN. Platelet dysfunction in patients with severe traumatic brain injury. J Neurotrauma. 2007;24:1699–706.

# Contribution to diagnosis and treatment of bone marrow aspirate results in critically ill patients undergoing bone marrow aspiration: a retrospective study of 193 consecutive patients

Laure Calvet[1*], Bruno Pereira[2], Anne-Françoise Sapin[3], Gabrielle Mareynat[3], Alexandre Lautrette[1,4] and Bertrand Souweine[1,4]

## Abstract

**Background:** The purpose of the work was to assess the contribution to diagnosis and/or treatment (CDT) of bone marrow aspiration (BMA) in the critically ill patient.

**Methods:** The retrospective study included 193 patients. On the basis of BMA findings, contribution to diagnosis was defined by one of four previously unestablished diagnoses (maturation arrest of granulocyte precursors, hemophagocytic lymphohistiocytosis, hematological malignancy, marrow infiltration with cancer cells) and to treatment as the initiation or withdrawal of a specific treatment including the decision to forgo life-sustaining treatment (DFLST).

**Results:** A CDT of BMA was observed in 40/193 patients (20.7%). BMA contributed to diagnosis in 37 cases (granulocyte precursor maturation arrest, $N = 10$; hemophagocytic lymphohistiocytosis, $N = 12$; hematological malignancy, $N = 15$) and to treatment in 14, including three DFLSTs. In multivariate analysis, the factors associated with a CDT were hematological malignancy, cancer or non-malignant hematological abnormality known on admission, indication for BMA excluding isolated thrombocytopenia, higher pre-BMA HScore (calculated prior to BMA), and higher SOFA score with or without platelet-count SOFA subscore. In the 160 patients without hematological malignancy or cancer known on admission, non-malignant hematological abnormality known on admission, indication for BMA excluding isolated thrombocytopenia, higher pre-BMA HScore, and higher SOFA score calculated with or without platelet-count SOFA subscore were independently associated with a CDT of BMA.

**Conclusion:** BMA can have a significant CDT in ICU patients with or without a known hematological malignancy or cancer on admission. An HScore calculated before BMA can be a valuable tool for predicting a CDT of BMA.

**Keywords:** Bone marrow, Hemophagocytic lymphohistiocytosis, Thrombocytopenia, Critically ill patient

* Correspondence: lcalvet@chu-clermontferrand.fr
[1]Service de Réanimation Médicale, Hôpital Gabriel Montpied, CHU de Clermont-Ferrand, BP 69, 63003 Clermont-Ferrand, Cedex 1, France
Full list of author information is available at the end of the article

## Background

Bone marrow aspiration (BMA) is mainly performed for cytomorphological examination of bone marrow cells, but also to proceed to other analyses such as immuno-phenotypic, flow cytometry, cytogenetic, molecular genetic, and microbiological tests. BMA is an important medical procedure for the diagnosis, staging, and follow-up of patients with hematological diseases and for investigating various non-hematological conditions including storage diseases, inborn errors of metabolism, metastatic cancer, and infection that has spread to the bone marrow.

BMA is easy to perform, and its examination often provides a reliable diagnosis within a matter of hours. However, it is invasive and painful requiring the administration of local anesthesia in patients not receiving general anesthetic sedation. Adverse events following BMA are rare but may result in severe complications [1, 2]. The indications for BMA are established in routine hematology practice [3].

Few reports have attempted to measure the contribution to diagnosis and/or treatment (CDT) of BMA in intensive care unit (ICU) patients, and most available data come from cohort studies of subgroups of patients with thrombocytopenia [4–6] or hemophagocytic lymphohistiocytosis (HLH) [7–9]. In ICU patients, BMA can be indicated for numerous conditions: as part of the follow-up of a malignancy previously known upon admission, for diagnostic purposes, and to guide treatment in patients with unexplained clinical features or laboratory or radiologic abnormalities such as lymphadenopathy, hepato-splenomegaly, osteolytic bone lesions, hypercalcemia, monoclonal proteins, cytopenia, cytosis, and the presence of immature or morphologically atypical cells in the peripheral blood. Dealing with these factors in the ICU is particularly difficult since these medical circumstances often result from multiple mechanisms caused by the severity of the acute illness, the underlying conditions, and their respective treatments. Because of the lack of information on BMA findings in the critically ill, the indications for the procedure are not standardized in the ICU and are highly dependent on local hospital practice and available technical expertise.

The aim of this retrospective study was therefore to assess the results of BMA performed in ICU patients and to determine the CDT of BMA in this subpopulation.

## Methods

### Setting and population

This retrospective study was carried out in the 10-bed medical ICU of the University Hospital of Clermont-Ferrand (France). All consecutive adult patients (age > 18 years) who underwent a BMA between 1 January 2010 and 31 October 2014 were screened. They were identified by electronic search in the database of the hematology department. Patients with no adequate bone marrow specimen because BMA had resulted in a dry tap or very dilute sample were excluded from the study. For patients with multiple ICU admissions over the study period, only the first ICU stay with a BMA yielding an adequate specimen was included in the analysis. For patients who had multiple adequate BMA specimens during the same ICU stay, only the first adequate specimen was taken into account in the analysis. At our institution, senior hematologists and intensivists are available 24 h a day 7 days a week and work together to indicate BMA. BMA is ordered to make a specific diagnosis, guide specific treatment, withhold potentially ineffective and/or harmful treatment, or provide important prognostic information. The data collected from the medical records are given in Additional file 1 [10–12] and the procedure of BMA in Additional file 2. The HScore was calculated for each patient before (pre-BMA HScore) and after (HScore) BMA results. The HScore is the first validated score to estimate individual risk of HLH. It was calculated from variables defined by a web-based Delphi study. The weight of each of the criteria was established by logistic regression modeling. The HScore is based on a set of nine weighted clinical, biological, and cytologic criteria. The minimum and maximum values of the pre-BMA HScore (before BMA results) are 0 and 302 points, respectively. The minimum and maximum values of the HScore are 0 and 337 points, respectively. The best diagnostic threshold of the HScore for HLH was 169 with a probability of HLH of 52%, corresponding to a sensitivity of 93%, a specificity of 86%, and an accurate classification of 90% of the patients [13].

Hematologists with knowledge of all clinical, radiologic, and laboratory tests analyze BMA samples. This study was approved by our institutional review board (Institutional review Board of Clermont-Ferrand South-East 6 – IRB00008526 number 2016/CE51) in accordance with French regulations. No consent was needed from patients.

### Definitions

The indications for BMA were divided into agranulocytosis, isolated thrombocytopenia, and suspicion of hemophagocytic lymphohistiocytosis (HLH), of hematological malignancy, and of cancer that had spread to the bone marrow. Agranulocytosis was considered as the indication for BMA when it was not associated with another indication. Isolated thrombocytopenia was considered as the indication for BMA when thrombocytopenia was the only indication for BMA. An adjudication committee (LC and BS) determined whether BMA made a CDT. Contribution to diagnosis was defined as a BMA result pointing to one of the

Contribution to diagnosis and treatment of bone marrow aspirate results in critically ill patients...

69

following previously unestablished diagnoses: maturation arrest of granulocyte precursors, HLH as defined by HScore calculation threshold $\geq 169$ [13], hematological malignancy, and infiltration with cancer cells. Contribution to therapy was defined as the initiation or discontinuation of a specific therapy strategy based on BMA findings, and the decision to forgo life-sustaining treatment (DFLST). Pre-BMA HScore was defined as HScore calculated with no points assigned for the variable "hemophagocytosis features on bone marrow aspirate." Post-BMA complications were bleeding or infection at the site of aspiration and other severe adverse events related to sternal aspiration such as manubrial separation and cardiac tamponade.

## Statistical analysis

Statistical analysis was performed with Stata software (version 13, StataCorp, TX). All tests were performed for a two-tailed type I error at 0.05. Quantitative data were expressed as mean ± standard deviation or median [interquartile range]. CDT was expressed in percentages (number of patients with a BMA yielding a CDT divided by number of patients in the study). Between-group comparisons were performed by chi-squared or Fisher's exact tests and Student's $t$ test or Mann-Whitney test if $t$ test conditions were not met. Relationships between quantitative parameters were studied by Pearson or Spearman correlation coefficients. Multivariable logistic regression was performed to predict CDT, with covariables determined according to univariate results and their clinical relevance. The results were expressed as odds ratios and 95% confidence intervals. The diagnostic accuracy of the pre-BMA HScore in predicting the CDT of BMA was evaluated with the area under the receiver-operating characteristic (AUC-ROC) curve. The optimal threshold was determined according to standard indices (Liu, Youden, and efficiency). A sensitivity analysis was performed on the subpopulation.

## Results

### Characteristics of patients and CDT of BMA

During the study period, 193 patients fulfilled the inclusion criteria (Fig. 1). The annual rate of ICU patients admitted with an adequate BMA did not differ over time ($p = 0.39$; Additional file 3). The characteristics of the study population are given in Table 1. The results of blood count and coagulation tests on the day of BMA are given in Additional file 4. The indications for, and

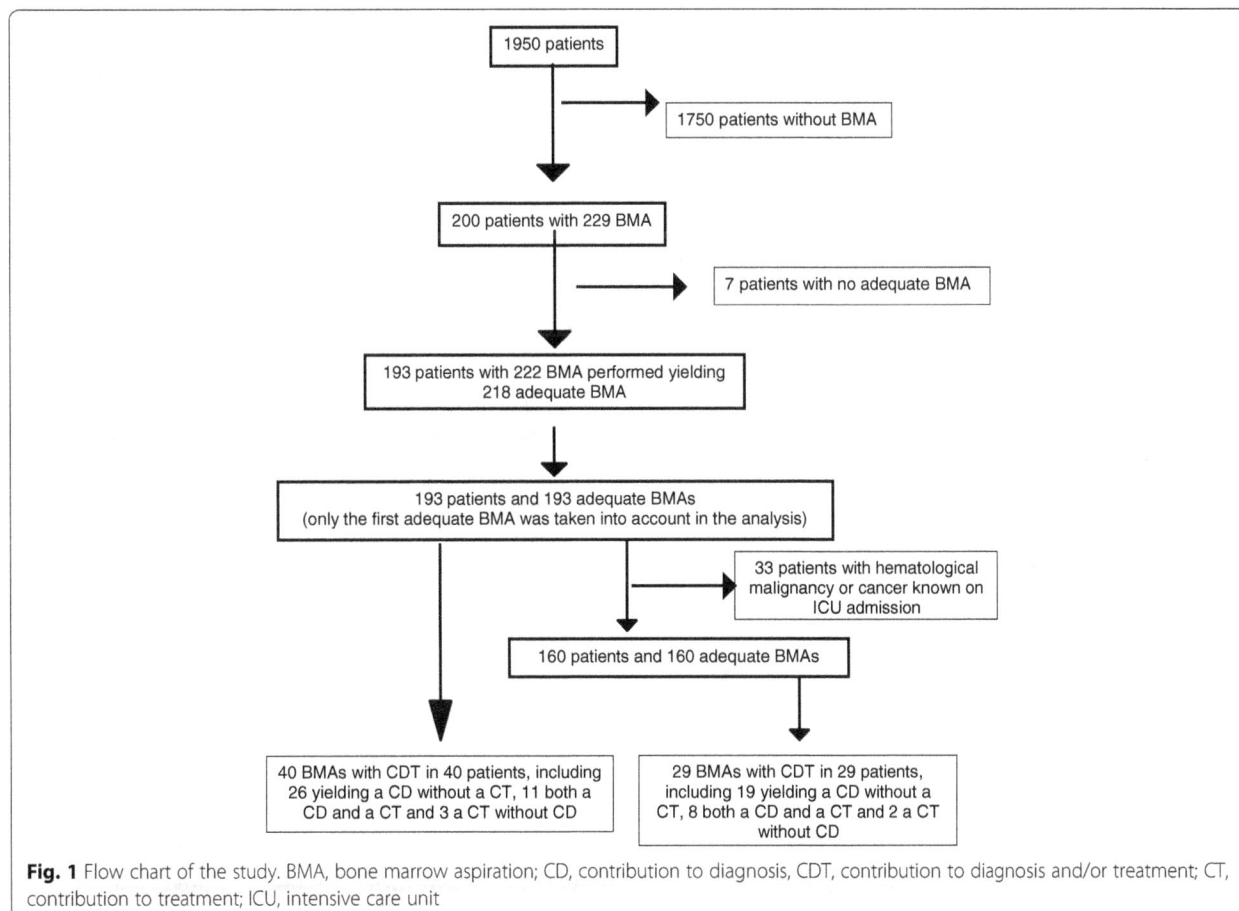

**Fig. 1** Flow chart of the study. BMA, bone marrow aspiration; CD, contribution to diagnosis, CDT, contribution to diagnosis and/or treatment; CT, contribution to treatment; ICU, intensive care unit

**Table 1** Characteristics of the study population

| Patients | n = 193 |
|---|---|
| Baseline characteristics | |
| Age (years)[a] | 66 ± 14 |
| Gender ratio (male/female) | 1.5 |
| Body mass index[a] | 26 ± 7 |
| SOFA on ICU admission[b] | 7 [5–11] |
| SAPS II on ICU admission[b] | 60 [40–72] |
| McCabe score 2[c,d] | 26 (13) |
| Hematological malignancy or cancer previously diagnosed[c] | 33 (17) |
| Nonmalignant hematological abnormality previously diagnosed[c,e] | 14 (7) |
| Reason for ICU admission[c] | |
| Acute respiratory failure | 67 (35) |
| Severe sepsis/septic shock | 50 (26) |
| Acute renal failure and metabolic disorder | 28 (14) |
| Coma | 19 (10) |
| Other[f] | 29 (15) |
| Vitamin B12 deficiency[c,g,h] | 2 (2) |
| Vitamin B9 deficiency[c,g,i] | 25 (36) |
| Days from admission to biopsy (days)[b] | 5 [3–8] |
| Characteristics on the day of BMA | |
| BMA at the sternal site[c] | 155 (80) |
| BMA at the iliac crest site | 38 (20) |
| Sepsis[c,j] | 124 (64) |
| Adenopathy[c,j] | 14 (7) |
| Splenomegaly[c] | 7 (4) |
| Monoclonal gammapathy[c] | 18 (9) |
| Anticoagulant agent[c,k] | 129 (67) |
| Prophylactic anticoagulation[c] | 87 (45) |
| Therapeutic anticoagulation[c] | 42 (22) |
| Antiplatelet agent[c] | 31 (16) |
| Proton-pump inhibitor agent[c] | 40 (21) |
| Anti-infectious agent with potential hematoxcicity[c] | 146 (76) |
| Other agent with potential hematoxcicity[c] | 76 (39) |
| Pre-BMA HScore | 62 [24–96] |
| SOFA[c] | 8 [5–11] |
| Invasive ventilation[c] | 52 (27) |
| Vasopressors[c] | 90 (47) |
| Renal replacement therapy | 31 (16) |
| ICU length of stay[b] | 14 [7–29] |
| ICU mortality[c] | 59 (31) |
| Hospital mortality[c] | 78 (40) |

*ICU* intensive care unit; *PreBMA HScore, SAPS II* simplified acute physiology score, *SOFA* Sequential Organ Failure Assessment score
[a]Mean ± SD
[b]Median [interquartile range]
[c]Number (percentage)
[d]Fatal outcome within 12 months
[e]Thrombocytopenia (n = 5), monoclonal gammapathy of undetermined significance (n = 3), polycythemia (n = 2), auto-immune cytopenia (n = 4)
[f]Cardiac arrest (N = 9), other shock (N = 8), thrombotic microangiopathy (N = 7), post-surgery surveillance (N = 5)
[g]Blood samples drawn between admission and BMA
[h]Eighty-two missing data
[i]One hundred twenty-four missing data
[j]In 48 patients, sepsis was unresolved since ICU admission
[k]Unfractionated heparin (N = 44), low-molecular-weight heparin (N = 78), danaparoid (N = 7)

pathological findings of, BMA are shown in Fig. 2 [14, 15]. BMA had a CDT in 40 patients (20.7%). It contributed to diagnosis in 37 patients and to treatment in 14 (Table 2). In the 10 patients with maturation arrest of granulocyte precursors, exposure to potentially hematotoxic agents within the preceding 7 days was identified in all cases, but corresponded to an immunosuppressive treatment in only one case (Additional file 5). Of the 12 patients with HLH, 7 were severely immunocompromised. Infection was the precipitating factors in 10 patients including herpesviridae infection in 5.

In the 14 patients with a BMA contributing to treatment, BMA findings resulted in initiation of treatment in 8, discontinuation in 3, and a DFLST in the other 3, established on the basis of the reported diagnosis (acute myeloid leukemia) against a background of worsening critical state (Table 2). No post-BMA complications were observed.

### Factors associated with BMA yielding a CDT

In the overall population, the factors associated with a CDT of BMA in univariate analysis are given in Additional file 6. In multivariate analysis, the factors significantly associated with a CDT of BMA were a known diagnosis on ICU admission of either cancer or hematological malignancy or non-malignant hematological abnormality; indication for BMA excluding isolated thrombocytopenia; higher pre-BMA HScore; and higher SOFA score calculated with or without platelet subscore on the day of BMA (Table 3). The AUC-ROC curve of pre-BMA HScore that predicted the CDT of BMA was 0.76 (95% confidence interval = 0.66–0.85). Youden's Index was maximal for a threshold of 76 with a sensitivity of 68% and a specificity of 73%. In a sensitive analysis performed in the subpopulation of 181 patients without HLH, a higher pre-BMA HScore was independently associated with a CDT of BMA (Additional file 7). CDT was more often observed in patients with hematological malignancy or cancer known on admission than in patients with no hematological malignancy or cancer known on admission (29/160 (18%) vs 11/33 (33%), $p = 0.05$).

In the 160 patients without hematological malignancy or cancer known on admission, the factors associated with a CDT of BMA in univariate analysis are given in Additional file 8. In multivariate analysis, the factors significantly associated with a CDT of BMA were as follows: a non-malignant hematological abnormality known on admission, indication of BMA excluding isolated thrombocytopenia, higher pre-BMA Hscore, and higher SOFA score calculated with or without platelet-count SOFA subscore on the day of BMA (Table 4). The AUC-ROC curve of pre-BMA HScore that predicted the CDT of BMA was 0.75 (95% confidence interval = 0.64–0.86).

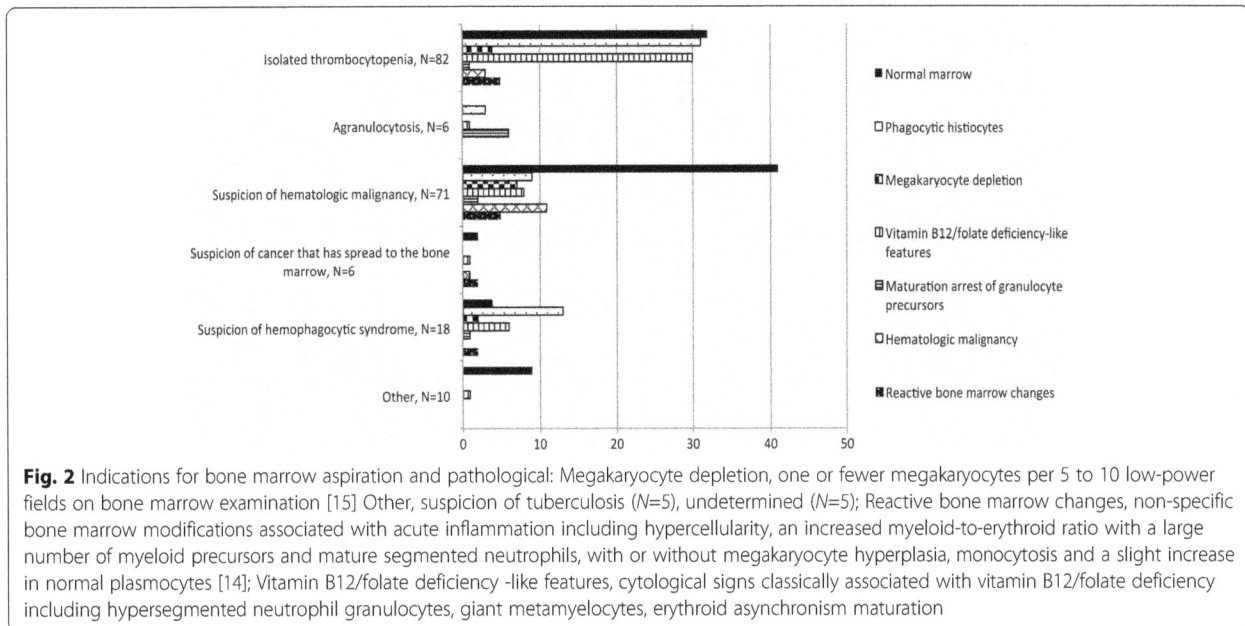

**Fig. 2** Indications for bone marrow aspiration and pathological: Megakaryocyte depletion, one or fewer megakaryocytes per 5 to 10 low-power fields on bone marrow examination [15] Other, suspicion of tuberculosis (N=5), undetermined (N=5); Reactive bone marrow changes, non-specific bone marrow modifications associated with acute inflammation including hypercellularity, an increased myeloid-to-erythroid ratio with a large number of myeloid precursors and mature segmented neutrophils, with or without megakaryocyte hyperplasia, monocytosis and a slight increase in normal plasmocytes [14]; Vitamin B12/folate deficiency -like features, cytological signs classically associated with vitamin B12/folate deficiency including hypersegmented neutrophil granulocytes, giant metamyelocytes, erythroid asynchronism maturation

Youden's Index was maximal for a threshold of 76 with a sensitivity of 69% and a specificity of 74%.

## Discussion

This study shows that in 21% of our ICU patients undergoing BMA, the results of the examination had a significant impact on diagnosis and management. We found a higher CDT in patients with higher values of SOFA scores calculated with or without platelet count subscore, in patients with higher values of pre-BMA HScore, and in patients with indication for BMA not restricted to isolated thrombocytopenia. These results were observed in our study population in patients both with and without hematological malignancy or cancer known on ICU admission.

Data on BMA in ICU patients are scant, and studies on this topic have focused on specific subpopulations, mostly of patients with thrombocytopenia [4–6] or with HLH [7–9]. To the best of our knowledge, our study is the first to report the CDT of bone marrow examination in an overall adult ICU population undergoing BMA for any reason.

The etiologies of thrombocytopenia in the ICU setting are classically multifactorial and mainly due to increased peripheral platelet destruction [16–18]. In a multicenter study involving 301 consecutive thrombocytopenic ICU patients, BMA findings yielded a previous unestablished diagnosis in 22% of patients and prompted a change in therapeutic management in 11% [6]. In our study, thrombocytopenia was present at the time of BMA in 128 patients and yielded a contribution to diagnosis in 32 (25%) and to treatment in 10 (8%). We found a higher CDT in patients undergoing BMA for indications

excluding isolated thrombocytopenia. This suggests that although cases of thrombocytopenia are currently due to multiple etiologies in the ICU setting, BMA should not be systematically performed on the basis of a single low platelet count. The decision to carry out a BMA in thrombocytopenic critically ill patients should include the presence of other features such as a detailed clinical history, physical examination, review of all medications, and results of other diagnostic procedures including blood test coagulation, blood cell counts, and peripheral blood smear examination.

Reactive HLH is a life threatening disorder. Its course may be improved by early etoposide administration. Several studies have reported the results of BMA in adult ICU patients with reactive HLH but used different definitions, which makes it difficult to compare their findings [7–9]. In our study, HLH was defined by the recently developed HScore [13], which includes variables defined by a web-based Delphi study [19], with the weight of each of the criteria established by logistic regression modeling.

The presence of hemophagocytosis on BMA specimens is not pathognomonic of HLH [8, 13] and is found, for instance, in severely ill patients with sepsis or after blood transfusion but with no proven HLH [7–9, 13, 20, 21]. In our study, hemophagocytosis on BMA examination was observed in 56 (29%) patients but corresponded to HLH in only 12. In addition, hemophagocytic activity may be absent during HLH particularly at the initial phases [22]. In a retrospective study performed in a medical ICU with HLH diagnosed according to criteria established by the International Histiocyte Society revised in 2004 [23], histological evidence of hemophagocytosis was not

**Table 2** Contribution of bone marrow aspiration to diagnosis and treatment

| Patient | Indication | Diagnostic contribution, $N = 37$ | Therapeutic contribution, $N = 14$ |
|---------|-----------|-----------------------------------|------------------------------------|
| 1 | b | Hemophagocytic syndrome | No |
| 2 (a) | b | Maturation arrest of granulocyte precursors | No |
| 3 (a) | c | Acute transformation of CMML | DFLST |
| 4 | d | Maturation arrest of granulocyte precursors | No |
| 5 (a) | c | Maturation arrest of granulocyte precursors | No |
| 6 | c | No (normal marrow) | Addition of erythropoietin |
| 7 | c | Marginal zone lymphoma | No |
| 8 (a) | c | No (normal marrow) | Addition of dasatinib |
| 9 (a) | e | Maturation arrest of granulocyte precursors | Discontinuation of TMP/SMX |
| 10 | e | Hemophagocytic syndrome | No |
| 11 | c | Lymphocytic lymphoma | No |
| 12 | e | No (presence of phagocytic histiocytes) | Addition of etoposide |
| 13 | e | Myelodysplastic syndrome | No |
| 14 | b | Hemophagocytic syndrome | No |
| 15 | c | Diffuse large B cell lymphoma | Addition of COP (g) |
| 16 | c | Marginal zone lymphoma | No |
| 17 | d | Maturation arrest of granulocyte precursors | No |
| 18 (a) | c | Acute monocytic leukemia | DFLST |
| 19 | c | Acute myeloid leukemia | DFLST |
| 20 | e | Hemophagocytic syndrome | No |
| 21 | e | Hemophagocytic syndrome | No |
| 22 | c | Myelodysplastic syndrome | No |
| 23 (a) | c | Relapsed multiple myeloma | No |
| 24 | e | Hemophagocytic syndrome | No |
| 25 | d | Maturation arrest of granulocyte precursors | Discontinuation of tacrolimus |
| 26 | e | Hemophagocytic syndrome | No |
| 27 (a) | c | Hemophagocytic syndrome | No |
| 28 | c | Multiple myeloma | No |
| 29 | e | Myelodysplastic syndrome | No |
| 30 | e | Myelodysplastic syndrome | No |
| 31 | b | Hemophagocytic syndrome | No |
| 32 | f | Diffuse large B cell lymphoma | Addition of COP (g) |
| 33 (a) | c | Myelodysplastic syndrome | No |
| 34 | e | Hemophagocytic syndrome | Addition of etoposide |
| 35 (a) | c | Hemophagocytic syndrome | No |
| 36 | e | Hemophagocytic syndrome | No |
| 37 | d | Maturation arrest of granulocyte precursors | Addition of lenogastrim |
| 38 | d | Maturation arrest of granulocyte precursors | Discontinuation of amoxicillin |
| 39 | d | Maturation arrest of granulocyte precursors | Addition of lenogastrim |
| 40 (a) | c | Maturation arrest of granulocyte precursors | No |

In patients 6, 8, and 12, BMA did not contribute to diagnosis but contributed to treatment
a, hematological malignancy or cancer already known upon ICU admission; b, suspicion of hemophagocytic lymphohistiocytosis; c, suspicion of hematological malignancy; d, agranulocytosis; e, thrombocytopenia; f, suspected cancer that has spread to the bone marrow; g, ultimately followed by DFLST; *CMML*, chronic myelomonocytic leukemia; *COP*, cyclophosphamide, vincristine, prednisone; *DFLST*, decision to forego life-sustaining treatment; *TMP/SMX*, trimethoprim/sulfamethoxazole

**Table 3** Multivariable analysis of factors associated with a CDT of BMA in the overall population ($N = 193$)

| Variable | Odds ratio | 95% confidence interval | P value |
|---|---|---|---|
| First model | | | |
| Hematological malignancy, cancer, or non-malignant hematological abnormality known on admission | 3.70 | [1.44–9.33] | 0.007 |
| Indication of BMA excluding isolated TP[a,b] | 3.69 | [1.46–9.30] | 0.006 |
| SOFA score[c] | 1.15 | [1.04–1.28] | 0.006 |
| Pre-BMA HScore[c,d] | 1.03 | [1.02–1.04] | < 0.001 |
| Second model | | | |
| Hematological malignancy, cancer, or non-malignant hematological abnormality known on admission | 3.21 | [1.78–8.76] | 0.023 |
| Indication of BMA excluding isolated TP[a,b] | 4.53 | [1.66–12.38] | 0.003 |
| SOFA—platelet-count SOFA subscore[c] | 1.15 | [1.03–1.29] | 0.013 |
| Pre-BMA HScore[c,d] | 1.03 | [1.02–1.04] | < 0.001 |
| Platelet count SOFA subscore 0 versus other groups[c] | 2.38 | [0.76-7.50] | 0.138 |

*BMA* bone marrow aspiration, *CDT* contribution to diagnosis and/or treatment, *Hscore* reactive hemophagocytic syndrome diagnostic score, *SOFA* sequential organ failure assessment, *TP* thrombocytopenia
[a]Thrombocytopenia may be present or absent in these patients
[b]Isolated thrombocytopenia, i.e., thrombocytopenia was the only indication for BMA
[c]Per point
[d]Calculated with no points assigned for the cytological variable

observed in 12/56 patients (22%) with HLH [8]. In a recent study performed in 98 adult ICU patients with BMA requested for suspicion of HLH and HLH diagnosed on an HScore threshold value higher than 169, hemophagocytosis on BMA examination was observed in 57/71 (83%) patients with HLH and in 21/27 (84%) without [9]. In our study, 12 patients had HLH defined by an HScore threshold value higher than 169, and hemophagocytosis on BMA examination was observed in all 12 cases. Infection was the predominant precipitating factor, as classically reported [22]. We found that a higher pre-BMA score was

associated with a CDT of BMA even in our subpopulation without HLH. This likely reflects the inclusion in the HScore of clinical and laboratory manifestations such as known underlying immunosuppression, fever, organomegaly (splenomegaly, hepatomegaly), and cytopenias, which were also commonly associated with diagnoses other than HLH defining a CDT of BMA in our study (maturation arrest of granulocyte precursors, hematological malignancy, and marrow infiltration with cancer cells). Thus, our study suggests that a single score, the HScore calculated either before BMA (pre-BMA HScore) or after,

**Table 4** Multivariable analysis of factors associated with a CDT of BMA in the subpopulation with no hematological malignancy or cancer known on admission ($N = 160$)

| Variable | Odds ratio | 95% confidence interval | P value |
|---|---|---|---|
| First model | | | |
| Non-malignant hematological abnormality known on admission | 7.75 | [1.77–34.02] | 0.007 |
| Indication of BMA excluding isolated TP[a,b] | 3.32 | [1.16–9.51] | 0.025 |
| SOFA score[c] | 1.19 | [1.06–1.34] | 0.003 |
| Pre-BMA HScore[c,d] | 1.03 | [1.01–1.04] | < 0.001 |
| Second model | | | |
| Non-malignant hematological abnormality known on admission | 6.76 | [1.51–30.38] | 0.013 |
| Indication of BMA excluding isolated TP[a,b] | 3.82 | [1.19–12.24] | 0.024 |
| SOFA—platelet-count SOFA subscore[c] | 1.19 | [1.04–1.35] | 0.009 |
| Pre-BMA HScore[c,d] | 1.03 | [1.01–1.04] | < 0.001 |
| Platelet count SOFA subscore 0 versus other groups | 2.14 | [0.60–7.62] | 0.239 |

*BMA* bone marrow aspiration, *CDT* contribution to diagnosis and/or treatment, *Hscore* reactive hemophagocytic syndrome diagnostic score, *SOFA* sequential organ failure assessment, *TP* thrombocytopenia
[a]Thrombocytopenia may be present or absent in these patients
[b]Isolated thrombocytopenia, i.e., thrombocytopenia was the only indication for BMA
[c]Per point
[d]Calculated with no points assigned for the cytological variable

could be a useful means of both predicting a CDT of BMA and establishing HLH diagnosis.

The incidence of BMA-related mechanical complications reported in the literature is lower than 0.4% [2, 6, 24, 25]. In our study, we observed no BMA procedure-related complications, which is in agreement with the results of a previous report [6]. We are aware that our study has several limitations. First, it was retrospective. Second, it involved only ICU patients undergoing BMA, and hence, the CDT of BMA in a general ICU population cannot be extrapolated from our results. Third, it was a single-center study performed in a medical ICU, and whether the results can be extrapolated to other ICUs remains questionable. Fourth, the indications for BMA were not pre-defined, although the year-on-year rates of patients who had a BMA did not differ over the period studied. Fifth, the definition of "contribution to diagnosis" did not account for factors such as the mechanism of thrombocytopenia or signs suggesting vitamin deficiency. The mechanism of thrombocytopenia was intentionally ruled out of the definition as all of the bone marrow examinations ordered to screen thrombocytopenia would have necessarily been diagnosis-contributive in some way given the "yes/no" output (absence or presence of megakaryocyte depletion). Likewise, the presence on bone marrow examination of signs pointing to vitamin B9 or B12 deficiency was not factored into the definition of contribution to diagnosis as signs like these are frequently found on ICU-patient aspirates yet only rarely associated with an actual deficit as evidenced in biological screening assays [6, 26]. Sixth, the definition of contribution to diagnosis did not include ongoing treatment when BMA yielded no abnormal findings. Normal BMA findings in a cytopenic patient can serve to rule out any potential myelotoxicity from certain drug therapies and thus allow them to continue. As our study was retrospective, we were unable to run this type of analysis. The latter two points may mean that we underestimated the CDT of the bone marrow examination here. In the intensive care setting, BMA is useful in cases of unexplained cytopenia, suspected HLH, suspected cancer that has spread to the bone marrow, or suspected hematological malignancy. The decision to perform a BMA in the ICU should be taken by a multidisciplinary team approach including intensivists and hematologists, and it requires the integration of various factors including clinical history, physical examination, peripheral blood film analysis, and other diagnostic procedure results, as recommended in other medical units [27]. In these conditions, BMA in the intensive care setting can yield the diagnosis of maturation arrest of granulocyte precursors, HLH or hematological malignancy, and bone marrow infiltration with cancer cells and also help in the decision to initiate or discontinue a specific therapy strategy. In some cases such as lymphomas, myeloproliferative neoplasms, or metastatic malignancies,

BMA cannot always establish the diagnosis and should then be combined with a trephine biopsy.

## Conclusion

BMA can be a valuable tool in critical care management, in patients both with and without hematological malignancy or cancer known on admission. The HScore may help to better define the population liable to benefit from BMA. Multicenter cohort studies should be performed to confirm these results and to determine the usefulness of BMA in an overall ICU population.

## Additional files

**Additional file 1:** Data collection. (DOCX 14 kb)

**Additional file 2:** Bone marrow aspiration procedures. (DOCX 11 kb)

**Additional file 3:** Annual rates of ICU admissions and adequate bone marrow aspirations. (DOCX 48 kb)

**Additional file 4:** Hematological parameters on the day of bone marrow aspiration in the overall population ($N = 193$) and in patients with BMA results yielding a CDT ($N = 40$). (DOCX 12 kb)

**Additional file 5:** Hematotoxic agents administered within the 7 days prior to bone marrow aspiration in the 10 patients with maturation arrest of granulocyte precursors observed on marrow aspirates. (DOCX 13 kb)

**Additional file 6:** Results of the univariate analysis in the overall population ($n = 193$ patients). (DOCX 14 kb)

**Additional file 7:** Multivariable analysis of factors associated with a CDT of BMA in the 181 patients without HLH. (DOCX 12 kb)

**Additional file 8:** Results of the univariate analysis in the 160 patients without hematological malignancy or cancer known on admission. (DOCX 14 kb)

**Abbreviations**
AUC-ROC: Area under the receiver-operating characteristic; BMA: Bone marrow aspiration; CDT: Contribution to diagnosis and/or treatment; DFLST: Decision to forgo life-sustaining treatment; HLH: Hemophagocytic lymphohistiocytosis; ICU: Intensive care unit; SOFA: Sequential organ failure assessment

**Acknowledgements**
The authors thank Jeffrey Watts for his help in preparing the manuscript.

**Funding**
No source of funding was received for the research.

**Authors' contributions**
LC and BS are the guarantor of the paper and takes responsibility for the integrity of the work as a whole, from inception to the published article. BP contributed to statistical analysis and to the interpretation of the data, critical revision of the manuscript, and final approval of the version to be published. AFS contributed to BMA samples analysis and to the interpretation of the data, critical revision of the manuscript, and final approval of the version to be published. GM contributed BMA samples analysis and to the interpretation of the data, critical revision of the manuscript, and final approval of the version to be published. AL contributed to the interpretation of the data, critical revision of the manuscript, and final approval of the version to be published. BS contributed to the interpretation of the data, critical revision of the manuscript, and final approval of the version to be published. All authors read and approved the final manuscript.

**Competing interests**

The authors declare that they have no competing interests.

**Author details**

[1]Service de Réanimation Médicale, Hôpital Gabriel Montpied, CHU de Clermont-Ferrand, BP 69, 63003 Clermont-Ferrand, Cedex 1, France. [2]Département de biostatistique, CHU de Clermont-Ferrand, Clermont-Ferrand, France. [3]Laboratoire d'hématologie, CHU de Clermont-Ferrand, Clermont-Ferrand, France. [4]Université Clermont Auvergne, CNRS, LMGE, F-63000 Clermont-Ferrand, France.

**References**

1.  Riley RS, Hogan TF, Pavot DR, et al. A pathologist's perspective on bone marrow aspiration and biopsy: I. Performing a bone marrow examination. J Clin Lab Anal. 2004;18(2):70–90.
2.  Bain BJ. Morbidity associated with bone marrow aspiration and trephine biopsy—a review of UK data for 2004. Haematologica. 2006;91(9):1293–4.
3.  Lee S-H, Erber WN, Porwit A, Tomonaga M, Peterson LC. International Council for Standardization In Hematology. ICSH guidelines for the standardization of bone marrow specimens and reports. Int J Lab Hematol. 2008;30(5):349–64.
4.  Stéphan F, Hollande J, Richard O, Cheffi A, Maier-Redelsperger M, Flahault A. Thrombocytopenia in a surgical ICU. Chest. 1999;115(5):1363–70.
5.  Baughman RP, Lower EE, Flessa HC, Tollerud DJ. Thrombocytopenia in the intensive care unit. Chest. 1993;104(4):1243–7.
6.  Thiolliere F, Serre-Sapin AF, Reignier J, et al. Epidemiology and outcome of thrombocytopenic patients in the intensive care unit: results of a prospective multicenter study. Intensive Care Med. 2013;39(8):1460–8.
7.  François B, Trimoreau F, Vignon P, Fixe P, Praloran V, Gastinne H. Thrombocytopenia in the sepsis syndrome: role of hemophagocytosis and macrophage colony-stimulating factor. Am J Med. 1997;103(2):114–20.
8.  Buyse S, Teixeira L, Galicier L, et al. Critical care management of patients with hemophagocytic lymphohistiocytosis. Intensive Care Med. 2010;36(10):1695–702.
9.  Barba T, Maucort-Boulch D, Iwaz J, et al. Hemophagocytic lymphohistiocytosis in intensive care unit: a 71-case strobe-compliant retrospective study. Medicine (Baltimore). 2015;94(51):e2318.
10. McCABE WR. Gram-negative bacteremia: I. Etiology and ecology. Arch Intern Med. 1962;110(6):847.
11. Vincent JL, Moreno R, Takala J, et al. The SOFA (Sepsis-related Organ Failure Assessment) score to describe organ dysfunction/failure. On behalf of the Working Group on Sepsis-Related Problems of the European Society of Intensive Care Medicine. Intensive Care Med. 1996;22(7):707–10.
12. Le Gall JR, Lemeshow S, Saulnier F. A new simplified acute physiology score (SAPS II) based on a European/North American multicenter study. JAMA 1993;270(24):2957–2963.
13. Fardet L, Galicier L, Lambotte O, et al. Development and validation of the HScore, a score for the diagnosis of reactive hemophagocytic syndrome. Arthritis Rheumatol Hoboken NJ. 2014;66(9):2613–20.
14. Diebold J, Molina T, Camilleri-Broët S, Le Tourneau A, Audouin J. Bone marrow manifestations of infections and systemic diseases observed in bone marrow trephine biopsy review. Histopathology. 2000;37(3):199–211.
15. Louwes H, Zeinali Lathori OA, Vellenga E, de Wolf JT. Platelet kinetic studies in patients with idiopathic thrombocytopenic purpura. Am J Med. 1999;106(4):430–4.
16. Vanderschueren S, De Weerdt A, Malbrain M, et al. Thrombocytopenia and prognosis in intensive care. Crit Care Med. 2000;28(6):1871–6.
17. Van der Linden T, Souweine B, Dupic L, Soufir L, Meyer P. Management of thrombocytopenia in the ICU (pregnancy excluded). Ann Intensive Care. 2012;2(1):42.
18. Pène F, Benoit DD. Thrombocytopenia in the critically ill: considering pathophysiology rather than looking for a magic threshold. Intensive Care Med. 2013;39(9):1656–9.
19. Hejblum G, Lambotte O, Galicier L, et al. A web-based delphi study for eliciting helpful criteria in the positive diagnosis of hemophagocytic syndrome in adult patients. PLoS One. 2014;9(4):e94024.
20. Suster S, Hilsenbeck S, Rywlin AM. Reactive histiocytic hyperplasia with hemophagocytosis in hematopoietic organs: a reevaluation of the benign hemophagocytic proliferations. Hum Pathol. 1988;19(6):705–12.
21. Strauss R, Wehler M, Mehler K, Kreutzer D, Koebnick C, Hahn EG. Thrombocytopenia in patients in the medical intensive care unit: bleeding prevalence, transfusion requirements, and outcome. Crit Care Med. 2002;30(8):1765–71.
22. Ramos-Casals M, Brito-Zerón P, López-Guillermo A, Khamashta MA, Bosch X. Adult haemophagocytic syndrome. Lancet Lond Engl. 2014;383(9927):1503–16.
23. Henter J-I, Horne A, Aricó M, et al. HLH-2004: diagnostic and therapeutic guidelines for hemophagocytic lymphohistiocytosis. Pediatr Blood Cancer. 2007;48(2):124–31.
24. Loctin A, Bailly F, Laroche D, Tavernier C, Maillefert J-F, Ornetti P. Clinical interest of bone marrow aspiration in rheumatology: a practice-based observational study of 257 bone marrow aspirations. Clin Rheumatol. 2013;32(1):115–21.
25. Bain BJ. Bone marrow biopsy morbidity and mortality. Br J Haematol. 2003;121(6):949–51.
26. Wickramasinghe SN. Diagnosis of megaloblastic anaemias. Blood Rev. 2006;20(6):299–318.
27. Bain BJ, Bailey K. Pitfalls in obtaining and interpreting bone marrow aspirates: to err is human. J Clin Pathol. 2011;64(5):373–9.

# 10

# Echocardiography for patients undergoing extracorporeal cardiopulmonary resuscitation: a primer for intensive care physicians

Zhongheng Zhang(iD)

**Abstract**

Echocardiography is an invaluable tool in the management of patients with extracorporeal cardiopulmonary resuscitation (ECPR) and subsequent extracorporeal membrane oxygenation (ECMO) support and weaning. At the very beginning, echocardiography can identify the etiology of cardiac arrest, such as massive pulmonary embolism and cardiac tamponade. Eliminating these culprits saves life and may avoid the initiation of extracorporeal cardiopulmonary resuscitation. If the underlying causes are not identified or intrinsic to the heart (e.g., such as those caused by cardiomyopathy and myocarditis), conventional cardiopulmonary resuscitation (CCPR) will continue to maintain cardiac output. The quality of CCPR can be monitored, and if cardiac output cannot be maintained, early institution of extracorporeal cardiopulmonary resuscitation may be reasonable. Cannulation is sometimes challenging for extracorporeal cardiopulmonary resuscitation patients. Fortunately, with the help of ultrasonography procedures including localization of vessels, selecting a cannula of appropriate size and confirmation of catheter tip may become easy under sophisticated hand. Monitoring of cardiac function and complications during extracorporeal membrane oxygenation support can be done with echocardiography. However, the cardiac parameters should be interpreted with understanding of hemodynamic configuration of extracorporeal membrane oxygenation. Thrombus and blood stasis can be identified with ultrasound, which may prompt mechanical and pharmacological interventions. The final step is extracorporeal membrane oxygenation weaning. A number of studies investigated the accuracy of some echocardiographic parameters in predicting success rate and demonstrated promising results. Parameters and threshold for successful weaning include aortic VTI ≥ 10 cm, LVEF > 20–25%, and lateral mitral annulus peak systolic velocity >6 cm/s. However, the effectiveness of echocardiography in ECPR patients cannot be determined in observational studies and requires randomized controlled trials in the future. The contents in this review are well known to echocardiography specialists; thus, it should be used as an educational material for emergency or intensive care physicians. There is a trend that focused echocardiography is performed by intensivists and emergency physicians.

**Keywords:** Echocardiography, Critical care, Extracorporeal cardiopulmonary resuscitation, Cardiac arrest, Thromboembolism

Correspondence: zh_zhang1984@hotmail.com
Department of Emergency Medicine, Sir Run-Run Shaw Hospital, Zhejiang University School of Medicine, No 3, East Qingchun Road, Hangzhou 310016, Zhejiang Province, China

## Background

Cardiac arrest is one of the most important causes of sudden death in general population. The causes of cardiac arrest include, but are not limited to, ischemic heart disease, trauma, sepsis, cardiac arrhythmia, acute respiratory insufficiency, hypotension, and stroke. The incidence of cardiac arrest is estimated to be 17–53 per million population per year [1–4]. Cardiopulmonary resuscitation (CPR) is the first-line therapy for these patients. In out-of-hospital cardiac arrest (OHCA), the major components of CPR include electronic defibrillation and chest compression, aiming to restore spontaneous circulation [5]. Although prompt and high-quality CPR is effective in rescuing a portion of cardiac arrest patients, the mortality of conventional CPR (CCPR) is unacceptably high and a significant number of patients require further advanced life support [6]. It has been reported that 44% of in-hospital cardiac arrest patients had a return of spontaneous circulation, and 17% survived to hospital discharge. However, if the initial pulseless arrhythmia was ventricular fibrillation, 58% patients had return of spontaneous circulation and 34% survived to discharge [6]. Extracorporeal cardiopulmonary resuscitation (ECPR) is considered to be an indispensible modality for those with refractory cardiac pump failure [7]. Extracorporeal membrane oxygenation is always needed after extracorporeal cardiopulmonary resuscitation; thus, we discuss on the use of echocardiography through the entire course of extracorporeal support. There is evidence supporting that extracorporeal cardiopulmonary resuscitation tends to be superior to conventional CPR in improving neurological outcome at 3–6 months in patients with out-of-hospital cardiac arrest (risk ratio, 4.65; 95% CI, 2–10.81) [8]. The same results have been

replicated in pediatric patients and in-hospital cardiac arrest [9]. It is recommended that the time for the decision of extracorporeal membrane oxygenation initiation and extracorporeal membrane oxygenation team activation should be shortened, particularly during the CPR of relatively young patients and in-hospital cardiac arrest (IHCA) patients [10]. In recent years, there is an increase in the use of extracorporeal membrane oxygenation for cardiac support, as well as extracorporeal membrane oxygenation for acute respiratory failure [11]. Therefore, the assessment before initiation of extracorporeal membrane oxygenation and the monitoring during extracorporeal membrane oxygenation performance are of critical importance [12]. Echocardiography provides a non-invasive, radiation-free modality for the assessment of patients undergoing extracorporeal cardiopulmonary resuscitation. There is a trend that focused echocardiography is performed by intensivists and emergency physicians. The concepts of critical care echocardiography indicate that the examination is performed and interpreted by the non-echocardiographer physician as an extension of the physical examination for hemodynamic assessment [13]. The present article aims to provide a comprehensive review of updated evidence on the use of echocardiography for assessment of extracorporeal cardiopulmonary resuscitation.

## Echocardiography in identification of pulmonary embolism

Massive pulmonary embolism is a common cause of cardiac arrest with a reported mortality rate between 20 and 50% [14, 15]. Epidemiological study suggested that incidence of pulmonary embolism increased from 0.03% in 1997 to 0.13% in 2008, but its case fatality is decreasing [16] (Fig. 1). This can be partly explained by increased

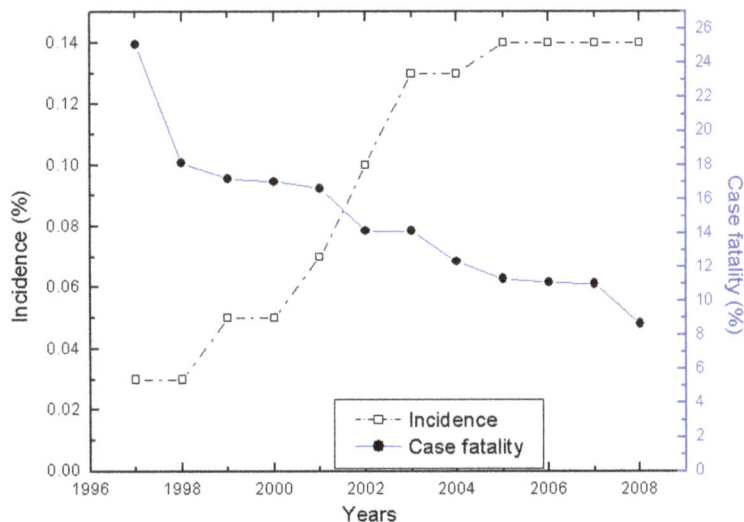

**Fig. 1** Incidence of pulmonary embolism increased from 0.03% in 1997 to 0.13% in 2008, but the case fatality rates decreased from 25 to 8% over the years [16].

awareness of this disease and extensive use of ultrasound for screening. Although there is no high-level evidence that echocardiography improves clinical outcome in cardiac arrest patients caused by pulmonary embolism, there are many case reports suggesting the potential role of echocardiography in management of such patients (Table 1). Focused echocardiography has been recommended for use to identify pulmonary embolism (PE), and the diagnostic performance is desirable [17, 18]. It is well known that computed tomography pulmonary angiography (CTPA) is the gold standard for the diagnosis of PE. However, the emergency setting of ECPR significantly limits the performance of CTPA. Thus, echocardiography can be the first modality in this particular setting. Typical findings of massive PE include marked dilation of the right heart and the compromised left ventricle (LV) (Fig. 2). Embolism can be noted for large portion of the population. However, in situations with disseminated microvascular embolism, imaging techniques including echocardiography and computed tomography angiography are usually unrevealing. The diagnosis was confirmed with necropsy [19]. These case series suggested that focused echocardiography performed by an emergency physician can be efficient in identifying massive PE, and appropriate interventions can be instituted including thrombolysis, extracorporeal mechanical support, and even the

underlying causes of pulmonary embolism [19–26]. However, evidence from the case series is subject to selection bias and thus the diagnostic utility of echocardiography in the condition of extracorporeal cardiopulmonary resuscitation is not well established. We recommend that focused echocardiography be performed in experienced centers.

Beyond the determination of PE, ultrasound monitoring during CPR is able to track the resolution of PE after thrombolytic therapy. Ramarapu reported that transesophageal echocardiography (TEE) monitoring during CPR revealed progressive resolution of the intracardiac, and after 45 min, complete resolution of thrombus was noted [27].

## Echocardiography in monitoring effectiveness of CCPR and transition to ECPR

A challenge in performing extracorporeal membrane oxygenation is the timing of extracorporeal membrane oxygenation initiation. There is some observational evidence that late initiation of extracorporeal membrane oxygenation results in poor neurological and mortality outcomes [28–32]. For example, Chen's study showed that patients who had conventional cardiopulmonary resuscitation for 45 min or less before extracorporeal cardiopulmonary resuscitation had higher rate of survival

**Table 1** Case reports of extracorporeal cardiopulmonary resuscitation caused by pulmonary embolism

| Cases (authors + year) | Age/gender | Condition | Type of cardiac arrest | Who performed ultrasound | Mode | Finding |
|---|---|---|---|---|---|---|
| Jeong et al 2015 [20] | 46/female | Large B cell lymphoma | PEA | Emergency physician | Transthoracic | Marked RA dilatation, a small LV, and abnormal inter-ventricular septal wall motion |
| Chowdhury et al. 2015 [21] | 63/male | Abdominal surgery | PEA | Not reported | Transthoracic | Enlarged RA with multiple thrombi, compressed LV with inter-ventricular septal shift |
| Swol et al. 2016 [22] | 5 cases (37–53 years) | Trauma and injury | Not reported | Not reported | Transthoracic | Thrombus of the inferior vena cava that extended to the RV |
| Northey et al. 2015 [23] | 34/female | No | Not reported | Not reported | Transthoracic | Severe RV dilatation with global systolic impairment and failure |
| Lu et al. 2004 [24] | 73/male | Fracture surgery | Not reported | Not reported | Transesophageal | Severely distended RA and RV, with a large embolus in the RA |
| Tsai et al. 1999 [25] | 58/female | Uterine cervix carcinoma | Not reported | Not reported | Transesophageal | Marked RA dilation, a small RV, and nearly empty chambers of the left heart, massive thromboembolism in the RA |
| Ilsaas et al 1998 [26] | 43/female | Cesarean section | Not reported | Not reported | Not reported | RV dilation, compressed LV and tricuspid insufficiency |
| Liang et al. 2011 [19] | 59/male | NSCLC | Not reported | Not reported | Transthoracic | Marked RV dilation; LVEF = 68% |

*Abbreviations:* PE pulmonary embolism, *RV* right ventricular, *RA* right atrium, *LV* left ventricle, *NSCLC* non-small cell lung cancer, *LVEF* left ventricular ejection fraction

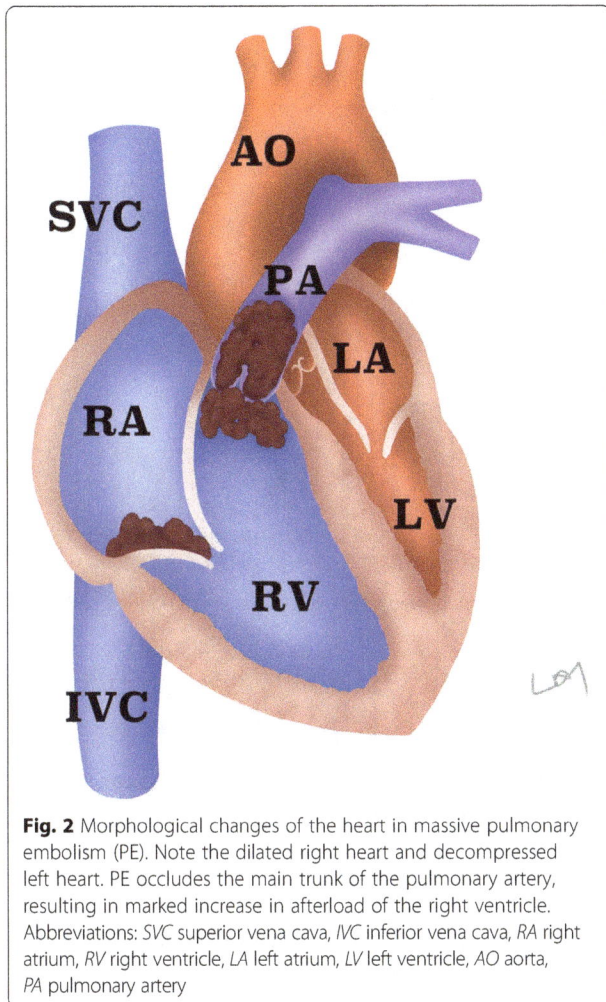

**Fig. 2** Morphological changes of the heart in massive pulmonary embolism (PE). Note the dilated right heart and decompressed left heart. PE occludes the main trunk of the pulmonary artery, resulting in marked increase in afterload of the right ventricle. Abbreviations: *SVC* superior vena cava, *IVC* inferior vena cava, *RA* right atrium, *RV* right ventricle, *LA* left atrium, *LV* left ventricle, *AO* aorta, *PA* pulmonary artery

to discharge than those who had conventional cardiopulmonary resuscitation greater than 45 min [32]. The reason may be that conventional cardiopulmonary resuscitation is associated with poor perfusion. There is evidence that even the best-performed chest compression during cardiopulmonary resuscitation provides inadequate cardiac output, ranging from 25 to 40% of the pre-arrest level [33, 34]. Furthermore, cardiopulmonary resuscitation with chest compression device was also associated with a period of "low-flow". Such low-flow period may dictate the initiation of extracorporeal cardiopulmonary resuscitation [35]. Otherwise, prolonged inadequate tissue perfusion will result in poor clinical outcome. Thus, extracorporeal cardiopulmonary resuscitation that is started too later after cardiac arrest will be futile. On the other hand, initiation of extracorporeal cardiopulmonary resuscitation cannot be too early because a substantial number of patients can have return of spontaneous circulation (ROSC) after a short time of conventional cardiopulmonary

resuscitation. These patients can have good clinical outcome, while avoiding catastrophic complications induced by extracorporeal membrane oxygenation.

Therefore, the key issue in transition from conventional cardiopulmonary resuscitation to extracorporeal membrane oxygenation is the identification of inadequate cardiac output. Unfortunately, there is no universal agreement on when to start extracorporeal membrane oxygenation from conventional cardiopulmonary resuscitation. The French guideline recommends initiation of extracorporeal cardiopulmonary resuscitation after 30-min conventional cardiopulmonary resuscitation without spontaneous circulation, and conventional cardiopulmonary resuscitation within 15 min are considered as the contraindication for extracorporeal cardiopulmonary resuscitation [36]. Kim and colleagues found that good neurological outcome appeared to decrease more sharply in the conventional cardiopulmonary resuscitation than in the extracorporeal cardiopulmonary resuscitation group with prolongation of conventional cardiopulmonary resuscitation duration [37]. The survival rate also showed a similar trend (Fig. 3). There are also other modalities to indicate when to transition to extracorporeal cardiopulmonary resuscitation. For example, end-tidal $CO_2 < 10$ mmHg after 20 min of CCPR is a good predictor of poor clinical outcome and thus may have potential role in deciding extracorporeal cardiopulmonary resuscitation initiation [38–40]. Other biomarkers include serum lactate, creatinine, phosphorous, pH value, and neuron-specific enolase [41–44]. Echocardiography may provide an alternative to monitor cardiac output during CCPR. Cardiac low-flow can be visualized using echocardiography [35]. Despite lack of evidence to support the use of echocardiography as a method to determine initiation of extracorporeal cardiopulmonary resuscitation, it is rational that if adequate cardiac output cannot be maintained with CCPR, extracorporeal cardiopulmonary resuscitation should be started as early as possible to avoid further neurological damage.

An interesting sign of echocardiography during cardiopulmonary resuscitation is the duration of cardiac standstill, which was defined as "the total duration of consecutive absence of cardiac motion when peri-resuscitation echocardiography was performed serially every 2 minutes" [45]. Kim et al.'s study found that patients with and without ROSC had significantly different standstill duration ($2.86 \pm 2.07$ min versus $20.30 \pm 8.42$ min, $p < 0.001$). Cardiac standstill >10 min was able to predict non-ROSC with 90% sensitivity and 100% specificity. Such a high diagnostic accuracy may help to triage patients into those who require extracorporeal cardiopulmonary resuscitation and those who do not. We propose that if cardiac standstill is persistent for one or two CPR cycle, ROSC is very unlikely within an expected time period and extracorporeal cardiopulmonary

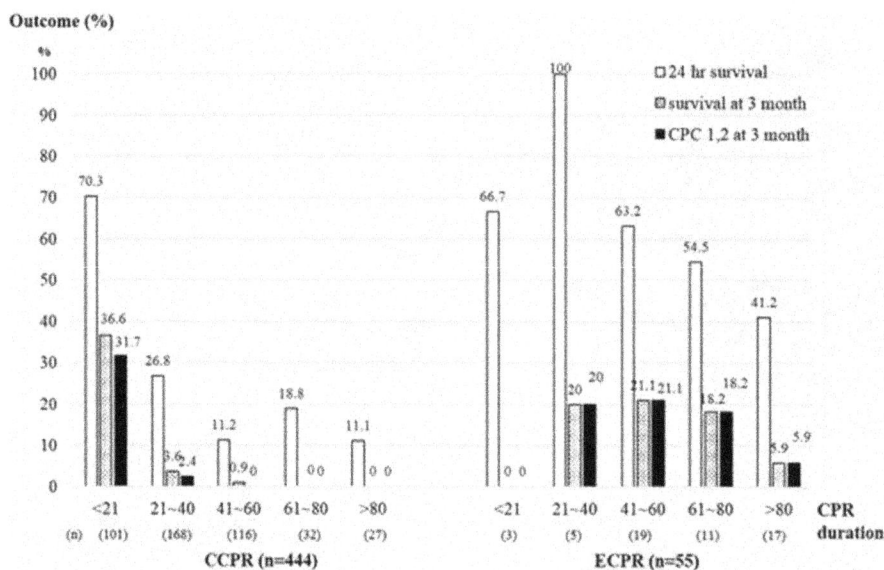

**Fig. 3** Twenty-four-hour survival, good neurological outcome, and survival rate at 3 months appeared to decrease more sharply in the CCPR than in the extracorporeal cardiopulmonary resuscitation group with prolongation of CPR duration [37].

resuscitation can be instituted, given that the underlying causes of the cardiac arrest is fully reversible.

The risk of performing echocardiography is the interruption of chest compression, and it is important not to intervene CPR. There have been extensive studies being conducted to explore the performance of echocardiography during CPR [46–48]. The subxiphoid window is the most commonly used because it will not intervene with the ongoing CPR (e.g., the placement of ultrasound probe is outside of the compression region). From this view, it is easy to observe ventricular wall motion, pericardial effusion, and tamponade [49].

## Ultrasonography for ECMO cannulation

Although the primary focus of the article is on echocardiography, here, we include ultrasonography for extracorporeal membrane oxygenation cannulation. For most instances, the cannulation can be performed without the help of ultrasound. However, ultrasound can help to reduce the rate of complications associated with cannulation such as hematoma, vascular injury, cardiac tamponade, and lower leg ischemia [50, 51]. In pediatric patients, the use of ultrasound was associated with significantly reduced rate of surgical repositioning of extracorporeal membrane oxygenation catheter [52].

Before cannulation, the diameter of the target vessels should be localized and measured with ultrasound. Some authors suggest that the diameter of the cannula should be less than two thirds of the diameter of the vessel [50]. Others suggest to choose a cannula that is at least 1–3F

sizes smaller than the vessel. The size of the cannula can be calculated as follows:

$$\text{Size}(F) = D\,(\text{mm}) \times 3$$

where $D$ is the diameter of the vessel. If the vessel is distorted by adjacent tissue, the size can be calculated by:

$$\text{Size}(F) = C\,(\text{mm})$$

where $C$ is the circumference of the distorted vessel. These two equations are very simple for clinical use [53]. The size of the cannula is particularly important for femoral artery because occlusion of it may cause lower extremity ischemia that requires amputation. The cannulation can be performed under real-time ultrasound guidance [54]. The tip position can also be identified by ultrasound, and there is evidence suggesting its superiority to chest radiography [55]. In VA-extracorporeal membrane oxygenation, the tip position of the cannula inserted in the femoral vein is important for reaching a target flow rate. Optimally, the cannula tip should be positioned at proximal inferior vena cava, above the hepatic vein [56] (Fig. 4). After successful cannulation, the heart should be scanned with ultrasound to exclude rare but catastrophic complication tamponade. Furthermore, the distal limb perfusion should be monitored with color-Doplar ultrasound. Percutaneous distal limb perfusion should be instituted in the presence of ischemic signs (Fig. 5) [54].

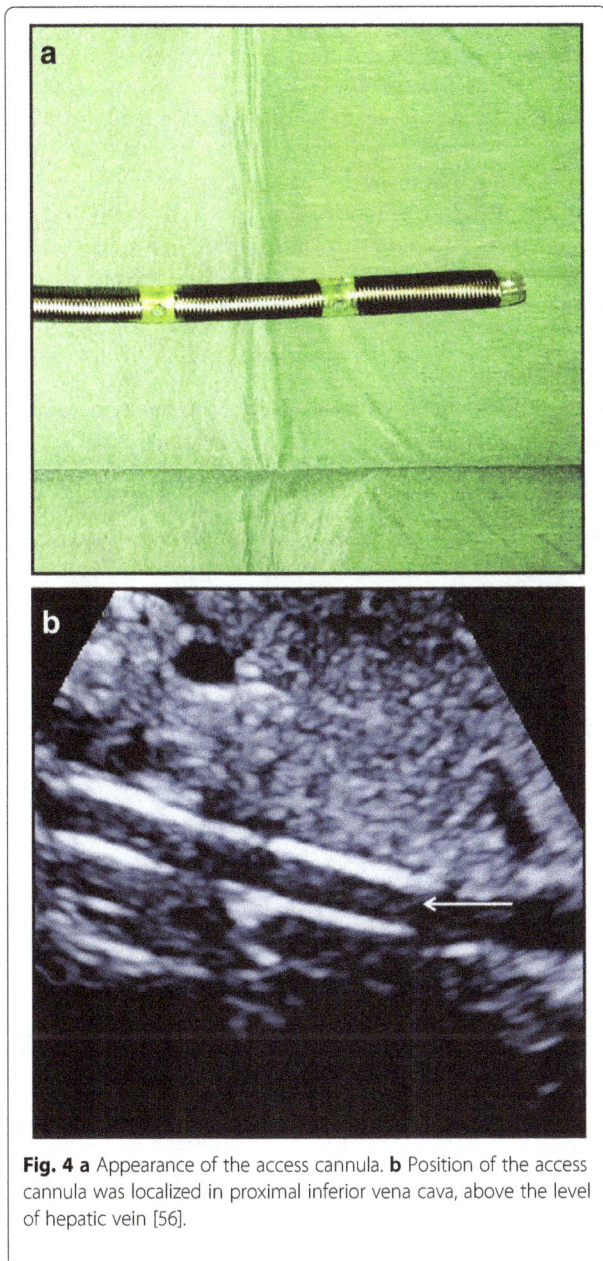

**Fig. 4 a** Appearance of the access cannula. **b** Position of the access cannula was localized in proximal inferior vena cava, above the level of hepatic vein [56].

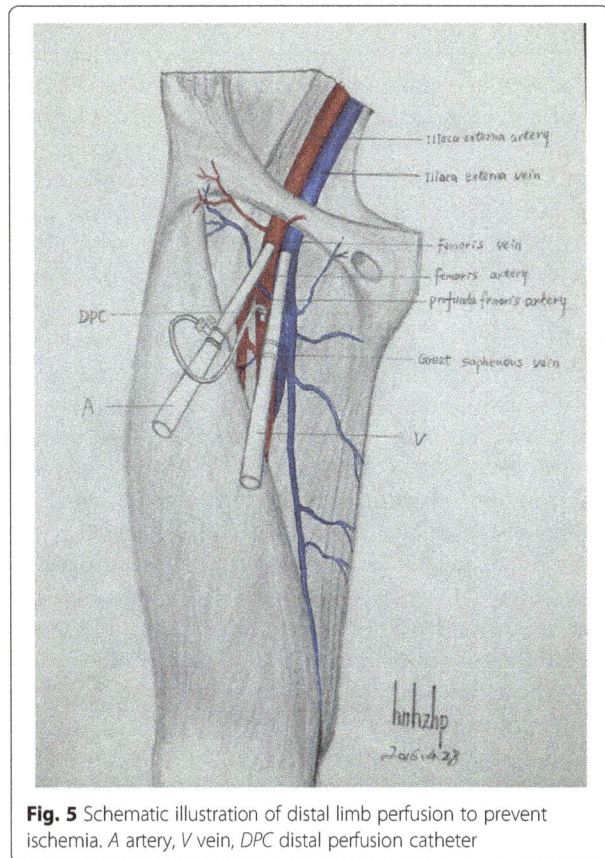

**Fig. 5** Schematic illustration of distal limb perfusion to prevent ischemia. *A* artery, *V* vein, *DPC* distal perfusion catheter

## Monitoring during ECMO performance

Cardiac function is one of the most important parameters that should be closely monitored during extracorporeal membrane oxygenation support after extracorporeal cardiopulmonary resuscitation. Echocardiography is a useful tool in this regard. Systolic function is assessed with conventional parameters such as the size of the left ventricle (LV), ejection fraction (EF), mitral regurgitation dP/dt, aortic velocity-time integral (VTI). The extracorporeal membrane oxygenation blood flow rate can be adjusted according to the global assessment of LV systolic function and cardiac preload. Aissaoui and colleagues have systematically investigated the effect of extracorporeal membrane oxygenation flow rate on changes in cardiac parameters [57]. A drop in the extracorporeal membrane oxygenation flow rate from 4 to 0.7 L/min leads to a 22% increase in E/Ea ratio (5.9 to 7.2; $p < 0.001$), 17% increase in EF (15 to 17.5%; $p < 0.001$), 12 and 45% increase in VTI (8 to 11.6 cm; $p < 0.001$), and 12% increase in left ventricular end-diastolic volume (95 to 108 mL; $p < 0.001$).

Another major issue in using echocardiography is to detect complications during extracorporeal membrane oxygenation running. As described previously, cardiac tamponade can happen when a passage of guide wire or cannula through myocardium. This complication is described in this section because anticoagulation during extracorporeal membrane oxygenation support may worsen pericardial effusion, and tamponade occurs hours or days after cannulation. Therefore, it requires continuous monitoring with echocardiography. What is worse is that conventional signs and symptoms of cardiac tamponade may be of limited use during extracorporeal membrane oxygenation running [58]. Fortunately, these complications can be readily detected using echocardiography [59].

Thrombosis is a major complication during extracorporeal membrane oxygenation support and can be catastrophic when embolism occurs in the brain. Many factors predispose the patient at increased risk of blood clotting. The passage of blood through extracorporeal circuit activates clotting cascade, which is compounded by obstruction of intravascular blood flow by the cannula. While evident thrombus is detectable with ultrasound, blood stasis is somewhat challenging to identify. The "spontaneous echo contrast" within cardiac chamber is a sign of blood stasis, which is considered as a harbinger of ensuing thrombosis [60–63]. Closed aortic valve and absence of pulsatile blood flow, which can be easily visualized with echocardiography, are also predictors of thrombosis [64–66]. On seeing this sign, some mechanical or pharmacological efforts could be make to promote forward blood flow. For example, reducing vascular resistance and extracorporeal membrane oxygenation flow rate may allow aortic valve opening and increase forward blood flow. Others recommend the use of intra-aortic balloon pump to facilitate blood flow [67–69]. Alternatively, the anticoagulation strategy can be strengthened.

Aortic and mitral regurgitation is a sign of increased in afterload produced by extracorporeal membrane oxygenation support. Theoretically, the increases in afterload may impair LV distention, ensuing subendocardial ischemia. These are risk factors for delayed recovery of cardiac function [70–72]. However, their clinical utility has been well established in extracorporeal membrane oxygenation setting, and further studies are warranted to clarify their association.

## Weaning from ECMO

The ultimate goal of extracorporeal membrane oxygenation management is to wean from it. Therefore, the prediction of successful weaning has long been an area of active research. Echocardiographic parameters have been shown to be good predictors of extracorporeal membrane oxygenation weaning [73]. If a patient is deemed suitable for weaning, extracorporeal membrane oxygenation weaning trial can be performed by reducing extracorporeal membrane oxygenation flow to less than 1.5 L/min. Parameters and threshold for successful weaning include aortic VTI ≥ 10 cm, LVEF > 20–25%, and lateral mitral annulus peak systolic velocity >6 cm/s [56, 74, 75]. By applying a standardized weaning protocol [76], Cavarocchi and coworkers developed an extracorporeal membrane oxygenation weaning protocol guided by echocardiography. The ability of ultrasound to detect left and right ventricular dysfunction was good, with a sensitivity of 100% (95% CI, 73.2–100%), specificity of 100% (95% CI, 56.1–100%), and positive predictive value of 100% (95% CI, 73–100%) [76]. In pediatric

patients undergoing VA-extracorporeal membrane oxygenation for cardiac support, a significant increase (0.0250 ± 0.269 m; $p = 0.03$) in VTI when extracorporeal membrane oxygenation flow rate was dropped from full support to minimal flow rate was an important predictor of those not requiring a heart transplant [77]. On the contrary, children without significant increase (0.0111 ± 0.283 m) in VTI during weaning trial were subjects that cannot be successfully weaned from extracorporeal membrane oxygenation.

## Conclusions

Echocardiography is an invaluable tool in the management of patients undergoing extracorporeal cardiopulmonary resuscitation and subsequent extracorporeal membrane oxygenation support and weaning. At the very beginning, echocardiography can identify the etiology of cardiac arrest, such as massive PE and cardiac tamponade. Eliminating these culprits saves life and may avoid the initiation of extracorporeal membrane oxygenation. If the underlying causes are not identified or intrinsic to the heart (e.g., such as those caused by cardiomyopathy, myocarditis), CCPR will continue to maintain cardiac output. The quality of CCPR can be monitored and if cardiac output cannot be maintained, early institution of extracorporeal cardiopulmonary resuscitation may be reasonable. Cannulation is sometimes challenging for extracorporeal cardiopulmonary resuscitation patients. Fortunately, with the help of ultrasonography procedures including localization of vessels, selecting a cannula of appropriate size, confirmation of catheter tip may become easy under sophisticated hand. Monitoring of cardiac function and complications during extracorporeal membrane oxygenation support can be done with echocardiography. However, the cardiac parameters should be interpreted with understanding of hemodynamic configuration of extracorporeal membrane oxygenation. Thrombus and blood stasis can be identified with ultrasound, which may prompt mechanical and pharmacological interventions. The final step is extracorporeal membrane oxygenation weaning. Some studies have investigated the accuracy of some echocardiographic parameters in predicting success rate. Although they showed promising results, the effectiveness of echocardiography on CPR survival cannot be determined. Further randomized controlled trials comparing the effects of echocardiography-guided CPR versus conventional CPR may be warranted.

**Acknowledgements**
We would like to thank Ms. Liu Xiaoyang and Dr. Zhiping Huang for providing medical illustrations.

**Funding**
There is no funding for this manuscript.

## Competing interests

The author declares that he has no competing interests.

## References

1. Gräsner J-T, Bossaert L. Epidemiology and management of cardiac arrest: what registries are revealing. Best Pract Res Clin Anaesthesiol. Elsevier; 2013;27:293–306

2. Nürnberger A, Sterz F, Malzer R, Warenits A, Girsa M, Stöckl M, et al. Out of hospital cardiac arrest in Vienna: incidence and outcome. Resuscitation. Elsevier; 2013;84:42–7

3. Rossano JW, Naim MY, Nadkarni VM, Berg RA. Epidemiology of pediatric cardiac arrest. pediatric and congenital cardiology, cardiac surgery and intensive care. London: Springer London; 2013. p. 1275–87.

4. De Maio VJ, Osmond MH, Stiell IG, Nadkarni V, Berg R, Cabanas JG. Epidemiology of out-of-hospital pediatric cardiac arrest due to trauma. Prehosp Emerg Care. 2011;16:230–6.

5. Travers AH, Perkins GD, Berg RA, Castren M, Considine J, Escalante R, et al. Part 3: adult basic life support and automated external defibrillation: 2015 International Consensus on Cardiopulmonary Resuscitation and Emergency Cardiovascular Care Science With Treatment Recommendations. Circulation. 2015;132(16 Suppl 1):S51–83.

6. Peberdy MA, Kaye W, Ornato JP, Larkin GL, Nadkarni V, Mancini ME, et al. Cardiopulmonary resuscitation of adults in the hospital: a report of 14720 cardiac arrests from the National Registry of Cardiopulmonary Resuscitation. Resuscitation. 2003;58:297–308.

7. Chai PJ, Jacobs JP, Dalton HJ, Costello JM, Cooper DS, Kirsch R, et al. Extracorporeal cardiopulmonary resuscitation for post-operative cardiac arrest: indications, techniques, controversies, and early results—what is known (and unknown). Cardiol Young. 2011;21 Suppl 2:109–17.

8. Kim SJ, Kim HJ, Lee HY, Ahn HS, Lee SW. Comparing extracorporeal cardiopulmonary resuscitation with conventional cardiopulmonary resuscitation: a meta-analysis. Resuscitation. 2016;103:106–16.

9. Lasa JJ, Rogers RS, Localio R, Shults J, Raymond T, Gaies M, et al. Extracorporeal cardiopulmonary resuscitation (E-CPR) during pediatric in-hospital cardiopulmonary arrest is associated with improved survival to discharge: a report from the American Heart Association's Get With The Guidelines-Resuscitation (GWTG-R) Registry. Circulation. Lippincott Williams & Wilkins; 2016;133:165–76.

10. Lee S-H, Jung J-S, Lee K-H, Kim H-J, Son H-S, Sun K. Comparison of extracorporeal cardiopulmonary resuscitation with conventional cardiopulmonary resuscitation: is extracorporeal cardiopulmonary resuscitation beneficial? Korean J Thorac Cardiovasc Surg. The Korean Society for Thoracic and Cardiovascular Surgery; 2015;48:318–27

11. Karagiannidis C, Brodie D, Strassmann S, Stoelben E, Philipp A, Bein T, et al. Extracorporeal membrane oxygenation: evolving epidemiology and mortality. Intensive Care Med. 2016;42:889–96.

12. Douflé G, Roscoe A, Billia F, Fan E. Echocardiography for adult patients supported with extracorporeal membrane oxygenation. Crit Care. BioMed Central; 2015;19:326

13. Gaspar HA, Morhy SS, Lianza AC, de Carvalho WB, Andrade JL, do Prado RR, et al. Focused cardiac ultrasound: a training course for pediatric intensivists and emergency physicians. BMC Med Ed. BioMed Central; 2014;14:25

14. Kucher N, Rossi E, De Rosa M, Goldhaber SZ. Massive pulmonary embolism. Circulation. Lippincott Williams & Wilkins; 2006;113:577–82

15. Goldhaber SZ, Visani L, De Rosa M. Acute pulmonary embolism: clinical outcomes in the International Cooperative Pulmonary Embolism Registry (ICOPER). Lancet. 1999;353:1386–9.

16. Yang Y, Liang L, Zhai Z, He H, Xie W, Peng X, et al. Pulmonary embolism incidence and fatality trends in Chinese hospitals from 1997 to 2008: a multicenter registration study. Cowling BJ, editor. PLoS ONE. Public Library of Science; 2011;6:e26861

17. Labovitz AJ, Noble VE, Bierig M, Goldstein SA, Jones R, Kort S, et al. Focused cardiac ultrasound in the emergent setting: a consensus statement of the American Society of Echocardiography and American College of Emergency Physicians. J Am Soc Echocardiogr. 2010. pp. 1225–30.

18. Squizzato A, Galli L, Gerdes VEA. Point-of-care ultrasound in the diagnosis of pulmonary embolism. Crit Ultrasound J. Springer Milan; 2015;7:7

19. Liang Y-H, Kuo S-W, Lin Y-L, Chang Y-L. Disseminated microvascular pulmonary tumor embolism from non-small cell lung cancer leading to pulmonary hypertension followed by sudden cardiac arrest. Lung Cancer. Elsevier; 2011;72:132 5

20. Jeong WJ, Lee JW, Yoo YH, Ryu S, Cho SW, Song KH, et al. Extracorporeal cardiopulmonary resuscitation in bedside echocardiography-diagnosed massive pulmonary embolism. Am J Emerg Med. 2015;33:1545. e1–2.

21. Chowdhury MA, Moza A, Siddiqui NS, Bonnell M, Cooper CJ. Emergent echocardiography and extracorporeal membrane oxygenation: lifesaving in massive pulmonary embolism. Heart Lung. Elsevier; 2015;44:344–6

22. Swol J, Buchwald D, Strauch J, Schildhauer TA. Extracorporeal life support (ECLS) for cardiopulmonary resuscitation (CPR) with pulmonary embolism in surgical patients—a case series. Perfusion. SAGE Publications; 2016;31:54–9

23. Northey LC, Shiraev T, Omari A. Salvage intraosseous thrombolysis and extracorporeal membrane oxygenation for massive pulmonary embolism. J Emerg Trauma Shock. Medknow Publications; 2015;8:55–7

24. Lu C-W, Chen Y-S, Wang M-J. Massive pulmonary embolism after application of an Esmarch bandage. Anesth Analg. 2004;98:1187–9. tableofcontents.

25. Tsai SK, Wang MJ, Ko WJ, Wang SJ. Emergent bedside transesophageal echocardiography in the resuscitation of sudden cardiac arrest after tricuspid inflow obstruction and pulmonary embolism. Anesth Analg. 1999;89:1406–8.

26. Ilsaas C, Husby P, Koller ME, Segadal L, Holst-Larsen H. Cardiac arrest due to massive pulmonary embolism following caesarean section. Successful resuscitation and pulmonary embolectomy. Acta Anaesthesiol Scand. 1998;42:264–6.

27. Ramarapu S. Complete neurological recovery after transesophageal echocardiography-guided diagnosis and management of prolonged cardiopulmonary resuscitation. A A Case Rep. 2015;5:192–4.

28. Mosca M, Weinberg A. The need to develop standardized protocols for the timing of extracorporeal membrane oxygenation initiation among adult patients in cardiac arrest: a case study. J Extra Corpor Technol. American Society of Extra-Corporeal Technology; 2014;46:305–9.

29. Krittayaphong R, Saengsung P, Chawaruechai T, Yindeengam A, Udompunturak S. Factors predicting outcome of cardiopulmonary resuscitation in a developing country: the Siriraj cardiopulmonary resuscitation registry. J Med Assoc Thai. 2009;92:618–23.

30. Nadkarni VM, Larkin GL, Peberdy MA, Carey SM, Kaye W, Mancini ME, et al. First documented rhythm and clinical outcome from in-hospital cardiac arrest among children and adults. JAMA. American Medical Association; 2006;295:50–7

31. Schultz SC, Cullinane DC, Pasquale MD, Magnant C, Evans SR. Predicting in-hospital mortality during cardiopulmonary resuscitation. Resuscitation. 1996;33:13–7.

32. Chen Y-S, Chao A, Yu H-Y, Ko W-J, Wu I-H, Chen RJ-C, et al. Analysis and results of prolonged resuscitation in cardiac arrest patients rescued by extracorporeal membrane oxygenation. J Am Coll Cardiol. 2003;41:197–203.

33. Andreka P, Frenneaux MP. Haemodynamics of cardiac arrest and resuscitation. Curr Opin Crit Care. 2006;12:198–203.

34. Rubertsson S, Grenvik A, Wiklund L. Blood flow and perfusion pressure during open-chest versus closed-chest cardiopulmonary resuscitation in pigs. Crit Care Med. 1995;23:715–25.

35. Giraud R, Siegenthaler N, Schussler O, Kalangos A, Müller H, Bendjelid K, et al. The LUCAS 2 chest compression device is not always efficient: an echographic confirmation. Ann Emerg Med Elsevier; 2015;65:23–6.

36. Conseil français de réanimation cardiopulmonaire, Société française d'anesthésie et de réanimation, Société française de cardiologie, Société française de chirurgie thoracique et cardiovasculaire, Société française de médecine d'urgence, Société française de pédiatrie, et al. Guidelines for indications for the use of extracorporeal life support in refractory cardiac arrest. French Ministry of Health. Ann Fr Anesth Reanim. 2009. pp. 182–90.

37. Kim SJ, Jung J-S, Park JH, Park JS, Hong YS, Lee SW. An optimal transition time to extracorporeal cardiopulmonary resuscitation for predicting good neurological outcome in patients with out-of-hospital cardiac arrest: a propensity-matched study. Crit Care. 2014;18:535.

38. Levine RL, Wayne MA, Miller CC. End-tidal carbon dioxide and outcome of out-of-hospital cardiac arrest. N. Engl. J. Med. Massachusetts Medical Society; 1997;337:301–6

39. Pantazopoulos C, Xanthos T, Pantazopoulos I, Papalois A, Kouskouni E, Iacovidou N. A review of carbon dioxide monitoring during adult cardiopulmonary resuscitation. Heart Lung Circ. Elsevier; 2015;24:1053–61

40. Eckstein M, Hatch L, Malleck J, McClung C, Henderson SO. End-tidal CO2 as a predictor of survival in out-of-hospital cardiac arrest. Prehosp Disaster Med. 2011;26:148–50.

41. Kelly RB, Harrison RE. Outcome predictors of pediatric extracorporeal cardiopulmonary resuscitation. Pediatr Cardiol. 2010;31:626–33.

42. Huang S-C, Wu E-T, Chen Y-S, Chang C-I, Chiu I-S, Wang S-S, et al. Extracorporeal membrane oxygenation rescue for cardiopulmonary resuscitation in pediatric patients. Crit Care Med. 2008;36:1607–13.

43. Kane DA, Thiagarajan RR, Wypij D, Scheurer MA, Fynn-Thompson F, Emani S, et al. Rapid-response extracorporeal membrane oxygenation to support cardiopulmonary resuscitation in children with cardiac disease. Circulation. Lippincott Williams & Wilkins; 2010;122:S241–8.

44. Böttiger BW, Möbes S, Glätzer R, Bauer H, Gries A, Bärtsch P, et al. Astroglial protein S-100 is an early and sensitive marker of hypoxic brain damage and outcome after cardiac arrest in humans. Circulation. 2001;103:2694–8.

45. Kim HB, Suh JY, Choi JH, Cho YS. Can serial focussed echocardiographic evaluation in life support (FEEL) predict resuscitation outcome or termination of resuscitation (TOR)? A pilot study. Resuscitation. Elsevier; 2016;101:21–6

46. Aichinger G, Zechner PM, Prause G, Sacherer F, Wildner G, Anderson CL, et al. Cardiac movement identified on prehospital echocardiography predicts outcome in cardiac arrest patients. Prehosp Emerg Care. 2012;16:251–5.

47. Chardoli M, Heidari F, Rabiee H, Sharif-Alhoseini M, Shokoohi H, Rahimi-Movaghar V. Echocardiography integrated ACLS protocol versus conventional cardiopulmonary resuscitation in patients with pulseless electrical activity cardiac arrest. Chin J Traumatol. 2012;15:284–7.

48. Wu J-P, Gu D-Y, Wang S, Zhang Z-J, Zhou J-C, Zhang R-F. Good neurological recovery after rescue thrombolysis of presumed pulmonary embolism despite prior 100 minutes CPR. J Thorac Dis. 2014;6:E289–93.

49. Ozen C, Salcin E, Akoglu H, Onur O, Denizbasi A. Assessment of ventricular wall motion with focused echocardiography during cardiac arrest to predict survival. Turk J Emerg Med. 2016;16:12–6.

50. Burns J, Cooper E, Salt G, Gillon S, Camporota L, Daly K, et al. A retrospective observational review of percutaneous cannulation for extracorporeal membrane oxygenation. ASAIO J. 2016;62(3):325–8.

51. Chung JH, Jung J-S, Son H-S, Lee SH. Transient limb ischaemia during extracorporeal membrane oxygenation: inappropriate venous cannula location. Interact Cardiovasc Thorac Surg. Oxford University Press; 2015;21:694–5

52. Kuenzler KA, Arthur LG, Burchard AE, Lawless ST, Wolfson PJ, Murphy SG. Intraoperative ultrasound reduces ECMO catheter malposition requiring surgical correction. J Pediatr Surg. 2002;37:691–4.

53. Conrad SA, Grier LR, Scott LK, Green R, Jordan M. Percutaneous cannulation for extracorporeal membrane oxygenation by intensivists: a retrospective single-institution case series. Crit Care Med. 2015;43:1010–5.

54. Benassi F, Vezzani A, Vignali L, Gherli T. Ultrasound guided femoral cannulation and percutaneous perfusion of the distal limb for VA ECMO. J Card Surg. 2014;29:427–9.

55. Thomas TH, Price R, Ramaciotti C, Thompson M, Megison S, Lemler MS. Echocardiography, not chest radiography, for evaluation of cannula placement during pediatric extracorporeal membrane oxygenation. Pediatr Crit Care Med. 2009;10:56–9.

56. Victor K, Barrett NA, Gillon S, Gowland A, Meadows CIS, Ioannou N. Critical care echo rounds: extracorporeal membrane oxygenation. Echo Res Pract. BioScientifica; 2015;2:D1–D11

57. Aissaoui N, Guerot E, Combes A, Delouche A, Chastre J, Leprince P, et al. Two-dimensional strain rate and Doppler tissue myocardial velocities: analysis by echocardiography of hemodynamic and functional changes of the failed left ventricle during different degrees of extracorporeal life support. J Am Soc Echocardiogr. 2012;25:632–40.

58. Yates AR, Duffy VL, Clark TD, Hayes D, Tobias JD, McConnell PI, et al. Cardiac tamponade: new technology masking an old nemesis. Ann. Thorac. Surg. Elsevier; 2014;97:1046–8

59. Hirose H, Yamane K, Marhefka G, Cavarocchi N. Right ventricular rupture and tamponade caused by malposition of the Avalon cannula for venovenous extracorporeal membrane oxygenation. J Cardiothorac Surg. BioMed Central; 2012;7:36.

60. Black IW, Hopkins AP, Lee LC, Walsh WF. Left atrial spontaneous echo contrast: a clinical and echocardiographic analysis. J Am Coll Cardiol. 1991;18:398–404.

61. Vincelj J, Sokol I, Jaksić O. Prevalence and clinical significance of left atrial spontaneous echo contrast detected by transesophageal echocardiography. Echocardiography. 2002;19:319–24.

62. Rittoo D, Sutherland GR, Currie P, Starkey IR, Shaw TR. A prospective study of left atrial spontaneous echo contrast and thrombus in 100 consecutive patients referred for balloon dilation of the mitral valve. J Am Soc Echocardiogr. 1994;7:516–27.

63. Ohtaka K, Takahashi Y, Uemura S, Shoji Y, Hayama S, Ichimura T, et al. Blood stasis may cause thrombosis in the left superior pulmonary vein stump after left upper lobectomy. J Cardiothorac Surg. BioMed Central; 2014;9:159.

64. Moubarak G, Weiss N, Leprince P, Luyt C-E. Massive intraventricular thrombus complicating extracorporeal membrane oxygenation support. Can J Cardiol. Pulsus Group; 2008;24:e1.

65. Madershahian N, Weber C, Scherner M, Langebartels G, Slottosch I, Wahlers T. Thrombosis of the aortic root and ascending aorta during extracorporeal membrane oxygenation. Intensive Care Med. Springer Berlin Heidelberg; 2014;40:432–3

66. Ramjee V, Shreenivas S, Rame JE, Kirkpatrick JN, Jagasia D. Complete spontaneous left heart and aortic thromboses on extracorporeal membrane oxygenation support. Echocardiography. 2013;30:E342–3.

67. Petroni T, Harrois A, Amour J, Lebreton G, Brechot N, Tanaka S, et al. Intra-aortic balloon pump effects on macrocirculation and microcirculation in cardiogenic shock patients supported by venoarterial extracorporeal membrane oxygenation*. Crit Care Med. 2014;42:2075–82.

68. Vlasselaers D, Desmet M, Desmet L, Meyns B, Dens J. Ventricular unloading with a miniature axial flow pump in combination with extracorporeal membrane oxygenation. Intensive Care Med. Springer-Verlag; 2006;32:329–33

69. Hu W, Liu C, Chen L, Hu W, Lu J, Zhu Y, et al. Combined intraaortic balloon counterpulsation and extracorporeal membrane oxygenation in 2 patients with fulminant myocarditis. Am J Emerg Med. Elsevier; 2015;33:736.e1–4.

70. Tverskaya MS, Sukhoparova VV, Karpova VV, Raksha AP, Kadyrova MK, Abdulkerimova NZ, et al. Pathomorphology of myocardial circulation: comparative study in increased left or right ventricle afterload. Bull Exp Biol Med. 2008;145:377–81.

71. Becker M, Kramann R, Dohmen G, Lückhoff A, Autschbach R, Kelm M, et al. Impact of left ventricular loading conditions on myocardial deformation parameters: analysis of early and late changes of myocardial deformation parameters after aortic valve replacement. J Am Soc Echocardiogr. Elsevier; 2007;20:681–9

72. Lucas SK, Schaff HV, Flaherty JT, Gott VL, Gardner TJ. The harmful effects of ventricular distention during postischemic reperfusion. Ann Thorac Surg. 1981;32:486–94.

73. Platts DG, Sedgwick JF, Burstow DJ, Mullany DV, Fraser JF. The role of echocardiography in the management of patients supported by extracorporeal membrane oxygenation. J Am Soc Echocardiogr. Elsevier; 2012;25:131–41

74. Aissaoui N, Luyt C-E, Leprince P, Trouillet J-L, Léger P, Pavie A, et al. Predictors of successful extracorporeal membrane oxygenation (ECMO) weaning after assistance for refractory cardiogenic shock. Intensive Care Med. Springer-Verlag; 2011;37:1738–45

75. Aissaoui N, El-Banayosy A, Combes A. How to wean a patient from veno-arterial extracorporeal membrane oxygenation. Intensive Care Med. 2015;41:902–5.

76. Cavarocchi NC, Pitcher HT, Yang Q, Karbowski P, Miessau J, Hastings HM, et al. Weaning of extracorporeal membrane oxygenation using continuous hemodynamic transesophageal echocardiography. J. Thorac. Cardiovasc. Surg. Elsevier; 2013;146:1474–9

77. Punn R, Axelrod DM, Sherman-Levine S, Roth SJ, Tacy TA. Predictors of mortality in pediatric patients on venoarterial extracorporeal membrane oxygenation. Pediatr Crit Care Med. 2014;15:870–7.

# 11

# Nicotine replacement therapy for agitation and delirium management in the intensive care unit

Melanie Kowalski[1,2,5*] , Andrew A. Udy[2,5], Hayden J. McRobbie[3,4] and Michael J. Dooley[1,5]

## Abstract

**Background:** Active smokers are prevalent within the intensive care setting and place a significant burden on healthcare systems. Nicotine withdrawal due to forced abstinence on admission may contribute to increased agitation and delirium in this patient group. The aim of this systematic review was to determine whether management of nicotine withdrawal, with nicotine replacement therapy (NRT), reduces agitation and delirium in critically ill patients admitted to the intensive care unit (ICU).

**Methods:** The following sources were used in this review: MEDLINE, EMBASE, and CINAHL Plus databases. Included studies reported delirium or agitation outcomes in current smokers, where NRT was used as management of nicotine withdrawal, in the intensive care setting. Studies were included regardless of design or number of participants. Data were extracted on ICU classification; study design; population baseline characteristics; allocation and dose of NRT; agitation and delirium assessment methods; and the frequency of agitation, delirium, and psychotropic medication use.

**Results:** Six studies were included. NRT was mostly prescribed for smokers with heavier smoking histories. Three studies reported an association between increased agitation or delirium and NRT use; one study could not find any significant benefit or harm from NRT use; and two described a reduction of symptomatic nicotine withdrawal. A lack of consistent and validated assessment measures, combined with limitations in the quality of reported data, contribute to conflicting results.

**Conclusions:** Current evidence for the use of NRT in agitation and delirium management in the ICU is inconclusive. An evaluation of risk versus benefit on an individual patient basis should be considered when prescribing NRT. Further studies that consider prognostic balance, adjust for confounders, and employ validated assessment tools are urgently needed.

**Keywords:** Nicotine replacement therapy, Nicotine withdrawal, Intensive care unit, Critical care, Delirium, Agitation

* Correspondence: m.kowalski@alfred.org.au
[1]Pharmacy Department, Alfred Health, 55 Commercial Road, Melbourne, VIC 3004, Australia
[2]Intensive Care Unit, Alfred Health, Melbourne, Australia
Full list of author information is available at the end of the article

## Background

Active tobacco smokers are highly represented among critically ill patients, placing a significant additional burden on healthcare systems. Smoking has been demonstrated to have dose-related adverse effects on length of stay and hospital mortality in the critically ill [1]. Moreover, clinical care can often be more complicated due the development of nicotine withdrawal. Symptoms of tobacco withdrawal include irritability, frustration, anger, anxiety, depressed mood, insomnia, and restlessness. Symptoms peak within the first week of smoking cessation and last around 2–4 weeks [2]. It has been proposed that tobacco withdrawal contributes to an increased risk of agitation and delirium in patients admitted to ICU [3, 4], the development of which has been independently associated with inferior clinical outcomes [4].

Delirium is an acute state of confusion. Diagnostic criteria comprise a relatively short onset disturbance in attention and awareness, associated with a fluctuating change in cognition [5]. ICU delirium is common, occurring in 11–80% of critically ill patients [6]. Agitation may exist on its own or in combination with delirium, with a reported frequency of 64% in smokers admitted to the ICU [3]. Development of delirium and/or agitation during admission are linked to adverse events, including a 10% increase in mortality for each additional day spent delirious [7]. Other negative associations include a greater length of time spent mechanically ventilated and in the ICU, increased nosocomial infection, and increased use of psychotropics [8, 9].

Symptoms of tobacco withdrawal have been effectively managed in ward-based and outpatient settings with the use of nicotine replacement therapy (NRT) [10]. NRT primarily acts to reduce the severity of the urge to smoke and other withdrawal symptoms. It is unclear how critically ill patients are affected by these symptoms; hence, there is uncertainty about the benefits of using NRT [11]. A recent systematic review concluded that NRT should only be considered in selected ICU patients, due to a lack of evidence regarding efficacy and safety; however, the primary endpoint of interest was mortality [12]. Rather, the aim of this systematic review was to determine whether management of nicotine withdrawal with NRT reduces agitation and delirium.

## Methods

### Search strategy

A systematic review was conducted of MEDLINE (1946 to July 2016), EMBASE (1974 to July 2016), and CINAHL Plus (1937 to July 2016) using the following terms: nicotine replacement therapy, tobacco use cessation products, smoking cessation, intensive care unit, critical care, nicotine withdrawal, delirium, and agitation. Keywords were combined using Boolean logic. The search was limited to adult human studies written in English. References of retrieved articles were also scanned to identify further studies.

### Study selection

Inclusion criteria required a study population of current smokers admitted to the ICU where NRT was used as part of management for nicotine withdrawal. Agitation and delirium was assessed by either quantitative or qualitative measures. Duplicate publications and review articles were excluded. The title or abstract of identified references were examined, and if deemed relevant, full text articles were retrieved and reviewed. A summary of the study selection strategy is illustrated in Fig. 1.

### Data extraction

A full text review was performed to establish if inclusion criteria were met. Data were extracted in a standardised manner. Information included ICU classification, study population baseline characteristics, baseline smoking status, allocation and dose of NRT used, agitation and delirium assessment methods, and frequency of agitation, delirium, and psychotropic medication use.

## Results

The initial search strategy identified 115 citations. A manual search of retrieved references identified one additional study. Duplicates were removed and 77 citations were excluded upon title and abstract review. Full text review was undertaken of the remaining 17 studies to determine eligibility. Eleven studies were excluded (see Fig. 1), leaving six studies eligible for systematic review [13–18]. Study design was of variable quality ranging from a case report [14] to a pilot randomised control trial (RCT) [17]. Study participants were all current smokers admitted either to a medical, surgical, or neurological ICU. Intervention groups, where present, were all prescribed a form of NRT, while studies with control groups received either placebo or no intervention. Mean patient age ranged from 41 to 57.4 years. Details of the included studies are summarised in Table 1.

### Assessment of current smoking status

Determination of baseline smoking status varied greatly (see Table 1), with two studies simply reporting all patients as "heavy" smokers [13, 14]. Pack year history could be derived from three studies [15–17]. Two of these studies also reported an average quantity of cigarettes smoked per day [16, 17], while the third study classified patients by those who smoked >10 cigarettes per day or not [15]. One study did not quantify smoking history [18]. The source of smoking history was either self or surrogate reported in three of the six studies [15–17], with one cohort study [16] also utilising a

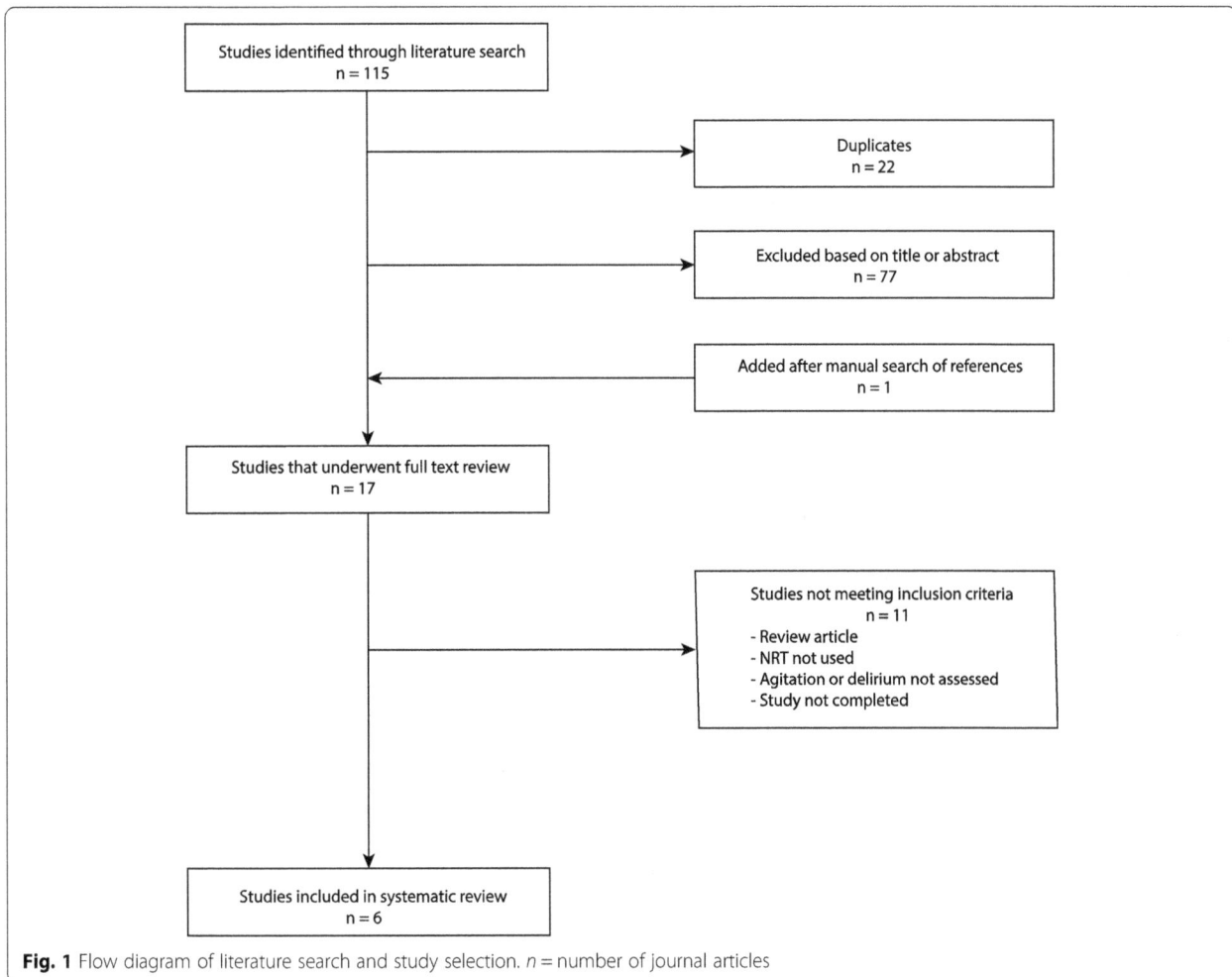

**Fig. 1** Flow diagram of literature search and study selection. *n* = number of journal articles

nurse-initiated tobacco assessment protocol. Another study [18] searched for smoking-related documentation via patient electronic medical records. Smoking history sources were not explicitly stated in the case report [14]; a family member reported smoking history for one of the case series [13].

### Allocation of nicotine replacement therapy
The allocation of NRT also varied between studies (Table 1). One study [17] randomised subjects, in a double-blinded manner, to receive either a 21-mg nicotine or placebo patch within 48 h of ICU admission. Another study [16] used a nurse-driven protocol to determine NRT prescribing, with patch doses adjusted for cigarette consumption. Two studies [15, 18] prescribed patients NRT at the clinicians' discretion. A patch strength of 21 mg was prescribed for all patients in one of these studies [15], while patch strength ranged from 10 to 30 mg/day in the other [18]. Two studies [13, 14] allocated nicotine patches to patients as treatment in response to suspected nicotine withdrawal.

Time to therapy initiation was mostly within 48 h of admission to ICU, although one study [15] included smokers with NRT commenced within 2 weeks of admission but did not specify median time to therapy. In the case series, NRT was commenced within 3–11 days, in response to symptoms of presumed nicotine withdrawal.

### Assessment of agitation or delirium
Agitation and delirium assessment methods ranged from validated tools to subjective description and surrogate markers (see Table 2). One study [16] used the Richmond Agitation-Sedation Scale (RASS) and Confusion Assessment Method for ICU (CAM-ICU) to assess agitation and delirium, respectively, both of which are validated tools with high sensitivity and specificity [19, 20]. The worst daily score for each tool was used to report median RASS score and number of days spent with delirium for each patient throughout the ICU admission. Use of physical restraints was also reported.

**Table 1** Study design and baseline characteristics

| First author, year (ref no.) | ICU type | Design, sample size | Mean age (years) | Gender Male % | APACHE II[a] | Mechanical ventilation % | Excessive alcohol intake | Smoking history | Source of smoking history |
|---|---|---|---|---|---|---|---|---|---|
| Mayer, 2001 [13] | Neurological ICU | Case series n = 5 | 52.6 | 60 | – | – | – | "Heavy" tobacco use | Surrogate n = 1 Not stated n = 4 |
| Honisett, 2001 [14] | Surgical ICU | Case report n = 1 | 41 | 100 | – | 100 | "Heavy" drinker | "Heavy" smoker | Not stated |
| Seder, 2010 [15] | Neurological ICU | Retrospective cohort NRT = 128 No NRT = 106 | NRT = 50 No NRT = 50 | NRT = 34 No NRT = 33 | NRT = 11.4 ± 7.4 No NRT = 10.7 ± 7.8 | – | NRT = 30% No NRT = 16% | >10 cigarettes/day NRT = 73% No NRT = 47% Pack year history[a] NRT = 34 ± 29 No NRT = 31 ± 34 | Patient/ surrogate reporting |
| Cartin-Ceba, 2011 [16] | Medical ICU | Prospective cohort NRT = 174 No NRT = 156 | NRT = 53.8 No NRT = 54.6 | NRT = 60.3 No NRT = 53.2 | APACHE III NRT = 50 (35–65.5) No NRT = 49 (38–62) | NRT = 69 No NRT = 44 | – | Cigarettes/day[b] NRT = 20 (10–30) No NRT = 15 (10–20) Pack year history[b] NRT = 30 (18–50) No NRT = 23 (10–45) | Patient/ surrogate reporting Tobacco assessment protocol |
| Gillies, 2012 [18] | Mixed medical/surgical ICU | Retrospective cohort NRT = 73 No NRT = 350 | NRT = 55.5 No NRT = 56.3 | NRT = 64.9 No NRT = 67.4 | NRT = 21.8 ± 15.5 No NRT = 27.2 ± 20.1 | – | NRT = 50% No NRT = 21.7% $p < 0.001$ | Not reported | Electronic medical records |
| Pathak, 2013 [17] | Mixed medical/surgical ICU | RCT double-blind pilot study NRT = 20 No NRT = 20 | NRT = 57.4 No NRT = 52.3 | 67.5 | NRT = 14.3 ± 9.7 No NRT = 13.8 ± 9.4 | NRT = 50 No NRT = 50 | – | Packs/day[a] NRT = 1.2 ± 0.5 No NRT = 1.0 ± 0.4 Years of smoking[a] NRT = 24.4 ± 10.2 No NRT = 23.3 ± 10.7 | Self report At time of written consent |

[a]Mean ± standard deviation
[b]Median (interquartile range)

**Table 2** Nicotine replacement therapy, agitation, delirium, and associated risk factors

| First author, year (ref no.) | Allocation of NRT | NRT dose and form | Time to NRT therapy (days) | Delirium and agitation assessment method | Incidence of delirium or agitation | Frequency and duration of assessment | New psychotropics prescribed |
|---|---|---|---|---|---|---|---|
| Mayer, 2001 [13] | Treatment response to suspected nicotine withdrawal | 21-mg patch | Range 3–11 | Subjective | NRT = 100% | – | Sedation, analgesia, or psychotropic use reported n = 4 |
| Honisett, 2001 [14] | Treatment response to suspected nicotine withdrawal | Patch dose not reported | <2 | Subjective description of agitation | NRT = 100% | – | Sedation and analgesia n = 1 |
| Seder, 2010 [15] | Clinician discretion | 21-mg patch | 1–14 | Delirium definition provided Assessment method not reported | NRT = 19% No NRT = 7% | – | – |
| Cartin-Ceba, 2011 [16] | Nurse-driven protocol | 21-mg patch (14–21 mg)[a] | <1 | RASS CAM-ICU Use of physical restraints | RASS[a] NRT = −1 (−4 to 0) No NRT = 0 (−2 to 0) Positive CAM-ICU days NRT = 23% (169/734) No NRT = 13.1% (75/131) Physical restraint days NRT = 38% (281/734) No NRT = 19.5% (112/573) | Worst daily assessment recorded | Fentanyl equivalence mcg[a] NRT = 50 (0–874.9) No NRT = 0 (0–472) $P < 0.001$ Lorazepam equivalence mg[a] NRT = 0.5 (0–11.5) No NRT = 0 (0–2.3) $P < 0.001$ More quetiapine in NRT group More dexmedetomidine and haloperidol in no NRT group |
| Gillies, 2012 [18] | Clinician discretion | 20-mg patch (range 10–30 mg) | 2.3 (1.5–5.0)[a] | Validated chart review with prescription of ≥2 anti-agitation drugs as surrogate marker | NRT = 25.7% No NRT = 7.1% | Once per patient | NRT = 25.7% No NRT = 7.1% Required ≥2 anti-agitation drugs $P < 0.001$ |
| Pathak, 2013 [17] | Randomised | NRT = 21-mg patch No NRT = placebo | ≤2 | Analgesia, sedation, and days on ventilator used as surrogate marker | Mechanical ventilation days[b] NRT = 1.9 ± 3.7 No NRT = 3.5 ± 5.3 | – | Sedation (days) NRT = 1.4 No NRT = 2.7 Analgesia (days) NRT = 1.1 No NRT = 2.1 |

[a]Median (interquartile range)
[b]Mean ± standard deviation

Another study [18] used a validated chart review to confirm the presence of an acute confusional state along with the prescription of two or more anti-agitation drugs as a marker for agitation or delirium.

The pilot RCT [17] compared use of analgesia, sedation, and days on mechanical ventilation as surrogate markers in order to comment on agitation or delirium. One study [15] provided a definition for delirium but did not describe a method of assessment. The case series and case report provided descriptions of either agitation or delirium but did not report a formal assessment method or frequency.

### Frequency of agitation and delirium
The case report subjectively describes the patient as agitated but does not comment on delirium status. Agitated behaviour is reported as markedly reduced after commencing a nicotine patch [14]. The case series documents five cases of agitated delirium, all of which completely resolve or markedly improve within 24 h of nicotine patch application [13].

One study [15] found delirium to be more prevalent in the group receiving NRT compared to smokers who were not prescribed NRT (NRT = 19% vs no NRT = 7% odds ratio (OR) 3.30; confidence interval (CI) 1.37–7.97; $P = 0.006$). Comparable results were noted in another study [18], with a greater percentage of patients who were prescribed NRT experiencing an episode of agitation or delirium (NRT = 25.7% vs no NRT = 7.1%; $P < 0.001$).

One study [16] found the group prescribed NRT required slightly heavier sedation with a median RASS = −1, compared to a RASS = 0 in the non-NRT group ($P = 0.02$). The percentage of positive CAM-ICU days was also greater for NRT users, with 23% of days spent in ICU with delirium versus 13.1% in those not receiving NRT ($P < 0.001$). Days spent in physical restraints were also significantly greater in the NRT group (NRT = 38% vs no NRT = 19.5%; $P < 0.001$).The pilot RCT [17] noted fewer days spent on mechanical ventilation with nicotine patches (NRT = 1.9 days vs placebo = 3.5 days).

### Psychotropic use
The case report describes post-operative weaning of sedation and patient-controlled morphine analgesia with agitation developing despite adequate analgesia [14]. Repeated doses of sedation, analgesia, and antipsychotics were reported to be required with limited effect in four out of five patients presented in the case series [13].

A cohort study [16] found greater median fentanyl equivalent analgesia use in the NRT group compared to the group without NRT ($P < 0.001$). Benzodiazepine use was also greater in the NRT group ($P < 0.001$). The group without NRT required larger doses of haloperidol and dexmedetomidine.

Another cohort study [18] did not specify quantities of psychotropic medications used, but reported that a higher proportion of NRT patients (26 vs 7% of the no NRT group, $P < 0.001$) required two or more anti-agitation drugs.

The pilot RCT [17] compared days spent in ICU with sedation or analgesia. The mean number of days on sedation was almost half in patients randomised to receive NRT (1.4 vs 2.7 days with placebo). Days receiving analgesia were also less in the NRT group (1.1 vs 2.1 days with placebo). $P$ values were non-significant due to inadequate sample size. The investigators comment that the finding of reduced sedation requirements may be linked with reduced agitation.

### Other risk factors for agitation or delirium
Overall reporting of other risk factors for agitation or delirium was poor. Possible confounders include age, severity of illness, and comorbid conditions such as hypertension, alcoholism, and cognitive impairment [4, 6, 9]. Excessive alcohol intake was the most commonly reported additional risk factor for agitation or delirium (Table 2).

One study [15] reported a greater percentage of heavy alcohol use in patients allocated NRT (30%) compared to smokers without NRT (16%). The case report stated the patient was a heavy drinker. The case series considered neurological causes of delirium. Alternative causes of delirium, including illicit drug use, were considered but not alcohol. The remaining studies did not report alcohol consumption or other specific risk factors for agitation or delirium.

### Discussion
Critically ill patients may develop delirium or agitation secondary to a range of causes. As agitation and delirium are associated with numerous adverse effects, it is therefore vital that modifiable risk factors are managed proactively. Nicotine dependence develops through desensitisation and upregulation of nicotinic acetylcholine receptors. This leads to significant changes in dopamine, glutamate, and gamma aminobutyric acid release in active smokers. Abrupt cessation of nicotine inhalation leads to a disruption of this new equilibrium (with previously desensitised receptors becoming unoccupied) and presents clinically as nicotine withdrawal [2, 21]. This systematic review assessed the evidence regarding the use of NRT for nicotine withdrawal within the ICU.

Our key finding is that there is a paucity of high-quality data informing this practice, with one underpowered pilot RCT providing the only interventional evidence. Equally, this review highlights that uncertainty remains regarding whether active smoking is truly a risk factor for ICU delirium, in part due to the deficiencies in identifying active smokers, quantifying baseline smoking status and risk of nicotine withdrawal [22].

The case report and case series describe promising results concerning NRT use in smokers experiencing acute agitated delirium. However, anecdotal reports are at risk of publication bias and should be used to guide clinical decision-making with caution. Further caution should also be applied when validated assessment tools are not used to determine patient outcomes.

Seder et al. [15] found delirium to be more common in the group receiving NRT. However, patients prescribed NRT would likely receive this therapy on the basis of a heavier smoking history. In addition, the method and frequency of cognitive assessment was not reported; hence, it is unclear if NRT was prescribed in response to the onset of agitation or delirium. Neither is it clear if delirium worsened or improved after NRT administration. The group receiving NRT also manifests heavier alcohol consumption. This and other unidentified confounding factors were not adjusted for in analysis; hence, causality cannot be determined.

Gillies et al. [18] have similar interpretive limitations. Specifically, baseline smoking status was not collected, so adjustment for this factor between groups cannot be performed. Robust methods of assessment were absent, meaning active smokers may have been misidentified, and delirium potentially under-reported.

Cartin-Ceba et al. [16] attempted to address these limitations. Allocating NRT using a nicotine dependence assessment protocol allows for appropriate prescribing on the basis of a high likelihood of nicotine withdrawal. This is supported by the observation that the median number of cigarettes smoked per day and years smoked was greater in those prescribed NRT. Of note, increased delirium and use of restraints were identified in the group prescribed NRT. However, baseline differences make causal interpretation difficult, with additional confounding factors, such as heavier sedation requirements, either not reported or not adjusted for. The outcome is further clouded by a trend towards greater antipsychotic requirements in those not prescribed NRT.

The pilot RCT by Pathak et al. [17] is the only publication to date which allows for an unbiased assessment of the effect of NRT in the ICU setting. Reported baseline prognostic factors were balanced due to randomisation. Fewer days requiring sedation, analgesia, and mechanical ventilation in those that received NRT support the hypothesis that this intervention may assist in reducing symptomatic nicotine withdrawal in the ICU, although these findings were not statistically significant due to the small sample size.

Sedatives and analgesics have been shown to increase the risk of delirium [6]. Thus, reducing agitation without having to increase use of sedatives or analgesics is desirable and associated with positive clinical outcomes [23, 24]. Determining whether the trends seen in the pilot RCT [17] also translate to a reduction in agitation or delirium will require a larger study. Assessments should be performed with validated tools rather than use of surrogate markers. An active RCT was identified during the literature search [25]; this may provide further insight into the role of NRT.

Measuring serum nicotine levels achieved with NRT has been validated within hospitalised patients and may support research findings. The critically ill population often have altered pharmacokinetics and augmented transdermal absorption and therefore may experience unexpected serum levels. Accuracy of smoking history assessments is challenging in the ICU population. The Fagerström Test for Nicotine Dependence is a commonly used validated tool, however, only for self-reporting [26]. The nature of ICU admission often deems this impossible and relies on surrogate information. Inaccuracies in this information may alter patient dependency classifications. These factors raise the question of using biochemical markers, such as cotinine, to support information provided from both patients and their families to identify smokers [27].

Overall, this review was not able to determine the true effect of NRT on agitation or delirium in the ICU. Different assessment methods, of varying quality, made interpretation and comparison of agitation and delirium levels difficult. Differences in baseline smoking status between study groups also cloud data interpretation. Reporting and adjusting for confounders was scarce. There is currently insufficient evidence to support prophylactic use of NRT in smokers admitted to the ICU. The decision to prescribe NRT may be considered in patients who are experiencing urges to smoke or who have developed agitation that is attributable to nicotine withdrawal.

## Conclusions

This systematic review was unable to definitively determine the role of NRT in agitation and delirium management in the intensive care setting. Further studies that balance baseline characteristics, adjust for confounders, and employ validated assessment tools are required. In current practice, an evaluation of risk versus benefit on an individual patient basis should be considered when prescribing NRT in the critically ill.

### Abbreviations

NRT: Nicotine replacement therapy; ICU: Intensive care unit; RCT: Randomised control trial; RASS: Richmond Agitation-Sedation Scale; CAM-ICU: Confusion Assessment Method for ICU

### Acknowledgements

Not applicable. Only the authors listed in the manuscript have contributed towards the article.

## Funding
No funding was received in relation to this review article.

## Authors' contributions
MK developed the concept, search strategy, and data extraction for this review. AU, HM, and MD provided guidance on the structure and content of the manuscript. All authors read and approved the final manuscript.

## Competing interests
The authors declare that they have no competing interests.

## Author details
[1]Pharmacy Department, Alfred Health, 55 Commercial Road, Melbourne, VIC 3004, Australia. [2]Intensive Care Unit, Alfred Health, Melbourne, Australia. [3]Wolfson Institute of Preventive Medicine, London, UK. [4]Queen Mary University of London, London, UK. [5]Monash University, Melbourne, Australia.

## References
1. Ho KM, et al. Dose-related effect of smoking on mortality in critically ill patients: a multicentre cohort study. Intensive Care Med. 2011;37(6):981–9.
2. Awissi DK, et al. Alcohol, nicotine, and iatrogenic withdrawals in the ICU. Crit Care Med. 2013;41(9 Suppl 1):S57–68.
3. Lucidarme O, et al. Nicotine withdrawal and agitation in ventilated critically ill patients. Crit Care. 2010;14(2):1–10.
4. Van Rompaey B, et al. Risk factors for delirium in intensive care patients: a prospective cohort study. Crit Care. 2009;13(3):R77.
5. American Psychiatric Association, Diagnostic and statistical manual of mental disorders : DSM-5. (Fifth ed.). 2013.
6. Ouimet S, et al. Incidence, risk factors and consequences of ICU delirium. Intensive Care Med. 2007;33(1):66–73.
7. Ely E, et al. Delirium as a predictor of mortality in mechanically ventilated patients in the intensive care unit. JAMA. 2004;291(14):1753–62.
8. Jaber S, et al. A prospective study of agitation in a medical-surgical ICU incidence, risk factors, and outcomes. CHEST J. 2005;128(4):2749–57.
9. Dubois MJ, et al. Delirium in an intensive care unit: a study of risk factors. Intensive Care Med. 2001;27(8):1297–304.
10. Rigotti NA, Munafo MR, Stead LF. Smoking cessation interventions for hospitalized smokers: a systematic review. Arch Intern Med. 2008;168(18): 1950–60.
11. Afessa B, Keegan M. Critical care support of patients with nicotine addiction. Crit Care. 2010;14(3):155.
12. Wilby KJ, Harder CK. Nicotine replacement therapy in the intensive care unit: a systematic review. J Intensive Care Med. 2014;29(1):22–30.
13. Mayer SA, et al. Delirium from nicotine withdrawal in neuro-ICU patients. Neurology. 2001;57(3):551–3.
14. Honisett TD. Nicotine replacement therapy for smokers admitted to intensive care. Intensive Crit Care Nurs. 2001;17(6):318–21.
15. Seder D, et al. Transdermal nicotine replacement therapy in cigarette smokers with acute subarachnoid hemorrhage. Neurocrit Care. 2011;14(1):77–83.
16. Cartin-Ceba R, et al. Nicotine replacement therapy in critically ill patients: a prospective observational cohort study. Crit Care Med. 2011;39(7):1635–40.
17. Pathak V, et al. Outcome of nicotine replacement therapy in patients admitted to ICU: a randomized controlled double-blind prospective pilot study. Respir Care. 2013;58(10):1625–9.
18. Gillies MA, et al. Safety of nicotine replacement therapy in critically ill smokers: a retrospective cohort study. Intensive Care Med. 2012;38(10):1683–8.
19. Ely EW, et al. Monitoring sedation status over time in ICU patients: reliability and validity of the Richmond Agitation-Sedation Scale (RASS). JAMA. 2003; 289(22):2983–91.
20. Ely EW, et al. Evaluation of delirium in critically ill patients: validation of the Confusion Assessment Method for the Intensive Care Unit (CAM-ICU). Crit Care Med. 2001;29(7):1370–9.
21. Paolini M, De Biasi M. Mechanistic insights into nicotine withdrawal. Biochem Pharmacol. 2011;82(8):996–1007.
22. Hsieh SJ, et al. Cigarette smoking as a risk factor for delirium in hospitalized and intensive care unit patients. Ann Am Thorac Soc. 2013;10(5):496–503.
23. Pandharipande P, Ely EW. Sedative and analgesic medications: risk factors for delirium and sleep disturbances in the critically ill. Critical Care Clinics. 2006;22(2): p. 313-27, vii.
24. Woods JC, et al. Severe agitation among ventilated medical intensive care unit patients: frequency, characteristics and outcomes. Intensive Care Med. 2004;30(6):1066–72.
25. Wageningen GVH. Nicotine replacement therapy in the intensive care unit. http://clinicaltrials.gov/show/NCT01362959. Accessed 25 Aug 2016.
26. Heatherton TF, et al. The Fagerström test for nicotine dependence: a revision of the Fagerstrom Tolerance Questionnaire. Br J Addict. 1991;86(9):1119–27.
27. Hsieh SJ, et al. Biomarkers increase detection of active smoking and secondhand smoke exposure in critically ill patients. Crit Care Med. 2011;39(1):40.

# 12

# Ventilator-associated respiratory infection in a resource-restricted setting: impact and etiology

Vu Dinh Phu[1,2†], Behzad Nadjm[2,3†], Nguyen Hoang Anh Duy[4], Dao Xuan Co[5], Nguyen Thi Hoang Mai[2,4,10], Dao Tuyet Trinh[1], James Campbell[2,3,10], Dong Phu Khiem[1], Tran Ngoc Quang[1], Huynh Thi Loan[4], Ha Son Binh[5], Quynh-Dao Dinh[2], Duong Bich Thuy[2,4,10], Huong Nguyen Phu Lan[2,4,10], Nguyen Hong Ha[1], Ana Bonell[2], Mattias Larsson[6], Hoang Minh Hoan[5], Đang Quoc Tuan[5], Hakan Hanberger[7], Hoang Nguyen Van Minh[3], Lam Minh Yen[2,10], Nguyen Van Hao[4,8], Nguyen Gia Binh[5], Nguyen Van Vinh Chau[4], Nguyen Van Kinh[1], Guy E. Thwaites[2,3,10], Heiman F. Wertheim[9], H. Rogier van Doorn[2,3] and C. Louise Thwaites[2,3,10*]

## Abstract

**Background:** Ventilator-associated respiratory infection (VARI) is a significant problem in resource-restricted intensive care units (ICUs), but differences in casemix and etiology means VARI in resource-restricted ICUs may be different from that found in resource-rich units. Data from these settings are vital to plan preventative interventions and assess their cost-effectiveness, but few are available.

**Methods:** We conducted a prospective observational study in four Vietnamese ICUs to assess the incidence and impact of VARI. Patients ≥ 16 years old and expected to be mechanically ventilated > 48 h were enrolled in the study and followed daily for 28 days following ICU admission.

**Results:** Four hundred fifty eligible patients were enrolled over 24 months, and after exclusions, 374 patients' data were analyzed. A total of 92/374 cases of VARI (21.7/1000 ventilator days) were diagnosed; 37 (9.9%) of these met ventilator-associated pneumonia (VAP) criteria (8.7/1000 ventilator days). Patients with any VARI, VAP, or VARI without VAP experienced increased hospital and ICU stay, ICU cost, and antibiotic use ($p < 0.01$ for all). This was also true for all VARI ($p < 0.01$ for all) with/without tetanus. There was no increased risk of in-hospital death in patients with VARI compared to those without (VAP HR 1.58, 95% CI 0.75–3.33, $p = 0.23$; VARI without VAP HR 0.40, 95% CI 0.14–1.17, $p = 0.09$). In patients with positive endotracheal aspirate cultures, most VARI was caused by Gram-negative organisms; the most frequent were *Acinetobacter baumannii* (32/73, 43.8%) *Klebsiella pneumoniae* (26/73, 35.6%), and *Pseudomonas aeruginosa* (24/73, 32.9%). 40/68 (58.8%) patients with positive cultures for these had carbapenem-resistant isolates. Patients with carbapenem-resistant VARI had significantly greater ICU costs than patients with carbapenem-susceptible isolates (6053 USD (IQR 3806–7824) vs 3131 USD (IQR 2108–7551), $p = 0.04$) and after correction for adequacy of initial antibiotics and APACHE II score, showed a trend towards increased risk of in-hospital death (HR 2.82, 95% CI 0.75–6.75, $p = 0.15$).

(Continued on next page)

---

* Correspondence: lthwaites@oucru.org
†Equal contributors
2Oxford University Clinical Research Unit, Hanoi, Vietnam
3Centre for Tropical Medicine and Global Health, University of Oxford, Oxford, UK
Full list of author information is available at the end of the article

(Continued from previous page)

**Conclusions:** VARI in a resource-restricted setting has limited impact on mortality, but shows significant association with increased patient costs, length of stay, and antibiotic use, particularly when caused by carbapenem-resistant bacteria. Evidence-based interventions to reduce VARI in these settings are urgently needed.

**Keywords:** Ventilator-associated respiratory infection, VARI, Ventilator-associated pneumonia, VAP, Ventilator-associated tracheobronchitis, Vat, Hospital-acquired infection, Resource-restricted, Vietnam, Carbapenem resistance, Antimicrobial resistance,

## Background

Ventilator-associated respiratory infection (VARI) is the commonest hospital-acquired infection in intensive care units (ICUs) [1, 2]. The condition includes both ventilator-associated tracheobronchitis (VAT) and ventilator-associated pneumonia (VAP) and has an incidence in resource-rich countries of 1–22 per 1000 ventilator days [3–6]. One reason for the variable incidence is the use of differing definitions, and there is increasing evidence to suggest that current definitions do not correlate well with real-world clinical practice [7–10].

In high-income settings, VARI has consistently been shown to be associated with increased hospital costs and length of ICU stay [11, 12], but estimating mortality attributable to VARI is difficult as patients requiring longer periods of ventilatory support are often the most severely ill patients and at increased risk of death. In an attempt to overcome this, a recent individual patient meta-analysis showed that the attributable mortality due to VAP was mainly associated with intermediate-severity underlying disease [13]. The relationship of VAT and mortality is even less clear, with some studies showing no deleterious effect on mortality [5, 14]. Nevertheless, a survey of physicians from 288 ICUs showed that 50% of physicians considered VAT to be associated with increased mortality [4].

There are fewer data concerning the occurrence of VARI in resource-restricted settings but it appears to be at least as common, if not more so, than in resource-rich settings [15–20]. However, estimating its true incidence is difficult and current surveillance definitions have been criticized as particularly inapplicable in resource-restricted settings [21]. VARI occurring in these locations is generally assumed to have similar impact to that occurring in high-income countries, but there are limited data to confirm this, and some studies have indicated significantly worse outcomes [17, 22]. Differences in underlying diagnoses, age, comorbidity, and nutritional status may all influence outcome in addition to variations in treatment facilities and staffing levels [23]. Studies suggest that in low- and middle-income countries (LMICs), infections are usually caused by multidrug-resistant Gram-negative organisms [24, 25]. Some studies, although not all, suggest poorer outcome

in these patients [17, 26, 27]. This combination of high rates of incidence and antibiotic resistance means VARI may also have an important influence on antibiotic use. A recent study from Vietnam reported that VARI is the most common reason for antibiotic use in ICU [16].

Understanding the nature and impact of VARI in low-resource settings is especially important as these are places where implementation of relatively simple preventative interventions could have a significant impact [17, 23]. In many ICUs, high rates of carbapenem-resistant pathogens necessitate increasing use of empiric regimes including colistin [16]. Identifying factors associated with antimicrobial resistance would therefore enable more effective prevention and treatment measures [17].

In this study, we performed a multicenter prospective study following patients receiving mechanical ventilation in four intensive care units in Vietnam with the aim of providing a comprehensive description of VARI in a resource-restricted setting. We examine the incidence, etiology, and outcome in addition to antibiotic usage and antimicrobial resistance to provide a complete clinical picture of VARI and its impact.

## Methods

This was a prospective observational study performed in four intensive care units of three tertiary referral hospitals in Vietnam between November 2013 and November 2015 (total 79 ICU beds). Three sites were ICUs in two specialist infectious disease hospitals: one serving northern Vietnam and the other southern Vietnam (combined capacity 800 beds). The fourth site was a mixed medical and surgical ICU of a 1900-bed teaching hospital. Patients were eligible for study entry if ≥ 16 years old and expected to be mechanically ventilated for at least 48 h. Patients intubated for more than 48 h prior to ICU admission were excluded. An initial sample size of 600 was calculated based on previous data to estimate VAP incidence of 30% with 95% confidence interval of 3.7% [16]. However, due to slow recruitment rate, recruitment was stopped after 2 years and enrollment of 450.

Baseline demographic and clinical data were recorded on admission to the study, and an endotracheal aspirate was taken as previously described [28]. Patients were followed for 28 days for development of VARI in two sites and until extubation in the remaining sites. Hospital outcome was recorded (death or discharge/transfer). Clinically suspected VAP was investigated with chest X-ray and endotracheal aspirate. VAP was diagnosed according to modified US Centers for Disease Control and Prevention (US CDC) criteria [29–31] as follows. Firstly, a deterioration in ventilation following a period of stability defined according to positive end expiratory pressure (PEEP): ≥ 2 days of stable or decreasing daily minimum PEEP followed by a rise in daily minimum PEEP of ≥ 3 cm $H_2O$, sustained ≥ 2 calendar days; or $F_iO_2$: ≥2 days of stable or decreasing daily minimum $F_iO_2$ followed by a rise in daily minimum $F_iO_2$ ≥ 0.15 points, sustained ≥ 2 calendar days. Secondly, systemic signs of fever > 38 °C or < 36 °C or white blood cell count > $12 \times 10^9$/L or < $4 \times 10^9$/L were required. Final criteria were increased/new purulent tracheobronchial secretions or ≥ 25 neutrophils per low power field (10 objective) on Gram stain of endotracheal aspirate and either new and persistent infiltrates, consolidation, or cavitation as read by two study physicians on chest X-ray, or the decision to commence new antibiotic therapy. VARI was defined as including those patients with VAP (defined as above) and patients meeting the following criteria (modified from Craven et al. [8]): clinically increased sputum volume or purulent sputum by microscopic examination (≥ 25 neutrophils per low power filed on Gram stain of endotracheal aspirate) and either systemic signs of infection (fever or white blood count as above) in addition to the clinician starting antibiotics within 2 days of these features developing. Thus, for the purposes of this paper, we use the term "VAP" to refer to patients fitting the above definition of VAP, "VARI" to describe all patients with either VAP or VARI as defined above, and "VARI without VAP" to refer to patients with VARI as above but not meeting full criteria for VAP. It can be considered that VARI would therefore encompass all patients with VAP and ventilator-associated tracheobronchitis (VAT).

The microbiological cause of VARI was determined by isolating at least one pathogenic organism from blood culture or from endotracheal aspirate ≥ $10^5$ colony forming units/ml or equivalent semi-quantitative culture. Microbiological methods varied by site in line with routine clinical microbiological work. Briefly, in all sites, the BACTEC (Becton Dickinson, Sparks, MD, USA) automated system for blood cultures was used with a single aerobic culture bottle inoculated in all suspected cases. Endotracheal aspirate samples were subjected to Ziehl-Neelsen and Gram staining prior to incubation on sheep blood in blood agar base (BioMérieux, Marcy l'Étoile, France), MacConkey, and chocolate blood agar. Colonies were identified using routine biochemical testing (involving VITEK2 and/or API test (BioMérieux) or MALDI-

TOF MS (Bruker Daltonics, Bremen, Germany)). Antimicrobial susceptibility testing was carried out by the Kirby/Bauer disc diffusion methods, including double disk diffusion for detection of extended spectrum beta-lactamases (ESBL), using cutoffs as per CLSI 2012 guidelines or using VITEK2 depending on site. In addition, CHROMagar (CHROMagar, Paris, France) for detection of methicillin-resistant *Staphylococcus aureus* (MRSA), ESBLs, *Amp*C beta-lactamase, and KPC carbapenemase were used in some sites.

Data were recorded onto a case record form and entered into a secure database. Data analysis used Stata Statistical Software, release 8 (Stata Corp LP, College Station, TX, USA). Data are given as median (interquartile range (IQR)). Comparison of medians was performed using Mann–Whitney $U$ test. Tests of proportion of categorical variables were carried out using chi-squared test. Days at risk of VARI were calculated as days of ventilation and limited to 28 days after enrollment for those not followed for VARI after 28 days. Risk of in-hospital death following VARI was assessed using Cox's proportional hazards model; those followed for VARI only until 28 days after enrollment were censored at 28 days. Patients with missing hospital discharge data were excluded from this analysis; those with missing APACHE_II data were allocated mean scores depending on admission diagnosis. Logistic regression models were used to evaluate the relationship between admission diagnosis and risk of VARI and relationship with antibiotic treatment. Relationship of ventilation length and admission diagnosis was assessed using Mann–Whitney $U$ test.

Antibiotic use was assessed using days of therapy (DOT) defined as the sum of all days on each antibiotic per 100 patient days. For the purpose of this analysis, only antibiotics for systemic use were included (i.e., topical preparations were not) and both metronidazole, which is used for treatment of tetanus, and anti-tuberculosis medications were excluded. Antibiotic therapy was defined as "adequate" if the pathogen showed in vitro susceptibility and "inadequate" if it showed intermediate or resistant results. Samples with no significant growth were excluded from these analyses. Cox models assessing effect of antibiotic resistance or adequacy of empiric therapy were constructed using time from VARI as time-to-event variable.

Economic analysis was limited to direct medical costs, derived from hospital bills and based on fees charged to the National Health Insurance and to the patients themselves combined.

## Results

Four hundred fifty patients were enrolled between November 2013 and November 2015. One patient withdrew from the study and 75 patients were excluded from analyses: 69 were ventilated for less than 48 h and 6 patients were transferred for extra-corporeal membrane oxygenation (ECMO). Thus, data from 374 patients were available for analysis.

A total of 37/374 (9.9%) patients were diagnosed with VAP with a total incidence density of 8.7/1000 ventilator days. A further 55/374 cases (14.7%), not fulfilling VAP criteria, were diagnosed with VARI, giving a total of 92/374 (24.6%) cases of VARI and an incidence density of 21.7/1000 ventilator days for all VARI. Median time from start of ventilation to developing VAP was 10 days (IQR 5.5–12) and 9 days (IQR 6–15) for cases of VARI without VAP.

### Risk factors for VARI

Baseline data for patients are given in Table 1. Baseline data by site are provided in Additional file 1: Table S1. Patients with both VAP and VARI without VAP experienced longer durations of mechanical ventilation than patients with no VARI. Median duration of ventilation for those with VAP was 22 days (IQR 17–31), 21 days with VARI without VAP (IQR 14–28 days), compared to 10 days (IQR 6–16) with no VARI ($p < 0.01$ for both) (Table 2 and Additional file 1: Table S2).

To identify baseline predictors of all VARI, admission diagnosis was examined. As this was significantly associated with risk of VARI (OR 1.23 95% CI 1.05–1.45 $p = 0.01$), different admission diagnoses were investigated. Patients with community-acquired pneumonia had the lowest risk of VARI with a risk of 9.6% (95% CI 3–17%). Compared to these, there was a significantly increased risk of VARI in patients with an admission diagnosis of tetanus (36.4%, 95%

CI 28.2–45.2%, $p < 0.01$) or "other diagnosis" category (26.7%, 95% CI 14.6–41.9%, $p = 0.02$) (Additional file 1: Table S3). Those with tetanus also had significantly longer duration of mechanical ventilation at a median 18 (IQR 13–24) days and lowest antibiotic use on admission compared to those with community-acquired pneumonia ($p < .01$ both) (Additional file 1: Table S4).

### Impact of VARI on outcomes

Patients with VARI experienced longer hospital and ICU stay, increased hospital, and ICU cost and increased antibiotic use in the first 28 days of study. This was true for both VAP and VARI without VAP (Table 2) ($p < 0.01$ all).

Compared to patients with no VARI, there were no significant differences in risk of in-hospital death with VARI (HR 0.88, 95% CI 0.44–1.73, $p = 0.70$). When VAP and VARI without VAP subgroups were analyzed, there was a trend towards higher risk of in-hospital death in patients with VAP compared to those with no VARI (HR 1.58, 95% CI 0.75–3.33, $p = 0.23$). However, there was a lower risk of in-hospital death in patients with VARI without VAP compared to those with no VARI (HR 0.40, 95% CI 0.14–1.17, $p = 0.09$) which was non-significant. After correction for APACHE II scores, these trends remained non-significant: VAP HR 1.67, 95% CI 0.78–3.55, $p = 0.18$ and VARI without VAP HR 0.46, 95% CI 0.15–1.39, ($p = 0.17$).

Due to the high proportion of patients with tetanus and its possible confounding, the effect of tetanus on the impact of VARI was specifically examined. Similar to the whole-sample analysis, in both patients with and without tetanus, patients with VARI experienced increased hospital and ICU length of stay, increased duration of

**Table 1** Baseline characteristics of patients with and without VARI

|  | All VARI ($n = 92$) | VAP ($n = 37$) | VARI without VAP ($n = 55$) | No VARI ($n = 286$) |
|---|---|---|---|---|
| Age | 48 (36–61.5) | 46 (37–62) | 50 (35–62) | 53 (40–65) |
| M:F | 70:22 | 25:12 | 45:10 | 197:85 |
| SOFA | 3 (2–6) | 5 (2–8) | 3 (1–3) | 4 (3–7) |
| APACHE | 8.5 (5–14) | 11 (5–15) | 7 (5–14) | 11 (7–15) |
| BMI | 21.97 (19.72–24.56) | 22.12 (21.12–24.61) | 21.97 (19.03–23.53) | 20.56 (18.69–23.48) |
| Comorbidity | 26 (28.3%) | 14 (37.9%) | 12 (21.8%) | 118 (42.1%) |
| Hospital previous 90 days† | 7 (7.6%) | 3 (8.1%) | 4 (7.3%) | 34 (12.1%) |
| Transferred for this illness | 69 (75%) | 27 (73.0%) | 42 (76.4%) | 212 (75.18) |
| Antibiotics in last 90 days | 4 (4.4%) | 3 (8.1%) | 1 (1.8%) | 21 (7.5%) |
| CNS infection | 11 (12.0%) | 1 (2.7%) | 10 (18.2%) | 49 (17.4%) |
| Dengue | 3 (3.3%) | 2 (5.4%) | 1 (1.8%) | 6 (2.1%) |
| Sepsis/septic shock | 11 (12.0%) | 6 (16.2%) | 5 (9.1%) | 44 (15.6%) |
| Tetanus | 48 (52.2%) | 14 (37.8%) | 34 (61.8%) | 84 (29.8%) |
| Pneumonia | 7 (7.6%) | 7 (18.9%) | 0 (0%) | 66 (23.4%) |

Values given are median (IQR) or count (percent)
†$n = 249$

**Table 2** Outcome of patients with VARI, VAP, other VARI, and no VARI

|  | All VARI (n = 92) | VAP (n = 37) | VARI without VAP (n = 55) | No VARI (n = 286) |
|---|---|---|---|---|
| ICU length of stay (days) | 27 (21–37) | 25 (19–37) | 27 (25–38) | 16 (10–28) |
| Days ventilated (days) | 22 (15.5–29.5) | 21 (14–28) | 22 (17–31) | 10 (6–16) |
| ICU cost (USD) * | 4723 (2778–7783) | 7213 (3011–8329) | 4196 (2726–7193) | 2534 (1493–4407) |
| Hospital length of stay (days) | 38 (26–49) | 31 (22–46) | 39.5 (29.5–49) | 25 (14–39) |
| Hospital cost (USD)** | 4434 (2656–7822) | 4522 (2716–7990) | 4167 (2658–6985) | 2639 (1555–4576) |
| Antibiotics use (DOT) | 31 (18–42.5) | 35 (21–45) | 30 (17–38) | 18 (10–28) |
| Antibiotics in hospital before VARI | 73/92 (79.4%) | 28/38 (75.6%) | 45/55 (87.7%) | 255/282 (90.43%) |
| In-hospital mortality | 17/91 (18.7%) | 13/37 (35.1%) | 4/54 (7.4%) | 54/277 (19.5%) |

Values given are median (IQR) or count (percent)

* n = 372; ** n = 313

ventilation, increased hospital and ICU costs, and increased antibiotic use within the 28-day study period (Additional file 1: Tables S5 and S6.). When tetanus status, Apache II, and interaction between tetanus and VARI were included in the cox model, there were no differences in the risk of in-hospital death following either VAP or other VARI (VAP HR 1.79, 95% CI 0.84–3.82, $p$ = 0.13; VARI without VAP HR 0.43, 95% CI 0.13–1.38, $p$ = 0.15).

## Microbiology of VARI

Of the 92 patients treated for VARI, 77 had endotracheal aspirates taken within 48 h of VARI diagnosis, 73 of which had positive cultures (Table 3). The predominant bacterium was *Acinetobacter baumannii* (32 patients) followed by *Klebsiella pneumoniae* (26 patients) and *Pseudomonas aeruginosa* (24 patients). 68/73 (92%) patients had specimens containing one or more of these three organisms.

## Antibiotic resistance and impact on outcomes

New antimicrobial therapy given within 48 h of VARI diagnosis is given in Additional file 1: Table S7. The majority of cases (49/92, 54.3%) were treated with a carbapenem; colistin was used in 25/92 (27.2%) cases and combination therapy was used in 36/92 (39.1%) cases. Adequacy of empiric initial antimicrobial therapy of VARI could be assessed in 71 cases and was inadequate in 20/71 (28%) cases. However, inadequate therapy was not associated with increased mortality (HR 0.1.11, 95% CI 0.34–3.66, $p$ = 0.86), nor were there differences in length of ICU stay or ICU costs (Table 4). Of note, all of the specimens from patients treated with inadequate antibiotic contained one or more carbapenem-resistant bacteria.

5/10 (50%) *Staphylococcus aureus* isolates were methicillin-resistant. 11/24 (46%) of *P. aeruginosa* isolates and 27/32 (84%) *A. baumannii* isolates were resistant to carbapenems, compared to only 6/26 (23%) of *K. pneumoniae*. In total, 40/68 (59%) patients with positive culture for *P. aeruginosa*, *A. baumannii*, or *K. pneumoniae* had carbapenem-resistant isolates. Patients with VARI attributed to these carbapenem-resistant bacteria had significantly greater ICU costs than patients with non-resistant isolates (6053 USD (IQR 3807–7824) vs 3131 USD (IQR 2109–7552), $p$ = 0.04). There were no differences between length of hospital or ICU stay but patients with carbapenem-resistant isolates had increased

**Table 3** Organisms isolated from initial endotracheal aspirates within 48 h of VARI diagnosis

|  | N (% isolates) | Carbapenem resistance N (%) |
|---|---|---|
| *Acinetobacter baumannii* | 32 (29.7%) | 27/32 (84.4%) |
| *Klebsiella pneumoniae* | 26 (24.1%) | 6/26 (23.1%) |
| *Pseudomonas aeruginosa* | 24 (22.2%) | 11/24 (45.8%) |
| *Staphylococcus aureus* | 10 (9.3%) | 5* (50%) |
| *Haemophilus influenza* | 5 (4.6%) | 0 (0%) |
| *Elizabethkingia meningoseptica* | 3 (2.8%) | 1 (33.3%) |
| *Stenotrophomonas maltophilia* | 3 (2.8%) | 3 (100%) |
| *Streptococcus pneumoniae* | 3 (2.8%) | 0* (0%) |
| *Escherichia coli* | 1 (0.9%) | 1 (100%) |
| *Proteus mirabilis* | 1 (0.9%) | 0 (0%) |

*Carbapenem susceptibility not formally assessed but carbapenem susceptibility assumed from penicillin or methicillin sensitivity

**Table 4** Adequacy of initial empiric antibiotic therapy for VARI

|                              | Adequate            | Inadequate           | p    |
|------------------------------|---------------------|----------------------|------|
| In-hospital mortality        | 9/51                | 4/20                 | 1.00 |
| ICU length of stay (days)    | 27 (22–37)          | 27.5 (25–37)         | 0.74 |
| Hospital length of stay (days) | 38 (26–49)        | 39 (28.5–44)         | 0.89 |
| ICU cost (USD)               | 4797 (2726–7806)    | 5485 (3541–7259)     | 0.88 |
| Hospital cost (USD)          | 4461 (2666–7883)    | 5549 (3843–7543)     | 0.54 |

Values given are median (IQR) or count (percent)

antibiotic use during the study period (37.5 (IQR 29.0–45.5) days of therapy (DOT) compared to 21 (IQR 15.5–33.0) DOT, $p < 0.01$) (Table 5). Additionally, patients with carbapenem-resistant isolates showed a trend towards increased in-hospital death (HR 2.82, 95% CI 0.75–6.75, $p = 0.15$) which remained when adequacy of initial empiric antibiotic therapy and APACHE II scores were taken into account (HR 2.82, 95% CI 0.87–9.19, $p = 0.09$).

In order to assess potential risk factors for development of VARI with carbapenem-resistant bacteria, treatment with carbapenems in ICU before diagnosis of VARI was examined. 22/39 (56%) patients with carbapenem-resistant isolates of *P. aeruginosa, A. baumannii,* or *K. pneumoniae* were treated with carbapenems between ICU admission and development of VARI, compared to only 2/26 (7.7%) of those with sensitive isolates ($p < 0.01$).

## Discussion

This study has shown that VARI is a common and important problem in resource-restricted ICUs and patients with VARI have an increased length of ICU stay, ICU cost, and antibiotic use. Calculating attributable mortality due to VARI is difficult due to difficulty identifying a control group and the numerous possible confounders. By using survival analysis, we aimed to account for differences in time at risk. In addition, by including a large subgroup of patients with tetanus, we have gained a unique insight into the impact of VARI on patient outcome. Patients with tetanus have little comorbidity or organ dysfunction in addition, and they lack features such as increased pulmonary vascular permeability that may confuse the diagnosis of VARI. In these patients, we observed increased risk of VARI but very low mortality, and there was no evidence

that risk of in-hospital death following VARI differed between patients with or without tetanus.

Although we did not observe any increased risk of in-hospital death in patients with either VAP or VARI without VAP, there was a trend towards improved outcome in patients with VARI without VAP and worse outcome in VAP. Similar findings have previously been reported in different populations. A large study of 2960 patients in Europe and South America reported mortality rates of 40% with VAP, 29% with VAT, and 30% with no VARI [5]. Similarly, a smaller observational study of patients in a single centre in France reported a mortality rate of 29% in VAT patients compared to 36% of controls without VARI [14]. VARI may be viewed as a continuum between VAT and VAP both in terms of severity and chronology: i.e., there is a progression from asymptomatic bacterial colonization of the respiratory tract through tracheobronchitis and eventually to pneumonia when chest X-ray changes become apparent [8, 32]. It is possible that patients meeting the full criteria for VAP have more severe disease, are diagnosed later, and therefore have worse outcome. This is supported by recent evidence that patients with VAP treated early with antibiotics showed higher response rates [33].

In 2013, as this study was being conceived, the CDC introduced a system of ventilator-associated event definitions, which encompassed criteria for ventilator-associated pneumonia. Our choice of definitions for use in this study was influenced by a desire to balance relevant, objective definitions with these new definitions. These definitions have now been widely criticized, and it has been recognized that they may need to be adjusted for specific patient groups [34]. The CDC explicitly states that some elements of the new framework

**Table 5** Impact of carbapenem-resistant bacteria causing VARI

|                           | Carbapenem-resistant Enterobacteriaceae/A. baumannii or P. aeruginosa | Carbapenem-sensitive Enterobacteriaceae/A. baumannii or P. aeruginosa | p      |
|---------------------------|----------------------|----------------------|--------|
| ICU length of stay (days) | 26 (20.5–33.5)       | 29.5 (23.5–39.5)     | 0.23   |
| ICU cost (USD)            | 6053 (3806–7824)     | 3131 (2108–7551)     | 0.04   |
| In-hospital mortality     | 10/40 (25%)          | 3/28 (10.7%)         | 0.14   |
| Antibiotic use (DOT)      | 37.5 (29–45.5)       | 21 (15.5–33)         | <0.01  |

Values given are median (IQR) or count (percent)

(probable VAP) are not suitable for public reporting or bench-marking [35]. For this reason, we chose to use the definitions we felt best reflected clinical practice and were relevant to the main issues of this study, namely the high use of broad-spectrum antibiotics in resource-restricted ICUs and outcome of patients treated for VARI. By using clear and consistent definitions throughout, we aimed to minimize bias when comparing these outcomes. As our main aim was to describe actual practice in resource-limited ICUs, and three out of four participating ICUs in our study were specialist infectious disease units, we deliberately chose to include patients with infections, including an admission diagnosis of pneumonia. An earlier pilot study had shown that not including patients with a possible pneumonia on admission led to patients with other primary diagnoses such as sepsis or meningitis being excluded from the study due to abnormal baseline chest X-rays. In view of this, we felt excluding these patients would introduce significant bias and reduce the relevance of this study for future practice.

Overall, compared to other studies in resource-restricted settings, we recorded a low incidence of VAP, but comparable levels of total VARI [16, 26, 36]. The low rate of VAP may be due to the insensitivity of VAP criteria used in our setting resulting in possible misclassification of cases. In our ICUs, low staffing levels, lack of ICU-specific training, and less frequent monitoring mean that higher ventilator settings are often used and ventilator settings are infrequently changed to reduce the risk of hypoxia. Thus, the demonstrable deterioration in ventilator settings (i.e., PEEP or $F_iO_2$) to diagnose VAP may be less likely to occur resulting in possible VAP cases classified as VARI without VAP. However, a strength of our study is that we have included all patients with VARI, thus patients not meeting VAP criteria, but treated for ventilator-related respiratory infection, have still been included in the analyses. The differences in VAP rates between ICUs included in our study may reflect differences in practices between ICUs as the overall VARI rates are similar.

Unlike VARI described in high-income settings, isolates associated with VARI were dominated by Gram-negative bacteria [37]. Of note, 92% of our patients had VARI attributable to one or more of the World Health Organization's three "critical" priority organisms: *K. pneumoniae*, *P. aeruginosa*, and *A. baumannii* [38]. We report high levels of antimicrobial resistance among these and also note that resistance to carbapenems was associated with a worse outcome and that prior use of carbapenems during hospital admission was a risk factor for isolation of carbapenem-resistant bacteria, suggesting a role for carbapenem-sparing agents in the management of severe infection. Furthermore, carbapenem resistance had a significant and substantial impact on costs and antibiotic use.

The lack of correlation between inadequate empiric therapy and mortality is in keeping with some of the literature from high-income countries, much of which comes from studies in sepsis and septic shock, yet is out of step with other studies [38–40]. In the context of this study, it most likely also relates to the behavior of clinicians faced with a single remaining option of colistin for treatment of increasingly resistant Gram-negative infections, reserving empiric treatment more likely to be adequate (i.e., colistin) for more severe cases. We have only analyzed the effects of adequate and inadequate therapy with respect to initial empiric therapy, and it is also possible that timely reporting of microbiological culture results enabled rapid rectification of inadequate regimes, hence limited impact on outcome measures.

Patient hospitalization costs were significantly and substantially higher in patients with VARI and approximately double for those with carbapenem-resistant organisms. In our setting, antibiotics such as carbapenems or colistin form a higher proportion of ICU cost than in resource-rich settings and treatment regimens for multidrug-resistant organisms include treatment with more expensive antibiotics for longer periods. A limitation of our study is that we have not been able to divide healthcare costs before and after VARI and as such may be subject to immortal time bias. Furthermore, we have only analyzed direct patient treatment costs and have not taken account of additional healthcare costs of staffing and equipment or indirect costs such as lost earnings, travel, and subsistence costs of patients and family members providing care. In a resource-restricted setting such as ours, where much of hospital care is provided by family members, these costs are likely to be substantial and an important additional burden.

Despite these limitations, we believe VARI remains an important problem in resource-restricted ICUs and clinicians working in these settings need locally relevant evidence demonstrating the efficacy and safety of interventions to reduce its incidence. Previous work aiming to prevent infection through patient positioning and hand hygiene have not shown benefit in our setting [24, 41], emphasizing the need for locally derived data. To this end, we are engaged in a randomized controlled trial of continuous cuff pressure to prevent ventilator-associated respiratory infections (ClinicalTrials.gov idn NCT02966392).

## Conclusions

VARI is a significant problem in a resource-restricted ICU setting. Despite no observed impact on mortality, there are significant and substantial cost implications related to occurrence of VARI, particularly that associated with carbapenem-resistant bacteria. Dealing with these high rates of carbapenem resistance needs to involve both antibiotic stewardship and infection prevention strategies.

## Additional file

> **Additional file 1: Table S1.** Baseline characteristics by site. **Table S2.** VARI and outcome by site. **Table S3.** Risk of VARI according to admission diagnosis. **Table S4.** Duration of ventilation and antibiotic use in patients according to admission diagnosis. **Table S5.** Impact of VARI in patients with and without tetanus. **Table S6.** Impact of VARI and other VARI in patients with and without tetanus. **Table S7.** Empiric antibiotic therapy for VARI (DOCX 16 kb)

## Abbreviations

CI: Confidence interval; DOT: Days of therapy; ECMO: Extra-corporeal membrane oxygenation; ESBL: Extended spectrum beta lactam; FiO2: Fraction of inspired oxygen; HR: Hazard ratio; ICU: Intensive care unit; IQR: Interquartile range; LMIC: low- and middle-income country; PEEP: Positive end expiratory pressure; USD: United States dollar; VAP: Ventilator-associated pneumonia; VARI: Ventilator-associated respiratory infection; VAT: Ventilator-associated tracheobronchitis

## Acknowledgements

We would like to thank the staff in the Biostatistics and Oxford University Clinical Research Unit, Centre for Tropical Medicine and Global Health, University of Oxford for the help and statistical advice.
We also thank all staff in ICUs at the National Hospital for Tropical Diseases, Hospital for Tropical Diseases, and Bach Mai Hospitals for their help with this study as well as the Clinical Trials Unit and Data Management Group at Oxford University Clinical Research Unit Ha Noi and Ho Chi Minh City.

## Funding

This study was funded by the Wellcome Trust UK, Swedish International Development Cooperation Agency (SIDA), and the Li Ka Shing Foundation.

## Authors' contributions

VDP and BN were involved in the conception/design, data acquisition, analysis/interpretation, and drafting/revising the manuscript. DZC, JC, DSB, HTL, MHM, LMY, NVH, and NGB were involved in the conception/design and data acquisition. NHAD and NTHM were involved in the conception/design, data acquisition, and analysis/interpretation. NTT, DPK, and TNQ were involved in the data acquisition. QDD, ML, and GET were involved in the conception/design and drafting/revising the manuscript. DBT and AB were involved in the data acquisition and revising the manuscript. HL, GQT, HNMV, LTDT, and GTA were involved in the data acquisition. NHH, HH, NVVC, and NVK were involved in the conception/design. RBG was involved in the data analysis/interpretation and drafting/ revising the manuscript. HRW, HRVD, and CLT were involved in the conception/design/data acquisition, analysis, and drafting/revising the manuscript. HFM was involved in conception/design of the study. DXC, DTT, HSB and DQT were involved in data acquisition. HFW contributed to conception, design and implementation DXC, DTT, HSB and DQT contributed to data collection. All authors read and approved the final manuscript.

Hanoi, and Hospital for Tropical Diseases, Ho Chi Minh City). The study was carried out according to the principals of the Declaration of Helsinki and all participants gave written informed consent to take part in the study.

## Competing interests

The authors declare that they have no competing interests.

## Author details

[1]National Hospital for Tropical Diseases, Hanoi, Vietnam. [2]Oxford University Clinical Research Unit, Hanoi, Vietnam. [3]Centre for Tropical Medicine and Global Health, University of Oxford, Oxford, UK. [4]Hospital for Tropical Diseases, Ho Chi Minh City, Vietnam. [5]Bach Mai Hospital, Hanoi, Vietnam. [6]Karolinska Institutet, Stockholm, Sweden. [7]Linköping University, Linköping, Sweden. [8]University of Medicine and Pharmacy, Ho Chi Minh City, Vietnam. [9]Department of Medical Microbiology and Radboud Center for Infectious Diseases, Radboudumc, Nijmegen, Netherlands. [10]Oxford University Clinical Research Unit, Ho Chi Minh City, Vietnam.

## References

1. Vincent J-L, Sakr Y, Sprung CL, et al. Sepsis in European intensive care units: results of the SOAP study. Crit Care Med. 2006;34:344–53.
2. Zarb P. The European Centre for Disease Prevention and Control (ECDC) pilot point prevalence survey of healthcare-associated infections and antimicrobial use. The European Centre for Disease Prevention and Control (ECDC) pilot point prevalence survey of health. Euro surveil 2012; 17:pii: 20316. https://ecdc.europa.eu/sites/portal/files/media/en/publications/Publications/healthcare-associated-infections-antimicrobial-use-PPS.pdf.
3. Dudeck MA, Weiner LM, Allen-Bridson K, et al. National Healthcare Safety Network (NHSN) report, data summary for 2012, device-associated module. Am J Infect Control. 2013;41:1148–66.
4. Rodríguez A, Póvoa P, Nseir S, et al. Incidence and diagnosis of ventilator-associated tracheobronchitis (VAT) in the intensive care unit: an international online survey. Crit Care. 2014;18:R32.
5. Martin-Loeches I, Povoa P, Rodríguez A, et al. Incidence and prognosis of ventilator-associated tracheobronchitis (TAVeM): a multicentre, prospective, observational study. Lancet Resp Med. 2015;3:859–68.
6. European Centre for Disease Prevention and Control. Surveillance of healthcare-associated infections in Europe 2007. Stock ECDC 2012. doi: https://doi.org/10.2900/18553.
7. Waltrick R, Possamai D, Perito de Aguair F, et al. Comparison between a clinical diagnosis method and the surveillance technique of the Center for Disease Control and Prevention for identification of mechanical ventilator-associated pneumonia. Rev Braz Ter Intensiva. 2015;27:260–5.
8. Craven DE, Lei Y, Ruthazer R, et al. Incidence and outcomes of ventilator-associated tracheobronchitis and pneumonia. Am J Med. 2013;126:542–9.
9. Murray CJL, Vos T, Lozano R, et al. Disability-adjusted life years (DALYs) for 291 diseases and injuries in 21 regions, 1990-2010: a systematic analysis for the Global Burden of Disease Study 2010. Lancet. 2012;380:2197–223.
10. Klompas M. Is a ventilator-associated pneumonia rate of zero really possible? Curr Opin Infect Dis. 2012;25:176–82.
11. Restrepo MI, Anzueto A, Arroliga AC, et al. Economic burden of ventilator-associated pneumonia based on total resource utilization. Infect Control Hosp Epidemiol. 2010;31:509–15.
12. Shahin J, Bielinski M, Guichon C, et al. Suspected ventilator-associated respiratory infection in severely ill patients: a prospective observational study. Crit Care. 2013;17:R251.
13. Melsen, Wilhelmina G Rovers MM, Groenwold RHH, Bergmans, Dennis C J J Camus C, et al. Attributable mortality of ventilator-associated pneumonia: a meta-analysis of individual patient data from randomised prevention studies. Lancet 2013; 13:665–671.
14. Nseir S, Di Pompeo C, Soubrier S, et al. Effect of ventilator-associated tracheobronchitis on outcome in patients without chronic respiratory failure: a case-control study. Crit Care. 2005;9:R238–45.

15. World Health Organization. The burden of health care-associated infection worldwide: a summary 2004. http://www.who.int/gpsc/country_work/summary_20100430_en.pdf

16. Phu VD, Wertheim HFL, Larsson M, et al. Burden of hospital acquired infections and antimicrobial use in Vietnamese adult intensive care units. PLoS One. 2016;11:1–15. https://doi.org/10.1371/journal.pone.0147544.

17. Arabi Y, Al-shirawi N, Memish Z, Anzueto A. Ventilator-associated pneumonia in adults in developing countries: a systematic review. Int J Infec Dis. 2008:505–12.

18. Bammigatti C, Doradla S, Narashimha B, et al. Healthcare associated infections in a resource limited setting. J Clin Diagn Res. 2017;11:5–8.

19. Salgado Yepez E, Bovera MM, Rosenthal VD, et al. Device-associated infection rates, mortality, length of stay and bacterial resistance in intensive care units in Ecuador: International Nosocomial Infection Control Consortium's findings. World J Biol Chem. 2017;8:95.

20. Ray U, Ramasubban S, Chakravarty C, et al. A prospective study of ventilator-associated tracheobronchitis: incidence and etiology in intensive care unit of a tertiary care hospital. Lung India. 2017;34:236–40.

21. Rrt HC, Chen C, Rrt SK, et al. Differences between novel and conventional surveillance paradigms of ventilator-associated pneumonia. Am J Infect Control. 2015;43:133–6.

22. Rosenthal VD, Maki DG, Salomao R, et al. Device-associated nosocomial infections in 55 intensive care units of 8 developing countries. Ann Intern Med. 2006;145:582–91.

23. Schultz MJ, Dunser MW, Dondorp AM, et al. Current challenges in the management of sepsis in ICUs in resource-poor settings and suggestions for the future. Intensive Care Med 2017. doi: https://doi.org/10.1007/s00134-017-4750-z.

24. Schultsz C, Bootsma MCJ, Loan HT, et al. Effects of infection control measures on acquisition of five antimicrobial drug-resistant microorganisms in a tetanus intensive care unit in Vietnam. Intensive Care Med. 2013;39:661–71.

25. Inchai J, Pothirat C, Liwsrisakun C, et al. Ventilator-associated pneumonia: epidemiology and prognostic indicators of 30-day mortality. Jpn J Infect Dis. 2015;68:181–6.

26. Mathai AS, Phillips A, Isaac R. Ventilator-associated pneumonia: a persistent healthcare problem in Indian intensive care units! Lung India. 2016;33:512–6.

27. Blot S, Koulenti D, Dimopoulos G, et al. Prevalence, risk factors, and mortality for ventilator-associated pneumonia in middle-aged, old, and very old critically ill patients*. Crit Care Med. 2014;42:601–9.

28. Loan HT, Parry J, Nga NTN, et al. Semi-recumbent body position fails to prevent healthcare-associated pneumonia in Vietnamese patients with severe tetanus. Trans R Soc Trop Med Hyg. 2012;106:90–7.

29. Centers for Disease Control and Prevention (CDC). Pneumonia (ventilator-associated [VAP] and non-ventilator-associated pneumonia [PNEU]) Event. http://www.cdc.gov/nhsn/pdfs/pscmanual/6pscvapcurrent.pdf

30. Klompas M, Kleinman K, Khan Y, et al. Rapid and reproducible surveillance for ventilator-associated pneumonia. Clin Infect Dis. 2012;54:370–7.

31. Johanson W, Pierce A, Sanford J, Thomas G. Nosocomial respiratory infections with gram-negative bacilli. The significance of colonization of the respiratory tract. Ann Int Med. 1971;77:701–6.

32. Craven DE, Hudcova J, Lei Y, et al. Pre-emptive antibiotic therapy to reduce ventilator-associated pneumonia: " thinking outside the box". Crit Care. 2016;20:300–12.

33. Ramirez P, Lopez-ferraz C, Gordon M, et al. From starting mechanical ventilation to ventilator-associated pneumonia, choosing the right moment to start antibiotic treatment. Crit Care 2017; 1–7. doi: https://doi.org/10.1186/s13054-016-1342-1

34. Spalding MC, Minshall CT. Ventilator-associated pneumonia: new definitions. Crit Care Clin. 2017;33(2):277–92.

35. Klompas M, Berra L. Should ventilator-associated events become a quality indicator for ICUs? Respir Care. 2016;61:723–36.

36. Allegranzi B, Nejad SB, Combescure C, et al. Burden of endemic health-care-associated infection in developing countries: systematic review and meta-analysis. Lancet. 2011;377:228–41.

37. Chastre J, Fagon J-Y. Ventilator-associated pneumonia. Am J Respir Crit Care Med. 2002;165:867–903.

38. WHO (2017) Global priority list of antibiotic-resistant bacteria to guide research, discovery, and development of new antibiotics. http://www.who.int/medicines/publications/WHO-PPL-Short_Summary_25Feb-ET_NM_WHO.pdf

39. Swanson J, Wells D. Empirical antibiotic therapy for ventilator-associated pneumonia. Antibiotics. 2013;2:339–51.

40. Thwaites CL, Lundeg G, Dondorp AM. Recommendations for infection management in patients with sepsis and septic shock in resource-limited settings. Intensive Care Med 2016. doi: https://doi.org/10.1007/s00134-016-4415-3

41. Thwaites CL, Yen LM, Nga NTN, et al. Impact of improved vaccination programme and intensive care facilities on incidence and outcome of tetanus in southern Vietnam, 1993-2002. Trans R Soc Trop Med Hyg. 2004;98:671–7.

# 13

# Risk factors and prognosis of pain events during mechanical ventilation

Ayahiro Yamashita[1], Masaki Yamasaki[1], Hiroki Matsuyama[1,2] and Fumimasa Amaya[1*]

## Abstract

**Background:** Pain assessment is highly recommended in patients receiving mechanical ventilation. However, pain intensity and its impact on outcomes in these patients remain obscure. We collected the results of routine pain assessments, utilizing the behavioral pain scale (BPS), from 151 patients receiving mechanical ventilation. Risk factors associated with a pain event, defined as BPS of >5, and its impact on patient outcomes were investigated.

**Methods:** A total of 151 consecutive adult patients receiving mechanical ventilation for more than 24 h in a single 10-bed ICU were enrolled in this study. The highest BPS within 48 h after the initiation of mechanical ventilation was collected, as well as information about the patients' characteristics and medication received. We also recorded patient outcomes, including time to successful weaning from mechanical ventilation, time to successful ICU discharge, and 30-day in-hospital mortality. Multivariate logistic regression analysis was used to determine factors independently associated with patients with a BPS of >5. Clinical outcomes were also assessed using multivariate logistic regression analysis, correcting for risk factors.

**Results:** We analyzed 151 patients. The median highest BPS was 4. The percentage of patients who recorded a BPS of >5 was 19.9% ($n = 30$). Multivariate logistic regression analysis revealed that the disuse of fentanyl and inotropic support was an independent predictor of pain event. Multivariable Cox regression analysis suggested that the development of a BPS of >5 was associated with increased mortality and a not statistically significant trend towards prolonged mechanical ventilation.

**Conclusions:** A significant proportion of ventilated patients experienced a BPS of >5 soon after the initiation of mechanical ventilation. Disuse of fentanyl and use of inotropic agents increased the risk of developing a BPS of >5 during mechanical ventilation. An association between adequate analgesia and improved patient outcomes provides a rationale for the assessment of pain during mechanical ventilation, with subsequent intervention if necessary.
Pain events were common among ventilated patients. In critical care settings, appropriate and adequate pain management is warranted, given the association with improved patient outcomes.

**Keyword:** Behavioral pain scale, Mechanical ventilation, Risk factors, Prognosis

* Correspondence: ama@koto.kpu-m.ac.jp
[1]Department of Anesthesiology, Kyoto Prefectural University of Medicine, Kajiicho 465, Kamigyo-Ku, Kyoto 602-8566, Japan
Full list of author information is available at the end of the article

## Background

In the critical care setting, routine pain assessment is associated with a decreased use of sedative agents, reduced duration of mechanical ventilation, a lower risk of nosocomial infection and reduced ICU stay [1, 2]. Clinical practice guidelines for the management of pain, agitation, and delirium in adult patients in the ICU (PAD guidelines) [3] recommend the implementation of pain assessment in the intensive care setting. The behavioral pain score (BPS) has been developed to measure the intensity of pain in patients receiving mechanical ventilation [4]. Reliability of the BPS has been demonstrated by the observation of increased scores during painful procedures [5–7].

Pain is considered to be common among critically ill patients [2, 8]. A previous study reported that 40% of ICU patients experienced "pain" defined as a BPS of >5, whereas 16% of ICU patients experienced "severe pain" defined as a BPS of >7 [1]. While there have been several attempts to develop pain treatment algorithms based on the BPS [9], the impact of an elevated BPS on patient outcomes remains unclear.

We hypothesized that pain event occurs within a distinctive subpopulation of patients during mechanical ventilation, and that this event is associated with poor clinical outcomes. To test this hypothesis, we retrospectively analyzed the results of routine BPS measurements during the first 48 h after the initiation of mechanical ventilation as well as patient characteristics. Based on these data, we identified risk factors for increased BPS condition during mechanical ventilation. In addition, we found an association between increased BPS and poor patient outcomes including increased mortality rate, increased duration of mechanical ventilation, and increased duration of ICU stay.

## Methods

This retrospective study was conducted in a 10-bed general ICU of a tertiary referral hospital. The study enrolled consecutive adult patients who received mechanical ventilation for more than 24 h in the ICU between September 2012 and June 2013. Patients were excluded if they were younger than 16 years old, had severe brain injury or quadriplegia, were in a deep coma before the mechanical ventilation, received surgery during the observational period, were treated with muscle relaxants, received noninvasive mechanical ventilation, or if there was any missing data in the patients' records. Approval for data collection was obtained from the hospital's institutional review board.

### ICU management

The patients were sedated with propofol, midazolam, or dexmedetomidine to achieve a Richmond agitation-sedation scale (RASS) score of 0 to −2. The intensivist in charge determined the target RASS level and selected the appropriate sedative regimen for each patient. Infusion rates were regulated by attending nursing staff, based on the observed RASS level. Fentanyl was used to maintain adequate analgesic condition. Adequate analgesic condition was determined by attending nursing staff. Agents were continuously infused intravenously. Protocoled regimens for sedatives/analgesics were determined for each patient. The BPS was recorded every 2–4 h in each patient who received mechanical ventilation. The score was evaluated by attending nurses trained in the use of the BPS. The BPS was evaluated when patients did not undergo any ICU related-procedure, such as tracheal suctioning or mobilization.

Mechanical ventilation was performed utilizing pressure-controlled, synchronized intermittent mandatory ventilation (SIMV) and/or pressure support ventilation (PSV). The fraction of inspired oxygen ($FiO_2$), level of positive end-expiratory pressure (PEEP), and respiratory rate were adjusted to maintain arterial oxygen partial pressure ($PaO_2$) between 80 and 120 mmHg and arterial carbon dioxide partial pressure ($PaCO_2$) between 35 and 50 mmHg. The decision to extubate was made after a trial of spontaneous breathing with low-level pressure support ventilation (7 $cmH_2O$ or less). Hemodynamic management was tailored according to the patient's clinical status, including appropriate volume expansion therapy and treatment with inotropes and/or vasopressors.

### Data collection

The highest BPS within 48 h after initiation of mechanical ventilation was recorded. Data collected included age, gender, body weight, height, surgery (cardiac or non-cardiac), and the acute physiology and chronic health evaluation II (APACHE II) score at admission. In addition, we recorded systolic blood pressure, P/F ratio as well as the use of fentanyl, propofol, dexmedetomidine, midazolam, and any kind of inotropic agents at the time of the highest BPS. Information regarding time to successful weaning from mechanical ventilation, time to successful ICU discharge, and 30-day in-hospital mortality was also collected.

Patients were divided into two groups: a pain event group in which the highest BPS exceeded 5 and a control group in which the highest BPS was 5 or under. A BPS of >5 was determined based on a previous study that defined a BPS of >5 as a "pain event" [1], and the description of a BPS of >5 as an "inadequate state" in the PAD guidelines [3]. In patients with a BPS of >5, the duration for which the BPS was >5 was collected.

The primary aim of our investigation was to determine the frequency and risk factors associated with a BPS of >5. Based on a previous study, we estimated that 40% of our patients would experience a BPS of >5. To ensure an adequate logistic regression analysis for the 6 explanatory variables, we considered that 60 observations would be required. We therefore selected 150 patients as our overall sample size.

### Risk factor assessment

Univariate logistic regression analysis was used to identify parameters associated with pain events in the pain event group. Normality was checked using the Kolmogorov-Smirnov test, while homogeneity of variance was checked by $F$ test. Student's $t$ test, the Welch test, or the Wilcoxon rank-sum test was used for continuous data as appropriate. Chi-square or Fisher's exact test were used for categorical variables. Thereafter, a multivariate logistic regression analysis was used to determine factors independently associated with pain events in the pain event group. Variables were entered into a model when they were associated with pain status. This was based on a univariate logistic regression analysis significance threshold of $p < 0.1$, and when there was no mutual correlation, based on a Spearman's correlation coefficient more than 0.7 or less than −0.7. The final model was constructed utilizing backward elimination of non-significant variables. Odds ratios and 95% confidence intervals (95%CI) were calculated based on the likelihood ratio statistic.

### Clinical outcome assessment

A comparison of the three components of the BPS was performed using Friedman's test followed by Dunn's multiple comparison test. Univariate analysis of clinical outcomes was performed for the time to successful weaning from mechanical ventilation, time to ICU discharge, as well as 30-day in-hospital mortality rate using the log-rank test. In addition to these univariate analyses, clinical outcomes were assessed using multivariate logistic regression analysis, correcting for risk factors that showed at least a trend toward significance ($p < 0.1$) in the univariate analysis. Parameters were checked for linearity, and nonlinear parameters were entered into the model as nominal variables. Odds ratios as well as 95%CI were calculated for the outcomes. All values resulted from two-sided statistical tests, and a $p$ value ≤ 0.05 was considered to be significant. R statistics (R, version 2.15.2) were used to analyze data.

Categorical data was expressed as a number (percentage). Continuous data was expressed with reference to the mean ± standard deviation (SD) or median (IQR), as appropriate.

## Results

During the study period, a total of 177 patients admitted to the ICU received mechanical ventilation for more than 24 h. Twenty-six patients were excluded from the study based on the defined exclusion criteria. We therefore analyzed 151 patients. The mean patient age was 68.5 ± 12.9 years. Overall, 66.9% were male. The median APACHE II score on admission was 19 (5–48). Fentanyl was used in 104 (68.9%) patients. All patients received at least one of the following sedatives: propofol [$n = 89$ (59.6%)], dexmedetomidine [$n = 46$ (30.5%)], and midazolam [$n = 18$ (11.9%)]. Half of the patients received inotropic support [$n = 75$ (49.7%)].

### Incidence and predictors of a BPS of >5 during mechanical ventilation

Figure 1 demonstrates the distribution of the highest BPS within 48 hours after the initiation of mechanical ventilation. The median highest BPS was 4.0 (range, 3.0–5.0). The overall incidence of patients who experienced a BPS of >5 was 19.9% ($n = 30$). The highest BPS was recorded on day 1 in 12.6% ($n = 19$) and on day 2 in 7.3% ($n = 11$) of patients. The median duration of the period in which the BPS was >5 was 2.0 h (range, 1.0–2.3 h). In more than 95% of patients, the BPS value declined to 5 or less at the next BPS measurement. The distribution of the three components of the BPS during the period in which the BPS was >5 is shown in Fig. 2. The score for "facial expression" was significantly higher than that for "compliance with ventilation". The RASS values recorded during the period in which the BPS was >5 are shown in Table 1. In 83.3% of the patients who experienced a BPS of >5, the RASS value was less than 0.

Univariate analysis of the differences in patient characteristics is shown in Table 2. Patients in the pain event group had a lower P/F ratio, a lower frequency of fentanyl use, and a higher frequency of inotropic support. Multivariate logistic regression analysis revealed the

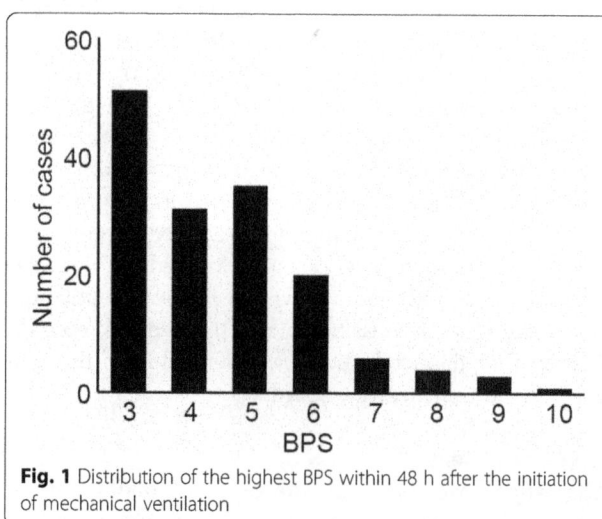

**Fig. 1** Distribution of the highest BPS within 48 h after the initiation of mechanical ventilation

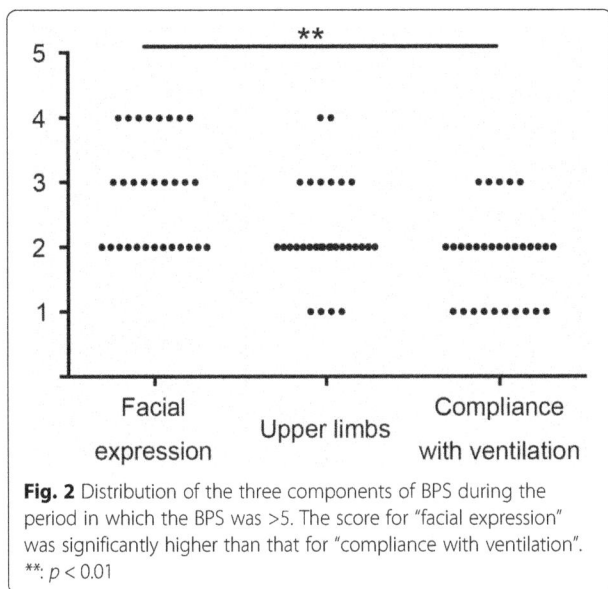

**Fig. 2** Distribution of the three components of BPS during the period in which the BPS was >5. The score for "facial expression" was significantly higher than that for "compliance with ventilation". **\*\***: $p < 0.01$

**Table 2** Univariate analysis of patient characteristics associated with pain event

|  | Pain event group | Control group | p value |
|---|---|---|---|
| Male sex | 21 (70.0) | 81 (66.1) | 0.686 |
| Age | 69.4 ± 10.2 | 68.2 ± 13.6 | 0.674 |
| Height (cm) | 158.0 ± 8.4 | 161.0 ± 10.2 | 0.226 |
| Body Weight (kg) | 55.8 ± 15.3 | 54.1 ± 11.3 | 0.501 |
| Cardiac surgery | 9 (30.0) | 43 (35.5) | 0.19 |
| Non-cardiac surgery | 7 (23.3) | 42 (34.7) | |
| No surgical intervention | 14 (46.7) | 36 (29.8) | |
| APACHE II score | 21.1 ± 9.51 | 19.8 ± 8.86 | 0.488 |
| Blood pressure | 109.0 ± 19.2 | 110.0 ± 19.8 | 0.883 |
| P/F ratio | 211 ± 121 | 272 ± 118 | 0.0123 |
| Fentanyl | 13 (43.3) | 91 (75.2) | <0.001 |
| Inotropic support | 24 (80.0) | 51 (42.1) | <0.001 |
| Propofol | 19 (63.3) | 70 (57.9) | 0.585 |
| Dexmedetomidine | 5 (16.7) | 41 (33.9) | 0.0666 |
| Midazolam | 7 (23.3) | 11 (9.09) | 0.0312 |

disuse of fentanyl (odds ratio = 0.35, 95%CI = 0.14–0.89) and the requirement of inotropic support (odds ratio = 4.74, 95%CI = 1.58–12.50) as independent predictors of the development of a BPS of >5 (Table 3). The mean Concordance Index was 0.789 (range, 0.709–0.869).

### Clinical outcomes of elevated BPS during mechanical ventilation

Figure 3a demonstrates Kaplan-Meier curves of patient outcomes after the initiation of mechanical ventilation. Thirty-day in-hospital mortality rate was 30.0% in the pain event group and 9.9% in the control group. The mortality rate was significantly higher in the pain event group compared to the control group (Fig. 3a, $p = 0.003$). Multivariable Cox regression analysis demonstrated that the pain event group had a 2.59 times greater risk of death, even after adjusting for APACHE II score, P/F ratio, surgical procedure, and the inotropic support and/or midazolam (Table 4). Median duration until successful weaning from mechanical ventilation was 4 days (2–11) in the pain event group and 3 days (2–7) in the control group. The duration of mechanical ventilation was significantly longer in the pain event group compared to the control group (Fig. 3b, $p = 0.046$). There was a non-significant association between the pain event group and a prolonged time to successful weaning from mechanical ventilation, after adjusting for APACHE II score, P/F ratio, surgical procedure, and the use of propofol, dexmedetomidine, and/or midazolam

(Table 4). The median duration of time to ICU discharge was 9 (4–17) days in the pain event group compared to 6 (4–12) days in the control group. Length of ICU stay did not differ between the severe and control groups (Fig. 3c). There was a non-significant association between BPS > 5 condition and duration of time to ICU discharge after adjusting for blood pressure, P/F ratio, surgical procedure, and the use of fentanyl, inotropic agents, propofol, dexmedetomidine, and/or midazolam (Table 4).

### Conclusions

We investigated the pain intensity in 151 patients receiving mechanical ventilation using the BPS. The percentage of patients who experienced a pain event, defined as BPS of >5, was 19.9%. The median duration of the period during which the BPS was >5 was 2 h, suggesting that pain event was not maintained for a long period. Inotropic support and fentanyl disuse were identified as independent risk factors for the development of a pain event. Patients who experienced pain event had a higher risk of in-hospital death and longer duration of ICU stay. An association between a pain event and poor clinical outcomes provides further rationale to support the important role of pain assessment and appropriate

**Table 1** RASS at the highest BPS in the pain event group

| RASS | −4 | −3 | −2 | −1 | 0 | 1 | 2 |
|---|---|---|---|---|---|---|---|
| Number (percentage) | 3 (10.0) | 2 (6.7) | 9(30.0) | 3 (10.0) | 8 (27.7) | 1 (3.3) | 4 (13.3) |

**Table 3** Logistic regression analysis for the pain event group

|  | Odds ratio | 95%CI | p value |
|---|---|---|---|
| Fentanyl | 0.350 | 0.140-0.890 | 0.027 |
| Inotropic support | 4.440 | 1.580-12.50 | 0.005 |

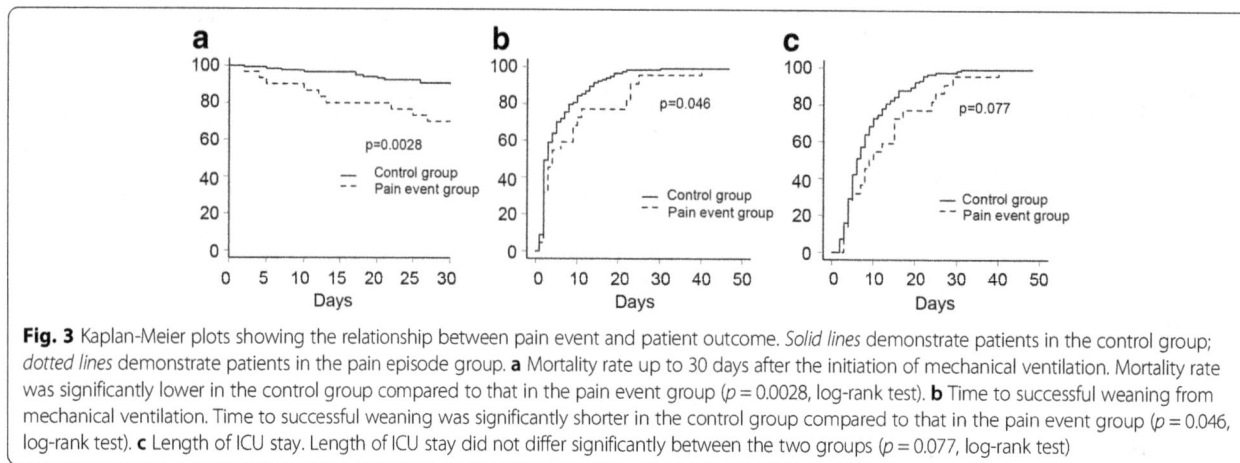

**Fig. 3** Kaplan-Meier plots showing the relationship between pain event and patient outcome. *Solid lines* demonstrate patients in the control group; *dotted lines* demonstrate patients in the pain episode group. **a** Mortality rate up to 30 days after the initiation of mechanical ventilation. Mortality rate was significantly lower in the control group compared to that in the pain event group ($p = 0.0028$, log-rank test). **b** Time to successful weaning from mechanical ventilation. Time to successful weaning was significantly shorter in the control group compared to that in the pain event group ($p = 0.046$, log-rank test). **c** Length of ICU stay. Length of ICU stay did not differ significantly between the two groups ($p = 0.077$, log-rank test)

intervention during mechanical ventilation, as recommended by the PAD guidelines [3].

We limited our observation of the BPS to 48 h after the initiation of mechanical ventilation. This decision was made taking into account the following factors: (1) our preliminary study demonstrated that more than 80% of patients had their highest BPS score recorded within 48 h after receiving mechanical ventilation, (2) early sedation after the initiation of mechanical ventilation is associated with long-term patient outcomes [10], and (3) observation periods exceeding the duration of mechanical ventilation [median = 3 days (2–10)] increases selection bias for the analysis of patient outcomes.

One of the major aims of our study was to document actual pain status during mechanical ventilation. Two evaluation tools, the BPS [4] and critical care pain observation tool (CPOT) [11], are available for evaluating pain intensity in patients who are unable to self-report [5–7]. In our ICU, the BPS is used because the BPS has a validated Japanese language version, but CPOT did not have a validated Japanese version during the observation period of this study, and because the medical staff in our institution are more familiar with the BPS than CPOT. The percentage of patients who experienced BPS > 5 was comparable to previous studies reporting that the incidence of pain during mechanical ventilation varies from 4% [12] to 30% [1]. Together, our results demonstrated that a significant percentage of ventilated patients experience pain at rest. Pain should be treated in a patient who requires critical care [3]. Our results, together with

those of previous reports [1, 8, 12, 13], however, demonstrate the difficulty of removing all minor pain from all critically ill patients. Such pain might be associated with such side effects of analgesic treatment as circulatory collapse, respiratory depression, and bowel movement inhibition.

Subgroup analysis of the three components of the BPS showed that patients experiencing a BPS of >5 typically show a mildly tightened or grimacing facial expression, partially bent upper limbs, and mild incompliance with ventilation and coughing. The wide distribution of RASS values during the period in which the pain event demonstrates that an elevated BPS is not always associated with an elevated RASS.

The presence or absence of surgical intervention did not affect the incidence of the development of pain event in our study, which is consistent with the results of a previous study [8]. Patients who require mechanical ventilation must remain immobilized in bed. Furthermore, they require vascular, urethral, and gastric catheters as well as tracheal tube insertion. All of these factors can be sources of pain or discomfort. In addition to the pain originating from mechanical ventilation, disease-associated pain is also common in both surgical and medical patients [8].

Opioids have been widely used for treating pain during mechanical ventilation [14]. We used fentanyl as a first-line opioid for mechanically ventilated patients and did not use other opioids throughout the study. Our findings demonstrated that the disuse of fentanyl increased the risk of increased BPS during mechanical ventilation. This is in accordance with a previous study showing the effect of opioids on the prevention of procedure-related increases in BPS [15], agitation [16], and reduction of pain intensity scores [17] during mechanical ventilation.

We identified inotropic support as another risk factor for the pain event during mechanical ventilation. It is

**Table 4** Multivariable analysis of clinical outcomes associated with pain event

|  | Hazard ratio | 95%CI | p value |
|---|---|---|---|
| Time to weaning from MV | 0.693 | 0.448–1.072 | 0.099 |
| Length of ICU stay | 0.668 | 0.420–1.061 | 0.087 |
| In-hospital mortality | 2.590 | 1.001–6.704 | 0.049 |

unclear whether the inotropic support has a direct effect on pain scores, or whether patient conditions requiring inotropic support are associated with a higher BPS. The correlation between inotropic support and disuse of fentanyl in this study was low ($r = 0.16$). An experimental animal study revealed that a higher blood catecholamine concentration is associated with increased pain sensitivity via the activation of $\beta$-adrenergic receptors in the peripheral sensory nerves [18].

Increased BPS occurring early after the initiation of mechanical ventilation was associated with lower survival rate. Pain increases sympathetic tone and evokes a stress response in ventilated patients [3]. Tachycardia, increased myocardial oxygen consumption [19], hypercoagulability [20], immunosuppression [21], and catabolism [22], are all associated with pain in critically ill patients and might partly explain the poor prognosis in patients who experienced a BPS of >5.

In our study, patients with pain event tended to be required longer duration of mechanical ventilation. Inadequate pain control is known to reduce patient-ventilator synchrony [23]. Patient-ventilator asynchrony may be a cause of ventilator-associated lung injury and may negatively affect prognosis [24, 25]. Severe pain is also associated with the development of agitation [26]. Agitation in ventilated patients negatively affects outcomes [27].

To the best of our knowledge, this is the first report describing an association between elevated BPS during mechanical ventilation and poor clinical outcomes. It may be worthwhile to investigate, therefore, whether analgesic intervention to prevent elevation of the BPS during mechanical ventilation can improve patient outcomes in a future prospective study.

There are several limitations to this study. This study was conducted in a retrospective manner and may have missed relevant clinically important confounders. Also, the study was conducted in a single ICU in a tertiary referral hospital which may have influenced the study sample. Furthermore, we used BPS instead of a subjective pain scale (such as the numerical rating scale or visual analog scale). Enrolled patients were not limited to those who were diagnosed as ARDS. Furthermore, since we did not routinely use neuromuscular blockade in these patients, those with severe ARDS could not be excluded from this study. Finally, we were not able to determine the exact reason for death.

In conclusion, we found that 20% of ventilated patients experienced a BPS of >5. An elevated BPS was associated with inotropic support and disuse of fentanyl, and was also associated with poor patient outcomes.

**Acknowledgements**
Not applicable.

**Funding**
FA and HM were supported by a Grant-in-Aid from the Japan Society for the Promotion of Science (KAKENHI, No. 15H04969, 26670692 and 26462760).

**Authors' contributions**
AY and HM collected the data. AY and MY performed the statistical analyses. FA designed the study and wrote the manuscript. All authors read and approved the final manuscript.

**Competing interests**
The authors declare that they have no competing interests.

**Author details**
[1]Department of Anesthesiology, Kyoto Prefectural University of Medicine, Kajiicho 465, Kamigyo-Ku, Kyoto 602-8566, Japan. [2]Department of Anesthesia, Japanese Red Cross Kyoto Daiichi Hospital, Kyoto, Japan.

**References**
1. Chanques G, Jaber S, Barbotte E, Violet S, Sebbane M, Perrigault PF, Mann C, Lefrant JY, Eledjam JJ. Impact of systematic evaluation of pain and agitation in an intensive care unit. Crit Care Med. 2006;34:1691–9.
2. Payen JF, Bosson JL, Chanques G, Mantz J, Labarere J, Investigators D. Pain assessment is associated with decreased duration of mechanical ventilation in the intensive care unit: a post hoc analysis of the DOLOREA study. Anesthesiology. 2009;111:1308–16.
3. Barr J, Fraser GL, Puntillo K, Ely EW, Gelinas C, Dasta JF, Davidson JE, Devlin JW, Kress JP, Joffe AM, et al. Clinical practice guidelines for the management of pain, agitation, and delirium in adult patients in the intensive care unit. Crit Care Med. 2013;41:263–306.
4. Payen JF, Bru O, Bosson JL, Lagrasta A, Novel E, Deschaux I, Lavagne P, Jacquot C. Assessing pain in critically ill sedated patients by using a behavioral pain scale. Crit Care Med. 2001;29:2258–63.
5. Ahlers SJ, van der Veen AM, van Dijk M, Tibboel D, Knibbe CA. The use of the behavioral pain scale to assess pain in conscious sedated patients. Anesth Analg. 2010;110:127–33.
6. Rahu MA, Grap MJ, Ferguson P, Joseph P, Sherman S, Elswick Jr RK. Validity and sensitivity of 6 pain scales in critically ill, intubated adults. Am J Crit Care. 2015;24:514–23.
7. Rijkenberg S, Stilma W, Endeman H, Bosman RJ, Oudemans-van Straaten HM. Pain measurement in mechanically ventilated critically ill patients: behavioral pain scale versus critical-care pain observation tool. J Crit Care. 2015;30:167–72.
8. Chanques G, Sebbane M, Barbotte E, Viel E, Eledjam JJ, Jaber S. A prospective study of pain at rest: incidence and characteristics of an unrecognized symptom in surgical and trauma versus medical intensive care unit patients. Anesthesiology. 2007;107:858–60.
9. Olsen BF, Rustoen T, Sandvik L, Miaskowski C, Jacobsen M, Valeberg BT. Development of a pain management algorithm for intensive care units. Heart Lung. 2015;44:521–7.
10. Shehabi Y, Bellomo R, Reade MC, Bailey M, Bass F, Howe B, McArthur C, Seppelt IM, Webb S, Weisbrodt L, et al. Early intensive care sedation predicts long-term mortality in ventilated critically ill patients. Am J Respir Crit Care Med. 2012;186:724–31.
11. Gelinas C, Harel F, Fillion L, Puntillo KA, Johnston CC. Sensitivity and specificity of the critical-care pain observation tool for the detection of pain in intubated adults after cardiac surgery. J Pain Symptom Manage. 2009;37:58–67.

12. Payen JF, Chanques G, Mantz J, Hercule C, Auriant I, Leguillou JL, Binhas M, Genty C, Rolland C, Bosson JL. Current practices in sedation and analgesia for mechanically ventilated critically ill patients: a prospective multicenter patient-based study. Anesthesiology. 2007;106:687–95. quiz 891-682.

13. Chanques G, Payen JF, Mercier G, de Lattre S, Viel E, Jung B, Cisse M, Lefrant JY, Jaber S. Assessing pain in non-intubated critically ill patients unable to self report: an adaptation of the behavioral pain scale. Intensive Care Med. 2009;35:2060–7.

14. Erstad BL, Puntillo K, Gilbert HC, Grap MJ, Li D, Medina J, Mularski RA, Pasero C, Varkey B, Sessler CN. Pain management principles in the critically ill. Chest. 2009;135:1075–86.

15. Robleda G, Roche-Campo F, Sendra MA, Navarro M, Castillo A, Rodriguez-Arias A, Juanes-Borrego E, Gich I, Urrutia G, Nicolas-Arfelis JM, et al. Fentanyl as pre-emptive treatment of pain associated with turning mechanically ventilated patients: a randomized controlled feasibility study. Intensive Care Med. 2016;42:183–91.

16. Muellejans B, Lopez A, Cross MH, Bonome C, Morrison L, Kirkham AJ. Remifentanil versus fentanyl for analgesia based sedation to provide patient comfort in the intensive care unit: a randomized, double-blind controlled trial [ISRCTN43755713]. Crit Care. 2004;8:R1–R11.

17. Egerod I, Jensen MB, Herling SF, Welling KL. Effect of an analgo-sedation protocol for neurointensive patients: a two-phase interventional non-randomized pilot study. Crit Care. 2010;14:R71.

18. Ciszek BP, O'Buckley SC, Nackley AG. Persistent catechol-O-methyltransferase-dependent pain is initiated by peripheral beta-adrenergic receptors. Anesthesiology. 2016;124:1122–35.

19. Lewis KS, Whipple JK, Michael KA, Quebbeman EJ. Effect of analgesic treatment on the physiological consequences of acute pain. Am J Hosp Pharm. 1994;51:1539–54.

20. Tuman KJ, McCarthy RJ, March RJ, DeLaria GA, Patel RV, Ivankovich AD. Effects of epidural anesthesia and analgesia on coagulation and outcome after major vascular surgery. Anesth Analg. 1991;73:696–704.

21. Desborough JP. The stress response to trauma and surgery. Br J Anaesth. 2000;85:109–17.

22. Schricker T, Meterissian S, Wykes L, Eberhart L, Lattermann R, Carli F. Postoperative protein sparing with epidural analgesia and hypocaloric dextrose. Ann Surg. 2004;240:916–21.

23. Richman PS, Baram D, Varela M, Glass PS. Sedation during mechanical ventilation: a trial of benzodiazepine and opiate in combination. Crit Care Med. 2006;34:1395–401.

24. Gogineni VK, Brimeyer R, Modrykamien A. Patterns of patient-ventilator asynchrony as predictors of prolonged mechanical ventilation. Anaesth Intensive Care. 2012;40:964–70.

25. Thille AW, Rodriguez P, Cabello B, Lellouche F, Brochard L. Patient-ventilator asynchrony during assisted mechanical ventilation. Intensive Care Med. 2006;32:1515–22.

26. Bennett S, Hurford WE. When should sedation or neuromuscular blockade be used during mechanical ventilation? Respir Care. 2011;56:168–76. discussion 176-180.

27. Woods JC, Mion LC, Connor JT, Viray F, Jahan L, Huber C, McHugh R, Gonzales JP, Stoller JK, Arroliga AC. Severe agitation among ventilated medical intensive care unit patients: frequency, characteristics and outcomes. Intensive Care Med. 2004;30:1066–72.

# 14

# Augmented renal clearance in Japanese intensive care unit patients

Yasumasa Kawano[*], Shinichi Morimoto, Yoshito Izutani, Kentaro Muranishi, Hironari Kaneyama, Kota Hoshino, Takeshi Nishida and Hiroyasu Ishikura

## Abstract

**Background:** Augmented renal clearance (ARC) of circulating solutes and drugs has been recently often reported in intensive care unit (ICU) patients. However, only few studies on ARC have been reported in Japan. The aims of this pilot study were to determine the prevalence and risk factors for ARC in Japanese ICU patients with normal serum creatinine levels and to evaluate the association between ARC and estimated glomerular filtration rate (eGFR) calculated using the Japanese equation.

**Methods:** We conducted a prospective observational study from May 2015 to April 2016 at the emergency ICU of a tertiary university hospital; 111 patients were enrolled (mean age, 67 years; interquartile range, 53–77 years). We measured 8-h creatinine clearance ($CL_{CR}$) within 24 h after admission, and ARC was defined as body surface area-adjusted $CL_{CR} \geq 130$ mL/min/1.73 m$^2$. Multiple logistic regression analysis was performed to identify the risk factors for ARC. Moreover, a receiver operating curve (ROC) analysis, including area under the receiver operating curve (AUROC) was performed to examine eGFR accuracy and other significant variables in predicting ARC.

**Results:** In total, 43 patients (38.7 %) manifested ARC. Multiple logistic regression analysis was performed for age, body weight, body height, history of diabetes mellitus, Acute Physiology and Chronic Health Evaluation II scores, admission categories of post-operative patients without sepsis and trauma, and serum albumin, and only age was identified as an independent risk factor for ARC (odds ratio, 0.95; 95 % confidence interval [CI], 0.91–0.98). Moreover, the AUROC of ARC for age and eGFR was 0.81 (95 % CI, 0.72–0.89) and 0.81 (95 % CI, 0.73–0.89), respectively. The optimal cutoff values for detecting ARC were age and eGFR of ≤63 years (sensitivity, 72.1 %; specificity, 82.4 %) and ≥76 mL/min/1.73 m$^2$ (sensitivity, 81.4 %; specificity, 72.1 %), respectively.

**Conclusions:** ARC is common in Japanese ICU patients, and age was an independent risk factor for ARC. In addition, age and eGFR calculated using the Japanese equation were suggested to be useful screening tools for identifying Japanese patients with ARC.

**Keywords:** Augmented renal clearance, Intensive care unit, Japan, Risk factor, eGFR

* Correspondence: kawano0301@cis.fukuoka-u.ac.jp
Department of Emergency and Critical Care Medicine, Fukuoka University Hospital, Faculty of Medicine, 7-45-1 Nanakuma, Jonan-ku, Fukuoka 8140180, Japan

## Background

Clinicians often modify drug prescriptions to a patient's glomerular filtration rate (GFR) because renal clearance influences the pharmacokinetics of many commonly prescribed agents [1]. Intensive care unit (ICU) patients in a critical condition with severe morbidity sometimes experience acute kidney injury (AKI) [2]. Clinicians usually reduce drug doses to prevent drug toxicity because drug elimination is impaired in these patients [3]. In contrast, recent studies [1, 4] reported that the phenomenon of increased renal blood flow due to an increased cardiac output might lead to an augmented renal clearance (ARC) of circulating solutes and drugs. Although creatinine clearance ($CL_{CR}$) is not a gold standard measurement of GFR (such as inulin clearance), a close correlation was found between the ARC phenomenon and $CL_{CR}$ [5, 6], and ARC phenomenon is characterized by $CL_{CR} \geq 130$ mL/min/1.73 m$^2$ [7]. ARC is potentially related to insufficient treatment and poor prognosis due to sub-therapeutic drug concentrations particularly in critically ill patients [5, 6, 8, 9]; therefore, ARC should be recognized in the ICU setting. However, ARC may occur in patients with normal serum creatinine ($S_{Cr}$) level [10, 11], and $CL_{CR}$ measurement is not routinely performed in the ICU for daily treatments; the accurate recognition of this phenomenon is difficult for clinicians. For this reason, previous studies [12, 13] verified the correlation between ARC and estimated glomerular filtration rate (eGFR), which was calculated using various formulas (such as Cockcroft–Gault equation [14], Modification of Diet in Renal Disease [MDRD] Study equation [15], Robert equation [16], and the Chronic Kidney Disease Epidemiology Collaboration [CKD-EPI] equation [17]) used in clinical practice worldwide. In contrast, few studies and discussions regarding ARC in Japan have been reported. To the best of our knowledge, no study has been reported on the correlation between ARC and eGFR calculated using the Japanese eGFR equation, which is used throughout Japan [18]. The aims of this pilot study were to determine the prevalence and risk factors for ARC in Japanese ICU patients with normal $S_{Cr}$ levels and to evaluate the association between ARC and eGFR calculated using the Japanese equation.

## Methods

### Setting

This prospective, single-center, observational study was conducted in a 32-bed emergency ICU of the Fukuoka University Hospital, a tertiary hospital in Japan, from May 2015 to April 2016. This study was approved by the institutional ethics committee (number 15-4-07), and informed consent was obtained from all participants or a surrogate decision maker.

### Study population

Patients who were expected to stay more than 24 h, with no evidence of renal impairment (admission $S_{Cr} > 1.1$ mg/dL) and no history of renal replacement therapy were enrolled. The exclusion criteria for study admission were as follows: age < 18 years, pregnancy, suspicion of rhabdomyolysis or admission $S_{Cr}$ kinase concentration >5000 IU/L, diagnosis of cardiopulmonary arrest on admission, and developing AKI as defined by the Risk, Injury, Failure, Loss of kidney function, End-Stage Kidney Disease criteria [19]. Moreover, patients treated without both an intra-arterial cannula, and an indwelling urinary catheter (IDC) were also excluded. In total, 111 patients were enrolled.

### Data collection and definition

Demographic and laboratory data, including age, sex, body measurements, cumulative number of systemic inflammatory response syndrome (SIRS) [20], medical history of diabetes mellitus, and the levels of serum albumin and blood glucose were recorded on admission. Information regarding ventilation variables, vasopressor or inotrope administration, diuretic use, and admission diagnosis was recorded after the first 24 h. In addition, the patients were divided into the following four groups based on the diagnosis on admission: sepsis, post-operative patients without sepsis, trauma (divided based on severity, injury severity score [ISS] $\geq 16$ or ISS < 16), and others.

Physiological and laboratory data needed to calculate the Acute Physiology and Chronic Health Evaluation (APACHE) II scores and Sequential Organ Failure Assessment (SOFA) scores were reported as the worst value within 24 h after hospital admission. The mean urine output (mL/kg/h) and fluid balance were recorded during the first hospital day. Because previous reports [21, 22] suggest that renal function can be measured most accurately using an 8-, 12-, or 24-h $CL_{CR}$ collection, the 8-h $CL_{CR}$ was measured in this study. Urinary volume was measured from the IDC within the first 24 h of admission, and the blood sampling for eGFR and $CL_{CR}$ measurement were performed simultaneously after the completion of the 8-h $CL_{CR}$ collection. The urinary creatinine ($U_{Cr}$) level and the $S_{Cr}$ were determined by laboratory analysis by using an enzymatic method.

We calculated eGFR by using a three-variable Japanese equation [18].

For males: eGFR (mL/min/1.73 m$^2$) = 194 × $[S_{Cr}$(mg/dL)$]^{-1.094}$ × age$^{-0.287}$

For females: eGFR (mL/min/1.73 m$^2$) = 194 × $[S_{Cr}$(mg/dL)$]^{-1.094}$ × age$^{-0.287}$ × 0.739

The $CL_{CR}$ was calculated by using the standard formula. $CL_{CR}$ values were subsequently normalized to a body surface area (BSA) of 1.73 m$^2$ as per convention.

$CL_{CR}$ and BSA were calculated based on the following formulae:

$$CL_{CR}(mL/min/1.73\ m^2) = [U_{Cr}\,(mg/dL)/S_{Cr}(mg/dL)$$
$$\times\ 8\text{-h urinary volume}(mL)/480$$
$$\times\ 1.73/BSA(m^2)]$$

$$BSA(m^2) = 0.007184 \times [\text{height (cm)}]^{0.725}$$
$$\times\ [\text{weight (kg)}]^{0.425}$$

Data collection began immediately after obtaining an informed consent and was discontinued at ICU discharge or death, development of severe renal impairment (measured $CL_{CR} < 30$ mL/min/1.73 m$^2$), initiation of renal replacement therapy, intra-arterial cannula or IDC removal, and patient consent withdrawal. ARC was defined as an 8-h $CL_{CR} \geq 130$ mL/min/1.73 m$^2$ [7].

## Statistical analysis

Continuous data were expressed as mean (standard deviation [SD]) or median (interquartile range [IQR]), and categorical data as percentage. The Student $t$ test or Mann–Whitney $U$ test and chi-square test were used for continuous and categorical data, respectively. Multiple logistic regression analysis was performed to identify the risk factors for ARC. Because serum albumin levels and diabetic conditions were shown to influence tubular creatinine secretion [23, 24], these factors were included as explanatory variables in multivariate analysis. Furthermore, the explanatory variables in this analysis were also determined from any variables with a $p$ value of less than 0.05 in the univariate analysis. The odds ratio (OR) and 95 % confidence interval (CI) were calculated. The correlations between the measured $CL_{CR}$ and eGFR were assessed by using Spearman correlation coefficient ($r$), and the Bland and Altman method [25] was used to

**Table 1** Demographic and laboratory data

| Variable | All patients ($n = 111$) | Patients with ARC ($n = 43$) | Patients without ARC ($n = 68$) | $p$ value[a] |
|---|---|---|---|---|
| Age, median (IQR) | 67 (53–77) | 55 (38–65) | 72 (66–79) | <0.05 |
| Male sex, $n$ (%) | 62 (55.9) | 22 (51.2) | 40 (58.8) | 0.44 |
| Body weight (kg), median (IQR) | 56.3 (49.9–68.2) | 60.7 (52.8–74.1) | 53.2 (47.9–62.5) | <0.05 |
| Body height (m), mean (SD) | 1.61 (0.1) | 1.64 (0.1) | 1.59 (0.09) | <0.05 |
| Body mass index (kg/m$^2$), mean (SD) | 22.7 (3.88) | 23.6 (3.75) | 22.1 (3.87) | <0.05 |
| Body surface area (m$^2$), median (IQR) | 1.57 (1.46–1.79) | 1.67 (1.54–1.85) | 1.55 (1.41–1.69) | <0.05 |
| Diabetes mellitus, $n$ (%) | 22 (19.8) | 5 (11.6) | 17 (25) | 0.09 |
| Mechanical ventilation, $n$ (%) | 21 (18.9) | 6 (14) | 15 (22.4) | 0.33 |
| Vasopressor, $n$ (%) | 2 (1.8) | 0 | 2 (2.9) | 0.52 |
| Inotrope, $n$ (%) | 8 (7.2) | 2 (4.6) | 6 (8.8) | 0.48 |
| Diuretic therapy, $n$ (%) | 6 (5.4) | 1 (2.3) | 5 (7.4) | 0.4 |
| APACHE II scores, median (IQR) | 14 (10.5–19.5) | 13 (8.5–15.5) | 16 (11.8–23) | <0.05 |
| SOFA scores, median (IQR) | 3 (2–5) | 3 (2–4) | 3 (2–5) | 0.33 |
| The cumulative number of SIRS, median (IQR) | 1 (1–2) | 1 (1–2) | 1 (1–2) | 0.96 |
| Admission category, $n$ (%) | | | | |
| Sepsis[b] | 3 (2.7) | 0 | 3 (4.4) | 0.28 |
| Post-operative patients without sepsis | 25 (22.5) | 4 (9.3) | 21 (30.9) | <0.05 |
| Trauma | 32 (28.8) | 20 (46.5) | 12 (17.6) | <0.05 |
| ISS $\geq$ 16 | 19 | 10 | 9 | |
| ISS < 16 | 13 | 10 | 3 | |
| Others | 51 (45.9) | 19 (44.2) | 32 (47.1) | 0.85 |
| Serum albumin (g/dL), median (IQR) | 3.9 (3.4–4.3) | 4.2 (3.7–4.4) | 3.8 (3.2–4.2) | <0.05 |
| Blood glucose (mg/dL), median (IQR) | 136 (115–160) | 128 (111–150) | 141 (118–168) | 0.12 |
| Mean urine output (mL/kg/h), median (IQR) | 0.92 (0.64–1.36) | 0.94 (0.7–1.4) | 0.77 (0.6–1.35) | 0.29 |
| Fluid balance (mL), median (IQR) | 739 (55.5–1290) | 993 (−70–1460) | 572 (81.3–1125) | 0.33 |

*ARC* augmented renal clearance, *IQR* interquartile range, *SD* standard deviation, *APACHE* Acute Physiology and Chronic Health Evaluation, *SOFA* Sequential Organ Failure Assessment, *SIRS* systemic inflammatory response syndrome, *ISS* injury severity score

[a] The $p$ values were evaluated by comparison between patients with and without ARC

[b] Sepsis was diagnosed based on evidence of infection along with the presence of SIRS

**Table 2** Multiple logistic regression analysis for augmented renal clearance

| Variables | OR (95 % CI) | p value |
|---|---|---|
| Age | 0.95 (0.91–0.98) | <0.05 |
| Body weight | 1.03 (0.98–1.09) | 0.25 |
| Body height | 0.96 (0.89–1.02) | 0.21 |
| Diabetes mellitus | 0.73 (0.20–2.73) | 0.64 |
| APACHE II scores | 0.95 (0.88–1.03) | 0.24 |
| Post-operative patients without sepsis | 0.28 (0.07–1.04) | 0.06 |
| Trauma | 1.83 (0.60–5.59) | 0.29 |
| Serum albumin | 1.36 (0.63–2.93) | 0.44 |

OR odds ratio, CI confidence interval, APACHE Acute Physiology and Chronic Health Evaluation

check the bias and limits of agreement between the measured $CL_{CR}$ and eGFR. Bias was defined as the mean difference between eGFR and measured $CL_{CR}$. The 95 % limits of agreement were calculated as the bias ±1.96 SD. Moreover, a receiver operating curve (ROC) analysis, including the area under the receiver operating curve (AUROC), was performed to examine the accuracy of the eGFR and other significant variables in predicting ARC. The ROC was plotted for each score by using sensitivity and specificity values for true prediction of ARC across the entire range of potential cutoff values to predict ARC. The AUROC was constructed and compared as described in a previous report [26]. All tests were two-tailed, and a $p$ value of <0.05 was considered statistically significant.

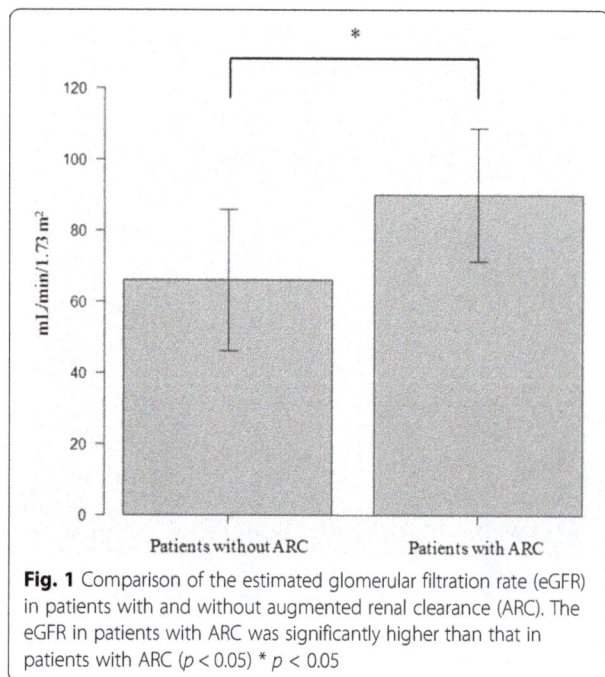

**Fig. 1** Comparison of the estimated glomerular filtration rate (eGFR) in patients with and without augmented renal clearance (ARC). The eGFR in patients with ARC was significantly higher than that in patients with ARC ($p < 0.05$) * $p < 0.05$

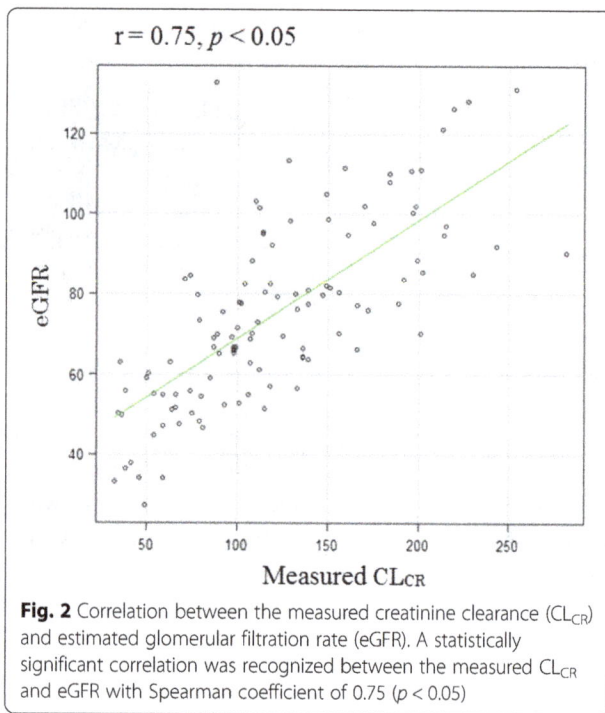

**Fig. 2** Correlation between the measured creatinine clearance ($CL_{CR}$) and estimated glomerular filtration rate (eGFR). A statistically significant correlation was recognized between the measured $CL_{CR}$ and eGFR with Spearman coefficient of 0.75 ($p < 0.05$)

All statistical analyses were performed by using the EZR software program (Saitama Medical Center, Jichi Medical University, Saitama, Japan) [27], which is a graphical user interface for the R software program (The R Foundation for Statistical Computing, Vienna, Austria). More precisely, it is a modified version of R commander, which was designed to add statistical functions frequently used in biostatistics.

## Results

### Baselines characteristics of study subjects

The characteristics of the enrolled patients are shown in Table 1.

We enrolled 111 patients in this study (mean age, 67 years [IQR, 53–77 years], 55.9 % male). Of these, 43 patients (38.7 %) were identified as manifesting ARC. In addition, ARC occurred more frequently in trauma patients (20/32, 62.5 %) and less frequently in post-operative patients without sepsis (4/25, 16.0 %), in comparison with the overall incidence of 38.7 % (43/111). The mean APACHE II score was 14 (IQR, 10.5–19.5), and the mean SOFA score was 3 (IQR, 2–5). Vasopressor and diuretic therapies were administered to a few patients in this study. Moreover, few patients had an admission diagnosis of sepsis (2.7 %), and only 59.4 % (19/32) were categorized as severe trauma patients (ISS ≥ 16).

### Risk factors for ARC

The following variables were significantly different between patients with and without ARC: age, body weight,

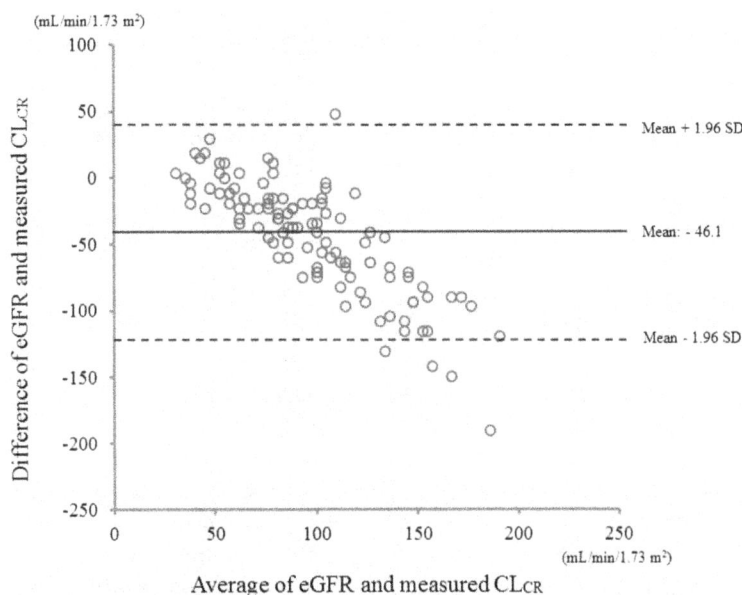

**Fig. 3** Measures of agreement between the measured creatinine clearance ($CL_{CR}$) and estimated glomerular filtration rate (eGFR). The *solid line* indicates the mean of the difference between the results of the eGFR and measured $CL_{CR}$. The *dashed line* shows the 95 % limits of agreement. Most parts of eGFR tended to underestimate the $CL_{CR}$. In addition, the difference between the eGFR and measured $CL_{CR}$ further increased when the kidney function of the patients improved

body height, body mass index, BSA, APACHE II scores, admission categories of post-operative patients without sepsis and trauma, and serum albumin (all $p < 0.05$). Multiple logistic regression analysis was performed for eight variables (such as age, body weight, body height, history of diabetes mellitus, APACHE II scores, admission categories of post-operative patients without sepsis and trauma, and serum albumin), and the result showed that only age is an independent risk factor for ARC (OR, 0.95; 95 % CI, 0.91–0.98) (Table 2).

**Evaluation of eGFR calculated using the Japanese equation**
Analysis to determine the correlation between ARC and eGFR revealed that the eGFR of patients with ARC was significantly higher than that of patients without ARC ($p < 0.05$) (Fig. 1). Moreover, a statistically significant correlation was found between measured $CL_{CR}$ and eGFR, with a Spearman coefficient ($r$) of 0.75 ($p < 0.05$) (Fig. 2). In contrast, the Bland–Altman plots showed that the bias of the two variables was –46.1 mL/min/1.73 m$^2$, and the 95 % limits of agreement were –128.9 to 36.7 mL/min/1.73 m$^2$.

Most parts of the eGFR tended to underestimate $CL_{CR}$. In addition, the difference between eGFR and measured $CL_{CR}$ further increased when the kidney function of the patients improved (Fig. 3).

**Prognostic value for ARC**
We performed the ROC analysis to evaluate the prognostic value of age and eGFR for ARC. The AUROC of age and eGFR was 0.81 (95 % CI, 0.72–0.89) and 0.81 (95 % CI, 0.73–0.89), respectively. The optimal cutoff value of each factor for ARC was age ≤63 years (sensitivity, 72.1 %; specificity, 82.4 %) and eGFR ≥ 76 mL/min/1.73 m$^2$ (sensitivity, 81.4 %; specificity, 72.1 %) (Table 3).

**Discussion**
To the best of our knowledge, this is the first study that investigated ARC in Japanese adult ICU patients. Our results demonstrate that approximately 40 % of patients who were admitted to our ICU with normal $S_{Cr}$ levels on the first hospital day manifested ARC, which was similar to a previous report [3]. Age was identified as an independent risk factor for ARC in multivariate logistic regression analysis in this study, and several previous

**Table 3** Augmented renal clearance prediction of age and estimated glomerular filtration rate using the receiver operating curves

| | AUROC | 95 % CI | Optimal cutoff values | Sensitivity (%) | Specificity (%) | PPV (%) | NPV (%) |
|---|---|---|---|---|---|---|---|
| Age (years) | 0.81 | 0.72–0.89 | 63 | 72.1 | 82.4 | 80.4 | 74.7 |
| eGFR (mL/min/1.73 m$^2$) | 0.81 | 0.73–0.89 | 76 | 81.4 | 72.1 | 74.5 | 79.5 |

*eGFR* estimated glomerular filtration rate, *AUROC* area under the receiver operating curve, *CI* confidence interval, *PPV* positive predictive value, *NPV* negative predictive value

studies [3, 12] have also shown that ARC is more common in younger patients.

In contrast, no relationship was found between urine output and ARC phenomenon, and the same trend on fluid balance was also shown in this report. We demonstrated that the ARC phenomenon was not simply related to ongoing fluid loading, and a previous study supported this statement [3]. Moreover, with regard to illness severity score, patients with ARC had significantly lower APACHE II scores on admission compared with patients without ARC in the univariate analysis. In contrast, we did not observe the same trend in SOFA scores. The result of the multivariate analysis showed that the different trends in the two severity scores could have been due to the influence of age. The APACHE II score evaluates the illness severity of patients based on physiologic measurements, age, and previous health status [28], whereas the SOFA score was assessed by grading organ dysfunction, not by age [29]. ARC was seen in the younger population; therefore, patients with ARC tend to obtain lower APACHE II scores compared with those of patients without ARC.

Previous studies [12, 30] showed that multi-trauma was a significant risk factor for ARC, but these findings were different from our results. The difference in these findings is likely related to the small sample of patients with severe trauma (only 19 patients) in this single-center study.

The eGFR in this report, which was calculated by using the Japanese equation, was significantly different between patients with and without ARC, and the correlations better represented the true relationship between the measured $CL_{CR}$ and eGFR, with a Spearman coefficient ($r$) of more than 0.7. Although a better correlation was recognized between these variables in this study, eGFR could not detect patients with ARC accurately; eGFR was not considered for ICU patients with severe conditions that influenced renal function because eGFR was principally designed for use in an ambulatory or ward-based setting initially [31, 32]. Therefore, previous reports [12, 13] showed that the derived values from several formulae (Cockcroft–Gault and MDRD) significantly underestimated the $CL_{CR}$, and no eGFR formula accurately identifies ARC in critically ill patients. However, given the better correlation between the measured $CL_{CR}$ and eGFR calculated using the Japanese equation, this study showed that eGFR might be a useful tool for screening Japanese patients with ARC. Because eGFR tended to underestimate the $CL_{CR}$ as shown in the Bland–Altman plots, the eGFR cutoff values for screening ARC were ≥76 mL/min/1.73 m$^2$, which was lower than 130 mL/min/1.73 m$^2$. In addition, age ≤63 years could also be evaluated for screening simultaneously. After screening patients with ARC, the $CL_{CR}$ should be measured through urine collection formally for modifying the drug dosage as necessary.

This study has some limitations. First, this was a single-center study including a limited number of study participants. Second, this study was not designed to assess ARC after the second hospital day. Although ARC on the first hospital day was strongly associated with higher clearances over a few days, ARC occurring after the second hospital day has been reported [3]. Third, the gold standard for the assessment of renal function is measurement of the urinary or plasma clearance of an ideal filtration marker (such as inulin) [33], but this measurement was not performed in this study. Fourth, because we did not evaluate eGFR, which was calculated by using various formulas (such as Cockcroft–Gault, MDRD, Robert, and CKD-EPI) used worldwide, for identifying ARC in the present study, the best equation for eGFR to identify Japanese patients with ARC is unclear. Fifth, although the creatinine levels were determined by an enzymatic method in the present study, the creatinine levels were determined by other methods such as the Jaffe method in a previous study, which was cited for the present ARC definition. The creatinine levels in serum and urine by the Jaffe method are higher than those by the enzyme method, and $CL_{CR}$ values are affected by these measurement methods [34]. Thus, ARC definition might need to be changed based on the measurement method for creatinine levels. Finally, because this report is a pilot study for ARC in the Japanese population, a validation of the predictive factors for ARC (such as age and eGFR) was not performed. Therefore, further studies are needed to address the limitations of this study.

## Conclusions

This study showed that ARC appeared to be common in Japanese ICU patients with normal $S_{Cr}$ levels on the first hospital day, and only age was an independent risk factor for ARC. In addition, not only age but also eGFR calculated using the Japanese equation might be useful as a screening tool for identifying Japanese patients with ARC. Further multicentre studies are needed to obtain precise data regarding ARC in the Japanese population.

**Abbreviations**
AKI: Acute kidney injury; APACHE: Acute Physiology and Chronic Health Evaluation; ARC: Augmented renal clearance; AUROC: Area under the receiver operating curve; BSA: Body surface area; CI: Confidence interval; $CL_{CR}$: Creatinine clearance; eGFR: Estimated glomerular filtration rate; GFR: Glomerular filtration rate; ICU: Intensive care unit; IDC: Indwelling urinary catheter; IQR: Interquartile range; ISS: Injury severity score; MDRD: Modification of Diet in Renal Disease; OR: Odds ratio; ROC: Receiver operating curve; $S_{Cr}$: Serum creatinine; SD: Standard deviation; SIRS: Systemic inflammatory response syndrome; SOFA: Sequential Organ Failure Assessment; $U_{Cr}$: Urinary creatinine

**Acknowledgements**
We sincerely thank Ms. Kanae Misumi of the Department of Emergency and Critical Care Medicine, Faculty of Medicine, Fukuoka University for her help in data encoding.

## Funding
None.

## Authors' contributions
YK drafted the manuscript, participated in the study design, and performed the statistical analysis. SM, YI, KM, HK, KH, TN, and HI helped draft the manuscript. All authors read and approved the final manuscript.

## Competing interests
The authors declare that they have no competing interests.

## References
1. Udy AA, Roberts JA, Boots RJ, Paterson DL, Lipman J. Augmented renal clearance: implications for antibacterial dosing in the critically ill. Clin Pharmacokinet. 2010; 49:1–16.
2. Doi K, Katagiri D, Negishi K, Hasegawa S, Hamasaki Y, Fujita T, et al. Mild elevation of urinary biomarkers in prerenal acute kidney injury. Kidney Int. 2012;82:1114–20.
3. Udy AA, Baptista JP, Lim NL, Joynt GM, Jarrett P, Wockner L, et al. Augmented renal clearance in the ICU: results of a multicenter observational study of renal function in critically ill patients with normal plasma creatinine concentrations*. Crit Care Med. 2014;42:520–7.
4. Roberts JA, Lipman J. Pharmacokinetic issues for antibiotics in the critically ill patient. Crit Care Med. 2009;37:840–51. quiz 859.
5. Conil JM, Georges B, Mimoz O, Dieye E, Ruiz S, Cougot P, et al. Influence of renal function on trough serum concentrations of piperacillin in intensive care unit patients. Intensive Care Med. 2006;32:2063–6.
6. Lipman J, Wallis SC, Boots RJ. Cefepime versus cefpirome: the importance of creatinine clearance. Anesth Analg. 2003;97:1149–54.
7. Udy AA, Varghese JM, Altukroni M, Briscoe S, McWhinney BC, Ungerer JP, et al. Subtherapeutic initial beta-lactam concentrations in select critically ill patients: association between augmented renal clearance and low trough drug concentrations. Chest. 2012;142:30–9.
8. Fuster-Lluch O, Geronimo-Pardo M, Peyro-Garcia R, Lizan-Garcia M. Glomerular hyperfiltration and albuminuria in critically ill patients. Anaesth Intensive Care. 2008;36:674–80.
9. Udy A, Boots R, Senthuran S, Stuart J, Deans R, Lassig-Smith M, et al. Augmented creatinine clearance in traumatic brain injury. Anesth Analg. 2010;111:1505–10.
10. Lipman J, Gous AG, Mathivha LR, Tshukotsoane S, Scribante J, Hon H, et al. Ciprofloxacin pharmacokinetic profiles in paediatric sepsis: how much ciprofloxacin is enough? Intensive Care Med. 2002;28:493–500.
11. Udy AA, Putt MT, Shanmugathasan S, Roberts JA, Lipman J. Augmented renal clearance in the intensive care unit: an illustrative case series. Int J Antimicrob Agents. 2010;35:606–8.
12. Ruiz S, Minville V, Asehnoune K, Virtos M, George B, Fourcade O, et al. Screening of patients with augmented renal clearance in ICU: taking into account the CKD-EPI equation, the age, and the cause of admission. Ann Intensive Care. 2015;5:49.
13. Baptista JP, Udy AA, Sousa E, Pimentel J, Wang L, Roberts JA, et al. A comparison of estimates of glomerular filtration in critically ill patients with augmented renal clearance. Crit Care. 2011;15:R139.
14. Cockcroft DW, Gault MH. Prediction of creatinine clearance from serum creatinine. Nephron. 1976;16:31–41.
15. Levey AS, Bosch JP, Lewis JB, Greene T, Rogers N, Roth D. A more accurate method to estimate glomerular filtration rate from serum creatinine: a new prediction equation. Modification of Diet in Renal Disease Study Group. Ann Intern Med. 1999;130:461–70.
16. Robert S, Zarowitz BJ, Peterson EL, Dumler F. Predictability of creatinine clearance estimates in critically ill patients. Crit Care Med. 1993;21:1487–95.
17. Levey AS, Stevens LA, Schmid CH, Zhang YL, Castro 3rd AF, Feldman HI, et al. A new equation to estimate glomerular filtration rate. Ann Intern Med. 2009;150:604–12.
18. Matsuo S, Imai E, Horio M, Yasuda Y, Tomita K, Nitta K, et al. Revised equations for estimated GFR from serum creatinine in Japan. Am J Kidney Dis. 2009;53:982–92.
19. Bellomo R, Ronco C, Kellum JA, Mehta RL, Palevsky P. Acute renal failure—definition, outcome measures, animal models, fluid therapy and information technology needs: the Second International Consensus Conference of the Acute Dialysis Quality Initiative (ADQI) Group. Crit Care. 2004;8:R204–12.
20. American College of Chest Physicians/Society of Critical Care Medicine Consensus Conference: definitions for sepsis and organ failure and guidelines for the use of innovative therapies in sepsis. Crit Care Med. 1992;20:864–74.
21. Pong S, Seto W, Abdolell M, Trope A, Wong K, Herridge J, et al. 12-hour versus 24-hour creatinine clearance in critically ill pediatric patients. Pediatr Res. 2005;58:83–8.
22. Wells M, Lipman J. Measurements of glomerular filtration in the intensive care unit are only a rough guide to renal function. S Afr J Surg. 1997;35:20–3.
23. Branten AJ, Vervoort G, Wetzels JF. Serum creatinine is a poor marker of GFR in nephrotic syndrome. Nephrol Dial Transplant. 2005;20:707–11.
24. Nakatani S, Ishimura E, Naganuma T, et al. Poor glycemic control and decreased renal function are associated with increased intrarenal RAS activity in type 2 diabetes mellitus. Diabetes Res Clin Pract. 2014;105:40–6.
25. Bland JM, Altman DG. Statistical methods for assessing agreement between two methods of clinical measurement. Lancet. 1986;1:307–10.
26. Hanley JA, McNeil BJ. The meaning and use of the area under a receiver operating characteristic (ROC) curve. Radiology. 1982;143:29–36.
27. Kanda Y. Investigation of the freely available easy-to-use software 'EZR' for medical statistics. Bone Marrow Transplant. 2013;48:452–8.
28. Knaus WA, Draper EA, Wagner DP, Zimmerman JE. APACHE II: a severity of disease classification system. Crit Care Med. 1985;13:818–29.
29. Vincent JL, Moreno R, Takala J, Willatts S, De Mendonca A, Bruining H, et al. The SOFA (Sepsis-related Organ Failure Assessment) score to describe organ dysfunction/failure. On behalf of the Working Group on Sepsis-Related Problems of the European Society of Intensive Care Medicine. Intensive Care Med. 1996;22:707–10.
30. Minville V, Asehnoune K, Ruiz S, Breden A, Georges B, Sequin T, et al. Increased creatinine clearance in polytrauma patients with normal serum creatinine: a retrospective observational study. Crit Care. 2011;15:R49.
31. Martin JH, Fay MF, Udy A, Roberts J, Kirkpatrick C, Ungerer J, et al. Pitfalls of using estimations of glomerular filtration rate in an intensive care population. Intern Med J. 2011;41:537–43.
32. Schetz M, Gunst J, Van den Berghe G. The impact of using estimated GFR versus creatinine clearance on the evaluation of recovery from acute kidney injury in the ICU. Intensive Care Med. 2014;40:1709–17.
33. Stevens LA, Coresh J, Greene T, Levey AS. Assessing kidney function—measured and estimated glomerular filtration rate. N Engl J Med. 2006;354:2473–83.
34. Horio M, Orita Y. Comparison of Jaffé rate assay and enzymatic method for the measurement of creatinine clearance. Jpn J Nephrol. 1996;38:296–9.

# 15

# Association between recurrence of acute kidney injury and mortality in intensive care unit patients with severe sepsis

Emilio Rodrigo[1]* (iD), Borja Suberviola[2], Miguel Santibáñez[3], Lara Belmar[1], Álvaro Castellanos[2], Milagros Heras[1], Juan Carlos Rodríguez-Borregán[2], Angel Luis Martín de Francisco[1] and Claudio Ronco[4]

## Abstract

**Background:** Acute kidney injury (AKI) occurs in more than half critically ill patients admitted in intensive care units (ICU) and increases the mortality risk. The main cause of AKI in ICU is sepsis. AKI severity and other related variables such as recurrence of AKI episodes may influence mortality risk. While AKI recurrence after hospital discharge has been recently related to an increased risk of mortality, little is known about the rate and consequences of AKI recurrence during the ICU stay. Our hypothesis is that AKI recurrence during ICU stay in septic patients may be associated to a higher mortality risk.

**Methods:** We prospectively enrolled all (405) adult patients admitted to the ICU of our hospital with the diagnosis of severe sepsis/septic shock for a period of 30 months. Serum creatinine was measured daily. 'In-ICU AKI recurrence' was defined as a new spontaneous rise of ≥0.3 mg/dl within 48 h from the lowest serum creatinine after the previous AKI episode.

**Results:** Excluding 5 patients who suffered the AKI after the initial admission to ICU, 331 patients out of the 400 patients (82.8%) developed at least one AKI while they remained in the ICU. Among them, 79 (19.8%) developed ≥2 AKI episodes.
Excluding 69 patients without AKI, in-hospital (adjusted HR = 2.48, 95% CI 1.47–4.19), 90-day (adjusted HR = 2.54, 95% CI 1.55–4.16) and end of follow-up (adjusted HR = 1.97, 95% CI 1.36–2.84) mortality rates were significantly higher in patients with recurrent AKI, independently of sex, age, mechanical ventilation necessity, APACHE score, baseline estimated glomerular filtration rate, complete recovery and KDIGO stage.

**Conclusions:** AKI recurred in about 20% of ICU patients after a first episode of sepsis-related AKI. This recurrence increases the mortality rate independently of sepsis severity and of the KDIGO stage of the initial AKI episode. ICU physicians must be aware of the risks related to AKI recurrence while multiple episodes of AKI should be highlighted in electronic medical records and included in the variables of clinical risk scores.

**Keywords:** Acute kidney injury, Mortality, Recurrence, Sepsis

* Correspondence: nefrce@humv.es
[1]Nephrology Service, IDIVAL-Hospital Marqués de Valdecilla, University of Cantabria, Santander, Spain
Full list of author information is available at the end of the article

## Background

Acute kidney injury (AKI) occurs in more than half critically ill patients admitted in intensive care units (ICU), being sepsis and septic shock the main causes of AKI in ICU patients [1, 2]. In the recently reported multinational AKI-EPI study, 57.3% of 1802 patients in ICU developed AKI [1]. Patients affected by AKI present higher risk of mortality, further chronic kidney disease (CKD) and end-stage renal disease (ESRD) [1, 3–5] and have a major impact on healthcare resources [6].

The important advance in AKI severity grading achieved by recent definitions and classification systems such as RIFLE, AKIN, KDIGO and creatinine kinetics has allowed identifying a specific metrics in epidemiology and outcome studies [7–10]. Furthermore, these four classifications have demonstrated the relationship between AKI severity and patient outcomes (mortality and hospital length of stay) and have improved our knowledge about AKI epidemiology [1, 11–15]. In these circumstances, the identification of all the AKI-related variables is quintessential to predict AKI occurrence, severity and outcome.

In fact, AKI severity is not the only factor influencing middle and long-term outcomes. Both AKI duration and recurrence could influence morbidity, mortality and healthcare cost associated to AKI. On the one hand, several authors have suggested that the duration of AKI is as important as severity with regard to outcomes [16–18]. On the other hand, some studies have demonstrated that AKI recurrence after hospital discharge can take place up to 30% after the initial AKI-related hospital admission and is associated to a higher risk of mortality and CKD [19, 20]. Although, currently no uniform definitions of AKI recovery and recurrence exist, there is a growing interest in increasing the knowledge about trajectories of recovery after an AKI episode [21, 22]. In this sense, a consensus conference was held in San Diego in 2015 focusing on 'Persistent AKI and renal recovery' [22]. Specifically, little is known about the rate and consequences of AKI recurrence during ICU and hospital stay. Our hypothesis was that AKI recurrence in septic patients during ICU stay is independently associated with mortality. To contrast this hypothesis, our first aim was to determine whether in-ICU AKI recurrence is an independent factor associated with mortality in comparison with patients without AKI and with patients who only suffered one AKI episode, showing a dose-response pattern. The second aim was to address the importance of AKI recurrence on the risk of mortality with independence of severity (KDIGO stage) of the first AKI. Last, our third objective was to determine the association between AKI recurrence and mortality in patients who recovered completely from their first AKI.

## Methods

A prospective observational cohort study was carried out in all patients (over 17 years of age) admitted to the ICU—of 'Marqués de Valdecilla' University Hospital in Santander (Spain)—with severe sepsis/septic shock according to the definitions proposed by the SCCM/ESICM/ACCP/ATS/SIS consensus conference (i.e. the presence of arterial hypotension and/or persistent signs of tissue hypoperfusion refractory to the intravenous administration of fluids [20 ml/kg], and requiring the infusion of vasoactive drugs) [23]. Enrollment occurred from April 2008 to September 2010. Patients with chronic kidney disease under renal replacement therapy or who had received a kidney transplant were excluded.

Clinical and demographic characteristics of all patients, including age, gender, previous diagnosis of hypertension, diabetes mellitus, chronic obstructive pulmonary disease (COPD), chronic heart failure (CHF) or cancer, immunosuppressive state (AIDS, neutropenia [neutrophil count $<1 \times 10^9$/L], exposure to glucocorticoids [>0.5 mg/kg for >30 days] and/or immunosuppressive or cytotoxic medications, solid organ transplantation, allogeneic or autologous stem cell transplantation, haematological malignancy or solid tumour), the source of infection, as well as Acute Physiology and Chronic Health Evaluation II score and Sequential Organ Failure Assessment score at ICU admission, mechanical ventilation necessity, use of vasopressors and length of ICU and hospital stay were recorded. Leukocyte number, lactate, C-reactive protein and procalcitonin values were collected at ICU admission. Serum creatinine was measured daily while the patients were in ICU. Baseline serum creatinine was defined by the most recent available value between 7 and 365 days before hospital admission. Baseline glomerular filtration rate (GFR) was estimated by 4-variable modification of diet in renal disease (MDRD) equation [24]. In 16 (4%) patients with no available baseline creatinine, it was calculated from the simplified MDRD formula assuming a GFR of 75 ml/min per 1.73 $m^2$ as recommended by the acute dialysis quality initiative (ADQI) workgroup [7]. We defined and staged AKI according to KDIGO serum creatinine criteria [9]. In-ICU recurrent AKI was defined as a new spontaneous rise of ≥0.3 mg/dl within 48 h from the lowest serum creatinine after the previous AKI episode, with partial or full recovery. We defined complete recovery when the patient serum creatinine returned to baseline creatinine or below. Partial recovery was defined when the patient was off renal replacement therapy and serum creatinine started to decrease after the peak value but failed to return to baseline creatinine. Rises of serum creatinine after renal replacement therapy withdrawal were not defined as AKI recurrences. In-hospital and at 90-day mortality were prospectively collected, and mortality at the end of follow-up was retrospectively collected in 2014, being analysed as dependent variables.

Categorical variables were expressed as percentages and continuous variables as median and interquartile rank (IQR). Statistical differences between groups were analysed by chi-square test or Fisher exact test when appropriate for categorical variables, and the non-parametric Mann-Whitney $U$ test was used for continuous variables.

We tested the equality of survival distributions for no AKI, one AKI existence and AKI recurrence by using the log-rank (Mantel-Cox) test and Kaplan-Meier survival curves. As KDIGO stage of the first AKI independently related to mortality, we additionally stratified by KDIGO stage after excluding patients without AKI, testing the equality of survival distributions for one AKI and AKI recurrence in patients with KDIGO 2 and 3 stages separately.

We estimated hazard ratios (HRs) to measure associations. We estimated adjusted HRs and their corresponding 95% confidence intervals (95%CI) using proportional hazards Cox regression models. We adjusted for the following variables: gender, age, mechanical ventilation necessity, APACHE score and baseline estimated GFR (ml/min/1.73 m$^2$). When patients without AKI were excluded from the analysis, KDIGO stage and 'complete recovery' were also included in the multivariable models. The alpha error was set at 0.05, and all $p$ values were two sided. We conducted all statistical analyses using IBM SPSS Statistics version 22.0.

## Results

Main characteristics of the 405 patients included in the cohort are shown in Table 1. Mean follow-up was 956 (IQR 28–1662) days. Throughout the study, they were no losses of follow-up during hospital stay. In 17 patients (4.25%), it was not possible a complete 'follow-up' up to 90 days after hospital discharge. In 25 patients, the follow-up was <1 year, and in 33 patients, the follow-up was <2 years. Five patients suffered AKI after the initial admission in ICU due to sepsis, and they were excluded from the analysis. Three hundred thirty-one patients out of the 400 patients (82.8%) developed at least one in-ICU acute kidney injury (AKI) according to KDIGO classification. Among them, 72, 6 and 1 patients suffered 2, 3 and 4 AKI episodes, respectively, so 79 out of 400 patients (19.8%) developed recurrent AKI episodes during their ICU stay. The flow chart of study population is shown in Fig. 1.

Variables related to AKI recurrence are also shown in Table 1. Patients with AKI recurrence were significantly older and with lower baseline estimated GFR. APACHE score was also higher. Crude mortality was 102/400

(25.5%) for in-hospital mortality, 110/400 (27.5%) at 90 days of follow-up and 188/400 (47%) at the end of follow-up. Ninety-day survival was 59.3, 44.0, 86.7 and 55.3% for patients with partial recovery without AKI recurrence, partial recovery with recurrence, complete recovery without recurrence and complete recovery with recurrence, respectively.

In relation to our first objective, statistically significant different survival distributions were observed when we ordinal categorised 'AKI existence' into 'patients without any AKI episode', 'only one AKI' and 'two or more AKI episodes (in-ICU recurrent AKI) (log rank $p < 0.001$) (Fig. 2, Table 1). By Cox regression analysis, significant dose-response patterns (adjusted $p$ trends ≤0.021) were also found. The greater the number of AKIs, the greater the association for 'intra-hospital', '90 days' and 'end of follow-up' mortality, with independence of sex, age, mechanical ventilation necessity, APACHE score and baseline estimated GFR (Table 2).

KDIGO stage of the first AKI, independently related to intra-hospital (adjusted HR per each increase of stage = 1.45, 95% CI 1.10–1.91), 90-day (adjusted HR per each stage increase of severity = 1.31, 95% CI 1.01–1.71) and end of follow-up mortality (adjusted HR per each increase = 1.28, 95% CI 1.05–1.57).

Regarding our second objective, a specific analysis was conducted with exclusion of non AKI patients, in order to address the importance of AKI recurrence with independence also of severity of the first AKI. Excluding 69 patients without AKI, in-hospital (adjusted HR 2.48, 95% CI 1.47–4.19), 90-day (adjusted HR 2.54, 95% CI 1.55–4.16) and end of follow-up (adjusted HR 1.97, 95% CI 1.36–2.84) mortality rates were significantly higher in patients with recurrent AKI, independently of the covariates above and KDIGO stage and 'complete recovery' (Table 2). Restricting to patients with KDIGO 2 or 3 stages in the first AKI, survival curves were also significantly lower for AKI recurrent patients in each KDIGO stage (log rank $p < 0.001$) (Fig. 3).

In relation to our third objective, 243 patients out of the 331 patients admitted in ICU due to sepsis with AKI recovered completely from their initial AKI episode. Analysing only this group of patients with complete recovery ($N = 243$), the recurrence of AKI remained as an independent risk factor for further mortality at 90 days (HR 3.21, 95% CI 1.74–5.92, $p < 0.001$) and at the end of follow-up (data not shown in tables).

## Discussion

The main finding of our study is that the development of a new episode of AKI during ICU stay after the first AKI episode related to sepsis is associated with a higher mortality rate and increases the mortality rate. The mortality risk rises more than double if the patient suffers

**Table 1** Baseline characteristic in all patients, and in relation to AKI recurrence risk

| | All patients | No AKI | Patients with in-ICU AKI | | |
| | | | AKI = 1 | AKI ≥2 (recurrent) | |
| | N = 405 | N = 69 | N = 252 | N = 79 | p value |
|---|---|---|---|---|---|
| Age (years), median [IQR] | 68.21 [56.52–77.70] | 55.84 [49.02–69.52] | 69.28 [58.07–78.23] | 74.29 [64.72–79.16] | 0.027 |
| Gender (male) | 68.9% | 56.5% | 71.0% | 72.2% | 0.848 |
| Hypertension | 47.7% | 27.5% | 50.8% | 58.2% | 0.248 |
| Diabetes mellitus | 18.3% | 4.3% | 22.6% | 17.9% | 0.380 |
| COPD | 14.8% | 13.0% | 14.3% | 19.0% | 0.313 |
| CHF | 6.4% | 4.3% | 7.1% | 6.3% | 0.804 |
| Cancer | 13.6% | 10.1% | 13.9% | 15.2% | 0.773 |
| Immunosuppressive state | 17.8% | 11.6% | 19.4% | 17.7% | 0.734 |
| Source of infection | | | | | 0.122 |
| Intra-abdominal | 30.9% | 29.0% | 31.0% | 32.9% | |
| Lung | 37.3% | 52.2% | 33.3% | 35.4% | |
| Endocarditis | 0.5% | 0.0% | 0.0% | 1.3% | |
| Line related | 1.5% | 1.4% | 2.0% | 0.0% | |
| Urinary tract | 12.3% | 8.7% | 15.5% | 6.3% | |
| Skin and soft infection | 2.0% | 0.0% | 2.0% | 3.8% | |
| Unknown/others | 15.6% | 8.7% | 16.3%% | 20.3% | |
| Leukocytes, median [IQR] | 13.60 [6.90–21.00] | 12.6 [5.15–23.55] | 13.60 [7.00–20.45] | 15.50 [7.35–21.58] | 0.441 |
| Lactate (mg/dl), median [IQR] | 23.0 [15.0–37.3] | [–] | 26.0 [16.0–41.0] | 26.0 [17.0–47.0] | 0.437 |
| Vasopresors | 84.3% | 83.8% | 85.6% | 79.7% | 0.214 |
| Septic shock | 85.4% | 85.5% | 86.4% | 82.3% | 0.366 |
| APACHE, median [IQR] | 20 [16–25] | 16 [12–19] | 20 [16–27] | 23 [19–27] | 0.032 |
| SOFA, median [IQR] | 8 [6–10] | 7 [5–8] | 9 [7–11] | 9 [6–11] | 0.952 |
| Mechanical ventilation | 51.1% | 54.4% | 49.4% | 51.9% | 0.699 |
| C-reactive protein (mg/l), median [IQR] | 19.4 [10.30–27.50] | 18.6 [7.85–25.45] | 20.4 [10.7–29.20] | 18.3 [11.05–27.55] | 0.673 |
| Procalcitonin (ng/l), median [IQR] | 10.24 [2.54–30.37] | 4.11 [1.25–10.91] | 13.11 [3.31–34.00] | 13.29 [2.32–41.90] | 0.749 |
| Baseline creatinine (mg/dl), median [IQR] | 0.97 [0.80–1.13] | 0.88 [0.72–1.00] | 0.95 [0.80–1.15] | 1.05 [0.90–1.20] | 0.022 |
| Baseline estimated GFR (ml/min/1.73 m$^2$), median [IQR] | 72.50 [58.36–87.86] | 81.91 [64.79–102.55] | 72.74 [57.23–86.47] | 66.18 [53.84–77.55] | 0.030 |
| ICU stay (days), median [IQR] | 4.99 [2.99–11.47] | 4.99 [1.99–8.48] | 3.98 [2.99–10.97] | 9.97 [4.99–17.95] | <0.001 |
| Hospital stay (days), median [IQR] | 16.95 [10.22–30.92] | 15.96 [10.97–32.41] | 15.96 [9.97–28.92] | 19.94 [13.96–34.90] | 0.003 |
| KDIGO AKI stages | | | | | 0.054 |
| 1, n (%) | 100 (24.7%) | – | 79 (31.3%) | 21 (26.6%) | |
| 2, n (%) | 121 (29.9%) | – | 98 (38.9%) | 23 (29.1%) | |
| 3, n (%) | 110 (27.2) | – | 75 (29.8%) | 35 (44.3%) | |
| Maximal creatinine (mg/dl), median [IQR] | 2.10 [1.40–3.16] | 1.00 [0.84–1.10] | 2.30 [1.70–3.19] | 2.99 [2.10–4.00] | <0.001 |
| Intra-hospital mortality, n (%) | 104 (25.7%) | 7 (10.1%) | 60 (23.8%) | 35 (44.3%) | <0.001 |
| 90-day mortality, n (%) | 112 (27.7%) | 8 (11.6%) | 64 (25.4%) | 38 (48.1%) | <0.001 |
| End of follow-up mortality, n (%) | 190 (46.9%) | 22 (31.9%) | 113 (44.8%) | 53 (67.1%) | 0.001 |

from two or more AKI episodes during the same admission. Similarly, Siew et al. reported that patients admitted to hospital with recurrent AKI—within 12 months of discharge from the previous hospitalization with AKI—near doubled the death rate [19]. It is known that diabetic patients with AKI recurrence after previous hospital discharge are at risk for stage 4 CKD. However, we did not analyse residual renal function in our study [20]. Obviously, in our cohort, this increment in mortality comes up after the first 5–10 days (Fig. 2) because AKI recurrence

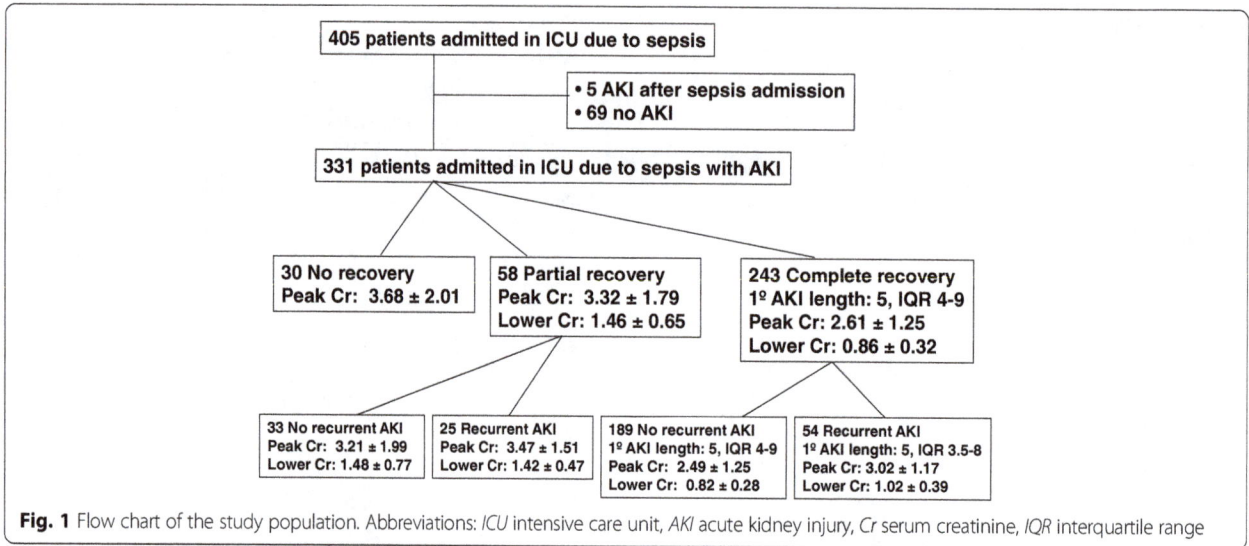

**Fig. 1** Flow chart of the study population. Abbreviations: *ICU* intensive care unit, *AKI* acute kidney injury, *Cr* serum creatinine, *IQR* interquartile range

takes some time to develop. As previously reported [15], KDIGO stages of the first AKI episode are independently related to mortality. Remarkably, using KDIGO serum creatinine criteria to define AKI, we found that such small elevations of creatinine as 0.3 mg/dl relate to a higher mortality risk when they appear after a first AKI event and this increment in mortality was independent of first episode KDIGO classification and severity of sepsis estimated by APACHE score [9].

Moreover, we found that in-ICU AKI recurrence was frequent, taking place in up to 20% of patients admitted due to sepsis. It is expected that the rate of recurrence after AKI related to different aetiologies should be lower because sepsis is the most frequent AKI cause [1]. AKI recurrence rate after hospital discharge is experienced by 25–30% patients, although in-hospital AKI recurrence rate has not been previously reported [19, 20]. In addition, some patients suffered a third and a fourth in-

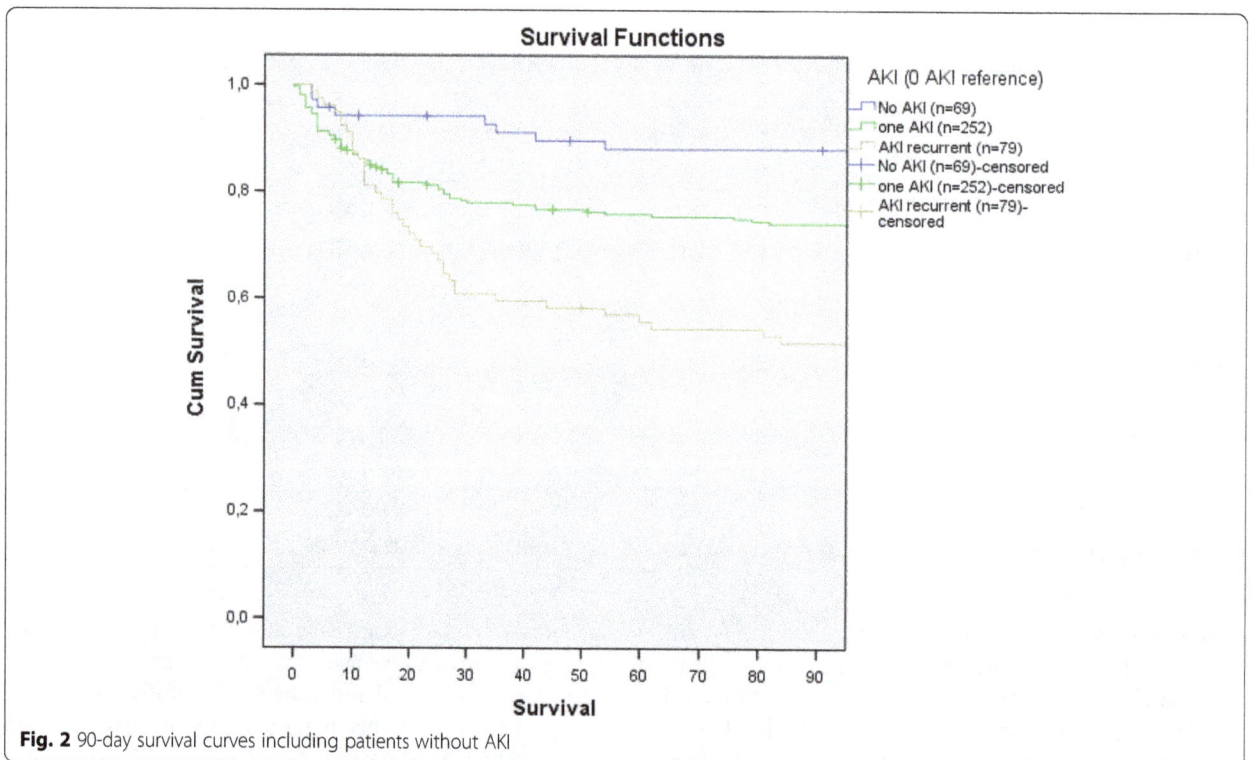

**Fig. 2** 90-day survival curves including patients without AKI

**Table 2** Hazard ratios for in-ICU AKI existence, in relation to mortality

| | Vital status (intra-hospital) | | | | Vital status (90-day) | | | | Vital status (end of follow-up) | | | |
|---|---|---|---|---|---|---|---|---|---|---|---|---|
| | Survival (N) | Death (N) | HR | (95% CI) | Survival (N) | Death (N) | HR | (95% CI) | Survival (N) | Death (N) | HR | (95% CI) |
| Including patients without AKI (N = 400) | 298 | 102 | | | 290 | 110 | | | 212 | 188 | | |
| No AKI (n = 69) | 62 | 7 | 1 | – | 61 | 8 | 1 | – | 47 | 22 | 1 | – |
| AKI = 1 (n = 252) | 192 | 60 | 1.68[a] | 0.74　3.82 | 188 | 64 | 1.54[a] | 0.71　3.34 | 139 | 113 | 1.00[a] | 0.61　1.63 |
| AKI ≥2 (n = 79) | 44 | 35 | 2.73[a] | 1.15　6.51 | 41 | 38 | 2.57[a] | 1.13　5.83 | 26 | 53 | 1.61[a] | 0.93　2.77 |
| *Linear p trend* | | | *0.006* | | | | *0.005* | | | | *0.021* | |
| Excluding patients without AKI (N = 331) | 236 | 95 | | | 229 | 102 | | | 165 | 166 | | |
| AKI = 1 (n = 252) | 192 | 60 | 1 | – | 188 | 64 | 1 | – | 139 | 113 | 1 | – |
| AKI ≥2 (n = 79) | 44 | 35 | 2.48[b] | 1.47　4.19 | 41 | 38 | 2.54[b] | 1.55　4.16 | 26 | 53 | 1.97[b] | 1.36　2.84 |

[a]HR = hazard ratio adjusted for sex, age, mechanical ventilation necessity, APACHE score, and baseline estimated glomerular filtration rate (GFR)
[b]HR = hazard ratio adjusted for sex, age, mechanical ventilation necessity, APACHE score, baseline estimated GFR, complete recovery and KDIGO stage

ICU AKI episode, which, in time, can even increase more the risk of death, although we could not confirm this case because only 7 patients developed so numerous AKI episodes.

As pointed out by Siew et al., in order to prevent further AKI recurrence, we need to identify patients at highest recurrence risk [19]. Age and baseline estimated GFR clearly related to a higher risk of recurrence in our cohort study, and both are well-known risk factors for AKI development [25]. By contrast, we did not find any

relationship between recurrence and gender or comorbid risk factors (Table 2). Siew et al. reported that age, baseline renal function and comorbid conditions such as congestive heart failure, advanced liver disease, dementia, diabetes and coronary artery disease were associated with recurrent AKI after discharge for initial hospital admission in 11,683 patients [19]. On the one hand, the lower number of patients included in our study can prevent us from detecting the influence of these risk factors. It is expected that older patients show more comorbid

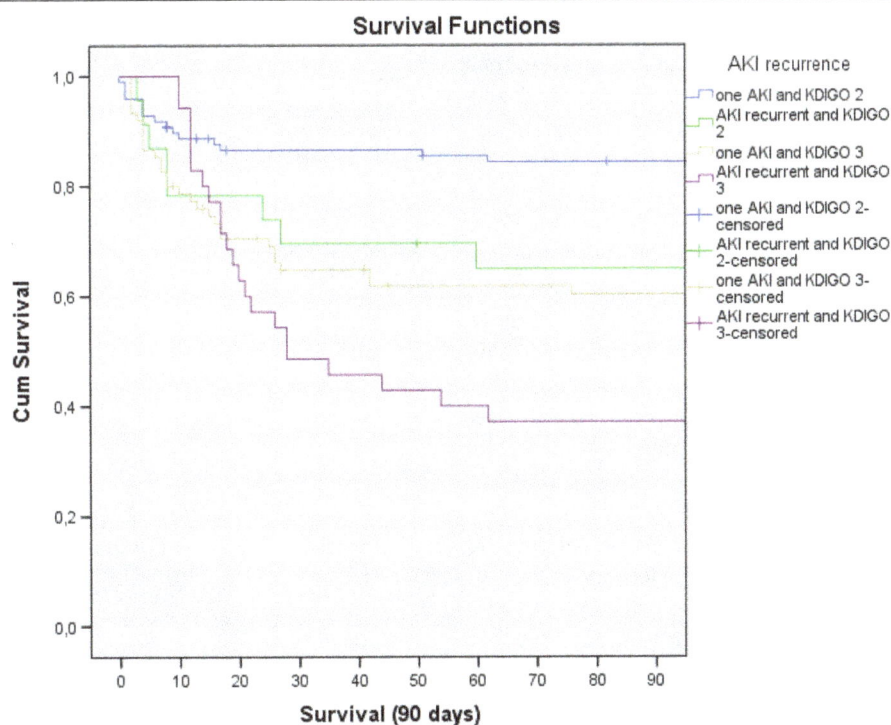

**Fig. 3** 90-day survival curves as a function of KDIGO stages, excluding patients without AKI and restricting to patients with KDIGO 2 or 3 stages

conditions that can place them at a higher risk for AKI recurrence. On the other hand, all our patients developed the first AKI episode due to sepsis and this can limit the influence of other comorbid risk factors.

In our study, severity of sepsis estimated by Sequential Organ Failure Assessment (SOFA), number of leukocytes, lactate, C-reactive protein, procalcitonin and use of vasopressors did not relate to AKI recurrence. Conversely, the severity of the first AKI episode was associated with a higher AKI recurrence as well as severity of sepsis as assessed by APACHE score. Although without reaching statistical significance, 44% patients with in-ICU recurrence had previously suffered a KDIGO stage 3 AKI episode, whereas only 30% patients without recurrence had shown a similar AKI stage. Maximal creatinine in the first AKI episode and baseline estimated GFR were also higher in patients with further recurrence. In this sense, older patients admitted in ICU due to sepsis, with higher APACHE scores and worse renal function and a more severe AKI episode can be identified as at a higher rate of AKI recurrence in our cohort.

The main advantage of our study was that we defined KDIGO stages and AKI recurrence analysing one-by-one daily creatinine for each patient. For example, a rise of creatinine ≥0.3 mg/dl after the initial AKI episode was only considered AKI recurrence when the previous AKI episode was recovering and not when it was due to continuous or intermittent renal replacement therapy withdrawal. AKI recurrence can be hard to record unless prospectively reported in the medical history of the patient or in electronic databases. Due to the association of AKI recurrence with mortality rate, we suggest that the ICU physicians must be aware to its risk and add this diagnosis in the clinical records and registers together with the AKI index episode.

Our study has several limitations. First, we performed a single-centre study and the number of patients included was not high enough to detect the influence of several risk factors previously related to AKI [19, 25]. Whereas one of the advantages of multicentre studies is the high number of patients that can be enrolled, studies carried out in single centres are more homogeneous with respect to inclusion criteria and type of care of the patients. In our case, all patients were included if they fulfilled severe sepsis/septic shock definition according to the SCCM/ESICM/ACCP/ATS/SIS consensus conference [23].

Second, we lost to follow up 4.25% of patients at 90 days because our ICU is part of a tertiary care hospital and some of these patients were discharged to different healthcare systems. We cannot rule out that this rate of follow-up losses had an impact on the reported results, but meaningfully, all the patients were followed up throughout the whole hospital admission until 'death' or 'discharge home' and there were no in-hospital losses.

Third, we did not use urine output to define AKI. Although urine volume rate is part of the AKI definition [9], most AKI staging studies are based on serum creatinine levels alone and do not include urine output data [26]. The course of ICU stay in patients with sepsis should be closely monitored in order to detect recurrent episodes of AKI [27–29].

## Conclusions

To conclude, we performed a single-centre observational study and detected that AKI can recur in up to 20% of patients who suffer a sepsis-related AKI during the initial hospital admission episode. This recurrence is associated with a higher mortality rate independently of several covariates such as initial AKI and sepsis severity, and the association between AKI recurrence and mortality seems to be also present in patients who recovered completely from their first AKI. If these findings are confirmed in larger subsequent multicenter studies, it may be advisable for ICU physicians to be aware of AKI recurrence risk and to add the number of AKI episodes along with their severity and duration in clinical and electronic records to establish the global influence of AKI episodes on patient outcome.

### Abbreviations
95%CI: 95% confidence intervals; ACCP: American College of Chest Physicians; ADQI: Acute dialysis quality initiative; AIDS: Acquired immune deficiency syndrome; AKI: Acute kidney injury; AKIN: Acute kidney Injury network; APACHE: Acute physiology and chronic health evaluation; ATS: American thoracic society; CHF: Chronic heart failure; CKD: Chronic kidney disease; COPD: Chronic obstructive pulmonary disease; ESICM: European Society of Intensive Care Medicine; ESRD: End-stage renal disease; GFR: Glomerular filtration rate; HR: Hazard ratio; ICU: Intensive care units; IQR: Interquartile range; KDIGO: Kidney Disease/Improving Global Outcomes; MDRD: Modification of diet in renal disease; RIFLE: Risk, injury, failure, loss of kidney function, and end-stage kidney disease; SCCM: Society of Critical Care Medicine; SIS: Surgical Infection Society; SOFA: Sequential Organ Failure Assessment

### Acknowledgements
We are indebted to Ania Szawczukiewicz for her linguistic assistance.

### Funding
No funding was received.

### Authors' contributions
ER and BS contributed to the conception and design of the study, to acquire the data and to analyse and interpret the data, and drafted and reviewed the manuscript. MS analysed and interpreted the data and drafted and reviewed the manuscript. LB, MH and JR contributed to acquire the data and reviewed the manuscript. AC contributed to the conception and design of the study, to acquire the data, and reviewed the manuscript. AM and CR contributed to the conception and design of the study and drafted and reviewed the manuscript critically for important intellectual content. All authors approved the final version of the manuscript.

### Competing interests
The authors declare that they have no competing interests.

**Author details**
[1]Nephrology Service, IDIVAL-Hospital Marqués de Valdecilla, University of Cantabria, Santander, Spain. [2]Intensive Care Unit, IDIVAL-Hospital Marqués de Valdecilla, University of Cantabria, Santander, Spain. [3]School of Nursing, IDIVAL-Hospital Marqués de Valdecilla, University of Cantabria, Santander, Spain. [4]Department of Nephrology Dialysis and Transplantation, International Renal Research Institute of Vicenza (IRRIV), San Bortolo Hospital, Vicenza, Italy.

**References**

1. Hoste EA, Bagshaw SM, Bellomo R, Cely CM, Colman R, Cruz DN, Edipidis K, Forni LG, Gomersall CD, Govil D, Honoré PM, Joannes-Boyau O, Joannidis M, Korhonen AM, Lavrentieva A, Mehta RL, Palevsky P, Roessler E, Ronco C, Uchino S, Vazquez JA, Vidal Andrade E, Webb S, Kellum JA. Epidemiology of acute kidney injury in critically ill patients: the multinational AKI-EPI study. Intensive Care Med. 2015;41:1411–23.

2. Bagshaw SM, Lapinsky S, Dial S, Arabi Y, Dodek P, Wood G, et al. Cooperative Antimicrobial Therapy of Septic Shock (CATSS) Database Research Group. Acute kidney injury in septic shock: clinical outcomes and impact of duration of hypotension prior to initiation of antimicrobial therapy. Intensive Care Med. 2009;35:871–81.

3. Coca SG, Yusuf B, Shlipak MG, Garg AX, Parikh CR. Long-term risk of mortality and other adverse outcomes after acute kidney injury: a systematic review and meta-analysis. Am J Kidney Dis. 2009;53:961–73.

4. Ishani A, Xue JL, Himmelfarb J, Eggers PW, Kimmel PL, Molitoris BA, Collins AJ. Acute kidney injury increases risk of ESRD among elderly. J Am Soc Nephrol. 2009;20:223–8.

5. Ruiz-Criado J, Ramos-Barron MA, Fernandez-Fresnedo G, Rodrigo E, De Francisco AL, et al. Long-term mortality among hospitalized non-ICU patients with acute kidney injury referred to nephrology. Nephron. 2015;131:23–33.

6. Clinical Guideline Centre (UK). Acute kidney injury: prevention, detection and management up to the point of renal replacement therapy. London: Royal College of Physicians (UK); 2013. http://www.ncbi.nlm.nih.gov/books/NBK247665/. Accessed Sept 2016.

7. Bellomo R, Ronco C, Kellum JA, Mehta RL, Palevsky P. Acute Dialysis Quality Initiative workgroup: acute renal failure—definition, outcome measures, animal models, fluid therapy and information technology needs: The Second International Consensus Conference of the Acute Dialysis Quality Initiative (ADQI) Group. Crit Care. 2004;8:R204–12.

8. Mehta RL, Kellum JA, Shah SV, Molitoris BA, Ronco C, et al. Acute kidney injury network: acute kidney injury network: report of an initiative to improve outcomes in acute kidney injury. Crit Care. 2007;11:R31.

9. Kidney Disease: Improving Global Outcomes (KDIGO) Acute Kidney Injury Work Group. KDIGO clinical practice guideline for acute kidney injury. Kidney Int Suppl. 2012;2:1–138.

10. Waikar SS, Bonventre JV. Creatinine kinetics and the definition of acute kidney injury. J Am Soc Nephrol. 2009;20:672–9.

11. Bagshaw SM, George C, Bellomo R, ANZICS Database Management Committe. A comparison of the RIFLE and AKIN criteria for acute kidney injury in critically ill patients. Nephrol Dial Transplant. 2008;23:1569–74.

12. Joannidis M, Metnitz B, Bauer P, Schusterschitz N, Moreno R, et al. Acute kidney injury in critically ill patients classified by AKIN versus RIFLE using the SAPS 3 database. Intensive Care Med. 2009;35:1692–702.

13. Lopes JA, Fernandes P, Jorge S, Gonçalves S, Alvarez A, Costa e Silva Z, França C, Prata MM. Acute kidney injury in intensive care unit patients: a comparison between the RIFLE and the Acute Kidney Injury Network classifications. Crit Care. 2008;12:R110.

14. Ostermann M, Chang RW. Challenges of defining acute kidney injury. QJM. 2011;104:237–43.

15. Zeng X, McMahon GM, Brunelli SM, Bates DW, Waikar SS. Incidence, outcomes, and comparisons across definitions of AKI in hospitalized individuals. Clin J Am Soc Nephrol. 2014;9:12–20.

16. Uchino S, Bellomo R, Bagshaw SM, Goldsmith D. Transient azotaemia is associated with a high risk of death in hospitalized patients. Nephrol Dial Transplant. 2010;25:1833–9.

17. Thakar CV, Christianson A, Freyberg R, Almenoff P, Render ML. Incidence and outcomes of acute kidney injury in intensive care units: a veterans administration study. Crit Care Med. 2009;37:2552–8.

18. Coca SG, King Jr JT, Rosenthal RA, Perkal MF, Parikh CR. The duration of postoperative acute kidney injury is an additional parameter predicting long-term survival in diabetic veterans. Kidney Int. 2010;78:926–33.

19. Siew ED, Parr SK, Abdel-Kader K, Eden SK, Peterson JF, Bansal N, Hung AM, Fly J, Speroff T, Ikizler TA, Matheny ME. Predictors of recurrent AKI. J Am Soc Nephrol. 2016;27:1190–200.

20. Thakar CV, Christianson A, Himmelfarb J, Leonard AC. Acute kidney injury episodes and chronic kidney disease risk in diabetes mellitus. Clin J Am Soc Nephrol. 2011;6:2567–72.

21. Kellum JA. How can we define recovery after acute kidney injury? Considerations from epidemiology and clinical trial design. Nephron Clin Pract. 2014;127:81–8.

22. Chawla LS, Bellomo R, Bihorac A, Goldstein SL, Siew ED, Bagshaw SM, Bittleman D, Cruz D, Endre Z, Fitzgerald RL, Forni L, Kane-Gill SL, Hoste E, Koyner J, Liu KD, Macedo E, Mehta R, Murray P, Nadim M, Ostermann M, Palevsky PM, Pannu N, Rosner M, Wald R, Zarbock A, Ronco C, Kellum JA, Acute Disease Quality Initiative Workgroup 16. Acute kidney disease and renal recovery: consensus report of the Acute Disease Quality Initiative (ADQI) 16 Workgroup. Nat Rev Nephrol. 2017;13:241–57.

23. Levy MM, Fink MP, Marshall JC, Abraham E, Angus D, Cook D, et al. International Sepsis Definitions Conference. 2001 SCCM/ESICM/ACCP/ATS/SIS International Sepsis Definitions Conference. Intensive Care Med. 2003;29:530–8.

24. Levey AS, Coresh J, Greene T, Marsh J, Stevens LA, Kusek JW, Van Lente F, Chronic Kidney Disease Epidemiology Collaboration. Expressing the modification of diet in renal disease study equation for estimating glomerular filtration rate with standardized serum creatinine values. Clin Chem. 2007;53:766–72.

25. Cartin-Ceba R, Kashiouris M, Plataki M, Kor DJ, Gajic O, Casey ET. Risk factors for development of acute kidney injury in critically ill patients: a systematic review and meta-analysis of observational studies. Crit Care Res Pract. 2012;2012:691013. doi:10.1155/2012/691013.

26. Thomas ME, Blaine C, Dawnay A, Devonald MA, Ftouh S, Laing C, Latchem S, Lewington A, Milford DV, Ostermann M. The definition of acute kidney injury and its use in practice. Kidney Int. 2015;87:62–73.

27. Camussi G, Ronco C, Montrucchio G, Piccoli G. Role of soluble mediators in sepsis and renal failure. Kidney Int. 1998;66:S38–42.

28. Uchino S, Bellomo R, Morimatsu H, Morgera S, Schetz M, Tan I, et al. Discontinuation of continuous renal replacement therapy: a post hoc analysis of a prospective multicenter observational study. Critical Care Med. 2009;37:2576–82.

29. Levin A, Warnock DG, Mehta RL, Kellum JA, Shah SV, Molitoris BA, et al. Improving outcomes from acute kidney injury: report of an initiative. Am J Kidney Dis. 2007;50:1–4.

# 16

# Hemodynamic effects of electrical muscle stimulation in the prophylaxis of deep vein thrombosis for intensive care unit patients

Masahiro Ojima[*], Ryosuke Takegawa, Tomoya Hirose, Mitsuo Ohnishi, Tadahiko Shiozaki and Takeshi Shimazu

## Abstract

**Background:** Deep vein thrombosis (DVT) is a major complication in critical care. There are various methods of prophylaxis, but none of them fully prevent DVT, and each method has adverse effects. Electrical muscle stimulation (EMS) could be a new effective approach to prevent DVT in intensive care unit (ICU) patients. We hypothesized that EMS increases the venous flow of the lower limbs and has a prophylactic effect against the formation of DVT.

**Methods:** This study included 26 patients admitted to a single ICU. We enrolled patients who could not move themselves due to spinal cord injury, head injury, central nervous system abnormalities, and sedation for mechanical ventilation. The patients were randomly allocated to either the EMS group or the control group. Patients in the EMS group received 30-min sessions of EMS applied to the bilateral lower extremities on arbitrary days within 14 days after admission. The control patients received no EMS. The peak flow velocity and diameter of the popliteal vein (Pop.V) and common femoral vein (CFV) were measured by ultrasound and then the volumes of venous flow were calculated using a formula.

**Results:** There were no statistically significant differences in patient characteristics between the two groups except for the mortality rate. In the EMS group, the median and interquartile range (IQR, 25th–75th percentile) of velocities of the Pop.V and CFV were higher during EMS compared with at rest: 10.6 (8.0–14.8) vs 24.5 (15.1–37.8) cm/s and 17.0 (12.3–23.8) vs 24.3 (17.0–33.0) cm/s, respectively ($p < 0.05$). The median (IQR) of volumes of venous flow of the Pop.V and CFV at rest and during EMS were 4.2 (2.7–7.2) vs 8.6 (5.4–16.1) $cm^3$/s and 12.9 (9.7–21.4) vs 20.8 (12.3–34.1) $cm^3$/s, respectively ($p < 0.05$). There were no major complications related to EMS.

**Conclusions:** EMS increased the venous flow of the lower limbs. EMS could be one potential method for venous thromboprophylaxis.

**Keywords:** Electrical muscle stimulation, Deep vein thrombosis, Hemodynamics, Thromboprophylaxis, Intensive care

* Correspondence: ojimarionet999@hp-emerg.med.osaka-u.ac.jp
Department of Traumatology and Acute Critical Medicine, Osaka University
Graduate School of Medicine, Suita, Osaka, Japan

## Background

Deep vein thrombosis (DVT) is one of the major complications in critical care and sometimes leads to fatal complication such as pulmonary embolism (PE). The in-hospital mortality rate associated with PE in 2010 in the USA was reported to be 4.4%, with 30-day and 6-month rates up to 9.1 and 19.6%, respectively [1]. To prevent accidental death by PE, it is important to prevent the formation of DVT of the lower limbs during the intensive care unit (ICU) stay.

Three factors are responsible for the formation of DVT: venous blood stasis, endothelial injury, and hypercoagulability [2]. Patients with trauma or severe diseases requiring mechanical ventilation are forced to be on long-term bed rest, which causes venous blood stasis of the lower limbs and puts them at high risk for DVT. It is well known that range of mobility exercises and early ambulation are important to prevent DVT. However, such exercises are difficult and sometimes impossible during intensive care. Most of the international guidelines recommend the use of intermittent pneumatic compression (IPC) or compression stockings, or early administration of anticoagulants to prevent DVT in high-risk patients [3]. However, these prophylactic methods cannot fully prevent DVT. A review suggested that critically ill patients commonly develop DVT with rates that vary from 10% to as high as 30% regardless of the prophylactic methods [4]. There are also several issues related to their use. IPC sometimes causes peroneal nerve palsy or compartment syndrome due to incorrect attachment [5], compression stockings sometimes cause hemodynamic complication through incorrect use [6], and anticoagulation involves a risk of major hemorrhage [7]. Thus, a more effective and safer approach to DVT prophylaxis is needed.

An electrical muscle stimulation (EMS) device has recently been used for the rehabilitation of immobilized people [8]. Circulating current between two electrodes generated by EMS causes cyclic contraction of muscles and results in rhythmic changes in venous blood flow, which is expected to have a prophylactic effect on DVT [9]. We have already shown that EMS prevented atrophy of muscles during prolonged bed rest [10]. Thus, we hypothesized that attaching EMS on the lower limbs might have a potential to produce a similar effect of exercise therapy even for the patients forced to be immobile for prolonged periods. Some reports suggest that EMS may have a preventive effect on DVT not only in healthy subjects [8] but also in total knee/hip arthroplasty patients [11, 12] and postoperative patients [13]. However, a report on EMS use in patients with major trauma failed to show a significant difference in the rate of DVT formation and venous flow parameters between the patients with and without EMS [14]. There are few reports on

EMS aimed at the prophylaxis of DVT in critical care settings, so the effect of EMS on the lower limbs is controversial. Additionally, there are major differences between patients in ICU setting and patients in another clinical settings; critically ill patients often were not able to move themselves voluntarily and could not have communication with others. They also have not only general risk factors but also specific ICU risk factors of DVT, like sedation, strong analgesia, vasopressors, or central venous catheter. We think these differences may have some effects on EMS. We hypothesized that EMS might increase the venous flow of the lower limbs and might have a prophylactic effect for formulating DVT even in critically ill patients.

The purpose of this study was to evaluate the short-term effects of EMS on venous blood flow of the lower limbs in ICU patients by ultrasonography.

## Methods

### Enrollment

This study was approved by the institutional review board of Osaka University Hospital (No. 13361-3), an academic urban tertiary referral hospital in Suita, Japan. The study was conducted in the ICU of the emergency department of Osaka University Hospital from April 2014 to May 2015. The ICU has 17 beds and treated 885 patients in 2014. Formal written consent for participation in this study was obtained from each patient or their next of kin.

We enrolled patients who could not voluntarily move their lower limbs, that is, (a) patients with limitation of lower limb motion due to traumatic brain injury, spinal cord injury or cerebral infarction, or hemorrhage and (b) sedated patients who were on mechanical ventilation for more than 3 days. Patients were excluded if they were under 16 years of age, were pregnant and parturient women, suffered from cardiac arrest on admission, were implanted with material containing metal parts, were on a life-support device such as extracorporeal membrane oxygenation, had a history of neurological disorder or present evidence of venous thrombosis of the lower limbs, received treatment for subarachnoid hemorrhage, were complicated with congestive heart failure, were in an unstable general condition, had local infection at the sites of electrode application, or required rest of the lower limbs because of fracture. We included 26 patients in this study.

### Study protocol

The risk of forming DVT was evaluated by the guideline at Osaka University Hospital. Patients are stratified into the high-risk group if they had a previous history of DVT or PE, have an advanced cancer located in the pelvis, had hip/knee replacement surgery or spinal surgery, or have antiphospholipid antibody syndrome. The risk factors of forming DVT are as follows: age over 60, presence of cancer not including advanced cancer located in the pelvis, presence of inflammatory bowel diseases, suffering from congestive heart failure or acute myocardial infarction, suffering from cerebral infarction or spinal cord injury, presence of nephrotic syndrome, pregnant women, obesity with body mass index (BMI) over 30 kg/m$^2$, oral contraceptive use, abnormality of clotting factors, tranexamic acid use, undergoing an operation in the dorsosacral position, undergoing thoracoscopic surgery, undergoing an operation of over 3 h in length, being forced to be on bed rest for over 3 days, or being immobilized in a plaster cast. Patients who had less than three risk factors were stratified into the low-risk group, those with three risk factors into the moderate-risk group, and those with four risk factors or more into the high-risk group.

Flowtron Excel (manufactured by ArjoHuntleigh, Malmö, Sweden) was used for IPC. Prevention of DVT by IPC was performed in the moderate- and high-risk patients if there were no contraindications such as arteriosclerosis obliterans. When a patient was evaluated as low-risk, the attending doctor decided to perform IPC or not. IPC was attached to the bilateral lower legs. The compression pressure was 40 mmHg. In this study, all patients were treated with IPC. Unfractionated heparin was also administered intravenously based on the attending doctor's decision for the high-risk patients. The dose of heparin was adjusted by

checking the activated partial thromboplastin time targeting 40 to 50 s. Compression stockings were not used in this study. The prevention of DVT was continued until the first ambulation or patient discharge. We assigned patients to the EMS group or the control group by drawing lots from a box containing 20 equally allocated lots.

### Electrical muscle stimulation

Patients in the EMS group were positioned in the supine position during EMS operation. We performed EMS only once a day on arbitrary days within 14 days after admission using the Torelete EM300 (distributed by Toray International, Inc., Tokyo, Japan; manufactured by ITO CO., LTD, Tokyo, Japan). EMS was performed at a time to suit researcher's convenience. The average number of EMS implementation was 6.6 times per each case during study period (total EMS implementation was 93 times). Two pairs of EMS electrodes (PALS Platinum, Axelgaard Manufacturing Co., Ltd., Fallbrook, CA) were placed on the posterior calves and anteromedial thighs of both extremities to deliver electricity to the calf and quadriceps muscles (Fig. 1) with two EMS machines. Stimulation from the two machines was administered at the same time. The patients received one 30-min session on each experimental day. The duration of stimulation included 2 min for warm-up (pulse frequency 5 Hz, pulse width 150 μs), 26 min for training (50 Hz, 200 μs), and 2 min for cool-down (6 Hz, 150 μs). During the

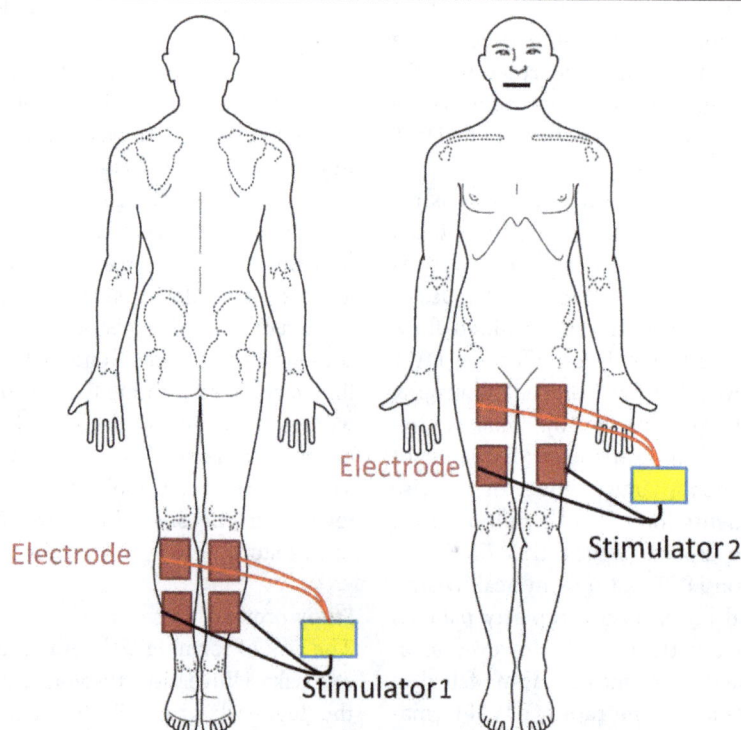

**Fig. 1** Position of the electrical muscle stimulation electrodes placed over the calf and quadriceps muscles

training time, muscle stimulation was set to a total cycle time of 19.2 s with an 8-s ON time, 8-s OFF time, 1.6-s ramp-up time, and 1.6-s ramp-down time. The output current of the device, which ranged from 20 to 50 mA, was set to obtain slight visual movement of the ankle in planter flexion. EMS was not conducted in the patients in the control group during the study period. IPC device was continuously activated between the EMS sessions in the EMS group.

## Doppler ultrasound measurements

The popliteal vein (Pop.V) and common femoral vein (CFV) were imaged in the short-axis view using a Philips CX50 CompactXtreme ultrasonic scanner (Philips Medical, Seattle, WA) and L12-3 broadband linear array transducer (Fig. 2). The measurements were taken at the popliteal fossa, just proximal to the venous confluence of the lower leg, and at the inguinal region, just below the inguinal ligament. The patients were positioned in the supine position with neutral positioning of the lower limbs when imaged of the CFV, while with externally rotated and mildly flexed knee when imaged of the Pop.V. In the EMS group, the peak venous blood flow velocity (cm/s) and the diameter (mm) of the Pop.V and CFV were recorded just before the application of EMS and 10 min after initiating EMS. The ultrasound probe was slightly angulated to face toward to obtain Doppler signal. The Doppler angle was fixed to 60 degrees during measurements of blood velocity. In the control group, the measurements were made similarly when the patient was at rest. All measurements were done by a single intensive care specialist well trained in ultrasound examination of the lower limbs.

After these measurements were obtained, we calculated the peak blood flow volume per second ($cm^3$/s) in the Pop.V and CFV by the following equation:

Peak blood flow volume per second ($cm^3$/s) = radius (cm) × radius (cm) × π (circular constant) × peak venous blood flow velocity (cm/s).

In this formula, "radius" refers to the radius of Pop.V or CFV, and "peak venous blood flow velocity" refers to the peak venous blood flow velocity of Pop.V or CFV.

## Patient data collection

Patient age, sex, height, body weight, BMI, Acute Physiology and Chronic Health Evaluation (APACHE II) score, Sequential Organ Failure Assessment (SOFA) score, Injury Severity Score (ISS), and diagnosis were recorded on admission. Each patient's final outcome, the duration of mechanical ventilation, and side effects experienced with EMS were archived as well. We also confirmed the presence or absence of DVT by echography.

## Statistical analysis

Patient baseline demographic and clinical variables are presented as median and interquartile range (IQR, 25th–75th percentile). Data on patient sex, mortality, and presence or absence of sedation and analgesia were compared between the control group and EMS group using Fisher's exact test. Data on the risk classification for DVT was compared between the control group and EMS group using Pearson's chi-square test. Data on patient age, BMI, APACHE II score, SOFA score, and ISS were compared between the control group and EMS group using the Mann-Whitney $U$ test. The differences in blood flow velocity, vessel diameter, and blood flow volume per second between the control

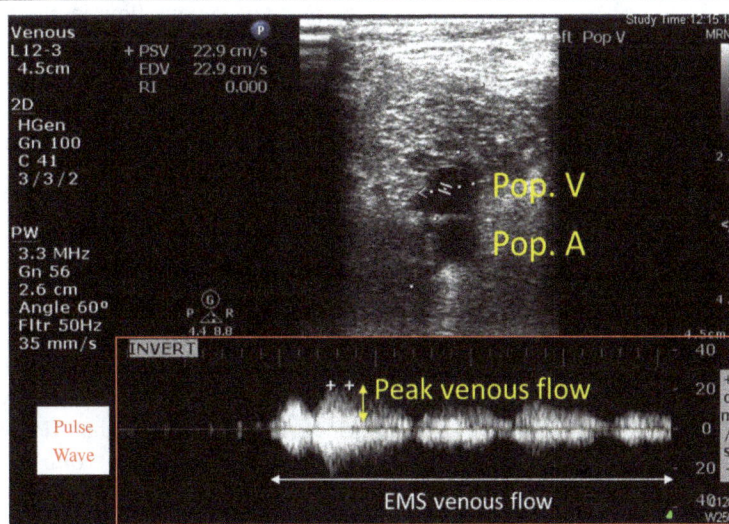

**Fig. 2** Representative screen shot from pulsed Doppler ultrasound for measurement of the peak venous velocity and diameter of the popliteal vein (Pop. V). Both were measured in the short-axis view. In this picture, the venous velocity was measured at the center of double line (denoted as *equal sign*) continuously and then the pulse wave was figured. The peak velocity was measured at the top of the pulse wave (denoted as *plus sign*)

group and the EMS group at rest and during EMS stimulation were analyzed using the Kruskal-Wallis test. Statistical analysis was performed using SPSS (version 22, SPSS, Chicago, IL). A *p* value of <0.05 was considered statistically significant.

## Results

Table 1 shows the patient characteristics of the two groups, which comprised 26 patients (52 legs, control group [*n* = 12], EMS group [*n* = 14]) and included 19 men and 7 women with a median (IQR) age of 70.0 (54.0–79.0) years. The diagnosis on admission was trauma in 12 patients, stroke in 6 patients, sepsis in 4 patients, and acute respiratory failure in 4 patients. Injuries in the 12 trauma patients were as follows: traumatic brain injury in 5, spinal cord injury in 5, pelvic injury in 1, and abdominal injury in 1. The median (IQR) of BMI, APACHE II score, SOFA score, and ISS on admission were 22.7 (20.9–24.5), 16.5 (9.0–22.0), 4.0 (2.0–5.0), and 25.0 (18.5–33.5), respectively. There were no statistical differences in these scores between the two groups. There was also no statistical difference in the probability of DVT between the two groups. The

**Table 1** Patient characteristics in the control group and EMS group

|  | Control (*n* = 12) | EMS (*n* = 14) | *p* value |
|---|---|---|---|
| Age (years) | 70.0 (61.0–79.0) | 70.0 (51.0–79.0) | 0.90 |
| Sex (male/female) | 9/3 | 10/4 | 1.00 |
| Body mass index (kg/m²) | 22.0 (20.2–24.2) | 24.1 (21.3–28.1) | 0.118 |
| APACHE II score | 20.0 (14.0–23.0) | 12.1 (9.0–20.0) | 0.27 |
| SOFA score | 4.0 (2.5–5.0) | 2.5 (1.0–4.0) | 0.40 |
| ISS (*n* = 12) | 25.0 (21.0–29.0) (*n* = 5) | 25.0 (18.5–31.5) (*n* = 7) | 0.76 |
| Mortality (%) | 5 (42) | 0 (0) | 0.012 |
| Sedation (%) | 11 (92) | 10 (71) | 0.33 |
| Analgesia (%) | 9 (75) | 10 (71) | 1.00 |
| Admitting diagnosis |  |  |  |
| Trauma | 5 | 7 |  |
| Stroke | 3 | 3 |  |
| Sepsis | 2 | 2 |  |
| Others | 2 | 2 |  |
| Risk classification for DVT |  |  | 0.71 |
| High risk | 4 | 3 |  |
| Moderate risk | 5 | 8 |  |
| Low risk | 3 | 3 |  |

Values are presented as median (IQR)

mortality rate was 19.2%, which was significantly higher in the control group.

The peak blood flow velocity, venous diameter, and the peak blood flow volume per second of the Pop.V and CFV are shown in Table 2. The data in the EMS group was the summary of all the 93 sessions of EMS. The data in the control group was the result of the 66 times measurements. The peak venous flow velocities and peak blood flow volume of the CFV and Pop.V in both of the lower extremities were higher during EMS than at rest in the EMS group patients. The peak venous flow velocity and blood flow volume of Pop.V tended to be lower in the EMS group patients than in the control group patients in the resting state, but the differences were not statistically significant without the peak venous flow velocity of right Pop.V. The peak venous flow velocity of CFV tended to be lower in the EMS group patients than in the control group patients in the resting state, but the differences were not statistically significant. The blood flow volume of CFV was significantly lower in the EMS group patients than in the control group patients in the resting state. No differences were identified in venous diameter between the control group patients and the EMS group patients at rest or during EMS.

There were no major complications related to EMS. There were no changes of blood pressure, heart rate, and respiratory status during EMS (data not shown). No patients complained of discomfort from application of EMS. DVT and PE were detected in 1 patient in the control group, but no instances of DVT or PE occurred in the EMS group.

## Discussion

This is the first report, to our knowledge, to show the increase of venous flow in the lower extremities during EMS in the ICU setting by using ultrasound assessment. We showed that the peak venous velocity and volume of the CFV and Pop.V were significantly increased by EMS. These findings may indicate that EMS could be a new alternative for the prevention of DVT of the lower extremities.

We observed increases in peak venous velocity of nearly 2.2-fold in the Pop.V and 1.4-fold in the CFV with EMS compared to those in the resting condition. The maximum blood flow volume of the Pop.V rose by nearly 2.2-fold and that of the CFV rose by 1.5-fold with EMS compared to those in the resting condition. A previous report showed that IPC produces similar influences on velocity and volume of venous flow in the lower limbs [15]. It has been thought that EMS activates muscle pumping by contracting the lower extremity skeletal muscles and thus produces more physiological hemodynamic forces than IPC or compression stocking [16, 17]. From this point of view, one report compared

**Table 2** Peak venous flow velocities, venous diameters, and peak blood flow volumes per second of Pop.V and CFV

| | Control (n = 66) | EMS (n = 93) | |
| --- | --- | --- | --- |
| | | At rest | During EMS |
| Peak venous flow velocity (cm/s) | | | |
| Right Pop.V | 15.3 (11.3–26.0) | 10.2 (7.6–14.0)# | 24.3 (15.1–40.8)*# |
| Left Pop.V | 13.3 (10.4–21.0) | 10.9 (8.2–16.4) | 24.9 (15.4–36.4)*# |
| Right CFV | 20.4 (15.8–27.0) | 16.3 (11.9–24.8) | 25.1 (17.0–32.6)* |
| Left CFV | 20.6 (16.2–28.6) | 17.3 (13.8–23.3) | 23.0 (18.2–34.3)* |
| Venous diameter (mm) | | | |
| Right Pop.V | 6.8 (6.0–7.7) | 6.9 (6.1–8.0) | 7.3 (6.1–7.8) |
| Left Pop.V | 6.9 (6.6–7.8) | 7.0 (6.0–7.8) | 7.2 (6.2–8.0) |
| Right CFV | 11.0 (10.0–12.8) | 10.2 (8.6–11.7)# | 10.3 (9.2–11.7) |
| Left CFV | 11.0 (9.8–12.7) | 10.4 (9.2–12.0) | 10.2 (8.9–12.0) |
| Blood flow volume (cm³/s) | | | |
| Right Pop.V | 5.5 (3.6–9.0) | 4.0 (2.5–7.2) | 9.3 (5.3–14.7)*# |
| Left Pop.V | 5.2 (3.4–8.2) | 4.7 (2.9–7.2) | 8.4 (5.5–16.9)*# |
| Right CFV | 20.0 (12.4–35.0) | 12.8 (9.4–19.6)# | 20.8 (12.2–32.3)* |
| Left CFV | 19.0 (12.7–35.4) | 13.0 (10.7–22.4)# | 20.9 (12.4–37.3)* |

*Abbreviations: CFV* common femoral vein, *EMS* electrical muscle stimulation, *Pop.V* popliteal vein

Values are presented as median (IQR)

*Statistical difference compared with at rest in the EMS group patients (p < 0.05)

#Statistical difference compared with control patients (p < 0.05)

EMS with IPC in terms of the influences of lower limb hemodynamics and showed that EMS led to more effective ejection of blood in conditions of venous stasis of the lower limbs [18]. It was shown that EMS had a potential for greater hemodynamic effect on the lower extremities than that of IPC. In addition, EMS did not influence the diameter of the Pop.V or CFV in this study. Another report addressed a similar finding in major trauma patients [14]. These findings imply that EMS intensifies the amount of venous return by activating muscle pumping without having a direct influence on major veins of the lower extremities.

There were a lot of EMS study, but most of them conducted EMS of calf muscles alone. Few reports addressing EMS effect with simultaneous stimulation of the thigh and calf muscles in clinical settings. A report was aimed to reveal EMS effect to reduce blood stasis during arthroplasty. The authors mentioned that EMS of calf muscles or thigh muscles alone was ineffective to put out venous-pooling blood from lower extremities to the central circulation [19]. We thought that simultaneous stimulation was important to maximize this effect and it would lead to prevent DVT more efficiently.

Blood flow velocity and the volume of Pop.V tended to be lower in the EMS group patients than in the control group patients in the resting state. These differences were possibly a result of the difference in BMI between

the two groups: BMI values indicated that the EMS group patients were more obese than the control group patients. Obesity is one of the major risk factors for DVT [20]. Several reports have shown that venous return in the inferior vena cava or in the femoral vein is reduced in obese patients due to obesity-induced increases in intra-abdominal pressure [21, 22]. Our results were comparable with the results on venous flow of the lower extremities in these reports.

There were no major complications related to EMS, and it was well tolerated by the patients in this study. EMS is reported to be a relatively safe procedure to use in adults with advanced diseases, such as cancer or chronic obstructive pulmonary disease, and even in critically ill patients. Some reports also revealed that it did not affect the patient's cardiorespiratory responses such as heart rate, blood pressure, oxygen saturation, and respiration rate. Compliance with its use is generally good, but it sometimes causes muscle discomfort, pain, or superficial burns, which may set limits to its use [23–25]. In intensive care settings, most of the patients are sedated and pain is controlled. This will relieve the pain associated with EMS and may make EMS more tolerable for ICU patients than non-ICU patients.

This study has several limitations. First, the efficacy of EMS to prevent DVT was not directly proven. High peak velocity and volume are not equal to better DVT protection. A large randomized controlled study is needed to elucidate this point. Second, blood inflow, i.e., arterial flow, in the lower extremities was not assessed in this study. It is possible for arterial flow to be influenced by EMS, which may have relevance to venous outflow. Arterial flow needs to be measured during EMS as well. Third, it was not clear which muscles should be stimulated, or when and how long and at what intensity muscles should be stimulated for DVT prophylaxis in ICU patients. These points also need to be assessed in future studies.

## Conclusions

EMS increased the venous flow of the lower limbs. This modality may have a prophylactic effect on DVT and could be one potential method for venous thromboprophylaxis, particularly in ICU patients. Further study is needed to confirm its optimal use.

**Abbreviations**

APACHE: Acute Physiology and Chronic Health Evaluation; BMI: Body mass index; CFV: Central femoral vein; DVT: Deep vein thrombosis; EMS: Electrical muscle stimulation; ICU: Intensive care unit; IPC: Intermittent pneumatic compression; IQR: Interquartile range; ISS: Injury Severity Score; PE: Pulmonary embolism; Pop.V: Popliteal vein; SOFA: Sequential Organ Failure Assessment

**Acknowledgements**

Not applicable.

## Funding

This work was supported by a medical research grant from ZENKYOREN (National Mutual Insurance Federation of Agricultural Cooperatives) and JSPS KAKENHI Grant Number JP15H05007.

## Authors' contributions

OMa participated in the conception and design of the study, acquisition of data, interpretation of data analysis, statistical analysis, and drafting of the manuscript. TR participated in the conception and design of the study and review of the manuscript. OMi and TShio participated in the conception and design of the study, interpretation of data analysis, and review of the manuscript. HT and TShima reviewed the manuscript. All authors read and approved the manuscript.

## Competing interests

The authors declare that they have no competing interests.

## References

1.  Minges KE, Bikdeli B, Wang Y, Kim N, Curtis JP, Desai MM, et al. National trends in pulmonary embolism hospitalization rates and outcomes for adults aged ≥65 years in the United States (1999 to 2010). Am J Cardiol. 2015;116:1436–42.
2.  Kumar DR, Hanlin E, Glurich I, Mazza JJ, Yale SH. Virchow's contribution to the understanding of thrombosis and cellular biology. Clin Med Res. 2010;8:168–
3.  Geerts WH, Pineo GF, Heit JA, Bergqvist D, Lassen MR, Colwell CW, et al. Prevention of venous thromboembolism: the Seventh ACCP Conference on Antithrombotic and Thrombolytic Therapy. Chest. 2004;126:338S–400.    72.
4.  Attia J, Ray JG, Cook DJ, Douketis J, Ginsberg JS, Geerts WH. Deep vein thrombosis and its prevention in critically ill adults. Arch Intern Med. 2001; 161:1268–79.
5.  Lachmann EA, Rook JL, Tunkel R, Nagler W. Complications associated with intermittent pneumatic compression. Arch Phys Med Rehabil. 1992;73:482–5.
6.  Collaboration CT, Dennis M, Sandercock PA, Reid J, Graham C, Murray G, et al. Effectiveness of thigh-length graduated compression stockings to reduce the risk of deep vein thrombosis after stroke (CLOTS trial 1): a multicentre, randomised controlled trial. Lancet. 2009;373:1958–65.
7.  Eppsteiner RW, Shin JJ, Johnson J, van Dam RM. Mechanical compression versus subcutaneous heparin therapy in postoperative and posttrauma patients: a systematic review and meta-analysis. World J Surg. 2010;34:10–
8.  Griffin M, Nicolaides AN, Bond D, Geroulakos G, Kalodiki E. The efficacy of a new stimulation technology to increase venous flow and prevent venous stasis. Eur J Vasc Endovasc Surg. 2010;40:766–71.    9.
9.  Stefanou C. Electrical muscle stimulation in thomboprophylaxis: review and a derived hypothesis about thrombogenesis—the 4th factor. Springerplus. 2016;5:884.
10. Hirose T, Shiozaki T, Shimizu K, Mouri T, Noguchi K, Ohnishi M, et al. The effect of electrical muscle stimulation on the prevention of disuse muscle atrophy in patients with consciousness disturbance in the intensive care unit. J Crit Care. 2013;28:536. e531–7.
11. Izumi M, Ikeuchi M, Aso K, Sugimura N, Kamimoto Y, Mitani T, et al. Less deep vein thrombosis due to transcutaneous fibular nerve stimulation in total knee arthroplasty: a randomized controlled trial. Knee Surg Sports Traumatol Arthrosc. 2015;23:3317–23.
12. Broderick BJ, Breathnach O, Condon F, Masterson E, Olaighin G. Haemodynamic performance of neuromuscular electrical stimulation (NMES) during recovery from total hip arthroplasty. J Orthop Surg Res. 2013;8:3.
13. Lobastov K, Barinov V, Laberko L, Obolensky V, Boyarintsev V, Rodoman G. Electrical calf muscle stimulation with Veinoplus device in postoperative venous thromboembolism prevention. Int Angiol. 2014;33:42–9.
14. Velmahos GC, Petrone P, Chan LS, Hanks SE, Brown CV, Demetriades D. Electrostimulation for the prevention of deep venous thrombosis in patients with major trauma: a prospective randomized study. Surgery. 2005;137:493–8.
15. Morris RJ, Woodcock JP. Evidence-based compression: prevention of stasis and deep vein thrombosis. Ann Surg. 2004;239:162–71.
16. Broderick BJ, O'Briain DE, Breen PP, Kearns SR, Olaighin G. A pilot evaluation of a neuromuscular electrical stimulation (NMES) based methodology for the prevention of venous stasis during bed rest. Med Eng Phys. 2010;32:349–55.
17. Lyons GM, Leane GE, Grace PA. The effect of electrical stimulation of the calf muscle and compression stocking on venous blood flow velocity. Eur J Vasc Endovasc Surg. 2002;23:564–6.
18. Broderick BJ, O'Connell S, Moloney S, O'Halloran K, Sheehan J, Quondamatteo F, et al. Comparative lower limb hemodynamics using neuromuscular electrical stimulation (NMES) versus intermittent pneumatic compression (IPC). Physiol Meas. 2014;35:1849–59.
19. Faghri PD, Van Meerdervort HF, Glaser RM, Figoni SF. Electrical stimulation-induced contraction to reduce blood stasis during arthroplasty. IEEE Trans Rehabil Eng. 1997;5:62–9.
20. Abdollahi M, Cushman M, Rosendaal FR. Obesity: risk of venous thrombosis and the interaction with coagulation factor levels and oral contraceptive use. Thromb Haemost. 2003;89:493–8.
21. Sterling SA, Jones AE, Coleman TG, Summers RL. Theoretical analysis of the relative impact of obesity on hemodynamic stability during acute hemorrhagic shock. Arch Trauma Res. 2015;4, e22602.
22. Willenberg T, Clemens R, Haegeli LM, Amann-Vesti B, Baumgartner I, Husmann M. The influence of abdominal pressure on lower extremity venous pressure and hemodynamics: a human in-vivo model simulating the effect of abdominal obesity. Eur J Vasc Endovasc Surg. 2011;41:849–55.
23. Williams N, Flynn M. A review of the efficacy of neuromuscular electrical stimulation in critically ill patients. Physiother Theory Pract. 2014;30:6–11.
24. Maddocks M, Gao W, Higginson IJ, Wilcock A. Neuromuscular electrical stimulation for muscle weakness in adults with advanced disease. Cochrane Database Syst Rev. 2013;1, CD009419.
25. Segers J, Hermans G, Bruyninckx F, Meyfroidt G, Langer D, Gosselink R. Feasibility of neuromuscular electrical stimulation in critically ill patients. J Crit Care. 2014;29:1082–8.

# 17

# Utility of SOFA score, management and outcomes of sepsis in Southeast Asia: a multinational multicenter prospective observational study

Khie Chen Lie[1], Chuen-Yen Lau[2], Nguyen Van Vinh Chau[3,4], T. Eoin West[5,6], Direk Limmathurotsakul[7,8,9*] (iD)
and for Southeast Asia Infectious Disease Clinical Research Network

## Abstract

**Background:** Sepsis is a global threat but insufficiently studied in Southeast Asia. The objective was to evaluate management, outcomes, adherence to sepsis bundles, and mortality prediction of maximum Sequential Organ Failure Assessment (SOFA) scores in patients with community-acquired sepsis in Southeast Asia.

**Methods:** We prospectively recruited hospitalized adults within 24 h of admission with community-acquired infection at nine public hospitals in Indonesia ($n = 3$), Thailand ($n = 3$), and Vietnam ($n = 3$). In patients with organ dysfunction (total SOFA score $\geq 2$), we analyzed sepsis management and outcomes and evaluated mortality prediction of the SOFA scores. Organ failure was defined as the maximum SOFA score $\geq 3$ for an individual organ system.

**Results:** From December 2013 to December 2015, 454 adult patients presenting with community-acquired sepsis due to diverse etiologies were enrolled. Compliance with sepsis bundles within 24 h of admission was low: broad-spectrum antibiotics in 76% (344/454), $\geq 1500$ mL fluid in 50% of patients with hypotension or lactate $\geq 4$ mmol/L (115/231), and adrenergic agents in 71% of patients with hypotension (135/191). Three hundred and fifty-five patients (78%) were managed outside of ICUs. Ninety-nine patients (22%) died. Total SOFA score on admission of those who subsequently died was significantly higher than that of those who survived (6.7 vs. 4.6, $p < 0.001$). The number of organ failures showed a significant correlation with 28-day mortality, which ranged from 7% in patients without any organ failure to 47% in those with failure of at least four organs ($p < 0.001$). The area under the receiver operating characteristic curve of the total SOFA score for discrimination of mortality was 0.68 (95% CI 0.62–0.74).

**Conclusions:** Community-acquired sepsis in Southeast Asia due to a variety of pathogens is usually managed outside the ICU and with poor compliance to sepsis bundles. In this population, calculation of SOFA scores is feasible and SOFA scores are associated with mortality.

**Keywords:** Sepsis, Asia, Southeastern, Organ dysfunction scores, Patient care bundles,

* Correspondence: direk@tropmedres.ac
[7]Centre for Tropical Medicine and Global Health, Nuffield Department of Medicine, University of Oxford, Oxford, UK
[8]Mahidol-Oxford Tropical Medicine Research Unit, Faculty of Tropical Medicine, Mahidol University, Bangkok, Thailand
Full list of author information is available at the end of the article

## Background

Sepsis, organ dysfunction due to a dysregulated host response to infection, is a major public health concern [1]. Sepsis is estimated to affect up to 20 million people around the world each year, and about 20–50% of people hospitalized with sepsis die [2]. Yet these estimates are extrapolations from high-income countries, home to only 13% of the world's population. Sepsis is understudied in the low- and middle-income countries (LMICs) that host over six billion people [3].

Identification of sepsis—in the absence of a gold standard test—may be challenging [4, 5]. Recently, an international taskforce suggested that "sepsis" should be defined as life-threatening organ dysfunction caused by a dysregulated host response to infection and that the term "severe sepsis" was redundant [1]. The taskforce emphasized the use of the Sequential (sepsis-related) Organ Failure Assessment (SOFA) score [1], and organ dysfunction can be represented by an increase in the SOFA score of 2 points or more. Nonetheless, the SOFA score was derived in and has been primarily evaluated for mortality prediction in high-income countries [6–8]. There are few data about the mortality prediction of the SOFA score in LMICs and in non-ICU settings [9, 10].

Following diagnosis, successful sepsis management hinges on prompt treatment of infection and correction of organ dysfunction. Sepsis bundles such as those derived from Surviving Sepsis Campaign (SSC) guidelines facilitate management but have been primarily evaluated in high-income countries [11–15]. Relatively little is known about adherence to recommended sepsis bundles in LMICs. Healthcare systems in LMICs in Southeast Asia also vary. Thailand, an upper middle-income country, has a universal healthcare system with reasonably adequate coverage for the poor [16], while the healthcare systems in Vietnam and Indonesia, lower middle-income countries, still provide limited critical care coverage for patients with sepsis [17, 18]. Therefore, it is possible that management and outcomes of sepsis patients are different within LMICs in Southeast Asia.

We recently reported the causes and outcomes of 815 adult patients presenting with community-acquired infection in nine hospitals in three middle-income countries in Southeast Asia: Indonesia, Thailand, and Vietnam [19]. Sepsis was identified on enrolment in 454 adult patients and was associated with increased mortality. We observed that infection in this cohort was caused by a wide range of known and emerging pathogens, including dengue viruses, *Leptospira* spp., *Rickettsia* spp., *Escherichia coli*, and influenza viruses [19]. The hosts, infecting pathogens, and clinical capacity in this study are markedly different from those populations and sites evaluated in most studies of sepsis to date. However, a better understanding of sepsis management and outcomes in these environments is critically important to reduce the global burden of this syndrome. Here, we report the management and adherence to sepsis care bundles and mortality prediction of the SOFA score in adult patients with community-acquired sepsis in Southeast Asia.

## Methods

### Study sites and populations

We conducted a prospective cohort study of community-acquired sepsis and severe sepsis [20] in patients in nine public hospitals in Indonesia ($n = 3$), Thailand ($n = 3$), and Vietnam ($n = 3$) (Additional file 1: Figure S1). All are tertiary public hospitals equipped with microbiology facilities and ICUs, with a median bed number of 1000 (range 760–2200). Children and adults were enrolled in the study; the present analysis is limited to adults. The term "severe sepsis" in the previous study was based on diagnostic criteria from SSC 2012 [20] and was not used in this study in accordance with the most updated sepsis definition (sepsis-3) [1].

### Study participants

We prospectively enrolled adult patients (age ≥ 18 years) who were admitted with a primary diagnosis of suspected or documented infection made by the attending physician, were within 24 h of hospital admission, and had at least three of 20 modified SSC 2012 sepsis diagnostic criteria documented in the medical record (Additional file 2: Table S1) [19]. We excluded patients who were suspected of having hospital-acquired infections, had a hospital stay within 30 days prior to this admission, were transferred from other hospitals with a total duration of hospitalization > 72 h, or were enrolled in other clinical studies. For this analysis, we defined organ dysfunction as total SOFA score ≥ 2 and analyzed individuals meeting this criterion [1].

### Study procedures

The study was initiated in December 2013 in Thailand, March 2014 in Vietnam, and March 2015 in Indonesia and completed at all sites in December 2015. On enrollment, the study team used a standardized case report form (CRF) to record clinical symptoms and their respective durations, known chronic conditions, vital signs, Glasgow Coma Scale (GCS), fluid challenge (if performed), administration of oxygen and other drugs documented in the medical charts, results of laboratory tests performed by the study hospital laboratories, and primary diagnoses made by attending clinicians. Then, study nurses visited enrolled patients daily to update clinical information captured and to record final diagnoses made by attending clinicians at discharge.

Per protocol, the following rapid diagnostic tests (RDTs) were performed immediately after enrollment: a whole blood lactate RDT (Lactate Pro 2, Arkray Global Business Inc., Australia), a whole blood glucose RDT (ACCU-CHECK Performa, Roche Diagnostic, Germany), a dengue RDT (NS1 and IgM, Standard Diagnostics, South Korea), and a leptospirosis RDT (Leptospira IgM/IgG, Standard Diagnostics). The results of all rapid tests were reported to the attending physicians immediately. Blood samples were collected for culture on site and for serological tests and molecular tests at reference laboratory centers of each country. Other diagnostic specimens and a set of reference diagnostic tests were performed for each patient according to clinical presentation as previously described [19].

The study did not involve any clinical interventions. All treatment was provided by attending physicians and their medical teams. The 28-day mortality was evaluated via telephone contact if subjects were no longer hospitalized and had been discharged alive.

### Statistical analysis

Data were entered into OpenClinica, Enterprise Edition (Waltham, USA), and all analyses were performed using STATA version 14.0 (StataCorp, College Station, USA). This was a secondary analysis; the sample size of the study was determined for the primary objective of ascertaining etiology of sepsis [19].

Maximum SOFA scores within 24 h of admission for each of six organ systems were determined as shown in Additional file 3: Table S2. The cardiovascular SOFA score was modified slightly as the study protocol was not designed to capture the dosage of adrenergic agents in units of micrograms per kilogram per minute: one for mean arterial pressure < 70, two if dopamine was administered, and three if epinephrine or norepinephrine were administered. For a missing value, we used the closest available value from the pre-transfer period to 24 h of admission. Where no value was available, the predictor was assumed to be normal and given a score of 0. The total SOFA score was then calculated by summing the maximum SOFA scores for each of the six organ systems. For patients who required mechanical ventilation, the total GCS was estimated by the formula previously described [21]. Differences in proportions were evaluated using Fisher's exact test and differences in medians by the Mann-Whitney test. The discriminative power of total SOFA score was defined by the area under the receiver operating characteristic curve (AUROC). We used logistic regression models stratified by study sites to evaluate the factors associated with mortality. Multivariable logistic regression models to evaluate the association between adherence to sepsis bundles and mortality were developed using purposeful selection

[22] and were adjusted for age and total SOFA score within 24 h of admission.

### Results

A total of 2093 adults presenting at nine study hospitals in three countries were screened by the study team (Fig. 1). The most common reasons for exclusion were hospitalization in the past 30 days (363, 14%) and suspicion or diagnosis of non-infectious conditions (262, 10%). Four hundred fifty-four adult patients had organ dysfunction as determined by total SOFA score ≥ 2. These patients were therefore deemed to have community-acquired sepsis and were included in the analysis (Table 1 and Additional file 4: Table S3). Of these, 219 patients (48%) were transferred from other hospitals.

Four hundred forty-four patients (98%) had lactate levels measured on enrollment as part of the study protocol (Table 2). Of 231 patients presenting with sepsis-induced hypotension or lactate ≥ 4 mmol/L, 172 (74%) received an initial fluid challenge within 24 h after admission and 115 (50%) received ≥ 1500 mL during the fluid challenge. Of 77 patients who received ≥ 1500 mL during the fluid challenge and had body weight recorded, the median volume of fluid received was 42 mL/kg (IQR 34–56 mL/kg; range 19–122 mL/kg). Of 191 patients who had hypotension, 135 (71%) received an adrenergic agent, and norepinephrine was the most common adrenergic agent used (86%; 116/135) (Additional file 5: Table S4).

Of 219 patients transferred from other hospitals, 137 (63%) had parenteral (intravenous or intramuscular) antibiotics administered prior to or during transfer. Another 207 patients had parenteral antibiotics

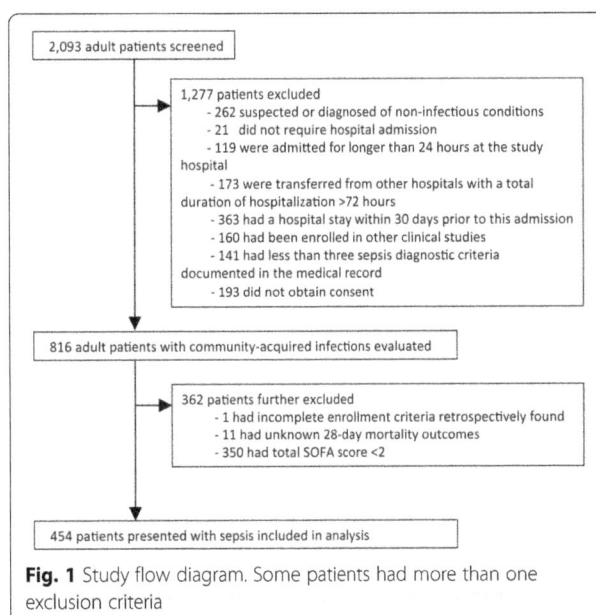

**Fig. 1** Study flow diagram. Some patients had more than one exclusion criteria

**Table 1** Baseline characteristics

| Characteristics | No. of patients (%, n = 454) |
|---|---|
| Sex, male | 287 (63%) |
| Age | |
| ≥ 18–< 40 years | 120 (26%) |
| ≥ 40–< 60 years | 169 (37%) |
| ≥ 60 years old | 165 (36%) |
| Country | |
| Indonesia | 51 (11%) |
| Thailand | 277 (61%) |
| Vietnam | 126 (27%) |
| Preexisting known conditions | |
| Diabetes | 88 (19%) |
| Hypertension | 127 (28%) |
| Chronic kidney disease | 45 (10%) |
| Chronic lung disease | 21 (5%) |
| HIV/AIDS | 0 |
| Clinical presentations* | |
| Acute respiratory tract infection | 243 (54%) |
| Acute diarrhea | 107 (24%) |
| Acute central nervous system (CNS) infection | 62 (14%) |
| Acute systematic infection | 128 (28%) |
| SOFA score (mean, SD)[†] | 5.0 ± 3.2 |

*The clinical presentations (in some cases, more than one) were defined based on the major presenting clinical symptoms. Acute respiratory tract infection was defined as manifestation of at least one respiratory symptom for no longer than 14 days. Acute diarrhea was defined as diarrhea for no longer than 14 days. Acute CNS infection was defined as manifestation of CNS symptoms for no longer than 14 days or the presence of signs of CNS infection on admission. Systemic infection was defined as the absence of acute respiratory infection, acute diarrhea, and acute CNS infection
[†]Total maximum SOFA scores from the pre-transfer period up to 24 h of admission

**Table 2** Adherence to Surviving Sepsis Campaign care bundles up to 24 h after admission

| Surviving Sepsis Campaign care bundles | Sepsis patients (n = 454)[†] |
|---|---|
| Measured lactate level | 444 (98%)[‡] |
| Obtained blood culture | 449 (99%)[‡] |
| Administered parenteral antibiotics | 344 (76%) |
| Administered ≥ 1500 mL fluid for hypotension or lactate ≥ 4 mmol/L | 115/231 (50%) |
| Administered adrenergic agent for hypotension | 135/191 (71%) |
| Re-measured lactate level for hypotension or lactate ≥ 4 mmol/L | 11/275 (4%) |

Adapted from Rhodes et al. [23]
[†]Denominator is total n unless otherwise specified
[‡]Measuring lactate level and obtaining blood culture were part of the study protocol

administered at the study hospitals within 24 h of admission. Overall, the most common antibiotics used were ceftriaxone (71%; 245/344), ceftazidime (13%; 44/344), and carbapenems (11%; 37/344). Per study protocol, 449 patients (99%) had blood culture on enrollment. Reference diagnostic tests identified bacteria in 39% of patients (176/454), viruses in 16% (71/454), and parasites in 2% (9/454, Additional file 6: Table S5). *Leptospira* spp. (n = 52, 11%), dengue viruses (n = 46, 10%), *Escherichia coli* (n = 33, 7%), rickettsial pathogens (n = 18, 4%), *Streptococcus suis* (n = 14, 3%), and *Klebsiella pneumoniae* (n = 10, 2%) were the pathogens most commonly identified (Additional file 6: Table S5). Pathogens were not identified in 212 patients (47%).

Additional file 7: Table S6 shows other supportive care provided up to 24 h after admission. Seventy of 454 study patients (15%) were admitted directly to an ICU, and additional 29 patients (6%) were admitted to an ICU within 24 h after admission. Of 219 patients who were transferred from other hospitals, 154 (62%) had a peripheral oxygen saturation ($SpO_2$) level documented at the outside facility, of whom 23 (15%) had a $SpO_2 < 90\%$ (median 97%; IQR 93 to 99; range 34 to 100%). On admission to the study hospital, 320 patients (70%) had a $SpO_2$ level noted in the medical records, of whom 56 (18%) had a $SpO_2 < 90\%$ (median 97%; IQR 92–99%; range 33 to 100%). Sixty-four patients (14%) were treated with mechanical ventilation. Per study protocol, 445 patients (98%) had whole blood glucose measured once on enrollment by the study team. Eight (2%) and 118 (26%) had severe hypoglycemia (blood glucose level < 40 mg/dL) and hyperglycemia (blood glucose level > 180 mg/dL), respectively.

The overall 28-day mortality was 22% (99/454). The 28-day mortality ranged from 7% (8/111) among those who had SOFA score = 2 to 39% among those who had SOFA score > 6 (Fig. 2). There were no clear differences for pathogens identified between survivors and non-survivors, except that *Leptospira* spp. and dengue viruses were more commonly identified in survivors (Additional file 8: Table S7). The mean total SOFA score was significantly higher in non-survivors than in survivors (6.7 vs. 4.6, OR 1.25; 95%CI 1.16–1.34, $p < 0.001$, Table 3). The odds of death increased with higher SOFA scores for all organ systems ($p < 0.01$ for all), except for the coagulation score ($p = 0.89$). The number of organ failures (where organ failure was defined as the maximum SOFA score ≥ 3 for an individual organ system) also showed a significant correlation with 28-day mortality, which ranged from 7% in patients without any organ failure to 47% in those with failure of at least four organs ($p < 0.001$; Additional file 9: Table S8). The AUROC of total SOFA score for discrimination of mortality was 0.68 (95% CI 0.62–0.74).

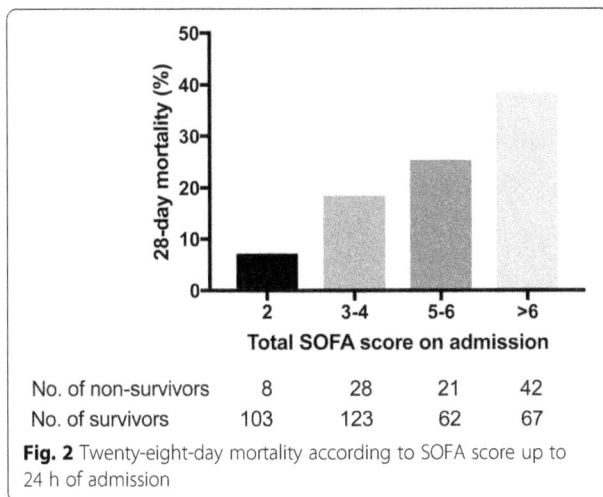

**Fig. 2** Twenty-eight-day mortality according to SOFA score up to 24 h of admission

| | 2 | 3-4 | 5-6 | >6 |
|---|---|---|---|---|
| No. of non-survivors | 8 | 28 | 21 | 42 |
| No. of survivors | 103 | 123 | 62 | 67 |

Determination of SOFA scores is based on both clinical and laboratory parameters [6, 7]. We found that some laboratory tests were not available or measured routinely for sepsis patients within 24 h after admission in our middle-income country settings. Most of the patients had both platelet ($n$ = 452, 99%) and creatinine ($n$ = 443, 98%) tests performed, while 65% ($n$ = 294) and 25% ($n$ = 113) had bilirubin and arterial blood gas tests performed, respectively (Additional file 10: Table S9). While every patient had vital signs documented, 64% ($n$ = 291) had GCS values documented in the medical charts prior to the enrollment.

In logistic regression models adjusted for age and SOFA score and stratified by study site (Table 4), we found that adherence to sepsis care bundles within 24 h was not associated with survival. Using tests for interactions, we found that relationships between SOFA score and mortality and between sepsis management and mortality were not significantly different among subgroup of patients with viruses or bacteria identified.

## Discussion

This prospective observational study characterized management and outcomes of patients with diverse etiologies of community-acquired sepsis in three middle-income countries in Southeast Asia. The main findings from this study are that adherence to SSC bundles even at the late time point of 24 h after admission is generally low. Most patients are not admitted to the ICU but are managed on the wards. The 28-day mortality is 22%. Despite incomplete laboratory and certain clinical data, calculation of SOFA scores with minor modifications is feasible and the total SOFA score within 24 h of admission is strongly correlated with mortality.

Sepsis care bundles have been developed to facilitate the implementation of core tenets of sepsis treatment guidelines [11, 23]. In middle-income countries, where resources are relatively limited compared to high-income countries, it is important to determine how sepsis care is provided as the applicability of or ability to implement these guidelines may be impaired [24, 25]. Our study only permitted assessment of adherence to bundles at 24 h, yet even at this late time point, sepsis care bundles were applied to patients presenting with community-acquired sepsis at variable rates. The high adherence of measuring lactates (98%) and obtaining blood culture (99%) was largely driven by the study protocol and may not reflect the current standard of care for community-acquired sepsis in Southeast Asia. Timely antimicrobial therapy is considered an essential component of sepsis treatment [20], but only 76% of patients received a parenteral antibiotic within the first 24 h. Notably, viruses, parasites, spirochetes, and rickettsial pathogens were identified in 33% of patients with sepsis. It is possible, for example, that if clinicians suspect or confirm by rapid diagnostic tests that the sepsis is caused by a virus such as dengue virus, antimicrobial therapies may not be administered [26]. However, distinguishing these patients based on clinical presentation is challenging and may result in inadequate treatment of bacterial infection. Intravenous fluid resuscitation in this study was generally restrictive.

Optimal fluid management of patients with sepsis in high-resource settings remains debated [27]. Intravenous

**Table 3** Maximum SOFA scores up to 24 h of admission for the six organ systems in sepsis patients

| System | Non-survivors*<br>($n$ = 99) | Survivors*<br>($n$ = 355) | Odds ratio | $p$ values[†] |
|---|---|---|---|---|
| Respiration | 1.2 (± 1.5) | 0.3 (± 0.9) | 1.70 (1.40–2.07) | < 0.001 |
| Coagulation | 1.1 (± 1.4) | 1.4 (± 1.3) | 1.01 (0.93–1.23) | 0.89 |
| Liver | 1.0 (± 1.4) | 0.6 (± 1.1) | 1.34 (1.10–1.63) | 0.004 |
| Cardiovascular | 1.2 (± 0.9) | 0.8 (± 0.9) | 1.80 (1.35–2.40) | < 0.001 |
| Central nervous system | 0.6 (± 0.6) | 0.3 (± 0.7) | 1.67 (1.24–2.25) | 0.001 |
| Renal | 1.6 (± 1.3) | 1.1 (± 1.3) | 1.27 (1.06–1.52) | 0.009 |
| Total SOFA score | 6.7 (± 3.8) | 4.6 (± 2.9) | 1.25 (1.16–1.34) | < 0.001 |

*Results are presented as mean (± standard deviation)
[†]$p$ value estimated by univariable logistic regression stratified by study site

**Table 4** Factors associated with 28-day mortality in adult patients with sepsis

| Factors | Outcome | | Odds ratio (95% CI)* | |
|---|---|---|---|---|
| | Non-survivors (n = 99)[‡] | Survivors (n = 355)[‡] | Univariable analysis | Multivariable analysis[†] |
| Admitted directly to ICU | 19 (19%) | 51 (14%) | 3.8 (1.8–8.1, p < 0.001) | 1.9 (0.8–4.5, p = 0.16) |
| Administered parenteral antibiotics | 87 (88%) | 257 (72%) | 3.4 (1.6–7.0, p = 0.001) | 1.7 (0.7–3.9, p = 0.22) |
| Administered ≥ 1500 mL fluid for hypotension or lactate ≥ 4 mmol/L | 32/72 (44%) | 83/159 (52%) | 0.9 (0.5–1.7, p = 0.73) | 0.8 (0.4–1.5, p = 0.43) |
| Administered adrenergic agent for hypotension | 40/52 (77%) | 95/139 (68%) | 1.7 (0.8–3.6, p = 0.20) | 1.4 (0.6–3.1, p = 0.45) |

*Stratified by study sites
[†]Adjusted for age and total SOFA score
[‡]Denominator is total n unless otherwise specified

fluid resuscitation in this study was generally restrictive. Of particular concern is the risk-benefit profile of fluid administration in low-resource settings [28, 29]. Despite the potential mortality benefits of following sepsis bundles, compliance has historically been low in many settings [23]. Proactive strategies for increasing compliance are necessary and may be uniquely challenging in limited resource settings. Approaches that may have benefit include educational campaigns, engaging a full-time intensivist, establishing nurse-driven protocols, and providing feedback to clinicians regarding specific performance metrics [14, 15]. Together, our findings underscore the importance of evaluating and prioritizing fundamental elements of sepsis care in Southeast Asia with an emphasis on efficacy, cost-effectiveness, and feasibility.

We found that performance of components of sepsis bundles within 24 h of admission was not associated with survival outcomes. It is possible that those therapies were not provided within 3 and 6 h, preferred benchmarks for sepsis treatment [23]; therefore, their benefits were not observed. The lack of benefit of administration of parenteral antibiotics and fluid challenge could also be due to residual confounding factors. Unfortunately, the information documented in the medical record in our settings was not adequate to estimate whether the bundles were performed within 3 or 6 h of admissions. While these findings should not be interpreted as indicating negative or no impact of sepsis care bundles in sepsis patients, they highlight the importance of understanding etiologies and evaluating management strategies for sepsis in different clinical environments.

SOFA scores permit the determination of organ dysfunction, using a combination of clinical and laboratory variables [6]. We found that, for the most part, SOFA scores can be measured with the available standard of care resources in middle-income countries in Southeast Asia. Nearly every patient presenting with sepsis had blood collected for platelet count and creatinine level on admission, whereas about half had bilirubin levels measured. Therefore, the additional cost for laboratory tests would be either minimal or moderate for middle-income countries. Cardiovascular and central nervous system scores—determined from clinical parameters—could be

readily measured without additional cost. Although our study did not capture doses of adrenergic agents—necessitating a modification of the cardiovascular SOFA score—this information is nonetheless available in clinical practice. However, the SOFA respiration score is based on the $PaO_2$ from an arterial blood gas (to calculate $PaO_2/FiO_2$). We observed that only 25% of our sepsis patients had arterial blood gas testing performed, perhaps reflecting the added complexity of arterial blood sampling or need for specialized testing equipment. This issue no doubt underestimated the severity of illness in many cases. For example, patients who required mechanical ventilation due to sepsis-associated hypoxemic respiratory failure, yet did not have an arterial blood gas drawn, received a respiratory SOFA score of 0. To overcome these challenges, reframing the SOFA respiratory score for LMICs by using $SpO_2/FiO_2$ [30] or simply based on a requirement for supplemental oxygen or respiratory support devices may be helpful.

In our study cohort, despite a weak AUROC for discrimination of 28-day mortality, total SOFA score was nonetheless robustly associated with 28-day mortality. This association was also valid for individual organ SOFA scores, with the exception of the coagulation score. This may be a spurious finding or due to the wide range of pathogens responsible for sepsis in our study. Previous studies evaluating the relationship of SOFA score with mortality have been performed in locations where most sepsis is attributed to bacterial infections [6, 9, 31]. Thrombocytopenia in those who have bacterial infections may be caused by disseminated intravascular coagulation and thus is highly associated with mortality [6, 9, 31]. It is possible that thrombocytopenia in those with viral infections, such as dengue, is not so strongly associated with mortality as that observed in those with bacterial infections. Thrombocytopenia is also common in leptospirosis patients [32], and overall mortality of leptospirosis (about 7% in the recent review [33] and 8% [4/52] in our study) is generally lower than in sepsis patients without *Leptospira* spp. identified (24% [95/402] in our study). Therefore, the limited predictability of thrombocytopenia observed in our study was possibly because dengue and leptospirosis were common, and mortality in patients in whom these pathogens were identified was lower than in patients with other pathogens (Additional file 8: Table S7). Tests for interaction [22] and our sample size may lack power to evaluate this phenomenon. Nonetheless, we raise the concern that the SOFA coagulation score for sepsis in tropical countries in Southeast Asia—where causes of infections are diverse [19, 34]—may not provide a linear contribution to the prediction of mortality as has been observed in other settings.

Our study has several potential limitations. First, the actual standard of care could be higher than what we observed due to lack of documentation in the medical records or lower due to observational bias. Second, we may have excluded some patients with organ dysfunction and the true SOFA score could be higher if arterial blood gas levels, bilirubin levels, dose of adrenergic agents in units of micrograms per kilogram per minute, and GCS were measured and documented in all patients; nonetheless, our results represent the real situation in middle-income countries in Southeast Asia.

## Conclusions

Our study characterizes the management and outcomes of sepsis due to a diversity of pathogens in public hospitals in Southeast Asia. We identify areas for improvement in sepsis care and show that the SOFA score is generally feasible to quantify the degree of organ dysfunction and determine the risk of death in these patients. To reduce mortality caused by sepsis in LMICs, the fundamental elements of sepsis care need to be tailored to and evaluated in these settings.

## Additional files

**Additional file 1: Figure S1.** Study sites. Red dots represent nine study areas. (1) Jakarta, (2) Yogyakarta and (3) Makassar in Indonesia; (4) Bangkok, (5) Chiang Rai and (6) Ubon Ratchathani in Thailand; and (7) Hanoi, (8) Hue and (9) Ho Chi Minh City in Vietnam. (TIFF 9143 kb)

**Additional file 2: Table S1.** Diagnostic criteria for sepsis in adult patients. (DOCX 63 kb)

**Additional file 3: Table S2.** Sequential (sepsis-related) Organ Failure Assessment Score. (DOCX 64 kb)

**Additional file 4: Table S3.** Baseline characteristics and mortality by country. (DOCX 65 kb)

**Additional file 5: Table S4.** Adherence to Surviving Sepsis Campaign care bundles up to 24 h after admission by country. (DOCX 62 kb)

**Additional file 6: Table S5.** Pathogens identified by country. (DOCX 72 kb)

**Additional file 7: Table S6.** Other supportive care provided from the pre-transfer period up to 24 h after admission by country. (DOCX 63 kb)

**Additional file 8: Table S7.** Pathogens identified in non-survivors and survivors. (DOCX 71 kb)

**Additional file 9: Table S8.** Number of organ system failures (maximum SOFA score ≥ 3 points) up to 24 h of admission and 28-day mortality in sepsis patients. (DOCX 61 kb)

**Additional file 10: Table S9.** Availability of tests to calculate SOFA scores up to 24 h of admission by country. (DOCX 61 kb)

### Acknowledgements

We gratefully acknowledge the support provided by the staff at all participating hospitals. We also thank the patients who participated in the study. This project was funded in part with federal funds from the National Cancer Institute, National Institutes of Health, under contract no. HHSN261200800001E. This research was also supported in part by the National Institute of Allergy and Infectious Diseases, National Institutes of Health, USA. The content of this publication does not necessarily reflect the views or policies of the Department of Health and Human Services, nor does mention of trade names, commercial products, or organizations that imply endorsement by the US Government. DL was supported by a Wellcome Trust Public Health and Tropical Medicine Intermediate Fellowship, grant reference no. 101103/Z/13/Z. Mahidol-Oxford Tropical Medicine Research Unit (MORU) in Thailand and Oxford University Clinical Research Unit (OUCRU) in Vietnam were supported by Wellcome Trust of Great Britain, grant reference nos. 106698/B/14/Z and 106680/B/14/Z, respectively. Southeast Asia Infectious Disease Clinical Research Network included Pratiwi Sudarmono (Cipto Mangunkusumo Hospital, Jakarta, Indonesia); Abu Tholib Aman (Sardjito Hospital, Yogyakarta, Indonesia); Mansyur Arif (Wahidin Soedirohusodo Hospital, Makassar, Indonesia); Armaji Kamaludi Syarif, Herman Kosasih, and Muhammad Karyana (National Institute of Health Research and Development (NIHRD), Jakarta, Indonesia); Tawee Chotpitayasunondh and Warunee Punpanich Vandepitte (Queen Sirikit National Institute of Child Health, Thailand); Adiratha Boonyasiri, Keswadee Lapphra, Kulkanya Chokephaibulkit, Pinyo Rattanaumpawan, and Visanu Thamlikitkul (Siriraj Hospital, Bangkok, Thailand); Achara Laongnualpanich (Chiang Rai Prachanukroh Hospital, Chiang Rai, Thailand); Prapit Teparrakkul and Pramot Srisamang (Sappasithiprasong Hospital, Ubon Ratchathani, Thailand); Phan Huu Phuc and Le Thanh Hai (National Hospital of Peaditrics, Hanoi, Vietnam); Nguyen Van Kinh (National Hospital of Tropical Diseases, Hanoi, Vietnam); Bui Duc Phu (Hue Central Hospital, Hue, Vietnam); Nguyen Thanh Hung and Tang Chi Thuong (Children's Hospital 1, Ho Chi Minh City, Vietnam); Ha Manh Tuan (Children's Hospital 2, Ho Chi Minh City, Vietnam); Lam Minh Yen and Nguyen Van Vinh Chau (Hospital for Tropical Diseases, Ho Chi Minh City, Vietnam); Direk Limmathurotsakul, Janjira Thaipadungpanit, Stuart Blacksell, and Nicholas Day (Mahidol-Oxford Tropical Medicine Research Unit (MORU), Bangkok, Thailand); Claire Ling (Shoklo Malaria Research Unit); Guy Thwaites, Heiman Wertheim, Le Van Tan, Motiur Rahman, and H. Rogier van Doorn (Oxford University Clinical Research Unit (OUCRU), Vietnam); and Chuen-Yen Lau (National Institute of Allergy and Infectious Diseases, National Institutes of Health, USA).

### Funding

This study was funded by the National Cancer Institute (HHSN261200800001E) and National Institute of Allergy and Infectious Diseases, National Institutes of Health, USA, and Wellcome Trust of Great Britain (106680/B/14/Z and 106698/B/14/Z).

### Authors' contributions

The SEAICRN executive committee conceived and supervised the study. The SEAICRN executive committee included Pratiwi Sudarmono, Abu Tholib Aman, Mansyur Arif, Tawee Chotpitayasunondh, Warunee Punpanich Vandepitte, Kulkanya Chokephaibulkit, Phan Huu Phuc, Nguyen Van Kinh, NVVC, Nicholas Day, Guy Thwaites, CYL, and DL. SEAICRN executive committee contributed to the conception and design. KCL, CYL, NVVC, TEW, and DL contributed to the analysis and interpretation. KCL, CYL, NVVC, TEW, and DL drafted the manuscript for important intellectual content. All authors approved the final version of the manuscript.

### Competing interests

The authors declare that they have no competing interests.

## Author details

[1]Department of Internal Medicine, Cipto Mangunkusumo Hospital, Jakarta, Indonesia. [2]Collaborative Clinical Research Branch, Division of Clinical Research, National Institute of Allergy and Infectious Diseases, National Institutes of Health, Bethesda, USA. [3]Department of Internal Medicine, Hospital for Tropical Diseases, Ho Chi Minh City, Vietnam. [4]Department of Internal Medicine, Oxford University Clinical Research Unit, Ho Chi Minh City, Vietnam. [5]Division of Pulmonary and Critical Care Medicine, Department of Medicine, University of Washington, Seattle, WA, USA. [6]Department of Global Health, University of Washington, Seattle, WA, USA. [7]Centre for Tropical Medicine and Global Health, Nuffield Department of Medicine, University of Oxford, Oxford, UK. [8]Mahidol-Oxford Tropical Medicine Research Unit, Faculty of Tropical Medicine, Mahidol University, Bangkok, Thailand. [9]Department of Tropical Hygiene, Faculty of Tropical Medicine, Mahidol University, 420/6 Rajvithi Road, Bangkok 10400, Thailand.

## References

1.  Singer M, Deutschman CS, Seymour CW, et al. The third international consensus definitions for sepsis and septic shock (sepsis-3). JAMA. 2016;315:801–10.
2.  Fleischmann C, Scherag A, Adhikari NK, et al. Assessment of global incidence and mortality of hospital-treated sepsis. Current estimates and limitations. Am J Respir Crit Care Med. 2016;193:259–72.
3.  Cheng AC, West TE, Peacock SJ. Surviving sepsis in developing countries. Crit Care Med. 2008;36:2487. author reply -8
4.  Angus DC, Seymour CW, Coopersmith CM, et al. A framework for the development and interpretation of different sepsis definitions and clinical criteria. Crit Care Med. 2016;44:e113–21.
5.  Seymour CW, Coopersmith CM, Deutschman CS, et al. Application of a framework to assess the usefulness of alternative sepsis criteria. Crit Care Med. 2016;44:e122–30.
6.  Vincent JL, Moreno R, Takala J, et al. The SOFA (Sepsis-related Organ Failure Assessment) score to describe organ dysfunction/failure. On behalf of the Working Group on Sepsis-Related Problems of the European Society of Intensive Care Medicine. Intensive Care Med 1996;22:707-710.
7.  Minne L, Abu-Hanna A, de Jonge E. Evaluation of SOFA-based models for predicting mortality in the ICU: a systematic review. Crit Care. 2008;12:R161.
8.  Seymour CW, Liu VX, Iwashyna TJ, et al. Assessment of clinical criteria for sepsis: for the Third International Consensus Definitions for Sepsis and Septic Shock (Sepsis-3). JAMA. 2016;315:762–74.
9.  Moreno R, Vincent JL, Matos R, et al. The use of maximum SOFA score to quantify organ dysfunction/failure in intensive care. Results of a prospective, multicentre study. Working Group on Sepsis related Problems of the ESICM. Intensive Care Med. 1999;25:686–96.
10. Papali A, Verceles AC, Augustin ME, et al. Sepsis in Haiti: prevalence, treatment, and outcomes in a Port-au-Prince referral hospital. J Crit Care. 2017;38:35–40.
11. Levy MM, Pronovost PJ, Dellinger RP, et al. Sepsis change bundles: converting guidelines into meaningful change in behavior and clinical outcome. Crit Care Med. 2004;32:S595–7.
12. Cardoso T, Carneiro AH, Ribeiro O, et al. Reducing mortality in severe sepsis with the implementation of a core 6-hour bundle: results from the Portuguese community-acquired sepsis study (SACiUCI study). Crit Care. 2010;14:R83.
13. Levy MM, Artigas A, Phillips GS, et al. Outcomes of the Surviving Sepsis Campaign in intensive care units in the USA and Europe: a prospective cohort study. Lancet Infect Dis. 2012;12:919–24.
14. Levy MM, Rhodes A, Phillips GS, et al. Surviving Sepsis Campaign: association between performance metrics and outcomes in a 7.5-year study. Crit Care Med. 2015;43:3–12.
15. Rhodes A, Phillips G, Beale R, et al. The Surviving Sepsis Campaign bundles and outcome: results from the International Multicentre Prevalence Study on Sepsis (the IMPreSS study). Intensive Care Med. 2015;41:1620–8.
16. Paek SC, Meemon N, Wan TT. Thailand's universal coverage scheme and its impact on health-seeking behavior. Springer Plus. 2016;5:1952.
17. Dat VQ, Long NT, Giang KB, et al. Healthcare infrastructure capacity to respond to severe acute respiratory infection (SARI) and sepsis in Vietnam: a low-middle income country. J Crit Care. 2017;42:109–15.
18. Rahmawati S. The implementation of Indonesian case-based groups (Ina-Cbg) of cesarean section patients in poor family health payment assurance in Undata Hospital of Central Sulawesi, Indonesia. IJHMT. 2016;1:56–78.
19. Southeast Asia Infectious Disease Clinical Research N. Causes and outcomes of sepsis in southeast Asia: a multinational multicentre cross-sectional study. Lancet Glob Health. 2017;5:e157–e67.
20. Dellinger RP, Levy MM, Rhodes A, et al. Surviving sepsis campaign: international guidelines for management of severe sepsis and septic shock: 2012. Crit Care Med. 2013;41:580–637.
21. Rutledge R, Lentz CW, Fakhry S, et al. Appropriate use of the Glasgow Coma Scale in intubated patients: a linear regression prediction of the Glasgow verbal score from the Glasgow eye and motor scores. J Trauma. 1996;41:514–22.
22. Hosmer DW, Lemeshow S. Applied logistic regression: Wiley Online Library; 2005. http://onlinelibrary.wiley.com/book/10.1002/0471722146. Accessed 30 Mar 2017.
23. Rhodes A, Evans LE, Alhazzani W, et al. Surviving sepsis campaign: international guidelines for management of sepsis and septic shock: 2016. Intensive Care Med. 2017;43(3):304–77.
24. Dunser MW, Festic E, Dondorp A, et al. Recommendations for sepsis management in resource-limited settings. Intensive Care Med. 2012;38:557–74.
25. Thwaites CL, Lundeg G, Dondorp AM, et al. Infection management in patients with sepsis and septic shock in resource-limited settings. Intensive Care Med. 2016;42:2117–8.
26. Teparrukkul P, Hantrakun V, Day NPJ, et al. Management and outcomes of severe dengue patients presenting with sepsis in a tropical country. PLoS One. 2017;12:e0176233.
27. Semler MW, Rice TW. Sepsis resuscitation: fluid choice and dose. Clin Chest Med. 2016;37:241–50.
28. Andrews B, Muchemwa L, Kelly P, et al. Simplified severe sepsis protocol: a randomized controlled trial of modified early goal-directed therapy in Zambia. Crit Care Med. 2014;42:2315–24.
29. Maitland K, Kiguli S, Opoka RO, et al. Mortality after fluid bolus in African children with severe infection. N Engl J Med. 2011;364:2483–95.
30. Brown SM, Grissom CK, Moss M, et al. Nonlinear imputation of Pao2/Fio2 from Spo2/Fio2 among patients with acute respiratory distress syndrome. Chest. 2016;150:307–13.
31. Vincent JL, Sakr Y, Sprung CL, et al. Sepsis in European intensive care units: results of the SOAP study. Crit Care Med. 2006;34:344–53.
32. Sharma J, Suryavanshi M. Thrombocytopenia in leptospirosis and role of platelet transfusion. Asian J Transfus Sci. 2007;1:52–5.
33. Costa F, Hagan JE, Calcagno J, et al. Global morbidity and mortality of leptospirosis: a systematic review. PLoS Negl Trop Dis. 2015;9:e0003898.
34. Prasad N, Murdoch DR, Reyburn H, et al. Etiology of severe febrile illness in low- and middle-income countries: a systematic review. PLoS One. 2015;10: e0127962.

# 18

# Monitoring of sedation depth in intensive care unit by therapeutic drug monitoring? A prospective observation study of medical intensive care patients

Richard J. Nies[1,6]* (iD), Carsten Müller[2], Roman Pfister[1], Philipp S. Binder[3], Nicole Nosseir[2], Felix S. Nettersheim[1], Kathrin Kuhr[4], Martin H. J. Wiesen[2], Matthias Kochanek[5] and Guido Michels[1]

## Abstract

**Background:** Analgosedation is a cornerstone therapy for mechanically ventilated patients in intensive care units (ICU). To avoid inadequate sedation and its complications, monitoring of analgosedation is of great importance. The aim of this study was to investigate whether monitoring of analgosedative drug concentrations (midazolam and sufentanil) might be beneficial to optimize analgosedation and whether drug serum concentrations correlate with the results of subjective (Richmond Agitation-Sedation Scale [RASS]/Ramsay Sedation Scale) and objective (bispectral (BIS) index) monitoring procedures.

**Methods:** Forty-nine intubated, ventilated, and analgosedated critically ill patients treated in ICU were clinically evaluated concerning the depth of sedation using RASS Score, Ramsay Score, and BIS index twice a day. Serum concentrations of midazolam and sufentanil were determined in blood samples drawn at the same time. Clinical and laboratory data were statistically analyzed for correlations using the Spearman's rank correlation coefficient rho ($\rho$).

**Results:** Average age of the population was 57.8 ± 16.0 years, 61% of the patients were males. Most frequent causes for ICU treatments were sepsis (22%), pneumonia (22%), or a combination of both (25%). Serum concentrations of midazolam correlated weakly with RASS ($\rho = -0.467$) and Ramsay Scores ($\rho = 0.476$). Serum concentrations of sufentanil correlated weakly with RASS ($\rho = -0.312$) and Ramsay Scores ($\rho = 0.295$). Correlations between BIS index and serum concentrations of midazolam ($\rho = -0.252$) and sufentanil ($\rho = -0.166$) were low.

**Conclusion:** Correlations between drug serum concentrations and clinical or neurophysiological monitoring procedures were weak. This might be due to intersubject variability, polypharmacy with drug-drug interactions, and complex metabolism, which can be altered in critically ill patients. Therapeutic drug monitoring is not beneficial to determine depth of sedation in ICU patients.

**Keywords:** Analgosedation, Intensive care, Richmond Agitation-Sedation Scale, Drug monitoring, Midazolam, Sufentanil

* Correspondence: richard.nies@uk-koeln.de
[1]Department III of Internal Medicine, Heart Center, University Hospital of
Cologne, Kerpener Str. 62, 50937 Cologne, Germany
[6]Department of Cardiology, University Hospital of Cologne, Kerpener Str. 62,
50937 Cologne, Germany
Full list of author information is available at the end of the article

# Background

Critically ill patients on intensive care units require regimens of analgosedation for several reasons such as mechanical ventilation. Finding the optimal treatment and sedation depth is often challenging because of multimorbidity and polypharmacy. High interindividual variability concerning pharmacokinetics as well as insufficient monitoring can lead to inadequate dosage of drugs, which might increase morbidity and mortality. Low states of analgosedation can cause hypercatabolism, immunosuppression, hypercoagulopathy, awareness and increased sympathetic activity, or inadvertent extubation, whereas deep sedation can be responsible for extended mechanical ventilation, higher risk of nosocomial pneumonia, increasing costs, and neuropsychological dysfunction [1–6]. Hence, monitoring of analgosedation is an elementary part of ICU procedures to avoid excessive sedation states, drug-induced delirium, and higher mortality [2, 4, 6]. According to the guidelines, the current state of analgesia, sedation, and delirium should therefore be measured every 8 h using validated monitoring procedures [4].

To improve individual treatment, clinical scores such as the Richmond Agitation-Sedation Scale (RASS) Score [7] and Ramsay Sedation Scale Score [8] (Additional files 1 and 2) as well as neurophysiological monitoring procedures such as BIS monitoring have been established. BIS monitoring is based on simplified electroencephalograms (EEG) and a consecutive spectral analysis [9, 10].

Gold standard for the assessment of sedation depth is the RASS Score in combination with physiological parameters like heart rate, blood pressure, mimic, gesture, lacrimation, and perspiration [4, 6]. Reliability and validity of the RASS Score have been analyzed in several studies [7, 11]. Particularly in deeper sedated patients, RASS Score is more precise than Ramsay Score, which is not recommended in the German AWMF guidelines anymore [4].

The BIS index is a unitless value ranging from 0 to 100, a value of 100 representing an adequate awake condition (Additional file 3) [12]. Several authors have shown that BIS index has a good validity and reliability regarding the RASS and the Ramsay Scores [3, 13–15].

The combination of benzodiazepines and opioids is a common regime in European ICUs, although nonbenzodiazepine sedatives should be preferred [4, 6]. In comparison with other benzodiazepines, the advantages of midazolam are its rapid metabolic inactivation, clearance, and comparatively short elimination half-time [16]. If the prolonged intravenous application is expected, sufentanil is superior to fentanyl because of its additional hypnotic potency [6, 17–19]. Sufentanil has a strong affinity to $\mu_1$-receptors causing a potent analgesic effect. Compared to other opioids, affinity to $\mu_2$-receptors, which induces respiratory depression, is lower [20]. Hence, both drugs are suitable for ICU therapy.

The correlations between serum concentrations and subjective monitoring procedures (RASS and Ramsay Scores) as well as objective monitoring procedures (BIS-monitoring) were investigated in this study. The aim of this study was to clarify whether or not therapeutic drug monitoring is useful to assess the sedation depth in intensive care patients.

# Methods

## Patient population

This study was performed between December 2012 and December 2014 in cooperation with the ICU of the Department of Internal Medicine and the Center of Pharmacology, University Hospital of Cologne. Intubated, artificially ventilated, and analgosedated intensive care patients, who agreed to this study by themselves or through legal representatives before intubation, were included. Exclusion criteria were age < 18 years, missing patient's consent, history of alcohol or drug abuse, history of neurological or psychiatric conditions, polytraumatization, conditions after CPR, and suspicion of hypoxic brain damage. RASS Score, Ramsay Score, BIS index, and serum concentrations of analgosedatives were measured twice a day (7:00 a.m. and 7:00 p.m.). Overall, 49 patients were included in the study, and 538 data points were determined. The maximal period under consideration was 10 days. Sepsis was defined according to the criteria by Bone et al. [21].

## Procedure of intubation and maintenance of analgosedation

After induction with fentanyl, etomidate and rocuronium orotracheal intubation was performed. Analgosedation was then maintained with midazolam (infusion rate of 0.03–0.2 mg/kg/h i.v.) and sufentanil (infusion rate of 0.1–1.0 µg/kg/h i.v.). According to the clinical presentation and sedation depth, the infusion rates were adapted.

## Assessment of depth of sedation

Sedation depth was evaluated by RASS Score, Ramsay Score, BIS monitoring, and measurements of serum concentrations of analgosedatives. To avoid artifacts, BIS index was recorded after 15 min of patients' rest, and averaging time was set at a maximum of 30 s. Afterwards, RASS and Ramsay Scores were assessed. Finally, blood samples were taken. For calculation of RASS Score, initially, the decision had to be made whether a patient was "awake" (positive values) or "sedated" (negative values). "Awake" patients were assessed regarding the reaction while the observer was entering the room. If the patient was considered to be "sedated," further evaluation was made using a fixed protocol in order to cause eye-opening or a change in facial expression: observer entering room, verbal contact, light physical contact, severe physical contact by shaking patient's shoulder, induction of light pain by pinching the back of patient's hand, and induction of severe pain by rubbing patient's sternum.

## Measurement of the drug serum concentrations

A liquid chromatography-tandem mass spectrometry (LC-MS/MS) method for quantitative serum concentration measurements of four analgosedatives (ketamine, lorazepam, midazolam, and sufentanil) frequently used in intensive care medicine has been previously developed and validated according to ICH Guidelines Q2 (R1) [22]. This technique was successfully applied on adult and critically ill patients and provides the basis for pharmacokinetic research projects. The results of this test are available within 2 to 4 h.

## Statistics

Statistical analysis and graphic design were performed using IBM SPSS Statistics version 22. Correlations were analyzed using Spearman's rank correlation coefficient rho ($\rho$). The value of $\rho$ was interpreted as follows: $0 \leq |\rho| < 0.1$—no or very weak correlation; $0.1 \leq |\rho| < 0.5$—weak correlation; $0.5 \leq |\rho| < 0.8$—moderate correlation; $0.8 \leq |\rho| \leq 1$—strong correlation. Box plots were used for graphic illustration.

## Results

### Patient population structure

Clinical data and baseline characteristics of the patient population are listed in Table 1. The average age of the study population was $57.8 \pm 16.0$ years. Sixty-one percent of the patients were males. About two thirds of the patients were suffering primarily from a hematooncologic condition. Indications for ICU treatments were manifold. Most frequent reasons were sepsis (22%), pneumonia (22%), or a combination of both (25%). Eight percent of the study population had no prior diseases and required ICU treatment due to an acute medical problem.

### Correlations between subjective monitoring procedures, objective monitoring procedures, and serum concentrations of analgosedatives

The correlation between RASS Score and serum concentrations of midazolam reached a $\rho$ value of $-0.467$ (Fig. 1a). A weak correlation was observed between RASS Score and serum concentrations of sufentanil ($\rho = -0.312$, Fig. 1b). Higher serum concentrations of analgosedatives are tendentiously associated with lower RASS Scores. Similar results were observed concerning Ramsay Score, which correlates also only weakly with midazolam serum concentrations ($\rho = 0.476$, Fig. 2a) and sufentanil serum concentrations ($\rho = 0.295$, Fig. 2b). Overall correlations between subjective monitoring procedures and serum concentrations of the investigated analgosedatives were low.

**Table 1** Clinical data and baseline characteristics of the study population

| Baseline data | | | |
|---|---|---|---|
| Total number of patients | $n = 49$ | | |
| Average age (years) ± SD (range) | $57.8 \pm 16.0$ | (20–83) | |
| Gender | 19 women/30 men | | |
| Weight (kg) ± SD (range) | $87.9 \pm 27.7$ | (60–210) | |
| APACHE II Score ± SD (range) | $13.1 \pm 6.7$ | (2–27) | |
| SOFA Score ± SD (range) | $17.8 \pm 3.5$ | (9–23) | |
| Endotracheal ventilation | $n = 49$ | | |
| Analgosedation with sufentanil and midazolam | $n = 49$ | | |
| Total number of blood samples | $n = 538$ | | |
| Number of blood samples per patient (range) | 11.0 | (3–20) | |
| Underlying disease | $n$ | % | |
| Hematooncology | 31 | 63.3 | |
| COPD | 7 | 14.3 | |
| Nephrology | 3 | 6.1 | |
| Infectiology | 2 | 4.1 | |
| Cardiology | 2 | 4.1 | |
| None | 4 | 8.2 | |
| Reason for ICU treatment | $n$ | % | |
| Pneumonia | 11 | 22.4 | |
| Sepsis | 11 | 22.4 | |
| Sepsis + pneumonia | 12 | 24.5 | |
| Sepsis + acute renal failure | 2 | 4.1 | |
| ARDS | 2 | 4.1 | |
| GvHD | 1 | 2.0 | |
| Acute renal failure | 3 | 6.1 | |
| Cardial decompensation | 2 | 4.1 | |
| Hb-relevant bleeding | 1 | 2.0 | |
| Pneumonia + acute pancreatitis | 1 | 2.0 | |
| Mesenterial ischemia | 1 | 2.0 | |
| Coecum perforation | 1 | 2.0 | |
| Pneumonia + upper intestinal bleeding | 1 | 2.0 | |

Correlations between BIS index and serum concentrations of midazolam ($\rho = -0.252$, Fig. 3a) and sufentanil ($\rho = -0.166$, Fig. 3b) were only weak. Nevertheless, higher blood levels of midazolam were observed with falling BIS index values.

## Discussion

Since light sedation levels are associated with improved clinical outcomes, monitoring procedures are part of the ongoing research. To avoid adverse clinical events due to excessively low or deep sedation, the purpose of this

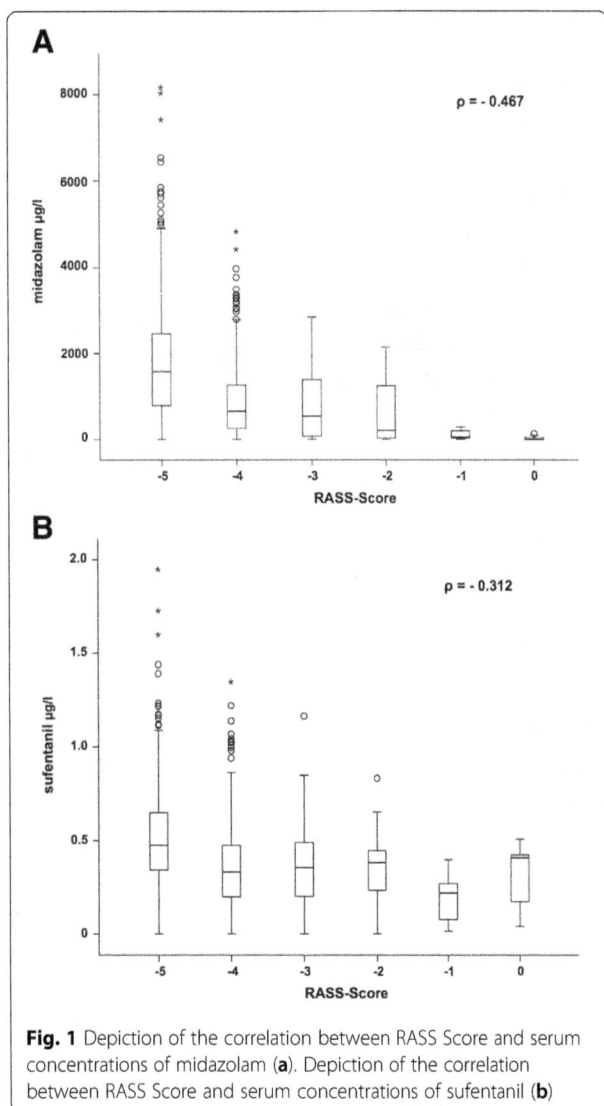

**Fig. 1** Depiction of the correlation between RASS Score and serum concentrations of midazolam (**a**). Depiction of the correlation between RASS Score and serum concentrations of sufentanil (**b**)

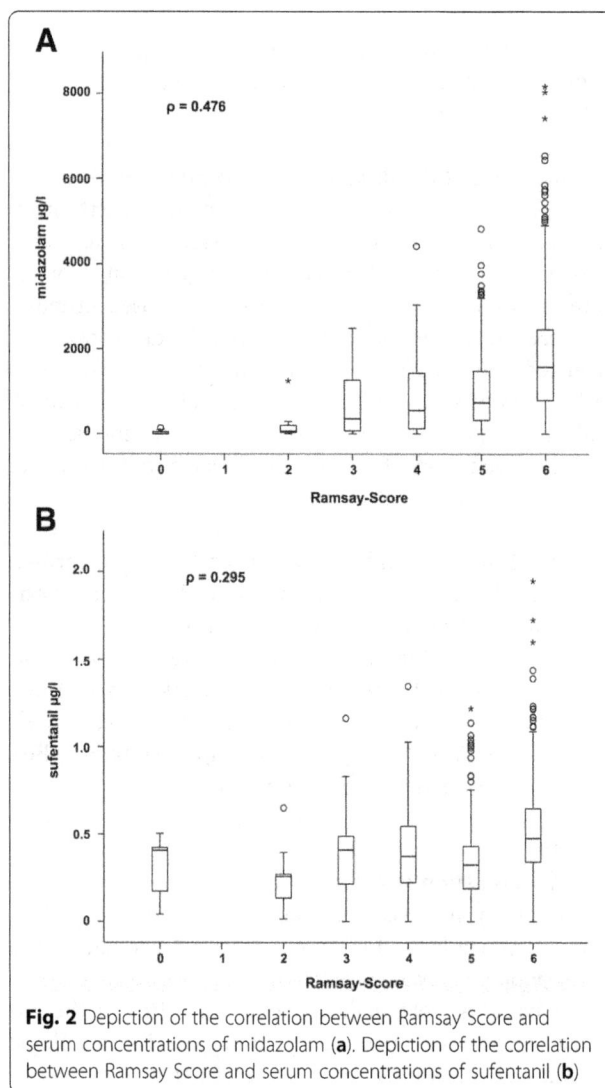

**Fig. 2** Depiction of the correlation between Ramsay Score and serum concentrations of midazolam (**a**). Depiction of the correlation between Ramsay Score and serum concentrations of sufentanil (**b**)

study was to analyze whether the measurement of drug serum concentrations might lead to a highly individual, drug concentration-guided analgosedation. Therefore, serum concentrations were compared to common monitoring procedures.

### Correlation between RASS/Ramsay Score and drug serum concentrations

Serum concentrations of sufentanil had only a weak correlation with RASS and Ramsay Scores, whereas serum concentrations of midazolam showed a better but still weak correlation. Bremer et al. [23] investigated 648 critically ill patients by therapeutic drug monitoring, who received a combination of fentanyl and midazolam when they had to be mechanically ventilated > 24 h. The authors found a strong correlation between midazolam plasma concentrations and sedation levels ($r^2 = 0.906$). A Ramsay Score of 6 was observed in patients with a median midazolam level of

594 ng/ml, and high intersubject variability was seen. Similar results were described by Glass et al. using the Observers' Assessment of Alertness/Sedation Scale (OAA/S Score; $r = 0.746$) [24].

In this study, serum midazolam levels correlated weakly with RASS and Ramsay Scores. A Ramsay Score of 6 was associated with a median midazolam concentration clearly above 1000 ng/ml, whereas the other patients showed median midazolam concentrations lower than that.

Bremer et al. [23] described a significant increase of midazolam plasma levels in critically ill patients within the first days due to reduced midazolam clearance mainly caused by impaired liver function. Park and Miller [25] found reduced cytochrome P450 3A4 (CYP3A4) activity in critically ill patients, which is a hepatic key enzyme for the midazolam pathway. Prolonged sedation additionally caused by an accumulation of conjugated 1-hydroxymidazolam was also observed in

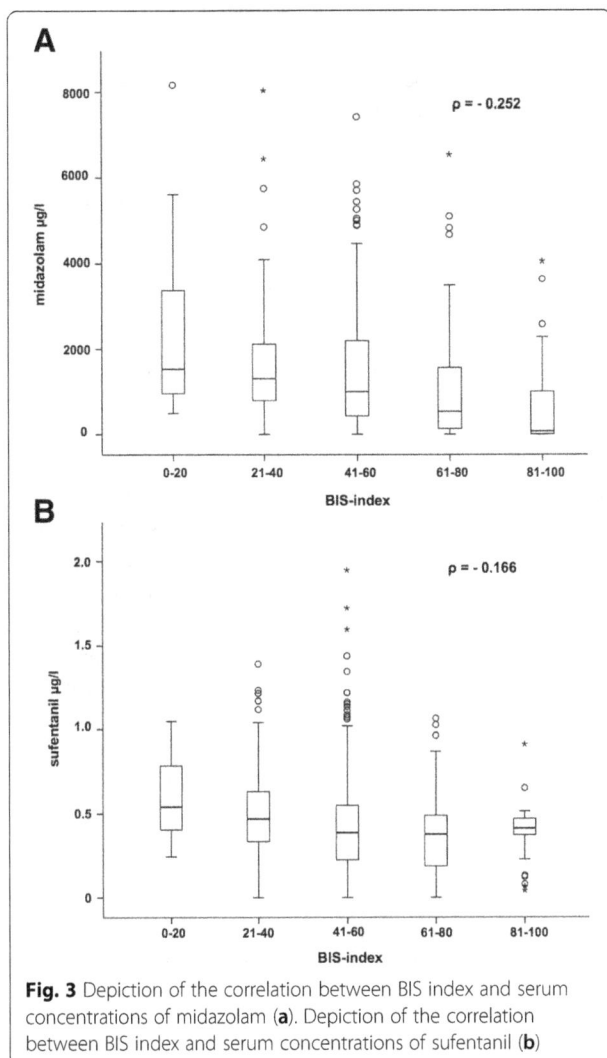

**Fig. 3** Depiction of the correlation between BIS index and serum concentrations of midazolam (**a**). Depiction of the correlation between BIS index and serum concentrations of sufentanil (**b**)

Ethuin et al. [31] analyzed the pharmacokinetics of long-term sufentanil infusion for analgosedation with midazolam in ten ICU patients. The mean sufentanil serum concentration to reach a Ramsay Score of at least 3 was $0.86 \pm 0.60$ ng/ml. In this study, median serum concentrations of sufentanil were between 0.25 and 0.5 ng/ml (Fig. 2b) independent of the sedation depth determined by Ramsay Score. Correlations between RASS/Ramsay Score and serum concentrations of sufentanil were weak. Since sufentanil is an analgesic drug with only a hypnotical side effect, it is not surprising that the correlations with clinical scales are lower than with midazolam, which is a primary sedative drug. In the study of Glass et al. [24], none of their patients lost consciousness (OAA/S Score, 0–2) receiving alfentanil solely. Because midazolam and sufentanil were given simultaneously, the analysis of the isolated clinical effect of each drug is limited and confounded. Wappler et al. [18] investigated the efficacy of a three-level regimen of analgosedation in patients during ICU treatment: sufentanil mono (short-stay, group 1), sufentanil + midazolam (long-term intubated patients, group 2), and sufentanil + midazolam + clonidin (group 3). Adequate sedation was defined by a Ramsay Score of 2–3, which was reached in all groups. However, sufentanil infusion rates were higher in groups 2 and 3, which showed that polypharmacy contributes to intersubject variability. Additionally, continuous drug infusion leads to longer elimination half-times of sufentanil compared with single bolus use caused by increased tissue distribution, changes in protein binding, and often impaired hepatic function in critically ill patients [31]. Hofbauer et al. [17] investigated sufentanil requirement of elderly patients undergoing ventilatory support in ICUs and concluded that no adjustements have to be made regarding the patients' age.

## Correlations between BIS index and drug serum concentrations

Miyake et al. [32] investigated the correlation between serum concentration of midazolam and BIS index in 24 orthopedic patients (ASA I/II). Patients were separated in a small dose ($0.2$ mg $kg^{-1}$) and a large dose midazolam group ($0.3$ mg $kg^{-1}$). After remifentanil, midazolam, and vecuronium were administered, intubation was performed, and eight blood samples were collected within 1 h before the operation. Although midazolam plasma concentrations were significantly higher in the large dose group, the authors found no differences concerning BIS index between the two groups. This indicates that there is no correlation between BIS index and serum concentrations of midazolam. In this study, BIS index and midazolam serum concentrations showed only a weak correlation ($\rho = -0.252$), which stands in line with the results of Miyake et al. [32]. A limitation of both studies

septic shock patients with severe renal failure [26, 27]. Bolon et al. [28] showed that in such cases, dialysis is rather effective in eliminating the conjugated metabolite than midazolam itself. Therefore, for patients needing dialysis, liver function plays a key role in midazolam clearance. Furthermore, Vinik et al. [29] observed a higher portion of unbound midazolam in patients with renal failure causing prolonged sedation, even when free drug clearance was unchanged.

Comedication with opioids could inhibit midazolam metabolism [30]. Moreover, the impact of age on the midazolam metabolism is commonly known, and the dosage has to be reduced in the elderly. However, surrogate parameters to guide the adaption of infusion rates such as serum bilirubin and serum creatinine levels rise with a delay of more than 10 days [23].

In this study, 57% of the patients suffered at least from sepsis or acute renal failure, which led to high intersubject variability (Figs. 1a and 2b) and a slight correlation.

is that concentrations of the active metabolite were not measured. Glass et al. [24] observed a decreasing BIS index at higher midazolam serum concentrations. Maximum midazolam serum concentration was around 800 ng/ml, whereas in this study, much higher concentrations were found (Fig. 3a). Concerning analgosedation, a BIS index between 55 and 70 seems to be adequate [14]. Several authors described that midazolam can only cause a decrease of BIS index to 65–70 [33, 34]. Miyake et al. [32] found a correlation between BIS index and the relative beta ratio in EEG, which indicates that BIS index is influenced by cerebral beta activity. Billard et al. [35] described that midazolam induces an increased EEG frequency and amplitude. Seven out of eight patients showed an increase in relative beta power in EEG. Bagchi et al. [34] detected a marked divergence between BIS index and a subjective monitoring evaluation (OAA/S Score) in sedation protocols with midazolam. Approximately 38% of their patients sedated with midazolam were deeply sedated based on OAA/S Score, whereas BIS index value remained at 70. The time to reach a BIS index of 70 was significantly longer in the midazolam group compared with a propofol group. Ibrahim et al. [33] also found that BIS index is a better predictor for sedation with propofol than with midazolam. However, in this study, BIS index below 70 occurred frequently (Fig. 3a), which might be explained by the combination of pharmacons. Ben-Shlomo et al. [36] showed that midazolam and opioids act as a supraadditve concerning sedation.

Conclusively, BIS index will reach its limits—especially as a primary monitoring of sedation depth—when the effect of midazolam is monitored because it does not further decrease although the patient is clinically sedated and plasma concentrations are higher than needed for adequate sedation.

Glass et al. [24] showed that BIS index correlated with hypnotic drug concentrations, whereas alfentanil at plasma concentrations < 300 ng/ml did not effect it. Despite increasing alfentanil serum concentrations (maximum, approximately 280 ng/ml), BIS index did not decrease and remained high. However, Billard et al. [35] showed that BIS index might be suppressed below 50 at higher doses of alfentanil. Guignard et al. [37] investigated how remifentanil levels influence BIS index in a pain-free steady state of propofol and during a painful intervention (orotracheal intubation). In all patients, BIS index remained stable before intubation, which means remifentanil did not influence BIS index. This might be explained by the fact that hypnotics have a higher impact on EEG than opioids, which unfold their effect through an inhibition of subcortical structures. Patients with lower remifentanil infusion rates showed an increase in heart rate, mean arterial pressure, and BIS index during intubation, which stand in line with the

observations made by Iselin-Chaves et al. [38], who described an inverse correlation between BIS index variability and level of analgesia. In contrast to that, Kato et al. [39] calculated clearly a better correlation between the RASS Score and the BIS index when low-dose remifentanil was administered in addition to propofol. In this study, high variable BIS index values were observed at almost the same serum concentrations of sufentanil (Fig. 3b).

**Limitations of the study**

This study was a single-center study with a relatively small population of 49 intubated patients. Moreover, BIS index values are very susceptible. For example, endotracheal or oral suctioning, body hygiene procedures, passive movements, and physical contact are able to influence BIS index without changing the sedation depth necessarily [10, 40]. To minimize this interference, BIS index was recorded after a period of patients' rest. Nevertheless, the level of noise in ICUs is significant and cannot be completely avoided to ensure the patients' safety. Pharmacokinetics of midazolam and sufentanil vary with disease severity such as sepsis with higher distribution volume and especially hypalbuminaemia due to capillary leaking. Septic shock patients often suffer from kidney and liver dysfunction, which lead to a dysregulated drug metabolism [27, 41]. CYP3A4 is a key enzyme for the midazolam and sufentanil metabolism. Its activity can be altered by CYP interactions caused by other drugs such as antibiotics, which were not monitored in this study. Further potential drug-drug interactions in ICUs are likely and often underestimated [42].

Delirium may influence the assessment of sedation. However, we did not screen our patients for delirium since Haenggi et al. [43] reported that even in patients with a RASS Score of – 2/– 3, delirium is overdiagnosed and difficult to be differentiated from sedation. Therefore, many factors contribute to an almost unpredictable interindividual variability of drug serum concentrations and its effects.

**Conclusion**

Correlations between drug serum concentrations (midazolam and sufentanil) and RASS Score, Ramsay Score, or BIS index were only weak, the results for midazolam being slightly better than those for sufentanil. This might be due to the intersubject variability, polypharmacy with drug-drug interactions, and complex metabolism, which can be altered especially in critically ill patients. Therefore, individual course of disease and patients' comorbidity have to be taken into account. Therapeutic drug monitoring is not beneficial to determine the depth of sedation in ICU patients. Analgosedation of patients in ICUs should therefore be guided by subjective monitoring procedures.

## Additional files

**Additional file 1:** Richmond Agitation Sedation Scale [7]. (PDF 50 kb)

**Additional file 2:** Ramsay Sedation Scale [8]. (PDF 44 kb)

**Additional file 3:** Monitoring the depth of sedation with BIS-monitoring [12]. (PDF 44 kb)

## Abbreviations

APACHE: Acute Physiology and Chronic Health Evaluation; ASA: American Society of Anesthesiologists; AWMF: Arbeitsgemeinschaft Wissenschaftlicher Medizinischer Fachgesellschaften; BIS: Bispectral index; CPR: Cardiopulmonary resuscitation; CYP3A4: Cytochrome P450 3A4; EEG: Electro encephalograms; IBM SPSS: International Business Machines Statistical Package for the Social Sciences; ICH: International Council for Harmonisation; ICU: Intensive care unit; LC-MS/MS: Liquid chromatography-tandem mass spectrometry; OAA/S: Observers' Assessment of Alertness/Sedation; RASS: Richmond Agitation-Sedation Scale; SOFA: Sequential Organ Failure Assessment

## Acknowledgements

The authors thank the medical and nursing staff of the two medical intensive care units. This paper includes the doctoral thesis of PSB.

## Authors' contributions

GM, RP, and MK were responsible for the study design. Clinical evaluation of the patients concerning depth of sedation was performed by PSB. CM, NN, and MHJW contributed to the study by their pharmacological expertise and determined the quantitative serum concentrations of the analgosedative drugs. KK was responsible for the statistical analysis. RN, PSB, and FN performed the data analysis. Furthermore, RN prepared the manuscript. All authors read, reviewed, and approved the final manuscript.

## Competing interests

The authors declare that they have no competing interests.

## Author details

[1]Department III of Internal Medicine, Heart Center, University Hospital of Cologne, Kerpener Str. 62, 50937 Cologne, Germany. [2]Center of Pharmacology, Department of Therapeutic Drug Monitoring, University Hospital of Cologne, Gleueler Str. 24, 50931 Cologne, Germany. [3]St. Katharinen-Hospital GmbH, Kapellenstrasse 1-5, 50226 Frechen, Germany. [4]Institute of Medical Statistics and Computational Biology, University of Cologne, Kerpener Str. 62, 50937 Cologne, Germany. [5]Department I of Internal Medicine, University Hospital of Cologne, Kerpener Str. 62, 50937 Cologne, Germany. [6]Department of Cardiology, University Hospital of Cologne, Kerpener Str. 62, 50937 Cologne, Germany.

## References

1. Jackson DL, Proudfoot CW, Cann KF, Walsh T. A systematic review of the impact of sedation practice in the ICU on resource use, costs and patient safety. Crit Care. 2010;14:R59.

2. Roberts DJ, Haroon B, Hall RI. Sedation for critically ill or injured adults in the intensive care unit: a shifting paradigm. Drugs. 2012;72:1881–916.

3. Consales G, Chelazzi C, Rinaldi S, De Gaudio AR. Bispectral index compared to Ramsay score for sedation monitoring in intensive care units. Minerva Anestesiol. 2006;72:329–36.

4. Taskforce DAS, Baron R, Binder A, Biniek R, Braune S, Buerkle H, et al. Evidence and consensus based guideline for the management of delirium, analgesia, and sedation in intensive care medicine. Revision 2015 (DAS-Guideline 2015) - short version. Ger Med Sci. 2015;13:Doc19.

5. Chanques G, Jaber S, Barbotte E, Violet S, Sebbane M, Perrigault PF, et al. Impact of systematic evaluation of pain and agitation in an intensive care unit. Crit Care Med. 2006;34:1691–9.

6. Barr J, Fraser GL, Puntillo K, Ely EW, Gelinas C, Dasta JF, et al. Clinical practice guidelines for the management of pain, agitation, and delirium in adult patients in the intensive care unit. Crit Care Med. 2013;41:263–306.

7. Sessler CN, Gosnell MS, Grap MJ, Brophy GM, O'Neal PV, Keane KA, et al. The Richmond Agitation-Sedation Scale: validity and reliability in adult intensive care unit patients. Am J Respir Crit Care Med. 2002;166:1338–44.

8. Ramsay MA, Savege TM, Simpson BR, Goodwin R. Controlled sedation with alphaxalone-alphadolone. Br Med J. 1974;2:656–9.

9. Rosow C, Manberg PJ. Bispectral index monitoring. Anesthesiol Clin North Am. 2001;19:947–66 xi.

10. Rampil IJ. A primer for EEG signal processing in anesthesia. Anesthesiology. 1998;89:980–1002.

11. Ely EW, Truman B, Shintani A, Thomason JW, Wheeler AP, Gordon S, et al. Monitoring sedation status over time in ICU patients: reliability and validity of the Richmond Agitation-Sedation Scale (RASS). JAMA. 2003;289:2983–91.

12. Johansen JW. Update on bispectral index monitoring. Best Pract Res Clin Anaesthesiol. 2006;20:81–99.

13. Jung YJ, Chung WY, Lee M, Lee KS, Park JH, Sheen SS, et al. The significance of sedation control in patients receiving mechanical ventilation. Tuberc Respir Dis (Seoul). 2012;73:151–61.

14. Karamchandani K, Rewari V, Trikha A, Batra RK. Bispectral index correlates well with Richmond Agitation Sedation Scale in mechanically ventilated critically ill patients. J Anesth. 2010;24:394–8.

15. Yaman F, Ozcan N, Ozcan A, Kaymak C, Basar H. Assesment of correlation between bispectral index and four common sedation scales used in mechanically ventilated patients in ICU. Eur Rev Med Pharmacol Sci. 2012; 16:660–6.

16. Gerecke M. Chemical structure and properties of midazolam compared with other benzodiazepines. Br J Clin Pharmacol. 1983;16(Suppl 1):11S–6S.

17. Hofbauer R, Tesinsky P, Hammerschmidt V, Kofler J, Staudinger T, Kordova H, et al. No reduction in the sufentanil requirement of elderly patients undergoing ventilatory support in the medical intensive care unit. Eur J Anaesthesiol. 1999;16:702–7.

18. Wappler F, Scholz J, Prause A, Mollenberg O, Bause H, Schulte am Esch J. Level concept of analgesic dosing in intensive care medicine with sufentanil. Anasthesiol Intensivmed Notfallmed Schmerzther. 1998;33:8–26.

19. Kroll W, List WF. Ils sufentanil suitable for long-term sedation of a critically ill patient? Anaesthesist. 1992;41:271–5.

20. Monk JP, Beresford R, Ward A. Sufentanil. A review of its pharmacological properties and therapeutic use. Drugs. 1988;36:286–313.

21. Bone RC, Balk RA, Cerra FB, Dellinger RP, Fein AM, Knaus WA, et al. Definitions for sepsis and organ failure and guidelines for the use of innovative therapies in sepsis. The ACCP/SCCM Consensus Conference Committee. American College of Chest Physicians/Society of Critical Care Medicine. Chest. 1992;101:1644–55.

22. Nosseir NS, Michels G, Binder P, Wiesen MH, Muller C. Simultaneous detection of ketamine, lorazepam, midazolam and sufentanil in human serum with liquid chromatography-tandem mass spectrometry for monitoring of analgosedation in critically ill patients. J Chromatogr B Analyt Technol Biomed Life Sci. 2014;973C:133–41.

23. Bremer F, Reulbach U, Schwilden H, Schuttler J. Midazolam therapeutic drug monitoring in intensive care sedation: a 5-year survey. Ther Drug Monit. 2004;26:643–9.

24. Glass PS, Bloom M, Kearse L, Rosow C, Sebel P, Manberg P. Bispectral analysis measures sedation and memory effects of propofol, midazolam, isoflurane, and alfentanil in healthy volunteers. Anesthesiology. 1997;86:836–47.

25. Park GR, Miller E. What changes drug metabolism in critically ill patients--III? Effect of pre-existing disease on the drug metabolism of midazolam. Anaesthesia. 1996;51:431–4.

26. Bauer TM, Ritz R, Haberthur C, Ha HR, Hunkeler W, Sleight AJ, et al. Prolonged sedation due to accumulation of conjugated metabolites of midazolam. Lancet. 1995;346:145–7.

27. Fragen RJ. Pharmacokinetics and pharmacodynamics of midazolam given via continuous intravenous infusion in intensive care units. Clin Ther. 1997; 19:405–19 discussion 367-408.

28. Bolon M, Bastien O, Flamens C, Paulus S, Boulieu R. Midazolam disposition in patients undergoing continuous venovenous hemodialysis. J Clin Pharmacol. 2001;41:959–62.

29. Vinik HR, Reves JG, Greenblatt DJ, Abernethy DR, Smith LR. The pharmacokinetics of midazolam in chronic renal failure patients. Anesthesiology. 1983;59:390–4.

30. Oda Y, Mizutani K, Hase I, Nakamoto T, Hamaoka N, Asada A. Fentanyl inhibits metabolism of midazolam: competitive inhibition of CYP3A4 in vitro. Br J Anaesth. 1999;82:900–3.

31. Ethuin F, Boudaoud S, Leblanc I, Troje C, Marie O, Levron JC, et al. Pharmacokinetics of long-term sufentanil infusion for sedation in ICU patients. Intensive Care Med. 2003;29:1916–20.

32. Miyake W, Oda Y, Ikeda Y, Hagihira S, Iwaki H, Asada A. Electroencephalographic response following midazolam-induced general anesthesia: relationship to plasma and effect-site midazolam concentrations. J Anesth. 2010;24:386–93.

33. Ibrahim AE, Taraday JK, Kharasch ED. Bispectral index monitoring during sedation with sevoflurane, midazolam, and propofol. Anesthesiology. 2001; 95:1151–9.

34. Bagchi D, Mandal MC, Das S, Basu SR, Sarkar S, Das J. Bispectral index score and observer's assessment of awareness/sedation score may manifest divergence during onset of sedation: study with midazolam and propofol. Indian J Anaesth. 2013;57:351–7.

35. Billard V, Gambus PL, Chamoun N, Stanski DR, Shafer SL. A comparison of spectral edge, delta power, and bispectral index as EEG measures of alfentanil, propofol, and midazolam drug effect. Clin Pharmacol Ther. 1997; 61:45–58.

36. Ben-Shlomo I, abd-el-Khalim H, Ezry J, Zohar S, Tverskoy M. Midazolam acts synergistically with fentanyl for induction of anaesthesia. Br J Anaesth. 1990; 64:45–7.

37. Guignard B, Menigaux C, Dupont X, Fletcher D, Chauvin M. The effect of remifentanil on the bispectral index change and hemodynamic responses after orotracheal intubation. Anesth Analg. 2000;90:161–7.

38. Iselin-Chaves IA, Flaishon R, Sebel PS, Howell S, Gan TJ, Sigl J, et al. The effect of the interaction of propofol and alfentanil on recall, loss of consciousness, and the bispectral index. Anesth Analg. 1998;87:949–55.

39. Kato T, Koitabashi T, Ouchi T, Serita R. The utility of bispectral index monitoring for sedated patients treated with low-dose remifentanil. J Clin Monit Comput. 2012;26:459–63.

40. LeBlanc JM, Dasta JF, Kane-Gill SL. Role of the bispectral index in sedation monitoring in the ICU. Ann Pharmacother. 2006;40:490–500.

41. Shelly MP, Mendel L, Park GR. Failure of critically ill patients to metabolise midazolam. Anaesthesia. 1987;42:619–26.

42. Vanham D, Spinewine A, Hantson P, Wittebole X, Wouters D, Sneyers B. Drug-drug interactions in the intensive care unit: do they really matter? J Crit Care. 2017;38:97–103.

43. Haenggi M, Blum S, Brechbuehl R, Brunello A, Jakob SM, Takala J. Effect of sedation level on the prevalence of delirium when assessed with CAM-ICU and ICDSC. Intensive Care Med. 2013;39:2171–9.

# 19

# Limitation of life support techniques at admission to the intensive care unit

Olga Rubio[1*], Anna Arnau[1], Sílvia Cano[1], Carles Subirà[1], Begoña Balerdi[2], María Eugenía Perea[3], Miguel Fernández-Vivas[4], María Barber[5], Noemí Llamas[6], Susana Altaba[7], Ana Prieto[8], Vicente Gómez[9], Mar Martin[10], Marta Paz[11], Belen Quesada[12], Valentí Español[13], Juan Carlos Montejo[14], José Manuel Gomez[15], Gloria Miro[16], Judith Xirgú[17], Ana Ortega[18], Pedro Rascado[19], Juan María Sánchez[20], Alfredo Marcos[21], Ana Tizon[22], Pablo Monedero[23], Elisabeth Zabala[24], Cristina Murcia[25], Ines Torrejon[26], Kenneth Planas[27], José Manuel Añon[28], Gonzalo Hernandez[29], María-del-Mar Fernandez[30], Consuelo Guía[31], Vanesa Arauzo[32], José Miguel Perez[33], Rosa Catalan[34], Javier Gonzalez[35], Rosa Poyo[36], Roser Tomas[37], Iñaki Saralegui[38], Jordi Mancebo[39], Charles Sprung[40] and Rafael Fernández[41]

## Abstract

**Purpose:** To determine the frequency of limitations on life support techniques (LLSTs) on admission to intensive care units (ICU), factors associated, and 30-day survival in patients with LLST on ICU admission.

**Methods:** This prospective observational study included all patients admitted to 39 ICUs in a 45-day period in 2011. We recorded hospitals' characteristics (availability of intermediate care units, usual availability of ICU beds, and financial model) and patients' characteristics (demographics, reason for admission, functional status, risk of death, and LLST on ICU admission (withholding/withdrawing; specific techniques affected)). The primary outcome was 30-day survival for patients with LLST on ICU admission. Statistical analysis included multilevel logistic regression models.

**Results:** We recruited 3042 patients (age 62.5 ± 16.1 years). Most ICUs (94.8%) admitted patients with LLST, but only 238 (7.8% [95% CI 7.0–8.8]) patients had LLST on ICU admission; this group had higher ICU mortality (44.5 vs. 9.4% in patients without LLST; $p < 0.001$). Multilevel logistic regression showed a contextual effect of the hospital in LLST on ICU admission (median OR = 2.30 [95% CI 1.59–2.96]) and identified the following patient-related variables as independent factors associated with LLST on ICU admission: age, reason for admission, risk of death, and functional status. In patients with LLST on ICU admission, 30-day survival was 38% (95% CI 31.7–44.5). Factors associated with survival were age, reason for admission, risk of death, and number of reasons for LLST on ICU admission.

**Conclusions:** The frequency of ICU admission with LLST is low but probably increasing; nearly one third of these patients survive for ≥ 30 days.

**Keywords:** Limitations on life support techniques, Palliative care, Critical care, Intensive care units

---

* Correspondence: orubio@althaia.cat
[1]Hospital Sant Joan De Déu, Fundació Althaia Xarxa Universitaria de Manresa, C/ Dr. Joan Soler s. n., 08243 Manresa, Spain
Full list of author information is available at the end of the article

## Background

Decisions to apply limitations on life support techniques (LLSTs) are common in intensive care units (ICUs) worldwide [1–5]. This practice is supported by adequate ethical consensus [1, 6–9] and is even considered an ICU quality indicator [10]. These decisions are usually taken when medical efforts become futile after ICU treatment for some time [11–13].

LLST can entail withholding new treatments, not increasing treatments being applied, or withdrawing treatments. LLSTs are applied in 13 to 34% of all patients admitted to ICUs [14–17] and in 40 to 90% of patients who died in ICUs [7]. LLSTs are associated with high mortality [1, 11, 18]. Lautrette et al. [11] found LLST in 13% of patients (treatments withheld in 39%, not increased in 26%, and withdrawn in 35%); 30-day mortality was 35% in patients in whom the treatment was withheld, 73% in those in whom in the treatment was not increased, and 94% in those in whom the treatment was withdrawn. Another study reported 99% mortality in patients in whom life support was withdrawn and 89% in those in whom further life support measures were withheld during the ICU stay [18].

The Ethicus study [1] of end-of-life practices in European ICUs found that the criteria for deciding LLSTs were patient age, diagnoses, ICU stay, and geographic and religious factors. In a large study, Azoulay et al. [5] found that a higher nurse-to-bed ratio was associated with an increased incidence of LLST, while the availability of an emergency department in the same hospital, full-time presence of intensivists, and presence of physicians during nights and weekends was associated with a decreased incidence of LLST.

In oncologic patients, early LLSTs are mainly related to cancer progression and functional stages; oncological treatment projects and complications leading to ICU admission have a major impact on LLST decisions [19].

In recent years, various authors have proposed that it could be useful to determine LLST on ICU admission for early integrated palliative care [19, 20]. Godfrey et al. [20] reported that 3.2% of patients were admitted to the ICU with orders to withhold life support; half of these survived the ICU stay, and one third were discharged home. More recently, Hart et al. [21] reported that 4.8% of patients had orders to withhold life support before ICU admission.

We aimed to determine the frequency of LLST on ICU admission, associated hospital- and patient-related characteristics, and 30-day survival in patients admitted with LLST. We also explored what types of LLST were applied under what conditions.

## Methods

This prospective observational study included all consecutive patients ≥ 18 years old admitted to 39 ICUs in Spain between 1 May 2011 and 15 June 2011. The ethics committees at each participating center approved the study.

LLST upon ICU admission were defined as orders to withhold or withdraw any life-sustaining treatment. The decisions to apply LLST were performed by a doctor during the guards and by the disciplinary team during the morning hours. Refusal of admission to the ICU was not considered LLST upon ICU admission. Informed consent was requested for the data collection.

We recorded the following characteristics of participating hospitals: number of hospital beds, number of ICU beds, number of step-down/intermediate care beds, funding (public or private), availability of ICU beds, use of restrictive criteria (based on age, previous comorbidity, and/or previous quality of life) for ICU admission, existence of ethics committee guidelines for LLST, and whether coronary and/or stroke patients were admitted.

At admission to the ICU, we recorded patients' age, sex, reason for admission, prior functional status (Knaus chronic health status score), and risk of death according to severity scales. We also recorded decisions to apply LLST (withhold new treatment, not increase current treatment, or withdraw treatment), the specific life support techniques to be limited (cardiopulmonary resuscitation, endotracheal intubation, noninvasive ventilation, vasopressor drugs, dialysis, and/or transfusion of blood products), and reason for LLST decision (age, severe chronic disease, prior functional limitations, unacceptable quality of life despite possible recovery from the acute process, advanced life directives, no expectation of surviving the hospital stay, and anticipated irreversibility of the current process within 24 h). We also recorded the reversal of LLST orders during the ICU stay.

On ICU discharge, we evaluated patients' clinical status and prognosis with the Sabadell score [22], which classifies patients into five groups: SS0 = good prognosis, SS1 = poor long-term (> 6 months) prognosis with no limits on ICU readmission, SS2 = poor short-term prognosis (< 6 months) with debatable ICU readmission, SS3 = death expected during hospitalization with ICU readmission not applicable, and SS4 = death in ICU.

The primary outcome was 30-day survival for patients with LLST on ICU admission. Secondary outcomes were decisions to withhold vs. withdraw life support at ICU admission, ICU length of stay, Sabadell score at ICU discharge, and in-hospital mortality.

## Statistical analysis

We summarize categorical variables as absolute and relative frequencies and continuous variables as means and standard deviations or medians and interquartile ranges. To compare patients with vs. without LLST, we used Student's $t$ tests for normally distributed continuous variables, nonparametric Mann-Whitney tests for non-normally distributed continuous variables, and chi-square tests, Fisher's exact tests, or the Monte Carlo method (in $2 \times 2$ contingency tables or $n \times 2$ when expected frequencies < 5) for categorical variables.

To determine whether the contextual effect of the hospital was related to LLST, we used a random-effects multilevel logistic regression model with the hospital as a second-level variable (random effect) and the patient and center characteristics that were associated with LLST in the bivariate analysis as first-level variables. We used odds ratios and median odds ratios (MOR) to measure the association between each covariate and LLST [23]. The MOR is a measure of the variation between the rates of LLST at different hospitals that is unexplained by the modeled risk factors; it is defined as the median of the set of odds ratios that could be obtained by comparing two patients with identical patient-level characteristics from two randomly chosen hospitals.

Survival was analyzed by Kaplan-Meier curves and compared by log-rank test. Crude and adjusted hazard ratios and 95% confidence intervals (CI) were calculated using Cox proportional regression models. We introduced covariates with $p \leq 0.20$ in the bivariate analysis or with evidence of an association in the literature into the multivariate regression model, using a researcher-controlled backward exclusion strategy. Proportionality of hazards was verified by examining Schoenfeld residual plots.

All tests were two-sided, and the significance was set at $p < 0.05$. For statistical analyses, we used IBM® SPSS® Statistics for Windows v.20 and Stata® v.10.

## Results

Of the 39 ICUs, 34 (87.2%) received public funding; the median number of hospital beds was 575 (360–800) and the median number of ICU beds was 17 (11–22). Beds were often available in 33 (84.6%) ICUs; 33 (84.6%) had restrictive admission policies, 37 (94.9%) had clinical ethics committees, and 13 (33%) had guidelines for LLST. Intermediate care units were available in 13 (33.3%) centers. (Additional file 1: Table S1).

During the study period, participating ICUs admitted 3042 patients (age, $62.5 \pm 16.1$ years; 1935 (63.6%) men). The reason for ICU admission was worsening of chronic disease in 353 (11.6%), coma/encephalopathy in 386 (12.7%), and sepsis in 411 (13.5%). The Knaus chronic health status score classified patients' prior functional status as class A in 57.4%, class B in 31.0%, class C in 9.4%, and class D in 2.1%. The median risk of death predicted by the severity scales was 14% [5.8–32.9%] (Additional file 1: Table S2).

Most ICUs (94.8%) accepted patients with LLST at ICU admission. A total of 238 (7.8%) [95% CI 7.0–8.8%] patients (age, $73.0 \pm 13.5$ years; 130 (55%) men) had

LLST on ICU admission, with a median predicted risk of death of 46.3% [24.0–63.9%].

Reasons for LLST were severe chronic disease ($n = 143$; 60.1%), prior functional limitations ($n = 110$; 46.2%), advanced age ($n = 90$; 37.8%), null expected survival ($n = 83$; 34.9%), unacceptable quality of life ($n = 63$; 26.5%), irreversibility within 24 h ($n = 50$; 21.0%), advanced life directives ($n = 12$; 5.0%), and others ($n = 15$; 6.3%); there were $2.4 \pm 1.1$ reasons recorded per patient (Additional file 1: Table S3).

Table 1 reports the life support techniques limited and the type of limitation on each. The most common type of LLST on ICU admission was withholding, especially for invasive treatments. Withholding or withdrawing is most commonly referred to invasive measures (cardiopulmonary resuscitation maneuvers, dialysis, and intubation). Decisions to limit noninvasive life support measures (vasoactive drugs, noninvasive ventilation, and transfusions) were less frequent and nearly always involved withholding rather than withdrawing treatment. Withdrawing life invasive support was very uncommon. LLST orders were reversed only in seven (2.9%) patients.

In the bivariate analysis, LLSTs were associated with older age (73.0 vs. 61.6 years; $p < 0.001$) and female sex (9.6% in women vs. 6.8% in men; $p = 0.006$) (Additional file 1: Tables S3 and S4). The most common reasons for ICU admission in patients with LLST were worsening of chronic disease (19.0%) and coma/encephalopathy (15.8%). Compared to patients without LLST, patients with LLST had a higher risk of death (46.3 vs. 12.0%; $p < 0.001$).Worsening prior functional status was associated with more LLST (from 46.0% in class D down to 2.1% in class A).

Table 2 shows the patient and hospital characteristics independently associated with LLST on ICU admission. Multilevel logistic regression found a contextual effect of hospital on LLST decisions on ICU admission (MOR = 2.30; model A; Table 2). Hospital characteristics associated with LLST were the lack of intermediate care units and

**Table 1** Life support techniques limited in patients with orders to limit life support on admission to the intensive care unit

| Technique | | Type of limitation | |
| --- | --- | --- | --- |
| | | Withhold | Withdraw |
| Invasive life support | | | |
| Cardiopulmonary resuscitation | 215 (91.5%) | 215 (91.5%) | 0 (0%) |
| Dialysis | 209 (89.3%) | 203 (86.8%) | 6 (2.6%) |
| Intubation | 147 (63.9%) | 126 (54.8%) | 21 (9.1%) |
| Noninvasive life support | | | |
| Vasopressors | 104 (45.0%) | 96 (41.5%) | 8 (3.5%) |
| Noninvasive ventilation | 61 (26.9%) | 60 (26.4%) | 1 (0.4%) |
| Blood transfusions | 59 (25.5%) | 55 (23.8%) | 4 (1.7%) |

**Table 2** Associations between limitations on life support on ICU admission and patient and hospital characteristics. Adjusted odds ratio (aOR) and 95% confidence interval (95% CI)

| | Limitations, n = 238 | No limitations, n = 2804 | Model A aOR (95% CI) | Model B aOR (95% CI) |
|---|---|---|---|---|
| Patient characteristics | | | | |
| Age | 73.0 ± 13.5 | 61.6 ± 16.0 | 1.04 (1.03–1.06) | 1.05 (1.03–1.06) |
| Female sex | 106 (44.5%) | 1000 (35.6%) | 1.30 (0.93–1.81) | 1.30 (0.92–1.78) |
| Reason for ICU admission | | | | |
| Other | 77 (32.3%) | 1816 (64.8%) | 1 | 1 |
| Sepsis | 33 (13.9%) | 377 (13.4%) | 0.94 (0.57–1.57) | 0.97 (0.58–1.62) |
| Coma or encephalopathy | 61 (25.6%) | 326 (11.6%) | 3.96 (2.50–6.30) | 3.88 (2.45–6.13) |
| Worsening of chronic disease | 67 (28.1%) | 285 (10.2%) | 2.34 (1.50–3.66) | 2.34 (1.50–3.66) |
| Predicted risk of death (%) | 46.3 [24.0–63.9] | 12.0 [5.1–29.0] | 1.03 (1.02–1.04) | 1.03 (1.02–1.04) |
| Prior functional Knaus status: | | | | |
| Class A | 37 (15.5%) | 1708 (60.9%) | 1 | 1 |
| Class B | 96 (40.3%) | 848 (30.2%) | 3.80 (2.44–5.92) | 3.71 (2.39–5.77) |
| Class C | 76 (31.9%) | 211 (7.5%) | 13.44 (8.00–22.58) | 13.30 (7.93–22.32) |
| Class D | 29 (12.2%) | 34 (1.2%) | 36.94 (17.34–78.71) | 36.77 (17.29–78.20) |
| Hospital characteristics | | | | |
| Intermediate care unit available | | | | |
| Yes | 43 (18.1%) | 826 (29.4%) | | 1 |
| No | 195 (81.9%) | 1978 (70.5%) | | 1.85 (1.00–3.44) |
| Patients with limitations on life support outside the ICU | | | | |
| Yes | 143 (60.1%) | 1928 (68.7%) | | 1 |
| No | 95 (39.9%) | 876 (31.2%) | | 2.57 (1.45–4.57) |
| Hospital variance (SE) | | | 0.765 (0.271) | 0.453 (0.191) |
| LR test; p value | | | 54.38; p < 0.001 | 24.69; p < 0.001 |
| Intraclass correlation coefficient | | | 0.189 | 0.121 |
| Median odds ratio (95% CI) | | | 2.30 (1.59–2.96) | 1.90 (1.31–2.38) |

Mean ± standard deviation; n (row %); median [interquartile range]; *SE* standard error

Model A—random effects multilevel logistic regression model with hospital as a second-level variable (random effect) and the patient characteristics as first-level variables

Model B—random effects multilevel logistic regression model with hospital as a second-level variable (random effect) and the patient and center characteristics as first-level variables

the incapability to treat severely ill patients with LLST outside the ICU (model B; Table 2). Patient characteristics independently associated with LLST were age; admission for coma, encephalopathy, or worsening of chronic disease; risk of death; and prior functional status class B, C, or D (Additional file 1: Table S5).

Median ICU stay was not different between patients with or without LLST at ICU admission. In LLST patients, the most common Sabadell score at ICU discharge was SS4 (death, 44.5%), followed by SS2 (poor short-term prognosis, 29.8%) and SS3 (expected survival null, 11.3%), while in patients without limitations, the most common was SS0 (good prognosis, 64.0%) (Table 3).

A greater proportion of patients with LLST on ICU admission died in the ICU (44.5 vs. 9.4% in those without; p < 0.001). Hospital mortality was higher in patients with LLST (59.2 vs. 12.7% in those without; p < 0.001) (Fig. 1).

Thirty-day survival in patients with LLST at ICU admission was 38% (95% CI 31.7–44.5). Independent predictors of worse 30-day survival were older age, ICU admission for coma/encephalopathy or sepsis, higher

predicted risk of death, and more reasons for LLST decision (Table 4).

Survival differed in function of whether both invasive and noninvasive or only noninvasive life support techniques were limited. Withholding and withdrawing noninvasive

**Table 3** Clinical outcome according to limitations on life support on ICU admission

| | Limitations, n = 238 | No limitations, n = 2804 | p value |
|---|---|---|---|
| ICU length of stay, days | 3 [1–6] | 3 [1–6] | 0.711[a] |
| Sabadell score at ICU discharge: | | | |
| SS0—good prognosis | 7 (2.9%) | 1794 (64.0%) | < 0.001[b] |
| SS1—poor long-term prognosis | 27 (11.3%) | 525 (18.7%) | |
| SS2—poor short-term prognosis | 71 (29.8%) | 182 (6.5%) | |
| SS3—expected to die | 27 (11.3%) | 37 (1.3%) | |
| SS4—died | 106 (44.5%) | 264 (9.4%) | |
| ICU mortality | 106 (44.5%) | 264 (9.4%) | < 0.001[b] |
| Ward mortality | 35 (14.7%) | 84 (3.1%) | < 0.001[b] |
| Hospital mortality | 141 (59.2%) | 348 (12.7%) | < 0.001[b] |

Median [interquartile range]; n (% of column)

[a]Mann-Whitney *U*

[b]Pearson chi-square

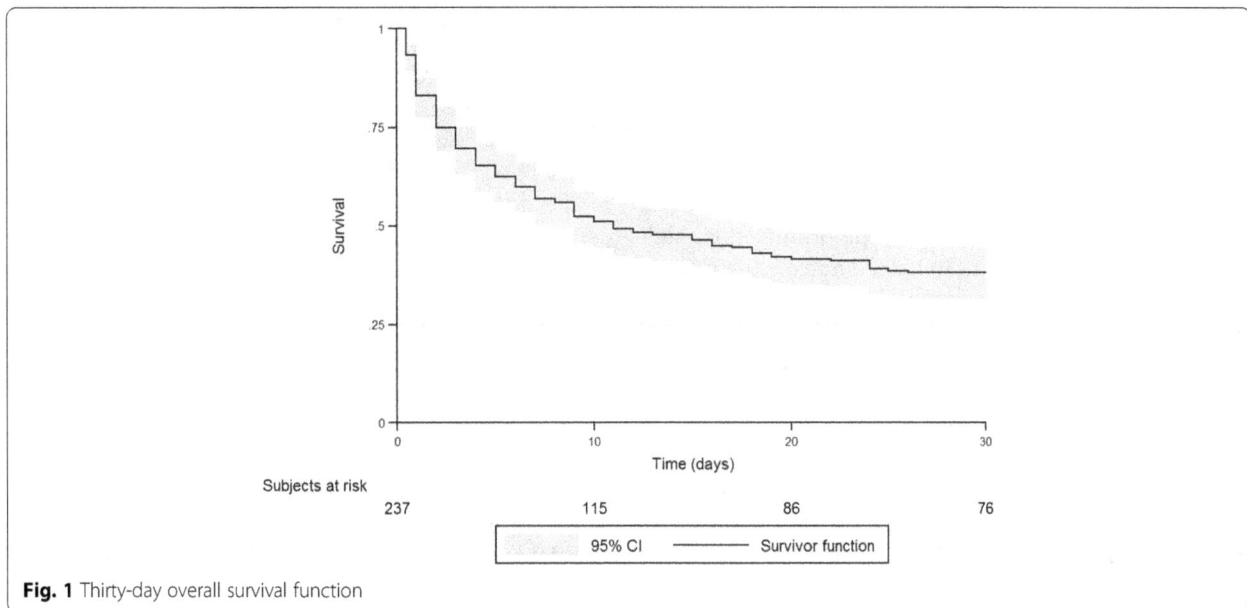

**Fig. 1** Thirty-day overall survival function

measures were both associated with lower survival. Not increasing the dose of vasoactive drugs was associated with greater survival than withdrawing them. Withholding invasive measures was associated with greater survival than withdrawing them, with the exception of intubation. Additional file 1: Figure S1 reports the survival related to the life support technique limited.

## Discussion

To our knowledge, this is the first prospective multicenter study to evaluate the clinical, structural, and demographic

factors associated with LLST decisions at ICU admission and their associations with survival.

Most centers admitted patients with LLST orders, and those patients accounted for 7.8% of all ICU admissions. This rate is somewhat higher than previously reported and may be influenced by the wide availability of ICU beds in the study period. Only two centers refused to admit LLST patients, and both had 100% occupancy rate. These two centers admitted more severe patients (median risk of death 40 vs. 22% in the other centers) and had step-down units (compared with only 3 3% of the other centers), so patients with LLST

**Table 4** Predictive factors for 30-day survival in patients with limitations on life support at ICU admission

|  | Died, n = 141 | Survived, n = 97 | Unadjusted HR (95% CI) | Adjusted HR (95% CI) |
|---|---|---|---|---|
| Age, year | 71.4 ± 12.2 | 75.2 ± 15.0 | 0.99 (0.98–0.99) | 0.98 (0.97–0.99) |
| Female sex | 58 (54.7%) | 48 (45.3%) | 1.16 (0.83–1.62) | 1.2 (0.85–1.71) |
| Reason for ICU admission |  |  |  |  |
| Worsening of chronic disease | 31 (46.3%) | 36 (53.7%) | 1 | 1 |
| Coma or encephalopathy | 48 (78.7%) | 13 (21.3%) | 2.51 (1.59–3.95) | 1.79 (1.10–2.91) |
| Sepsis | 22 (66.7%) | 11 (33.3%) | 1.80 (1.04–3.11) | 1.64 (0.90–2.97) |
| Other | 40 (51.9%) | 37 (48.1%) | 1.23 (0.77–1.97) | 1.23 (0.68–1.97) |
| Predicted risk of death, % | 54.6 [38.9–72.0] | 24.0 [12.0–45.0] | 1.03 (1.02–1.03) | 1.02 (1.02–1.03) |
| Prior functional Knaus status |  |  |  |  |
| Class A | 26 (70.3%) | 11 (29.7%) | 1 | 1 |
| Class B | 55 (57.3%) | 41 (42.7%) | 0.78 (0.49–1.25) | 0.83 (0.49–1.38) |
| Class C | 45 (59.2%) | 31 (40.8%) | 0.83 (0.51–1.34) | 0.56 (0.31–1.02) |
| Class D | 15 (51.7%) | 14 (48.3%) | 0.71 (0.38–1.35) | 0.45 (0.22–0.92) |
| Criteria for limitations, number | 2 [2–3] | 2 [1–3] | 1.33 (1.14–1.55) | 1.45 (1.22–1.76) |
| Limited techniques, number | 3 [2–5] | 3 [2–4] | 1.16 (1.03–1.31) | 1.10 (0.97–1.25) |

Mean (SD); n (% of the row); median [interquartile range]

in these two centers were probably admitted to step-down units.

Although LLST patients were sicker, their 30-day survival was 38%. LLST at ICU admission were related to patient factors (age, comorbidities, functional status, and predicted risk of death) and hospital factors. Survival was affected by the same patient-related factors and by the number of reasons for LLST, the type of limitation, and the specific life support techniques limited. A study in Brazil found 9.8% of patients admitted to the ICU had limitations on advanced life support, and LLST decisions were associated with older age, clinical diagnosis, Karnofsky performance status score < 40%, and SAPS3 score > 49 points [24]. As in our study, Godfrey et al. [20] found that older age, more comorbid disease, and more acute physiological disturbance were associated with mortality in patients with LLST at admission; moreover, 30% were discharged directly to their homes.

Our findings suggest a trend toward an increase in LLST at ICU admission; whereas earlier studies found limitations in only 1 to 3% of patients [20, 25], we found limitations in nearly 8%. This trend may be related to patients' increasing age and complexity (associated comorbidities and frailty) due to increased life expectancy, changes in patterns of end-of-life trajectories [26], changes in ICU admission criteria, and advanced life directives in patients with advanced cancer and organ failure [24]. Thus, many patients (oncological, hematologic, and geriatric patients) are admitted to ICUs for therapeutic tests or conditioning treatments because ICU admission seems to improve outcomes in these situations; for example, in cancer patients requiring mechanical ventilation are widely viewed as poor candidates for intensive care unit (ICU) admission. One study of patients has demonstrated that if patients were admitted at the earliest phase of the malignancy (diagnosis < 30 days) without any restriction, the survival was 40% in mechanically ventilated cancer patients who survived to day 5 and 21.8% overall. All patients were prospectively included in The ICU Trial, consisting of a full-code ICU admission followed by reappraisal of the level of care on day 5. It would be interesting to conduct efficiency studies in these case [27–30]. Nevertheless, although the frequency of LLST at ICU admission is increasing, it is still lower than the frequency of limitations applied during the ICU stay (13–34%) [3, 17].

In the univariate analysis, hospital mortality was associated with the reason for admission, previous poor functional status, LLST at admission, age, and risk of death. In the multivariate analysis, hospital mortality was associated with age, reason for admission type II/III, predicted risk of death, poor functional status (C and D), and LLST at admission.

Decision-making about LLST is affected by patient-related factors and factors related to health professionals [1]. Pathophysiological factors often preclude ICU patients from making decisions, and the burden of decision-making falls on their relatives or legal representatives. However, up to half of ICU patients' relatives do not want to participate in the decision-making about LLST [5]. Trends toward patient empowerment in the near future through more active participation and shared decision-making models will likely influence decisions to limit life support before ICU admission [31, 32]. Factors related to professionals also affect LLST decisions and account for some of the variability in decision-making [33].

On average, more than two reasons were given for LLST decisions; the most common were directly related to preexisting chronic disease and prior functional status, whereas poor quality of life was rarely considered. We found that LLSTs were more prevalent in patients admitted for worsening of severe chronic disease, as suggested by Godfrey et al. [20], who reported that chronic disease was the reason LLST in 77%. Prognosticating in these patients is more straightforward, so it is easier to establish LLST in advance.

We do not know if the decisions were proposed by the patient, the family, or unilaterally by the doctor on duty or the medical team (that it could be a point of interest for future research), but all the decisions were endorsed later in the clinical session.

We found that LLST decisions at ICU admission usually entailed withholding invasive life support measures. By contrast, LLST decisions made during the ICU stay more often involved withdrawing measures when they proved futile [34]. This is probably due to the different profiles of patients admitted with LLST and those without. The EPIPUSE study [35] showed that patients with LLST decided during the ICU stay were younger and rarely admitted for worsening of chronic disease or coma/encephalopathy; the risk of death predicted by severity scores in the EPIPUSE study was also notably lower than in our study [36].

The life support measure most often limited to ICU admission was cardiopulmonary resuscitation, commonly associated with the decision not to increase life support [37]. These findings also differ from LLST decided during the ICU stay, where most decisions are not to increase life support or to withdraw life support after they prove futile [3].

At ICU discharge, patients admitted with LLST had a worse prognosis, and the mortality in this group was approximately fourfold that of patients admitted without LLST, unsurprisingly, given the difference in severity at ICU admission [38].

In line with Godfrey et al. [20], ICU and in-hospital mortality were higher in patients with LLST at ICU admission in our study, due to both LLST and greater severity.

Nevertheless, our 30-day survival in patients with LLST on ICU admission was 38%, slightly higher than the 30% previously reported [20].

Interestingly, mortality is lower (up to 90%) when LLSTs are decided on ICU admission than when decided during the ICU stay [11], most likely because patients in the latter group are sicker and because LLSTs are decided after therapy failure and more often entail withdrawing rather than withholding life support. Furthermore, survival differed with the type of LLST at admission; survival was greater in patients in whom life support measures were withheld than in those in whom they were withdrawn similar to what happens when the decision is taken during the ICU stay [11, 15].

Regarding survival curves according to the type of limited life support, two limitations must be taken into account for correct reading; one is that we do not know the patient's previous starting point (we do not know if he was intubated on admission before making decisions), and the second is that for each patient with decisions could be marked several limited life supports at once but the analysis has been done in isolation for each life support without taking into account their interrelation. Therefore, the results should always be interpreted with caution.

It seems paradoxical that life support intubation has better survival in the form not start than the nonlimitation and withdrawal when the other vital supports are the opposite. An explanation could lie in the fact that some patients are intubated at home by the urgent prehospital care and that after arriving at the hospital and before being admitted to the ICU they are cataloged as LLST.

The factors independently associated with LLST decisions at ICU admission in our study agree with those reported in other studies [20], although the contextual effect of hospital on LLST decisions in our study is new. The factors independently associated with survival in patients with LLST at ICU admission were related to the underlying chronic disease, better prior functional status, less severe disease, and fewer reasons for the LLST decision.

Nevertheless, further studies are needed to define how these decisions are made at admission, and how this affects patients' outcomes, about the validation of tools to quantify frailty and about comorbidity and performance status [39]. Furthermore, studies should assess survivors' quality of life and satisfaction to evaluate the efficiency of ICU admission in these patients.

### Limitations of the study

Not including patients with LLST decided outside the ICU and therefore not admitted may have underestimated the global incidence of LLST. Our sample (about six patients with LLST on ICU admission per center) precluded an analysis of the contextual effect of hospital on survival, although a systematic review found LLST varied among countries and regions [40]. Finally, we cannot rule out a seasonal bias, as the study took place during a 6-week period in late spring, but LLST has never been associated with seasonal bias.

### Conclusions

Most ICUs admitted patients with LLST. The frequency of such admissions is low but probably increasing; nearly one third of these patients survive for 30 days. The main factors associated with LLST decisions at ICU admission and with 30-day survival in patients with these limitations are age, reason for ICU admission, and predicted risk of death.

### Appendix
#### LLST investigators and centers
ANDALUCIA: José Miguel Pérez-Villares (Hospital Virgen Nieves de Granada). ASTURIAS: Valentín Español-Boren (Hospital Universitario central de Asturias). ISLAS BALEARES: Rosa Poyo-Guerrero (Hospital Son Llatzer). CANARIAS: Mar Martín-Velasco (Hospital Candelaria Tenerife). CASTILLA Y LEON: María Eugenia Perea-Rodríguez (Complejo Asistencial Universitario de Burgos. Hospital General Yagué), Alfredo Marcos-Gutiérrez (Hospital Virgen de la Concha de Zamora), Mercedes Lara-Calvo (Hospital Rio Hortega de Valladolid), José Manuel Añon-Elizalde (Hospital Virgen de la Luz de Cuenca), Marta Paz-Pérez (Hospital Clínico Universitario de Salamanca). CATALUÑA: Gloria Miro-Andreu (Hospital de Mataró), Juan María Sánchez-Segura (Hospital de la Santa Creu i Sant Pau de Barcelona), Elisabeth Zabala-Jiménez (Hospital Clínico Barcelona UCI quirúrgica), Roser Tomas-Puig (Hospital General Cataluña en Sant Cugat), Cristina Murcia-Gubianes (Hospital de Girona), Kenneth Planas (Hospital de Sant Joan Despí Moises Broggi), Judith Xirgú-Cortacans (Hospital Universitario de Granollers), Mar Fernández-Fernández (Hospital Universitario Mútua de Terrassa), Consuelo Guía-Rambla (Hospital de Sabadell), Vanesa Arauzo-Rojo (Hospital de Terrassa), Rosa Catalan-Ibars (Hospital Universitari de Vic), Javier Gónzalez-Robledo (Hospital Virgen de la Vega de Salamanca). GALICIA: Ana Ortega-Montes (Hospital Montecelo de Pontevedra), Pedro Rascado-Sedes (CHU Santiago Compostela), Ana Tizón-Varela (Complejo Hospital Xeral Cíes de Vigo), Pedro Rascado-Sedes (Hospital Santiago de Compostela). COMUNIDAD DE MADRID: Juan Carlos Montejo-González (Hospital 12 de octubre), José Manuel Gómez-García (Hospital Gregorio Marañón), Inés Torrejón-Pérez (Hospital de Henares), Gonzalo Hernández-González (Hospital Infanta Sofía). REGIÓN DE MURCIA: Noemí Llamas-Fernández (Hospital Morales Meseguer de Murcia), Miguel Fernández-Vivas (Hospital Virgen de la Arrixaca de Murcia). COMUNIDAD FORAL DE NAVARRA: Pablo Monedero-Rodríguez

(Clínica Universitaria de Navarra), María Barber-Ansón (Hospital de Navarra), Belén Quesada-Bellber (Fundación Jiménez Díaz), Vicente Gómez-Tello (Hospital de la Moncloa). PAIS VASCO: Iñaki Saralegui-Reta (Hospital Santiago Apóstol de Álava). COMUNIDAD VALENCIANA: Susana Altaba-Tena (Hospital General de Castellón), Begoña Balerdi-Pérez (Hospital la Fe de Valencia).

## Additional file

Additional file 1: Table S1. Hospital characteristics. Table S2. Patient characteristics. Table S3. Reasons for limitations on life support at admission to the ICU. Table S4. Bivariate analysis. Patient characteristics associated with LLST. Crude odds ratio (OR) and 95% confidence interval. Table S5. Bivariate analysis. Hospital characteristics associated with LLST. Crude odds ratio (OR) and 95% confidence interval. Figure S1. Thirty-day overall survival function according to the specific support measures limited and the type of limitation. (RTF 56201 kb)

## Abbreviations

ICU: Intensive care unit; LLST: Limitations on life support technique; MOR: Median odds ratio; SS: Sabadell score

## Acknowledgements

The authors thank the members of the Althaia Research Department for their statistical help.

## Funding

No source of funding was received for the research.

## Authors' contributions

RO and FR are the guarantor of the paper and takes responsibility for the integrity of the work as a whole, from inception to the published article. AA contributed to the statistical analysis and to the interpretation of the data, critical revision of the manuscript, and final approval of the version to be published. All authors have participated in the data collection, and they have read and approved the final manuscript. CS and JM have revised the text and made methodological contributions, and they have given the expert's point of view.

## Competing interests

The authors declare that they have no competing interests.

## Author details

[1]Hospital Sant Joan De Déu, Fundació Althaia Xarxa Universitaria de Manresa, C/ Dr. Joan Soler s. n., 08243 Manresa, Spain. [2]Hospital la Fe de Valencia, Valencia, Spain. [3]Hospital General Yagué de Burgos, Burgos, Spain. [4]Hospital Virgen Arrixaca Murcia, Murcia, Spain. [5]Hospital de Navarra, Pamplona, Spain. [6]Hospital Morales Messeguer, Murcia, Spain. [7]Hospital Universitario de Castellon, Castellon de la Plana, Spain. [8]Hospital Rio Hortega, Valladolid, Spain. [9]Hospital la Moncloa, Madrid, Spain. [10]Hospital Candelaria de Tenerife,

Santa Cruz de Tenerife, Spain. [11]Hospital Clínico Universitario de Salamanca, Salamanca, Spain. [12]Fundación Jiménez Díaz, Madrid, Spain. [13]Hospital Central de Asturias, Oviedo, Spain. [14]Hospital Universitario Doce de Octubre, Madrid, Spain. [15]Hospital Gregorio Marañon, Madrid, Spain. [16]Hospital Mataro, Mataro, Spain. [17]Hospital de Granollers, Granollers, Spain. [18]Hospital Montecelo Pontevedra, Pontevedra, Spain. [19]Centro Hospitalario Universitario Santiago Compostela, Santiago de Compostela, Spain. [20]Hospital de la Sant Creu i Sant Pau, Barcelona, Spain. [21]Hospital Virgen de la Concha, Zamora, Spain. [22]Hospital Xeral Cíes Vigo, Vigo, Spain. [23]Clínica Universitaria de Navarra, Pamplona, Spain. [24]Hospital Clínico Universitario de Barcelona, Barcelona, Spain. [25]Hospital Josep Trueta, Girona, Spain. [26]Hospital de Henares, Coslada, Spain. [27]Hospital Moisses Broggi, Sant Joan Despí, Spain. [28]Hospital Virgen de la Luz, Cuenca, Spain. [29]Hospital Infanta Sofía, San Sebastián de los Reyes, Spain. [30]Hospital Mútua de Terrassa, Terrassa, Spain. [31]Hospital Parc Tauli, Sabadell, Spain. [32]Hospital de Terrassa, Terrassa, Spain. [33]Hospital Virgen de las Nieves, Granada, Spain. [34]Hospital General de Vic, Vic, Spain. [35]Hospital Virgen Vega Salamanca, Salamanca, Spain. [36]Hospital Son Llátzer, Palma, Spain. [37]Hospital General de Catalunya, Sant Cugat del Valles, Spain. [38]Hospital de Áraba, Vitoria-Gasteiz, Spain. [39]Hospital de la Santa Creu i Sant Pau, Barcelona, Spain. [40]Hadassh Hebrew University Medical Center, Jerusalem, Israel. [41]Hospital Sant Joan de Deu, Fundació Althaia Xarxa Universitaria de Manresa, Manresa, Spain.

## References

1. Sprung CL, Cohen SL, Sjokvist P, et al. End-of-life practices in European intensive care units: the Ethicus Study. JAMA. 2003;6:790–7.
2. Ho KM, Liang J. Withholding and withdrawal of therapy in New Zealand intensive care units (ICUs): a survey of clinical directors. Anaesth Intensive Care. 2004;32:781–6.
3. Lesieur O, Leloup M, Gonzalez F, et al. Withholding or withdrawal of treatment under French rules: a study performed in 43 intensive care units. Ann Intensive Care. 2015;5:56.
4. Prendergast TJ, Claessens MT, Luce JM. A national survey of end-of-life care for critically ill patients. Am J Respir Crit Care Med. 1998;158:1163–7.
5. Azoulay E, Metnitz B, Sprung CL, et al. End-of-life practices in 282 intensive care units: data from the SAPS 3 database. Intensive Care Med. 2009;35:623–30.
6. Sprung CL, Truog RD, Curtis JR, et al. Seeking worldwide professional consensus on the principles of end-of-life care for the critically ill: the consensus for worldwide end-of-life practice for patients in intensive care units (WELPICUS) study. Am J Respir Crit Care Med. 2014;190:855–66.
7. Eidelman LA, Jakobson DJ, Pizov R, et al. Forgoing life-sustaining treatment in an Israeli ICU. Intensive Care Med. 1998;24:162–6.
8. Cabré L, Solsona JF. Limitación del esfuerzo terapéutico en medicina intensiva. Med Int. 2002;26:304–11.
9. Truog RD, Campbell ML, Curtis JR, et al. Recommendations for end-of-life care in the intensive care unit: a consensus statement by the American College of Critical Care Medicine. Crit Care Med. 2008;36:953–63.
10. Martin MC, Cabre L, Ruiz J, et al. Indicators of quality in the critical patient. Med Int. 2008;32:23–32.
11. Lautrette A, Garrouste-Orgeas M, Bertrand PM, et al. Respective impact of no escalation of treatment, withholding and withdrawal of life-sustaining treatment on ICU patients prognosis: a multicenter study of the Outcomerea Research Group. Intensive Care Med. 2015;41:1763–72.
12. Loncan P, Gisbert A, Fernandez C, et al. Palliative care and intensive medicine in health care at the end of life in the XXI century. An Sist Sanit Navarra. 2007;30:113–28.
13. Nates JL, Nunnally M, Kleinpell R, et al. ICU admission, discharge, and triage guidelines: a framework to enhance clinical operations, development of institutional policies, and further research. Crit Care Med. 2016;44:1553–602.
14. Jensen HI, Ammentorp J, Ãrding H. Withholding or withdrawing therapy in Danish regional ICUs: frequency, patient characteristics and decision process. Acta Anaesthesiol Scand. 2011;55:344–51.
15. Ferrand E, Robert R, Ingrand P, et al. Withholding and withdrawal of life support in intensive care units in France: a prospective survey. Lancet. 2001;357:9–14.
16. Yazigi A, Riachi M, Dabbar G. Withholding and withdrawal of life-sustaining treatment in a Lebanese intensive care unit: a prospective observational study. Intensive Care Med. 2005;31:562–7.

17. Esteban A, Gordo F, Solsona JF, et al. Withdrawing and withholding life support in the intensive care unit: a Spanish prospective multi-centre observational study. Intensive Care Med. 2001;27:1744–9.

18. Curtis JR, Vincent JL. Ethics and end-of-life care for adults in the intensive care unit. Lancet. 2010;376:1347–53.

19. Meert AP, Dept S, Th B, et al. Causes of death and incidence of life-support techniques limitations in oncological patients dying in the ICU: a retrospective study. J Palliat Care Med. 2012;2:107–11.

20. Godfrey G, Pilcher D, Hilton A, et al. Treatment limitations at admission to intensive care units in Australia and New Zealand: prevalence, outcomes, and resource use. Crit Care Med. 2012;40:2082–9.

21. Hart JL, Harhay MO, Gabler NB, et al. Variability among US intensive care units in managing the care of patients admitted with preexisting limits on life-sustaining therapies. JAMA Intern Med. 2015;175:1019–26.

22. Fernandez R, Serrano JM, Umaran I, et al. Ward mortality after ICU discharge: a multicenter validation of the Sabadell score. Intensive Care Med. 2010;36: 1196–201.

23. Merlo J, Chaix B, Ohlsson H, et al. A brief conceptual tutorial of multilevel analysis in social epidemiology: using measures of clustering in multilevel logistic regression to investigate contextual phenomena. J Epidemiol Community Health. 2006;60:290–7.

24. Mazutti S, Nascimento A, Fumis R. Limitation to advanced life support in patients admitted to intensive care unit with integrated palliative care. Rev Bras Ter Intensiva. 2016;28:294–300.

25. Fernandez R, Baigorri F, Artigas A. Limitación del esfuerzo terapéutico en Cuidados Intensivos. ¿Ha cambiado en el siglo XXI? Med Int. 2005;29:338–41.

26. Murray S, Kendall M, Sheikh A. Illness trajectories and palliative care. BMJ. 2005;7498:1007–11.

27. Sprung CL, Artigas A, Kesecioglu J, et al. The Eldicus prospective, observational study of triage decision making in European intensive care units. Part II. Crit Care Med. 2012;40:132–8.

28. Boumendil A, Somme D, Garrouste-Orgeas M, et al. Should elderly patients be admitted to the intensive care unit? Intensive Care Med. 2007;33:1252–62.

29. Añon JM, Gómez-Tello V, González-Higueras E, et al. Pronóstico de los ancianos ventilados mecánicamente en la UCI. Med Int. 2013;37:149–55.

30. Lecuyer L, Chevret S, Thiery G, et al. The ICU trial: a new admission policy for cancer patients requiring mechanical ventilation. Crit Care Med. 2007;35:808–14.

31. Oshima Lee E, Emanuel EJ. Shared decision making to improve care and reduce costs. N Engl J Med. 2013;368:6–8.

32. Graw JA, Spies CD, Kork F, et al. End-of-life decisions in intensive care medicine-shared decision-making and intensive care unit length of stay. World J Surg. 2015;39:644–51.

33. Frost DW, Cook DJ, Heyland DK, et al. Patient and healthcare professional factors influencing end-of-life decision-making during critical illness: a systematic review. Crit Care Med. 2011;39:1174–89.

34. Iribarren S, Latorre K, Muñoz T, et al. Limitation of therapeutic effort after ICU admission. Analysis of related factors. Med Int. 2007;31:68–72.

35. Hernández-Tejedor A, Cabré-Pericas L, Martín-Delgado MC, et al. Evolution and prognosis of long intensive care unit stay patients suffering a deterioration: a multicenter study. J Crit Care. 2015;30:654e1–7.

36. Hernández-Tejedor A, Martín Delgado MC, Cabré Pericas L, et al. Limitation of life-sustaining treatment in patients with prolonged admission to the ICU. Current situation in Spain as seen from the EPIPUSE study. Med Int. 2015;39:395–404.

37. Monzon JL, Saralegui I, Molina R, et al. Ethics of the cardiopulmonary resuscitation decisions. Med Int. 2010;34:534–49.

38. Fuchs L, Chronaki CE, Park S, et al. ICU admission characteristics and mortality rates among elderly and very elderly patients. Intensive Care Med. 2012;38:1654–61.

39. Capuzzo M, Moreno RP, Jordan B, et al. Predictors of early recovery of health status after intensive care. Intensive Care Med. 2006;32:1832–8.

40. Mark NM, Rayner SG, Lee NJ, et al. Global variability in withholding and withdrawal of life-sustaining treatment in the intensive care unit: a systematic review. Intensive Care Med. 2015;41:1572–85.

# 20

# Recruitment maneuver does not provide any mortality benefit over lung protective strategy ventilation in adult patients with acute respiratory distress syndrome

Sulagna Bhattacharjee[1], Kapil D. Soni[2] and Souvik Maitra[1*] ⓘD

## Abstract

**Background:** Clinical benefits of recruitment maneuver in ARDS patients are controversial. A number of previous studies showed possible benefits; a large recent study reported that recruitment maneuver and PEEP titration may even be harmful. This meta-analysis was designed to compare the clinical utility of recruitment maneuver with low tidal volume ventilation in adult patients with ARDS.

**Methods:** Randomized controlled trials comparing recruitment maneuver and lung protective ventilation strategy with lung protective strategy ventilation protocol alone in adult patients with ARDS has been included in this meta-analysis. PubMed and Cochrane Central Register of Controlled Trials were searched from inception to 10 November 2017 to identify potentially eligible trials. Pooled risk ratio (RR) and standardized mean difference (SMD) were calculated for binary and continuous variables respectively.

**Results:** Data of 2480 patients from 7 randomized controlled trials have been included in this meta-analysis and systemic review. Reported mortality at the longest available follow-up [RR (95% CI) 0.93 (0.80, 1.08); $p = 0.33$], ICU mortality [RR (95% CI) 0.91 (0.76, 1.10); $p = 0.33$] and in-hospital mortality [RR (95% CI) 0.95 (0.83, 1.08); $p = 0.45$] were similar between recruitment maneuver group and standard lung protective ventilation group. Duration of hospital stay [SMD (95% CI) 0.00 (− 0.09, 0.10); $p = 0.92$] and duration of ICU stays [SMD (95% CI) 0.05 (− 0.09, 0.19); $p = 0.49$] were also similar between recruitment maneuver group and standard lung protective ventilation group. Risk of barotrauma was also similar.

**Conclusion:** Use of recruitment maneuver along with co-interventions such as PEEP titration does not provide any benefit in terms of mortality, length of ICU, and hospital stay in ARDS patients.

**Keywords:** ARDS, Recruitment maneuver, Open lung, PEEP titration

* Correspondence: souvikmaitra@live.com
[1]Department of Anaesthesiology, Pain Medicine and Critical Care, All India Institute of Medical Sciences, Room No. 5011, 5th Floor Teaching block, Ansari Nagar New Delhi 110029, India
Full list of author information is available at the end of the article

# Background

Acute respiratory distress syndrome (ARDS) is a potentially life-threatening hypoxic respiratory failure, characterized by arterial hypoxemia ($PaO_2/FiO_2 < 200$), pulmonary congestion, and decreased respiratory compliance [1] Single centric studies reported a wide range of incidence of ARDS in intensive care unit (ICU) patients [2]. A large international multicenter observation study [3] in 2016 reported that incidence of ARDS was more than 10% in all ICU patients, and it was over 23% in all patients requiring mechanical ventilation. Reported unadjusted ICU mortality and hospital mortality in that study were 35.3 and 40%, respectively.

Atelectasis from alveolar or interstitial edema and consolidation and intra-pulmonary shunt are important pathophysiologic basis hypoxemia in ARDS patients [4]. Increased pulmonary capillary permeability from a variety of pulmonary and extra-pulmonary insults causes pulmonary edema in these patients [5]. Atelectasis contributes to the ventilator-induced lung injury by reducing the amount of functional aerated lung unit and repeated recruitment and de-recruitment of the small alveoli increases sheer stress leading to atelectotrauma [6]. Recruitment maneuver includes elevations of applied airway pressure for short duration aiming to recruit the collapsed alveoli and increase the number of alveolar units participating in tidal ventilation [7]. Positive end-expiratory pressure (PEEP) helps to keep the recruited lung unit 'open' and thereby reduces atelectasis and improves oxygenation [8]. Recruitment maneuver is usually used along with other methods of open lung approach such as high PEEP. Recruitment maneuver provides short-term improvement in oxygenation and lung compliances; on the contrary, it may be associated with barotrauma from increased airway pressure and hemodynamic compromise [6].

We designed this systematic review and meta-analysis of randomized controlled trials to know the clinical benefits of recruitment maneuver alone or along with other therapeutic modalities of open lung approach such as high PEEP or PEEP titration in adult patients with ARDS.

# Methods

This meta-analysis follows the recommendations of Preferred Reporting Items for Systematic Review and Meta-Analysis Protocols (PRISMA- P) statement [9]. A protocol of this meta-analysis has not been registered.

## Eligibility criteria

Published prospective randomized controlled trials comparing recruitment maneuver and lung protective ventilation strategy with lung protective strategy ventilation protocol in adult patients with ARDS has been included in this meta-analysis. Trials where PEEP titration was used following recruitment maneuver were also considered for inclusion in this meta-analysis. Trials of those that did not report mortality data for at least a one-time point and where a lung protective ventilation strategy has not been used have been considered to be included in this meta-analysis.

## Information sources

PubMed and The Cochrane Library databases (CENTRAL) were searched for potentially eligible trials from inception to 10 November 2016. We have not imposed any language restriction or date restriction in search strategy. References of the previously published meta-analyses were also searched for eligible trials.

## Search strategy

The following keywords were used to search database: "ARDS, acute respiratory distress syndrome, acute lung injury, acute hypoxemic respiratory failure, recruitment maneuver, recruitment manoeuvre, lung recruitment, open lung." Details of PubMed search strategy have been provided in Additional file 1.

## Study selection

Two authors (SM and KDS) independently searched title and abstract of the potentially eligible articles. Finally, full text of the possible articles was retrieved and assessed for eligibility. Any disputes between the two authors were solved by discussion and consultation with a third author (SB).

## Data collection process

Two authors (SM and SB) independently retrieved required data from the eligible RCTs, and all data were initially tabulated in a Microsoft Excel™ (Microsoft Corp., Redmond, WA) data sheet. Another author crosschecked these data before analysis (KDS).

## Data items

The following data were retrieved from the full text for all studies: first author, year of publication, country where work was done, sample size, characteristics of included patients, respiratory goals (oxyhemoglobin saturation, arterial oxygen, and $PaO_2/FiO_2$), details of recruitment maneuver (method application, any associated therapeutic modality, timing of recruitment maneuver and duration, details of rescue therapy, if any), details of mechanical ventilation, and clinical outcome (reported complications, organ dysfunction, length of hospital and ICU stay, and mortality at different time points).

### Risk of bias in individual studies

Two authors (SM and SB) independently assessed the methodological quality of the included studies. The following methodological questions were searched from the studies as per the Cochrane methodology: method of randomization, allocation concealment, blinding of the participants and personnel, blinding of outcome assessment, incomplete data reporting, selective reporting, and any other bias. For each area of bias, we will designate the trials as low risk of bias, unclear risk of bias, or high risk of bias. Risk of bias at individual study level will be graphically presented in the review.

### Summary measures and synthesis of results

Primary outcome of this meta-analysis is 'mortality at longest available follow-up' in the included patients. Secondary outcomes are ICU mortality rate, in-hospital mortality rate, incidence of barotrauma after randomization, incidence of hemodynamic compromise after randomization and length of hospital and ICU stay.

For continuous variables, mean and standard deviation (SD) values were extracted for both groups, a standardized mean difference (SMD) was computed at the study level, and a weighted mean difference was computed in order to pool the results across all studies. If the values were reported as median and an inter-quartile range or total range of values, the mean value was estimated using the median and the low and high end of the range for samples smaller than 25; for samples greater than 25, the median itself was used. The standard deviation (SD) was estimated from the median, and the low and high end of the range for samples smaller than 15, as range/4 for samples from 15 to 70, and as range/6 for samples more than 70. If only an inter-quartile range was available, SD was estimated as inter-quartile range/1.35 [10].

For binary outcomes, we calculated the following: [1] the risk ratio (RR) for each trial; [2] the pooled RR using the inverse variance method; [3] the number needed to treat (NNT) where a statistical significance was found, i.e., the number of patients who must be treated for one patient to benefit from the intervention. NNT was calculated from OR in Visual Rx online software (Visual Rx version 3.0, Dr. Chris Cates, http://www.nntonline.net/visualrx/). All statistical variables were calculated with 95% confidence interval (95% CI). The Q-test was used to analyze heterogeneity of trials. Considering possible clinical heterogeneity due to study design and patients' population, we used a random effect model for all pooled analysis. Pooled analysis was done in RevMan software (Review Manager (RevMan) [Computer program]. Version 5.3. Copenhagen: The Nordic Cochrane Centre, The Cochrane Collaboration, 2014). Publication bias was assessed by visual inspection of funnel plot. A meta-regression was planned by *metareg* command in

STATA version 13.0 (STATA SE 13.0, Stata Corp, College Station, TX, USA) in case of more than 10 trials is found for any outcome.

## Results

Initial searching of database revealed 9558 articles, and searching of the other sources revealed another 114 articles. After duplicate removal, 540 articles were assessed and 12 articles were screened from

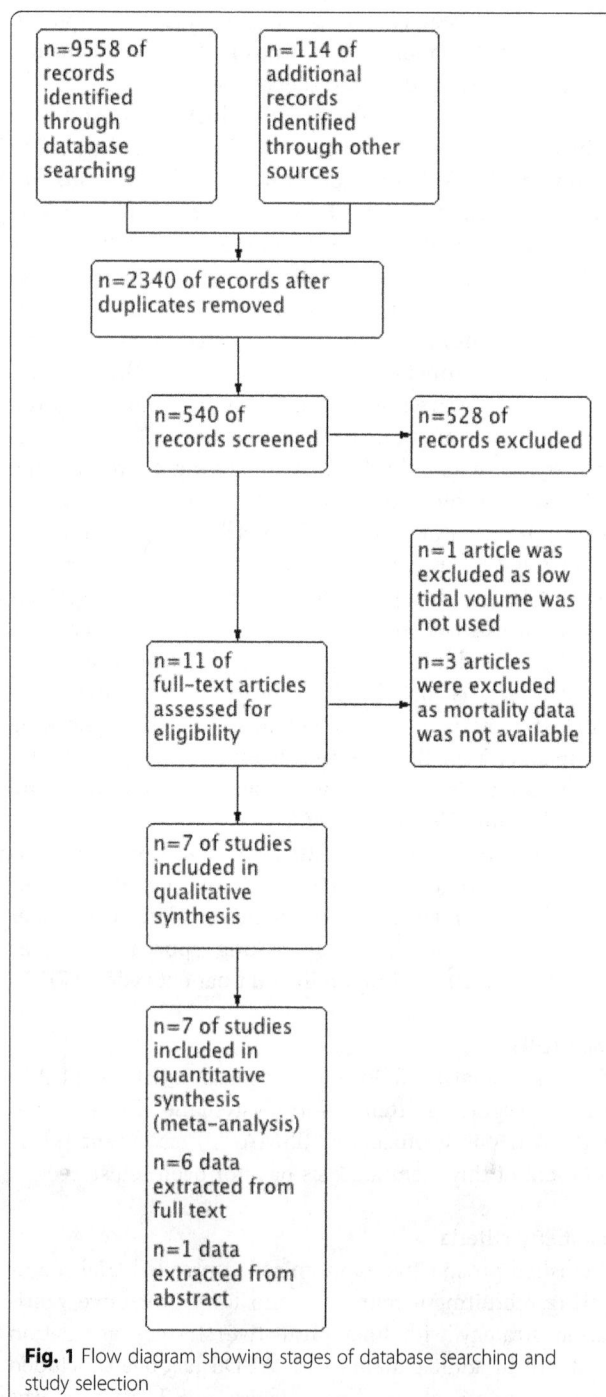

**Fig. 1** Flow diagram showing stages of database searching and study selection

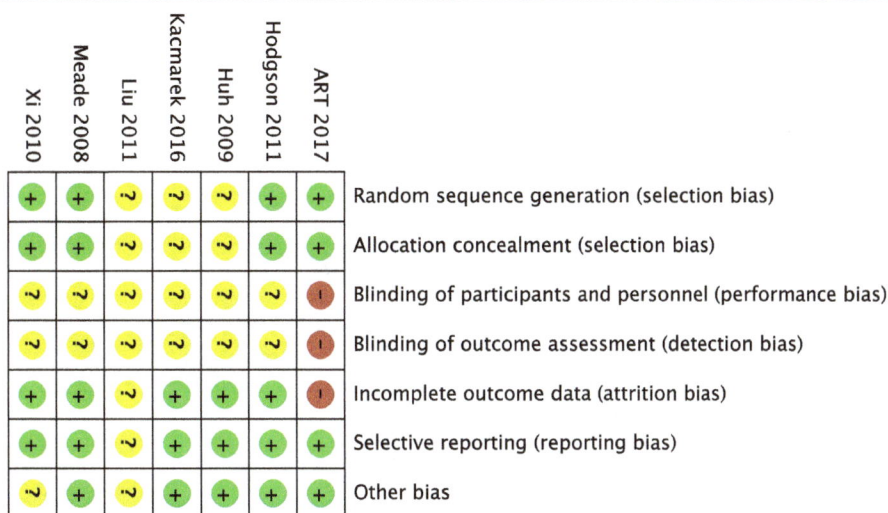

**Fig. 2** A summary of risk of biases showing review authors' judgments about each risk of bias item for each included study

title and abstract to identify potentially eligible trials. Finally, data of 2480 patients from 7 randomized controlled trials from published full text [11–16] and abstract [17] have been included in this meta-analysis and systemic review. A flow diagram showing stages of database searching and study selection has been provided in Fig. 1. One RCT [18] was excluded as lung protective ventilation was not used in control group and three trials [19–21] were excluded, as they did not report mortality data. Risk of biases in the individual studies have been reported in Fig. 2. Characteristics of the individual studies have been reported in Table 1.

**Mortality**

Reported mortality at the longest available follow-up [RR (95% CI) 0.93 (0.80, 1.08); $p = 0.33$; $I^2 = 43\%$; $n = 2480$], ICU mortality [RR (95% CI) 0.91 (0.76, 1.10); $p = 0.33$; $I^2 = 58\%$; $n = 2359$] and in-hospital mortality [RR (95% CI) 0.95 (0.83, 1.08); $p = 0.45$, $I^2 = 33\%$; $n = 2378$] were similar between recruitment maneuver group and standard lung protective ventilation group. A forest plot for odds ratio of mortality at different time points at individual study level and pooled analysis level has been provided in Fig. 3. Visual inspection of funnel plot for publication bias revealed that included trials are near the apex of the arbitrary triangle; hence, possibilities of

**Table 1** Characteristics of the included studies

| Author | Participants | Intervention | Control |
|---|---|---|---|
| ART investigators 2017 | Patients receiving invasive mechanical ventilation with moderate to severe ARDS (AECC definition) of < 72 h duration | LRM with incremental PEEP levels, followed by decremental PEEP titration according to the best respiratory system Cs and by a second LRM | Low PEEP strategy |
| Hodgson 2011 | Adult patients (age > 15years) with $PaO_2/FiO_2 < 200$ | LRM to $P_{peak}$ of 55 cm $H_2O$ and decremental PEEP titration to determine optimal PEEP | ARDSnet protocol |
| Kacmarek 2016 | ARDS patients with $PaO_2/FiO_2 < 200$ at $FiO_2 \geq 0.5$ and PEEP $\geq 10$ | LRM to $P_{peak}$ of $\leq 60$ cm $H_2O$ for 2 min and decremental PEEP titration to determine optimal PEEP. | ARDSnet protocol |
| Liu 2011 | Adult patients with ARDS ($PaO_2/FiO_2 \leq$ 250 mmHg) with $FiO_2 \geq 0.5$ and PEEP $\geq 10$ cm $H_2O$) at least 30 min | LRM with PEEP 35 cm $H_2O$ and $P_{peak}$ up to 50 cm $H_2O$ maintained for 2 min, then PEEP was set higher at 2 cm $H_2O$ above closing pressure | Lung protective ventilation strategy |
| Xi 2010 | Adult patients with ARDS ($PaO_2 \leq 200$ mmHg at $FiO_2$ 1.0 and PEEP $\geq 10$ cm $H_2O$) | LRM with CPAP 40 cm $H_2O$ for 40 s | Lung protective ventilation strategy |
| Meade 2008 | Adult patients with ARDS ($PaO_2/FiO_2 < 250$) | LRM by CPAP of 40 cm $H_2O$ for 40 s with $FiO_2$ 1.0. PEEP was adjusted as per $FiO_2$ requirement. | Low tidal volume ventilation with standard PEEP |
| Huh 2009 | ARDS patients with $PaO_2/FiO_2 < 200$ | LRM to $P_{peak}$ of 55 cm $H_2O$ and 25% tidal volume reduction and decremental PEEP titration to determine optimal PEEP | ARDSnet protocol |

*ARDS* acute respiratory distress syndrome, *AECC* American European Consensus Conference Criteria, *PaO₂* arterial oxygen tension, *FiO₂* fraction of oxygen in inspiration, *PEEP* positive end-expiratory pressure, *P_peak* peak airway pressure, *LRM* lung recruitment maneuver, *CPAP* continuous positive airway pressure

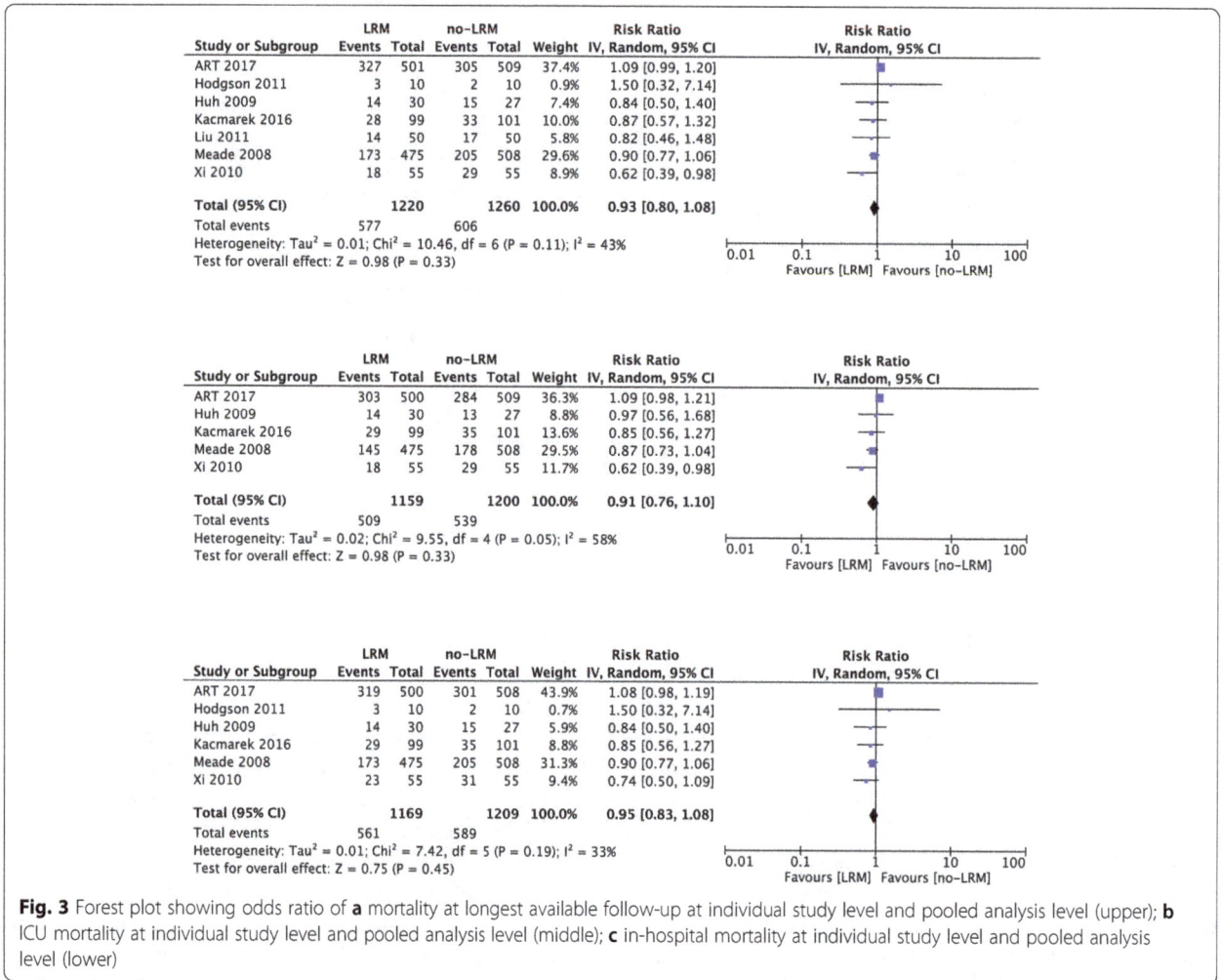

**Fig. 3** Forest plot showing odds ratio of **a** mortality at longest available follow-up at individual study level and pooled analysis level (upper); **b** ICU mortality at individual study level and pooled analysis level (middle); **c** in-hospital mortality at individual study level and pooled analysis level (lower)

publication bias cannot be excluded here. Similar results were obtained when the trial by Xi et al. [16] was excluded as PEEP titration was not used along with recruitment maneuver in that study.

### Length of stay

Duration of hospital stay [SMD (95% CI) 0.00 (− 0.09, 0.10); $p = 0.92$, $I^2 = 11\%$; $n = 2323$] and duration of ICU stays [SMD (95% CI) 0.05 (− 0.09, 0.19); $p = 0.49$, $I^2 = 47\%$; $n = 2380$] were similar between recruitment maneuver group and standard lung protective ventilation group. A forest plot for SMD in length of ICU stay and length of hospital stay at individual study level and pooled analysis level has been provided in Fig. 4. Similar results were obtained even after exclusion of the trial by Xi et al. [16].

### Complications

Only four trials reported incidence of barotrauma from recruitment maneuver, and it was found to be similar

with standard lung protective ventilation group [RR (95% CI) 1.27 (0.68, 2.36); $p = 0.45$, $I^2 = 57\%$, $n = 2350$].

### Discussion

Principal findings of this meta-analysis and systematic review are that recruitment maneuver neither provides any mortality benefit nor reduces length of hospital and ICU stays in adult patients with ARDS. Findings of this meta-analysis contradicts the reported mortality benefits of recruitment maneuver by Goligher et al. [6] in a meta-analysis of randomized controlled trials that included 1423 patients from 6 trials. However, the authors did not include a recent large trial [11], and on the other hand, they included another trial, which did not use lung protective ventilation strategy in the control group [18]. In the light of present clinical knowledge, we believe that lung protective ventilation strategy is an integral part of ARDS management and studies those are not using it is at significant high risk of bias.

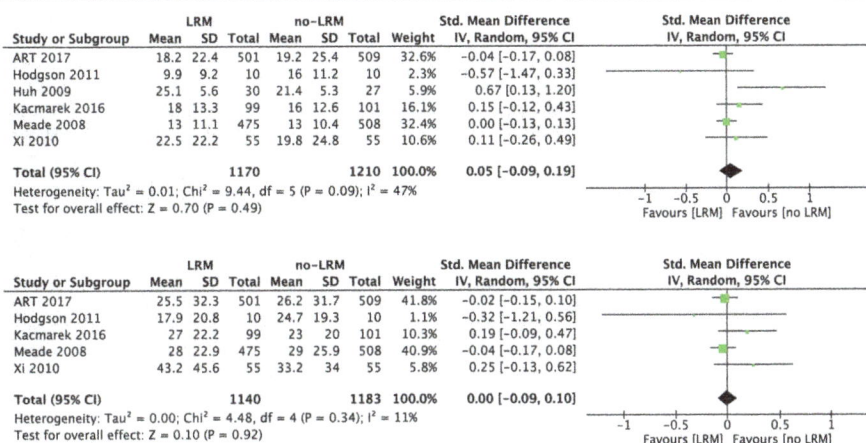

**Fig. 4** Forest plot showing standardized mean difference of **a** length of ICU stay (upper) and **b** length of hospital stay (lower) in two groups at individual study level and at the pooled analysis level

Another Cochrane database systematic review [22] reported a reduction in ICU mortality rate from a pooled analysis of data of 1370 patients from 5 trials. However, the authors did not report reduction in mortality in any other time points. Authors of that review of graded the quality of evidence as 'low' because of 4 of the included trials used various co-interventions along with recruitment maneuver. Though the co-interventions such as high PEEP or PEEP titration, used in various trials have the potential to interfere with the clinical outcome; from a physiological point of view, co-interventions to keep the recruited alveoli 'open' is an integral part of this approach. PEEP applied after recruitment maneuver expected to reduce sheer stress generated the collapsed and open alveoli interface from repeated recruitment and de-recruitment [23]. A higher PEEP with lung protective ventilation strategy may be beneficial in patients with ARDS [24].

Observational studies have found benefits of recruitment maneuver in ARDS patients in terms of oxygenation and lung compliance [25, 26]. An optimum PEEP and sigh maneuver also increases efficacy of recruitment maneuver in ARDS patients [27]. Toth et al. in 2007 suggested that improvement in oxygenation after recruitment maneuver and PEEP is due to primarily reduction in atelectasis rather than reduction in extra-vascular lung water [28]. However, success of recruitment maneuver may be dependent upon the amount of lung tissue available for recruitment and which is variable between patient and patient. In early ARDS, it may be possible to recruit lung and reverse hypoxemia in most of the patients [7]. Success of PEEP-induced recruitment may also depend upon the regional distribution and character-

istics of the atelectasis and it may be greater in case of inflammatory atelectasis at the lower lobes [29].

In this meta-analysis, we have found that recruitment maneuver used along with or without PEEP titration does not provide any mortality benefit at any time points. Our results remain essentially similar even when the trial by Xi et al. [16] excluded, as they did not use any co-intervention along with recruitment maneuver. However, the Xi et al. reported a reduction in ICU mortality but not in hospital mortality with the standalone use of recruitment maneuver. These findings suggest that recruitment maneuver without PEEP titration might have some beneficial effect in ARDS patients.

### Limitations

Our meta-analysis has several limitations. We have found significant amount of statistical heterogeneity most of the all analyses which is probably due to a heterogeneity in patients' selection and in the methods of recruitment maneuver application across the studies. As the number of the included trials were small in our meta-analysis, a meta-regression analysis was not possible. A visual inspection of the funnel plot also suggested that publication biases might also be present.

### Conclusion

Recruitment maneuver along with co-interventions such as PEEP titration does not provide any benefit in terms of mortality, length of ICU and hospital stay. Further studies are required to know the clinical benefits of recruitment maneuver without PEEP titration in ARDS patients.

## Abbreviations

95% CI: 95% confidence interval; ARDS: Acute respiratory distress syndrome; CENTRAL: The Cochrane Central Register of controlled trials; ICU: Intensive care unit; NNT: Number needed to treat; OR: Odds ratio; $PaO_2/FiO_2$: Ratio of arterial partial pressure of oxygen to fractional-inspired oxygen content; PEEP: Positive end-expiratory pressure; RCT: Randomized controlled trial; SD: Standard deviation; SMD: Standardized mean difference

## Acknowledgements

B B Dixit Library, All India Institute of Medical Sciences, New Delhi for providing access for database searching.

## Authors' contributions

KDS and SM contributed to the study design. SB and SM helped in the data collection and data analysis. SB, KDS, and SM helped in manuscript preparation. All authors read and approved the final manuscript.

## Competing interests

The authors declare that they have no competing interests.

## Author details

[1]Department of Anaesthesiology, Pain Medicine and Critical Care, All India Institute of Medical Sciences, Room No. 5011, 5th Floor Teaching block, Ansari Nagar New Delhi 110029, India. [2]Department of Trauma Critical Care, Jai Prakash Narayan Apex Trauma Centre, All India Institute Medical Sciences, New Delhi, India.

## References

1. Maitra S, Bhattacharjee S, Khanna P, Baidya DK. High-frequency ventilation does not provide mortality benefit in comparison with conventional lung-protective ventilation in acute respiratory distress syndrome: a meta-analysis of the randomized controlled trials. Anesthesiology. 2015;122:841–51.
2. McNicholas BA, Rooney GM, Laffey JG. Lessons to learn from epidemiologic studies in ARDS. Curr Opin Crit Care. 2018;24:41–8.
3. Bellani G, Laffey JG, Pham T, Fan E, Brochard L, Esteban A, Gattinoni L, van Haren F, Larsson A, McAuley DF, Ranieri M, Rubenfeld G, Thompson BT, Wrigge H, Slutsky AS. Pesenti A; LUNG SAFE Investigators; ESICM Trials Group. Epidemiology, patterns of care, and mortality for patients with acute respiratory distress syndrome in intensive care units in 50 countries. JAMA. 2016;315:788–800.
4. Albert RK. The role of ventilation-induced surfactant dysfunction and atelectasis in causing acute respiratory distress syndrome. Am J Respir Crit Care Med. 2012;185:702–8.
5. Pierrakos C, Karanikolas M, Scolletta S, Karamouzos V, Velissaris D. Acute respiratory distress syndrome: pathophysiology and therapeutic options. J Clin Med Res. 2012;4:7–16.
6. Goligher EC, Hodgson CL, Adhikari NKJ, Meade MO, Wunsch H, Uleryk E, Gajic O, Amato MPB, Ferguson ND, Rubenfeld GD, Fan E. Lung recruitment maneuvers for adult patients with acute respiratory distress syndrome. A systematic review and meta-analysis. Ann Am Thorac Soc. 2017;14:S304–11.
7. Borges JB, Okamoto VN, Matos GF, Caramez MP, Arantes PR, Barros F, Souza CE, Victorino JA, Kacmarek RM, Barbas CS, Carvalho CR, Amato MB. Reversibility of lung collapse and hypoxemia in early acute respiratory distress syndrome. Am J Respir Crit Care Med. 2006;174:268–78.
8. Guo L, Wang W, Zhao N, Guo L, Chi C, Hou W, Wu A, Tong H, Wang Y, Wang C, Li E. Mechanical ventilation strategies for intensive care unit patients without acute lung injury or acute respiratory distress syndrome: a systematic review and network meta-analysis. Crit Care. 2016;20:226.
9. Liberati A, Altman DG, Tetzlaff J, Mulrow C, Gøtzsche PC, Ioannidis JP, Clarke M, Devereaux PJ, Kleijnen J, Moher D. The PRISMA statement for reporting systematic reviews and meta-analyses of studies that evaluate health care interventions: explanation and elaboration. J Clin Epidemiol. 2009;62:e1–34.
10. Hozo SP, Djulbegovic B, Hozo I. Estimating the mean and variance from the median, range, and the size of a sample. BMC Med Res Methodol. 2005;5:13.
11. Writing Group for the Alveolar Recruitment for Acute Respiratory Distress Syndrome Trial (ART) Investigators, Cavalcanti AB, Suzumura ÉA, Laranjeira LN, Paisani DM, Damiani LP, Guimarães HP, Romano ER, Regenga MM, LNT T, Teixeira C, Pinheiro de Oliveira R, Machado FR, Diaz-Quijano FA, MSA F, Maia IS, Caser EB, Filho WO, Borges MC, Martins PA, Matsui M, Ospina-Tascón GA, Giancursi TS, Giraldo-Ramirez ND, SRR V, MDGPL A, Hasan MS, Szczeklik W, Rios F, MBP A, Berwanger O, Ribeiro de Carvalho CR. Effect of lung recruitment and titrated positive end-expiratory pressure (PEEP) vs low PEEP on mortality in patients with acute respiratory distress syndrome: a randomized clinical trial. JAMA. 2017;318(14):1335–45.
12. Kacmarek RM, Villar J, Sulemanji D, Montiel R, Ferrando C, Blanco J, Koh Y, Soler JA, Martínez D, Hernández M, Tucci M, Borges JB, Lubillo S, Santos A, Araujo JB, Amato MB, Suárez-Sipmann F. Open lung approach network. Open lung approach for the acute respiratory distress syndrome: a pilot, randomized controlled trial. Crit Care Med. 2016;44(1):32–42.
13. Hodgson CL, Tuxen DV, Davies AR, Bailey MJ, Higgins AM, Holland AE, Keating JL, Pilcher DV, Westbrook AJ, Cooper DJ, Nichol AD. A randomised controlled trial of an open lung strategy with staircase recruitment, titrated PEEP and targeted low airway pressures in patients with acute respiratory distress syndrome. Crit Care. 2011;15:R133.
14. Meade MO, Cook DJ, Guyatt GH, Slutsky AS, Arabi YM, Cooper DJ, Davies AR, Hand LE, Zhou Q, Thabane L, Austin P, Lapinsky S, Baxter A, Russell J, Skrobik Y, Ronco JJ, Stewart TE. Lung Open Ventilation Study Investigators. Ventilation strategy using low tidal volumes, recruitment maneuvers, and high positive end-expiratory pressure for acute lung injury and acute respiratory distress syndrome: a randomized controlled trial. JAMA. 2008;299(6):637–45.
15. Huh JW, Jung H, Choi HS, Hong SB, Lim CM, Koh Y. Efficacy of positive end-expiratory pressure titration after the alveolar recruitment manoeuvre in patients with acute respiratory distress syndrome. Crit Care. 2009;13:R22.
16. Xi XM, Jiang L, Zhu B, RM group. Clinical efficacy and safety of recruitment maneuver in patients with acute respiratory distress syndrome using low tidal volume ventilation: a multicenter randomized controlled clinical trial. Chin Med J (Engl). 2010;123:3100–5.
17. Liu W-L, Wang C-M, Chen W-L. Effects of recruitment maneuvers in patients with early acute lung injury and acute respiratory distress syndrome. Respirology. 2011;16(Suppl 2):1–326.
18. Amato MB, Barbas CS, Medeiros DM, Magaldi RB, Schettino GP, Lorenzi-Filho G, Kairalla RA, Deheinzelin D, Munoz C, Oliveira R, Takagaki TY, Carvalho CR. Effect of a protective-ventilation strategy on mortality in the acute respiratory distress syndrome. N Engl J Med. 1998;338:347–54.
19. Oczenski W, Hörmann C, Keller C, Lorenzl N, Kepka A, Schwarz S, Fitzgerald RD. Recruitment maneuvers after a positive end-expiratory pressure trial do not induce sustained effects in early adult respiratory distress syndrome. Anesthesiology. 2004;101(3):620–5.
20. Wang Z, Zhu X, Li H, Wang T, Yao G. A study on the effect of recruitment maneuver imposed on extravascular lung water in patients with acute respiratory distress syndrome. Chinese Critical Care Medicine. 2009;21(10):604–8.
21. Yang G, Wang C, Ning R. Effects of high positive end-expiratory pressure combined with recruitment maneuvers in patients with acute respiratory distress syndrome. Chinese Critical Care Med. 2011;21(1):28–31.
22. Hodgson C, Goligher EC, Young ME, Keating JL, Holland AE, Romero L, Bradley SJ, Tuxen D. Recruitment manoeuvres for adults with acute respiratory distress syndrome receiving mechanical ventilation. Cochrane Database Syst Rev. 2016;11:CD006667.
23. Slutsky AS. Lung injury caused by mechanical ventilation. Chest. 1999 Jul; 116(1 Suppl):9S–15S.
24. Briel M, Meade M, Mercat A, Brower RG, Talmor D, Walter SD, Slutsky AS, Pullenayegum E, Zhou Q, Cook D, Brochard L, Richard JC, Lamontagne F, Bhatnagar N, Stewart TE, Guyatt G. Higher vs lower positive end-expiratory pressure in patients with acute lung injury and acute respiratory distress syndrome: systematic review and meta-analysis. JAMA. 2010;303:865–73.

25. Póvoa P, Almeida E, Fernandes A, Mealha R, Moreira P, Sabino H. Evaluation of a recruitment maneuver with positive inspiratory pressure and high PEEP in patients with severe ARDS. Acta Anaesthesiol Scand. 2004;48:287–93.

26. Gernoth C, Wagner G, Pelosi P, Luecke T. Respiratory and haemodynamic changes during decremental open lung positive end-expiratory pressure titration in patients with acute respiratory distress syndrome. Crit Care. 2009;13:R59.

27. Badet M, Bayle F, Richard JC, Guérin C. Comparison of optimal positive end-expiratory pressure and recruitment maneuvers during lung-protective mechanical ventilation in patients with acute lung injury/acute respiratory distress syndrome. Respir Care. 2009;54:847–54.

28. Toth I, Leiner T, Mikor A, Szakmany T, Bogar L, Molnar Z. Hemodynamic and respiratory changes during lung recruitment and descending optimal positive end-expiratory pressure titration in patients with acute respiratory distress syndrome. Crit Care Med. 2007;35:787–93.

29. Puybasset L, Gusman P, Muller JC, Cluzel P, Coriat P, Rouby JJ. Regional distribution of gas and tissue in acute respiratory distress syndrome. III. Consequences for the effects of positive end-expiratory pressure. CT scan ARDS study group. Adult respiratory distress syndrome. Intensive Care Med. 2000;26:1215–27.

# 21

# Serial change of C1 inhibitor in patients with sepsis

Tomoya Hirose[*], Hiroshi Ogura, Hiroki Takahashi, Masahiro Ojima, Kang Jinkoo, Youhei Nakamura, Takashi Kojima and Takeshi Shimazu

## Abstract

**Background:** C1 inhibitor (C1-INH), which belongs to the superfamily of serine protease inhibitors, regulates the complement system and also the plasma kallikrein-kinin, fibrinolytic, and coagulation systems. The biologic activities of C1-INH can be divided into the regulation of vascular permeability and anti-inflammatory functions. The objective of this study was to clarify the serial change of C1-INH in patients with sepsis and evaluate the relationship with the shock severity.

**Methods:** This was a single-center, prospective, observational study. We serially examined C1-INH activity values (normal range 70–130%) in patients with sepsis admitted into the intensive care unit of the Trauma and Acute Critical Care Center at Osaka University Hospital (Osaka, Japan) during the period between January 2014 and August 2015. We defined "refractory shock" as septic shock unresponsive to conventional therapy such as adequate fluid resuscitation and vasopressor therapy to maintain hemodynamics.

**Results:** Serial changes of C1-INH were evaluated in 40 patients with sepsis (30 men, 10 women; 30 survivors, 10 non-survivors; mean age, $70 \pm 13.5$ years). We divided the patients into three groups: non-shock group ($n = 14$), non-refractory shock group ($n = 13$), and refractory shock group ($n = 13$: 3 survivors, 10 non-survivors). In the non-shock group, C1-INH was $107.3 \pm 26.5\%$ on admission and $104.2 \pm 22.3\%$ on day 1, and it increased thereafter to $128.1 \pm 26.4\%$ on day 3, $138.3 \pm 21.2\%$ on day 7, and $140.3 \pm 12.5\%$ on day 14 ($p < 0.0001$). In the non-refractory shock group, C1-INH was $113.9 \pm 19.2\%$ on admission, $120.2 \pm 23.0\%$ on day 1, $135.7 \pm 19.9\%$ on day 3, $138.8 \pm 17.2\%$ on day 7, and $137.7 \pm 10.7\%$ on day 14 ($p < 0.0001$). In the refractory shock group, C1-INH was $96.7 \pm 15.9\%$ on admission, $88.9 \pm 22.3\%$ on day 1, $119.8 \pm 39.6\%$ on day 3, $144.4 \pm 21.1\%$ on day 7, and $140.5 \pm 24.5\%$ on day 14 ($p < 0.0001$). The difference between these three groups was statistically significant ($p < 0.0001$). C1-INH in non-survivors did not increase significantly during their clinical course ($p = 0.0690$).

**Conclusions:** In refractory shock patients with sepsis, the values of C1-INH activity were lower (especially in non-survivors) on admission and day 1 as compared with non-shock and non-refractory shock patients.

**Keywords:** C1 inhibitor (C1-INH), Sepsis, Vascular permeability, Shock

* Correspondence: htomoya1979@hp-emerg.med.osaka-u.ac.jp
Department of Traumatology and Acute Critical Medicine, Osaka University
Graduate School of Medicine, 2-15 Yamadaoka, Suita, Osaka 565-0871, Japan

# Background

C1 inhibitor (C1-INH), which belongs to the superfamily of serine protease inhibitors, regulates not only the complement system but also the plasma kallikrein-kinin, fibrinolytic, and coagulation systems [1, 2].The biologic activities of C1-INH can be divided into the regulation of vascular permeability and anti-inflammatory functions [1]. Hereditary angioedema (HAE), caused by an inherited deficiency of C1-INH, has been a focus in recent years [3]. During attacks of HAE, vascular permeability increases markedly, which leads to angioedema [4, 5].

The detailed pathology underlying increased vascular hyperpermeability in patients with HAE is not completely understood. Bradykinin is the main mediator of increased vascular permeability in patients with HAE [6] [7] During acute attacks of HAE, kallikrein is insufficiently inhibited because of the deficiency in C1-INH, the kallikrein-kinin system becomes activated, and at the end of the cascade, an increased amount of bradykinin is produced that results in the edema seen in patients with HAE.

In sepsis, significant vascular hyperpermeability is similarly observed systemically; however, the mechanism of vascular hyperpermeability in sepsis has not been completely elucidated [8, 9]. Cytokines and other inflammatory mediators induce gaps between endothelial cells by disassembly of intercellular junctions, by altering the cellular cytoskeletal structure, or by directly damaging the cell monolayer, and this creation of gaps can result in microvascular leakage and tissue edema, which are characteristic of sepsis [10]. Endothelial hyperpermeability is the key in the progression from sepsis to organ failure [9], but the role of C1-INH in the pathogenesis has not been clarified. In 1985, Kalter et al. [11] reported that C1-INH levels are significantly increased in uncomplicated bacteremia, moderately increased in patients with nonfatal episodes of bacterial shock, and not increased in those with fatal episodes. However, they did not evaluate the serial change of C1-INH levels, and the timing of blood sampling was unclear. Recently, in a preliminary report, we noted that C1-INH activity was not enhanced in two refractory shock patients with sepsis (one survivor and one non-survivor) on admission to hospital. The surviving patient's general condition had improved with increases in C1-INH activity, and enhancement of C1-INH activity was also observed in three non-refractory shock patients with sepsis [12, 13].

Thus, the objectives of this study were to prospectively evaluate the serial changes of C1-INH activity in a larger population of patients with sepsis under the current standard treatment policy and to evaluate the relationship with the shock severity.

# Methods

## Patients and setting

This was a single-center, prospective, observational study that was approved by the Ethics Committee of Osaka University Graduate School of Medicine. From January 2014 to August 2015, we examined blood samples collected from patients with sepsis admitted into the intensive care unit of the Trauma and Acute Critical Care Center at Osaka University Hospital (Osaka, Japan). Sepsis and septic shock were diagnosed according to the "Surviving Sepsis Campaign: International Guidelines for Management of Severe Sepsis and Septic Shock: 2012" [14]. Exclusion criteria were age < 15 year and end stage of malignant disease.

Our principle therapeutic policy regarding circulation management for sepsis is as follows. Initial resuscitation is performed according to the "Surviving Sepsis Campaign: International Guidelines for Management of Severe Sepsis and Septic Shock: 2012" [14]. Even with adequate fluid resuscitation and vasopressor therapy (noradrenalin of > 0.1 μg/kg/min div. for more than at least 1 h), if the arterial systolic pressure is < 90 mmHg, we administer intravenous hydrocortisone (initial dose 100-mg bolus intravenously and then 200 mg per day via continuous intravenous administration).

We defined "refractory shock" as septic shock unresponsive to conventional therapy such as adequate fluid resuscitation and vasopressor therapy to maintain hemodynamics. We divided the patients into three groups: the non-shock group, the non-refractory shock group, and the refractory shock group. We obtained all necessary consents from all patients and their kin involved in this study.

## Evaluation of clinical background and C1-INH activity

The patients' clinical background and course including age, sex, Acute Physiological and Chronic Health Evaluation (APACHE) II score, Sequential Organ Failure Assessment (SOFA) score, prognosis, infusion volume, catecholamine administration, and steroid administration were recorded. We serially examined C1-INH activity values (normal range 70–130%) in patients with sepsis. The timing of sampling was day 0 (at admission), 1, 3, 5, 7, 10, and 14. The blood samples were stored at − 80°C until C1-INH activity values were measured in plasma samples using a Berichrom C1-INHibitor kit (Siemens Healthcare Diagnostics, Deerfield, IL) according to the manufacturer's instructions.

## Statistical analysis

All data are presented as the mean ± standard deviation (SD) except that in the figure captions, which are the mean ± standard error of the mean (SEM). To compare the baseline characteristics of the subjects in the three groups, analysis of variance (ANOVA) was used for the continuous values. Differences in longitudinal data between the groups were tested by repeated measures ANOVA. A $p$ value $> 0.05$ was considered to indicate statistical significance. All statistical analyses were performed using JMP Pro 11.2.0 (SAS Institute Inc., Cary, NC).

## Results

### Patient characteristics

The serial changes of C1-INH activity values were evaluated in 40 patients with sepsis (30 men and 10 women; 30 survivors and 10 non-survivors; mean age, $70.0 \pm 13.5$ years): the non-shock group ($n = 14$), the non-refractory shock group ($n = 13$), and the refractory shock group ($n = 13$: 3 survivors, 10 non-survivors). The characteristics of these groups are shown in Table 1. Among the three groups, the volume of infusion required during the first 48 h after admission to maintain hemodynamics was the greatest in the refractory shock group. The relationship between infusion volume required during the first 48 h and C1-INH activity at day 0 was not statistically significant ($p = 0.1104$).

### Comparison of serial changes of C1-INH activity between groups

A comparison of the serial changes of C1-INH activity values between the three groups is shown in Fig. 1. In the non-shock group, C1-INH was $107.3 \pm 26.5\%$ on admission and $104.2 \pm 22.3\%$ on day 1. Thereafter, it increased

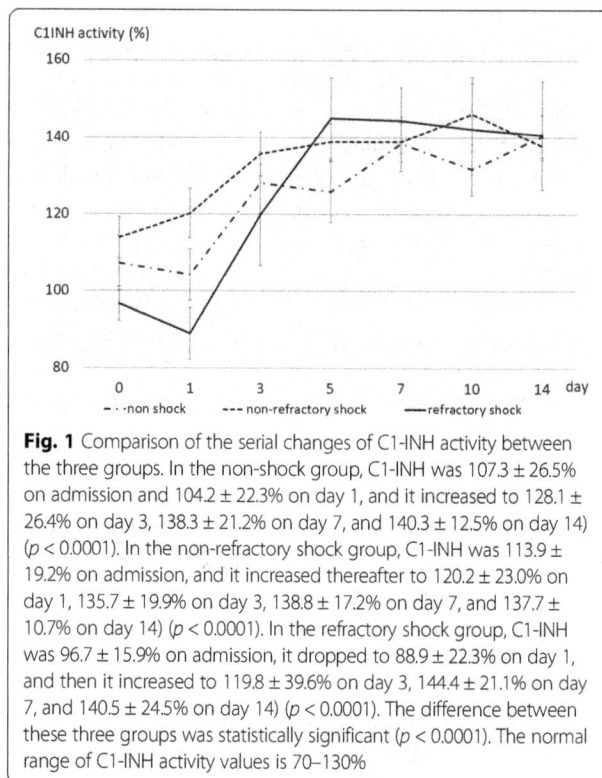

**Fig. 1** Comparison of the serial changes of C1-INH activity between the three groups. In the non-shock group, C1-INH was $107.3 \pm 26.5\%$ on admission and $104.2 \pm 22.3\%$ on day 1, and it increased to $128.1 \pm 26.4\%$ on day 3, $138.3 \pm 21.2\%$ on day 7, and $140.3 \pm 12.5\%$ on day 14) ($p < 0.0001$). In the non-refractory shock group, C1-INH was $113.9 \pm 19.2\%$ on admission, and it increased thereafter to $120.2 \pm 23.0\%$ on day 1, $135.7 \pm 19.9\%$ on day 3, $138.8 \pm 17.2\%$ on day 7, and $137.7 \pm 10.7\%$ on day 14) ($p < 0.0001$). In the refractory shock group, C1-INH was $96.7 \pm 15.9\%$ on admission, it dropped to $88.9 \pm 22.3\%$ on day 1, and then it increased to $119.8 \pm 39.6\%$ on day 3, $144.4 \pm 21.1\%$ on day 7, and $140.5 \pm 24.5\%$ on day 14) ($p < 0.0001$). The difference between these three groups was statistically significant ($p < 0.0001$). The normal range of C1-INH activity values is 70–130%

**Table 1** Patient characteristics

| Characteristic | Non-shock | Non-refractory shock | Refractory shock | $p$ |
|---|---|---|---|---|
| $N$ | 14 | 13 | 13 | |
| Age ($\pm$ SD) (years) | $66.8 \pm 17.1$ | $72.5 \pm 10.4$ | $71.0 \pm 12.2$ | 0.5346 |
| Male (%) | 11 (78.6) | 9 (69.2) | 10 (76.9) | 0.8388 |
| Survivor $n$ (%) | 14 (100) | 13 (100) | 3 (23.1) | $< .0001$ |
| APACHE II score | $13.1 \pm 5.9$ | $25.5 \pm 5.7$ | $27.9 \pm 10.2$ | $< .0001$ |
| SOFA score | $4.3 \pm 0.9$ | $9.4 \pm 0.9$ | $9.7 \pm 0.9$ | 0.0001 |
| Volume of infusion over the first 48 h after admission ($\pm$ SD) (mL) | $9735.5 \pm 6852.9$ | $11,765.2 \pm 6369.4$ | $18,390.7 \pm 8908.8$ | 0.0127 |
| Mean volume of infusion/h over the first 48 h after admission ($\pm$ SD) (mL/h) | $204.3 \pm 140.6$ | $263.9 \pm 146.2$ | $484.0 \pm 146.3$ | $< .0001$ |
| Diagnosis ($n$) | | | | |
| Pneumonia | 1 | 3 | 3 | |
| Urinary tract infection | 2 | 2 | 3 | |
| Gas gangrene | 3 | 1 | 2 | |
| Abdominal infection | 3 | 5 | 2 | |
| CNS infection | 1 | 1 | 0 | |
| Infective endocarditis | 1 | 0 | 0 | |
| Cellulitis | 1 | 1 | 3 | |
| Others | 2 | 0 | 0 | |

*APACHE* Acute Physiological and Chronic Health Evaluation, *CNS* central nervous system, *SD* standard deviation, *SOFA* Sequential Organ Failure Assessment

to $128.1 \pm 26.4\%$ on day 3, $138.3 \pm 21.2\%$ on day 7, and $140.3 \pm 12.5\%$ on day 14 ($p < 0.0001$). In the non-refractory shock group, C1-INH was $113.9 \pm 19.2\%$ on admission, and it increased thereafter to $120.2 \pm 23.0\%$ on day 1, $135.7 \pm 19.9\%$ on day 3, $138.8 \pm 17.2\%$ on day 7, and $137.7 \pm 10.7\%$ on day 14 ($p < 0.0001$). In the refractory shock group, C1-INH was $96.7 \pm 15.9\%$ on admission, it dropped to $88.9 \pm 22.3\%$ on day 1, and then increased to $119.8 \pm 39.6\%$ on day 3, $144.4 \pm 21.1\%$ on day 7, and $140.5 \pm 24.5\%$ on day 14 ($p < 0.0001$). The difference between these three groups was statistically significant ($p < 0.0001$).

## Serial change of C1-INH activity in each patient in the refractory shock group

Serial changes of C1-INH activity values in each patient in the refractory shock group are shown in Fig. 2. C1-INH activity increased after admission in the three survivors, but it did not necessarily increase after admission in the non-survivors. Some patients died because hemodynamics could not be maintained during the first few days after admission, and others died because of multiple organ failure at more than 1 week after admission.

## Comparison of serial changes of C1-INH activity between survivors and non-survivors in the refractory shock group

Serial changes of C1-INH activity between the survivors and non-survivors in the refractory shock group are compared in Fig. 3. Over the clinical courses, C1-INH increased significantly in the survivors ($p < 0.0001$) but did not increase significantly in the non-survivors ($p = 0.0690$).

## Discussion

In this study, we showed the serial changes of C1-INH activity values in patients with sepsis. Septic patients are reported to often exhibit a relative deficiency of

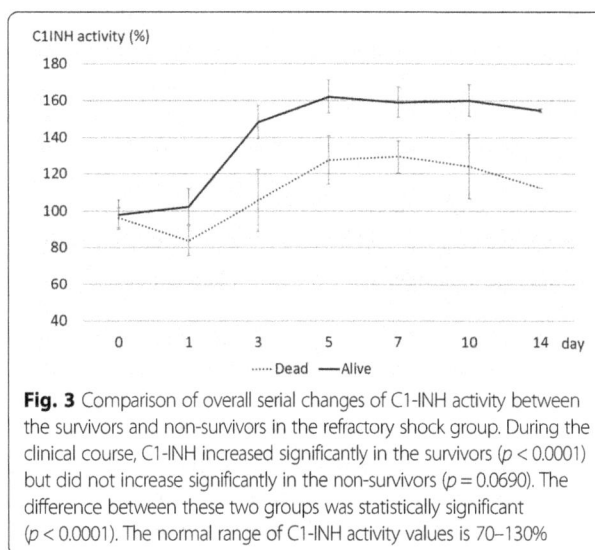

**Fig. 3** Comparison of overall serial changes of C1-INH activity between the survivors and non-survivors in the refractory shock group. During the clinical course, C1-INH increased significantly in the survivors ($p < 0.0001$) but did not increase significantly in the non-survivors ($p = 0.0690$). The difference between these two groups was statistically significant ($p < 0.0001$). The normal range of C1-INH activity values is 70–130%

C1-INH [15, 16]. The findings in our previous preliminary study suggested that C1-INH activity may be suppressed in patients with refractory shock due to the enhanced consumption or suppressed production of C1-INH [12, 13].

In sepsis, significant endothelial hyperpermeability similar to that of HAE is observed systemically [8]. In the present study, the highest values of C1-INH activity were found in the non-refractory shock group, followed by those in the non-shock group and those in the refractory shock group, especially on days 0 and 1 (Fig. 1). We thought that C1-INH works to suppress vascular permeability; thus, the C1-INH activity values in the non-refractory shock group increased, whereas those in the refractory shock group decreased due to the enhanced consumption or suppressed production of C1-INH. As a result, the patients in the refractory shock group required a high volume of fluid resuscitation (Table 1), and these patients might develop a relative deficiency of C1-INH. It is presently not clear how high the C1-INH activity value should be throughout sepsis treatment, especially in refractory shock patients. Further study is required to evaluate this point.

Animal studies showed that C1-INH administration improves vascular permeability [17, 18]. Schmidt et al. [17] revealed that pretreatment with C1-INH attenuates macromolecular leakage in postcapillary venules of rat mesentery, and Liu et al. [18] reported that C1-INH suppresses the systemic lipopolysaccharide-induced increase in microvascular permeability in mice. In CLP (cecal ligation and puncture) models of sepsis, treatment with a single dose of C1-INH improved survival as reported by Liu et al. [19]. Some validity for the administration of C1-INH in the treatment of sepsis has been shown by animal models such as these [20].

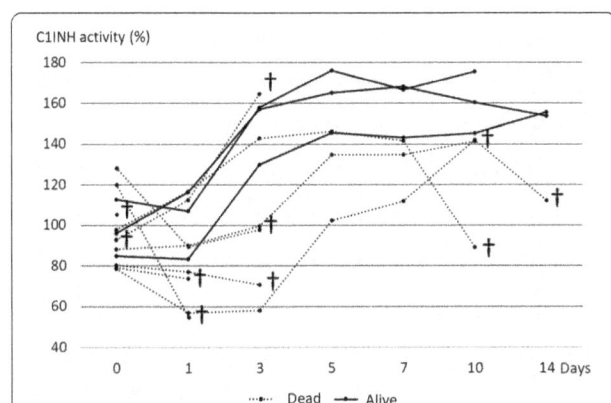

**Fig. 2** Serial changes of C1-INH activity in the 13 patients in the refractory shock group (3 survivors, 10 non-survivors). C1-INH activity increased in all survivors after admission, but in the non-survivors, it did not necessarily increase after admission. †Dead. The normal range of C1-INH activity values is 70–130%

In contrast, there is very little clinical data on C1-INH administration in patients with sepsis [20]. Recently, Igonin et al. [21] reported that C1-INH infusion increased survival rates for patients with sepsis in an open-label, randomized, controlled study. C1-INH administration in patients with sepsis was associated with reduced all-cause mortality (12 vs. 45% in the control, $p = 0.008$) and sepsis-related mortality (8 vs. 45% in the control, $p = 0.001$) assessed over 28 days. However, their study population was small (C1-INH group: $n = 42$, control group: $n = 20$), one of their inclusion criteria was that patients begin treatment within 48 h of sepsis onset, and C1-INH activity values were not evaluated. We thought that the inclusion criteria of their study on C1-INH replacement therapy in patients with sepsis may have been focused on refractory shock cases. Further study is required to evaluate the effect of C1-INH replacement therapy in sepsis.

In sepsis, the complement system including C1-INH has an important role in the host defense against bacterial infection, and activation of the complement system through the classic, alternative, and lectin pathways leads to inflammatory host response [15, 20]. These pathways include various component factors such as C1, C2, C3, C4, C5, C6, C7, C8, C9, MBL (mannose-binding lectin), and MASP2 (MBL-associated serine proteases) [20]. C1-INH regulates the complement system such as C1r, C1s, and MASP2 [1]. We only evaluated C1-INH activity in the present study. Therefore, the evaluation of serial changes in the other complemental factors is also needed to clarify the role of C1-INH regulation of hyperpermeability in human sepsis patients.

Our study has some limitations. First, we only evaluated C1-INH over the first 2 weeks after admission, and the long-term change in C1-INH was not clarified. Second, complement factors other than C1-INH were not evaluated. Third, we only evaluated fluid volume and did not evaluate markers of vascular endothelial dysfunction such as glycocalyx injury or changes in bradykinin concentration. Fourth, we may have to consider the effect of dilution by fluid infusion. Fifth, the sample size was small. Finally, we only evaluated C1-INH activity, not C1-INH quantitative values, in the present study. In our previous study, C1-INH quantitative values were low on admission in refractory shock patients even though they had normal C1-INH activity values [12, 13]. Because we have no data on C1-INH quantitative values in the present study, further evaluation is required on this point.

Further prospective, randomized, control studies to validate C1-INH replacement therapy including the evaluation of C1-INH and other complement factors in a larger population with sepsis are needed.

## Conclusions

In refractory shock patients with sepsis, the values of C1-INH activity were lower (especially in non-survivors) on admission and day 1 as compared with non-shock and non-refractory shock patients.

## Abbreviations
APACHE: Acute Physiological and Chronic Health Evaluation; C1-INH: C1 inhibitor; HAE: Hereditary angioedema; SD: Standard deviation; SEM: Standard error of the mean

## Acknowledgements
We gratefully acknowledge the devoted cooperation of the medical staff in the Trauma and Acute Critical Care Center at Osaka University Hospital.

## Funding
This study was supported by a medical research grant on traffic accidents from The General Insurance Association of Japan.

## Authors' contributions
TH designed the study. TH, HT, MO, KJ, and YN collected and generated the data. TK measured C1-INH activity values. TH wrote the first draft. TH, HO, HT, and MO analyzed the data. HO and TS helped to draft the manuscript. All of the authors read and approved the final manuscript.

## Competing interests
The authors declare that they have no competing interests.

## References
1. Davis AE 3rd, Mejia P, Lu F. Biological activities of C1 inhibitor. Mol Immunol. 2008;45:4057–63.
2. Davis AE 3rd, Lu F, Mejia P. C1 inhibitor, a multi-functional serine protease inhibitor. Thromb Haemost. 2010;104:886–93.
3. Bowen T, Cicardi M, Farkas H, Bork K, Longhurst HJ, Zuraw B, et al. 2010 International consensus algorithm for the diagnosis, therapy and management of hereditary angioedema. Allergy Asthma Clin Immunol. 2010;6:24.
4. Bork K. Recurrent angioedema and the threat of asphyxiation. Dtsch Arztebl Int. 2010;107:408–14.
5. Bork K, Meng G, Staubach P, Hardt J. Hereditary angioedema: new findings concerning symptoms, affected organs, and course. Am J Med. 2006;119:267–74.
6. Björkqvist J, Sala-Cunill A, Renné T. Hereditary angioedema: a bradykinin-mediated swelling disorder. Thromb Haemost. 2013;109:368–74.
7. Craig TJ, Bernstein JA, Farkas H, Bouillet L, Boccon-Gibod I. Diagnosis and treatment of bradykinin-mediated angioedema: outcomes from an angioedema expert consensus meeting. Int Arch Allergy Immunol. 2014; 165:119–27.

8.  Smedegård G, Cui LX, Hugli TE. Endotoxin-induced shock in the rat. A role for C5a. Am J Pathol. 1989;135:489–97.
9.  Ince C, Mayeux PR, Nguyen T, Gomez H, Kellum JA, Ospina-Tascón GA, et al. The endothelium in sepsis. Shock. 2016;45:259–70.
10. Lee WL, Slutsky AS. Sepsis and endothelial permeability. N Engl J Med. 2010;363:689–91.
11. Kalter ES, Daha MR, ten Cate JW, Verhoef J, Bouma BN. Activation and inhibition of Hageman factor-dependent pathways and the complement system in uncomplicated bacteremia or bacterial shock. J Infect Dis. 1985; 151:1019–27.
12. Hirose T, Ogura H, Kang J, Nakamura Y, Hosotsubo H, Kitano E, et al. Serial change of C1 inhibitor in patients with sepsis—a preliminary report. Am J Emerg Med. 2016;34:594–8.
13. Hirose T, Ogura H, Kang J, Nakamura Y, Hosotsubo H, Kitano E, et al. Erratum to "Serial change of C1 inhibitor in patients with sepsis—a preliminary report" [Volume 34, Issue 3, March 2016, pages 594–598]. Am J Emerg Med. 2016;34:1741–2.
14. Dellinger RP, Levy MM, Rhodes A, Annane D, Gerlach H, Opal SM, et al. Surviving sepsis campaign: international guidelines for management of severe sepsis and septic shock: 2012. Crit Care Med. 2013;41:580–637.
15. Charchaflieh J, Wei J, Labaze G, Hou YJ, Babarsh B, Stutz H, et al. The role of complement system in septic shock. Clin Dev Immunol. 2012;2012:407324.
16. Hack CE, Ogilvie AC, Eisele B, Eerenberg AJ, Wagstaff J, Thijs LG. C1-inhibitor substitution therapy in septic shock and in the vascular leak syndrome induced by high doses of interleukin-2. Intensive Care Med. 1993;19(1):S19–28.
17. Schmidt W, Stenzel K, Gebhard MM, Martin E, Schmidt H. C1-esterase inhibitor and its effects on endotoxin-induced leukocyte adherence and plasma extravasation in postcapillary venules. Surgery. 1999;125:280–7.
18. Liu D, Zhang D, Scafidi J, Wu X, Cramer CC, Davis AE 3rd. C1 inhibitor prevents Gram-negative bacterial lipopolysaccharide-induced vascular permeability. Blood. 2005;105:2350–5.
19. Liu D, Lu F, Qin G, Fernandes SM, Li J, Davis AE 3rd. C1 inhibitor-mediated protection from sepsis. J Immunol. 2007;179:3966–72.
20. Singer M, Jones AM. Bench-to-bedside review: the role of C1-esterase inhibitor in sepsis and other critical illnesses. Crit Care. 2011;15:203.
21. Igonin AA, Protsenko DN, Galstyan GM, Vlasenko AV, Khachatryan NN, Nekhaev IV, et al. C1-esterase inhibitor infusion increases survival rates for patients with sepsis*. Crit Care Med. 2012;40:770–7.

# 22

# The safety of a novel early mobilization protocol conducted by ICU physicians

Keibun Liu[1]*[iD], Takayuki Ogura[1], Kunihiko Takahashi[2], Mitsunobu Nakamura[2], Hiroaki Ohtake[3], Kenji Fujiduka[1], Emi Abe[4], Hitoshi Oosaki[3], Dai Miyazaki[1], Hiroyuki Suzuki[1], Mitsuaki Nishikimi[1], Alan Kawarai Lefor[5] and Takashi Mato[6]

## Abstract

**Background:** There are numerous barriers to early mobilization (EM) in a resource-limited intensive care unit (ICU) without a specialized team or an EM culture, regarding patient stability while critically ill or in the presence of medical devices. We hypothesized that ICU physicians can overcome these barriers. The aim of this study was to investigate the safety of EM according to the Maebashi EM protocol conducted by ICU physicians.

**Methods:** This was a single-center prospective observational study. All consecutive patients with an unplanned emergency admission were included in this study, according to the exclusion criteria. The observation period was from June 2015 to June 2016. Data regarding adverse events, medical devices in place during rehabilitation, protocol adherence, and rehabilitation outcomes were collected. The primary outcome was safety.

**Results:** A total of 232 consecutively enrolled patients underwent 587 rehabilitation sessions. Thirteen adverse events occurred (2.2%; 95% confidence interval, 1.2–3.8%) and no specific treatment was needed. There were no instances of dislodgement or obstruction of medical devices, tubes, or lines. The incidence of adverse events associated with mechanical ventilation or extracorporeal membrane oxygenation (ECMO) was 2.4 and 3.6%, respectively. Of 587 sessions, 387 (66%) sessions were performed at the active rehabilitation level, including sitting out of the bed, active transfer to a chair, standing, marching, and ambulating. ICU physicians attended over 95% of these active rehabilitation sessions. Of all patients, 143 (62%) got out of bed within 2 days (median 1.2 days; interquartile range 0.1–2.0).

**Conclusions:** EM according to the Maebashi EM protocol conducted by ICU physicians, without a specialized team or EM culture, was performed at a level of safety similar to previous studies performed by specialized teams, even with medical devices in place, including mechanical ventilation or ECMO. Protocolized EM led by ICU physicians can be initiated in the acute phase of critical illness without serious adverse events requiring additional treatment.

**Keywords:** Early mobilization, Protocol, Safety, ICU physicians, Medical devices, Acute phase

* Correspondence: keiliu0406@gmail.com
[1]Advanced Medical Emergency Department and Critical Care Center, Japan Red Cross Maebashi Hospital, 3-21-36 Asahi-cho, Maebashi, Gunma 371-0014, Japan
Full list of author information is available at the end of the article

## Background

After surviving a critical illness, many patients suffer long-term cognitive and physical dysfunction, and reduced health-related quality of life [1–6]. Several studies have shown that about half of patients cannot return to work [7, 8]. This has a major impact on patients, their families, and society. Recently, early mobilization (EM) in the intensive care unit (ICU) has been recommended to prevent or limit cognitive and physical dysfunction [9]. EM provides many benefits, such as reducing the duration of delirium, improved muscle strength, and improved quality of life [10–14]. EM can decrease both ICU and hospital length of stay [10, 13, 15], increase ventilator-free days [11], and improve the rate of discharge to home [11]. The safety, feasibility, and effectiveness of EM have been extensively reported [11, 14, 16–18]. EM has become an evidence-based practice and should be incorporated in daily practice, starting in the early phase of critical illness in the ICU [19].

However, many studies of EM, showing the successive introduction of active mobilization in ICU, were conducted at universities and hospitals in Europe and the USA which have specialized EM personnel or teams and have developed an "EM culture" in the ICU [10–18]. There are barriers to conducting EM as routine practice in the ICU, where there are few specialized EM teams and EM is not yet routine practice. The lack of a formalized mobilization program, an environment without a priority for EM, lack of available medical or personnel, the need for a specialized team, and the lack of specialists to lead the effort have been reported as barriers to implement EM [19–23]. In Japan, many hospitals are faced with these barriers [22] and there are few reports of the introduction of active EM in the ICU. It is unknown whether EM can be safely initiated and performed in Japanese ICUs in hospitals without a specialized team or an EM culture.

Referring to existing EM protocols reported in prior studies [9, 11, 12, 14–16, 19, 24–26], we developed a novel EM program, the Maebashi EM protocol, which is conducted at the bedside by ICU physicians in our closed mixed ICU. The EM protocol is a novel system, with the ICU physician as the key person to manage EM safely. The purpose of this study is to investigate whether EM according to this ICU physician-conducted protocol can be safely performed in the ICU without a specialized EM team or an EM culture, even though the patients have undergone the placement of a variety of medical devices. Another aspect of the study is to evaluate whether EM led by an ICU physician can be initiated in the acute phase of critical illness.

## Methods

### Study design

This is a single center prospective observational study. The study was approved by the ethics committee of the Japan Red Cross Maebashi Hospital and followed the STROBE guidelines [27]. This study is registered in UMIN (ID: 00002289).

### Hospital setting

Japan Red Cross Maebashi Hospital is a tertiary care hospital (560-bed general hospital in Gunma prefecture, Japan), with a 12-bed closed-mixed ICU. Admission sources to the ICU are the emergency room and hospital wards. Admissions from the emergency room to the ICU are all due to unplanned emergency critical illness and from the hospital wards are due to planned post-operative or unplanned emergency conditions which develop in the ward. ICU physicians and nurses (the nurse-to-patient ratio is 1:2) are present in the ICU, but there are no physical therapists assigned to the ICU. ICU physician staff includes one ICU consultant (attending physician), three ICU fellows, and one junior resident. None of them are specialized in rehabilitation. The fellows and resident treat patients with an appropriate level of supervision by the ICU consultant.

### Patients

All consecutive patients 18 years of age or older with an unplanned admission to the ICU from June 2015 to June 2016 are included in this study. Patients with planned post-operative, acute cardiovascular, acute cerebrovascular disease, progressive neuromuscular disease, post cardiopulmonary arrest syndrome, or a condition limiting mobilization such as an unstable pelvic fracture were excluded. Informed consent was obtained from all enrolled patients, if they were conscious, or from family members if the patient was unconscious.

### The Maebashi early mobilization protocol

An EM working group was formed to discuss how to promote EM in the ICU. The working group included two ICU physicians and three ICU nurses, who are not specialized in EM, and one rehabilitation doctor and three physical therapists, who are not also specialized in EM and do not usually engage in ICU rehabilitation. Non-specialized means that they are not trained specifically to provide rehabilitation for critically ill ICU patients with ICU-related medical devices in place, in the acute phase of critical illness. The EM working group confirmed that the staff who participated in this study and provided rehabilitation had no specific training in rehabilitation before this study. The EM working group sent ICU physicians, ICU nurses, and physical therapists a questionnaire to investigate barriers to care in the ICU [see Additional file 1]. After summarizing the results of the questionnaire, this group reviewed available literature and created the Maebashi EM protocol in May 2015 [see Additional file 2], which was specifically developed to be used in this ICU. A 1-month training period was used to teach ICU physicians, ICU nurses, and physical therapists how to conduct the protocol. The details of conducting rehabilitation sessions were taught by using charts at each rehabilitation level made by the EM working group [see Additional file 3].

The Maebashi EM protocol consists of three steps and includes five levels of rehabilitation. The details of the steps and rehabilitation levels are shown in Figs. 1 and 2. The five levels of rehabilitation are as follows: (1) no mobilization or bed exercise (2) sitting position in bed, including using a cycling ergometer and active range of motion (3) sitting on the edge of the bed, (4) active transfer to the chair, and (5) standing, stepping in place, or ambulating. Although all patients are supposed to receive one rehabilitation session each day for 20 min, the actual rehabilitation period was determined by ICU physicians based on the patient's clinical condition. The role of the ICU physician during active rehabilitation sessions was to monitor the hemodynamic and respiratory status of the patient and to maintain vigilance over the central venous catheter, ECMO

cannula, or endotracheal tube. Discontinuation criteria are defined as follows: a fall to the knees or ground, tachycardia (> 130/min) or bradycardia(< 40/min), hypertension (systolic blood pressure > 180 mmHg), hypotension (systolic blood pressure < 80 mmHg), symptomatic orthostatic hypotension, arrhythmias except a pre-existing arrhythmia, myocardial infarction-associated symptoms, desaturation (peripheral capillary oxygen saturation < 88%), abnormal respiratory rate (> 40/min or < 5/min), asynchrony with mechanical ventilation, patient's intolerance to request to stop rehabilitation, cardiopulmonary arrest, bleeding, unexpected/inadvertent removal of medical devices (an endotracheal tube, feeding tube, chest tube, abdominal drain, urinary catheter, arterial catheter, peripheral or central venous catheter, or hemodialysis catheter.)

If an event meets any of the discontinuation criteria, the patient stops the rehabilitation session and rests. If the patient recovers, the rehabilitation session is reinitiated at the same rehabilitation level or at a lower level based on the judgment of the ICU physician. If the patient could not recover or requests to discontinue the session, it is stopped immediately and counted as an adverse event. A serious adverse event was defined as an adverse event requiring additional treatment.

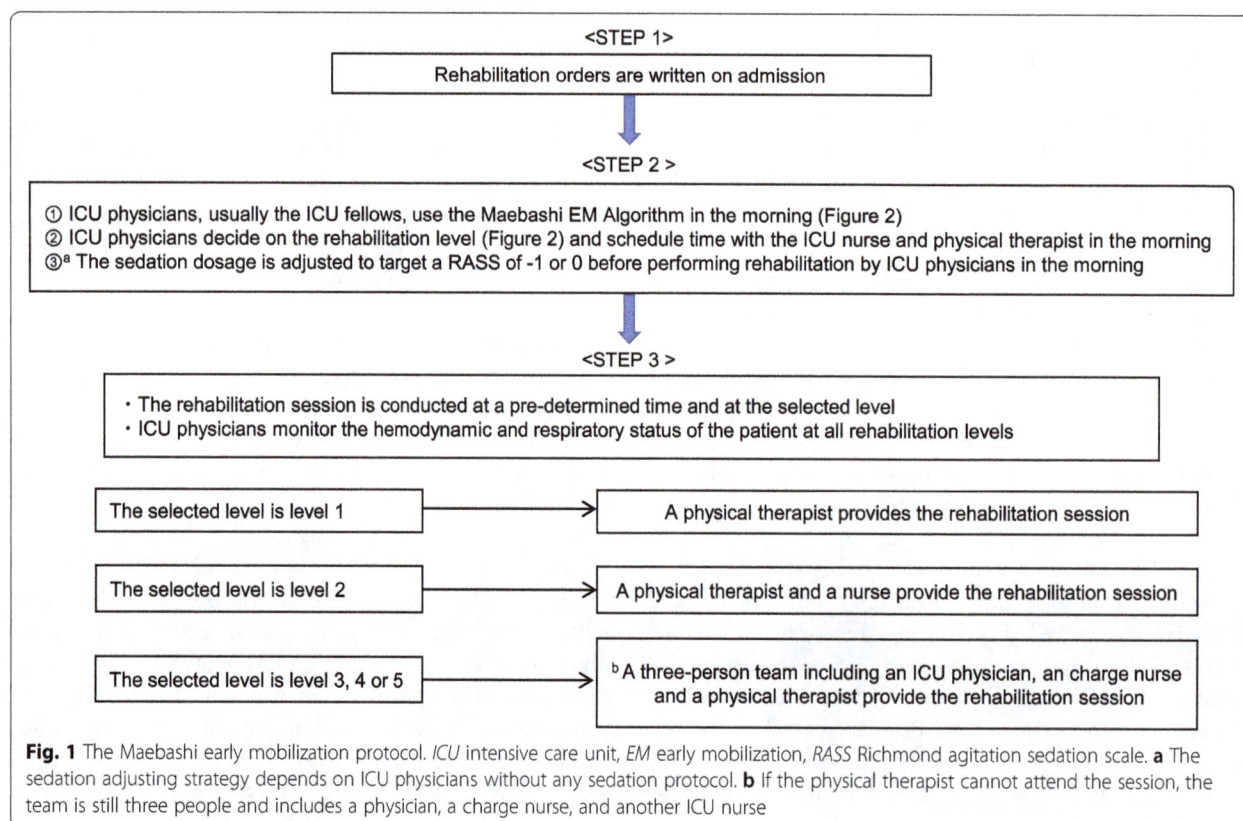

**Fig. 1** The Maebashi early mobilization protocol. *ICU* intensive care unit, *EM* early mobilization, *RASS* Richmond agitation sedation scale. **a** The sedation adjusting strategy depends on ICU physicians without any sedation protocol. **b** If the physical therapist cannot attend the session, the team is still three people and includes a physician, a charge nurse, and another ICU nurse

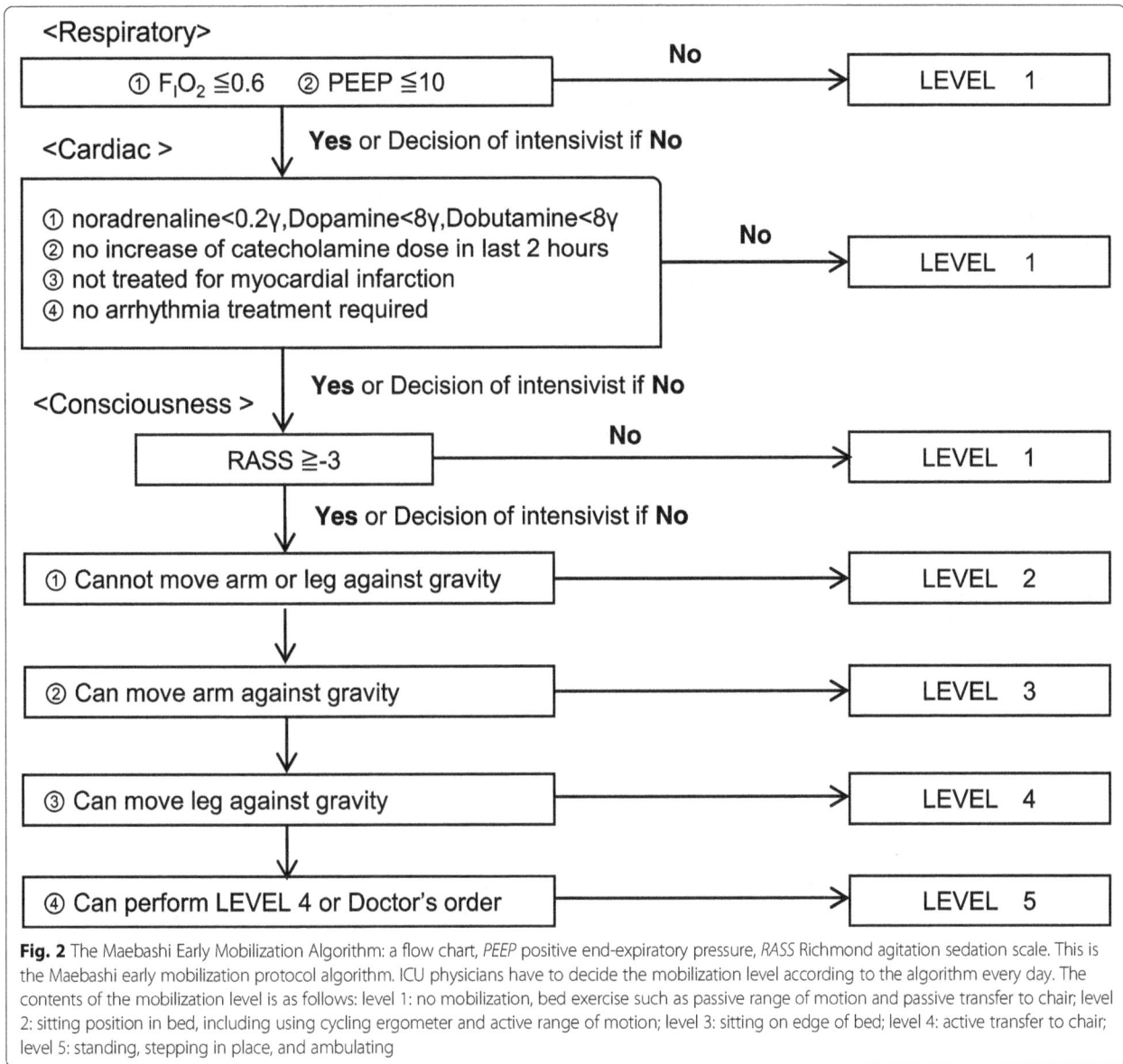

**Fig. 2** The Maebashi Early Mobilization Algorithm: a flow chart, *PEEP* positive end-expiratory pressure, *RASS* Richmond agitation sedation scale. This is the Maebashi early mobilization protocol algorithm. ICU physicians have to decide the mobilization level according to the algorithm every day. The contents of the mobilization level is as follows: level 1: no mobilization, bed exercise such as passive range of motion and passive transfer to chair; level 2: sitting position in bed, including using cycling ergometer and active range of motion; level 3: sitting on edge of bed; level 4: active transfer to chair; level 5: standing, stepping in place, and ambulating

## Study outcomes

The primary outcome was the safety of EM conducted according to the Maebashi EM protocol. The safety objective was the incidence rate of adverse events in all rehabilitation sessions. Rehabilitation levels and the types of adverse events were recorded and reviewed to evaluate the safety of EM. Medical devices in place during rehabilitation sessions were also reviewed to investigate any possible relationship between adverse events and equipment.

Secondary outcomes include the number of days to first rehabilitation and the number of days to progress to higher rehabilitation levels. Other outcomes of rehabilitation sessions, including the percentage of patients who got out of bed, standing, or ambulating, were also collected. The active rehabilitation level was defined to be sitting out of the bed, active transfer to a chair, standing, marching, and ambulating.

## Data collection

Baseline medical characteristics of all enrolled patients were collected on admission, and during the course of the ICU stay, including age, gender, body mass index (BMI), the ability to ambulate prior to ICU admission, admission source, reason for admission to the ICU, Acute Physiology and Chronic Health Evaluation II (APACHE II) score, Sequential Organ Failure Assessment (SOFA) score on admission, the need for mechanical ventilation, Extracorporeal Membrane Oxygenation (ECMO), continuous analgesia, continuous sedation, vasopressors, corticosteroids, neuromuscular blocking agents, or dialysis. Other information such as ICU length of stay, hospital length of stay, mechanical ventilation periods, ability to ambulate at hospital discharge, mortality, and where the patient went after leaving the hospital were recorded at the time of discharge.

Rehabilitation information was recorded immediately after the session on that day, including the highest level of rehabilitation which continued for at least 5 min, medical devices in place during the session, the site of each medical device, any event which met the criteria for discontinuing the session, whether the session was conducted according to protocol, and if there were any protocol violations.

There are no missing data in this study. All data were collected prospectively and sent to personnel uninvolved with the EM working group. After data collection, rehabilitation outcomes were summarized, and the relationships between adverse events and the rehabilitation level, or adverse events and medical devices were examined.

### Subgroup analysis and sensitivity analysis

To reduce the influence of the patients who had mild critical illnesses and were discharged from the ICU early, a subgroup analysis was conducted as a post hoc study, focusing on rehabilitation outcomes. Data from patients who stayed in the ICU for more than 72 h were analyzed. In the main analysis, rehabilitation information, including the number of rehabilitation sessions performed at each level, the number and rate of adverse events, the percentage of patients who got out of bed, standing or ambulating in the ICU, number of days to first rehabilitation, and number of days to progress to higher levels of rehabilitation, were summarized.

### Statistical analysis

Distributed continuous variables without a normal distribution are presented as median and interquartile range (IQR). Categorical data are summarized using numbers or percentages. The Wilcoxon rank sum test was used for comparing continuous variables, and the chi-squared test was used for categorical data. Same statistic measures were used for the sub-group analysis.

In this study, the primary outcome was set as the incidence rate of adverse events among all rehabilitation sessions, following previous study designs of safety [10, 16, 25]. The sample size was calculated at a 95% confidence level. The assumed rate of adverse events was set at 3.0% (0.03), and the expected confidence interval was 0.03, based on the rate of adverse events of the prior studies [12, 14, 16, 17, 25, 26, 28]. According to a power calculation, a total sample size of 497 rehabilitation sessions are needed to assess the safety of EM according to the Maebashi EM protocol driven by ICU physicians. To enhance

the internal validity of the safety, the incidence rate of adverse events for active rehabilitation levels (levels 3, 4, and 5) and non-active rehabilitation levels (levels 1 and 2) were compared by the chi-squared test, as done in a prior study [16]. All statistical analyses were conducted using EZR (Saitama Medical Center, Jichi Medical University, Saitama, Japan), which is a graphical user interface for R (The R Foundation for Statistical Computing, Vienna, Austria) [29]. Statistical tests were two sided and statistical significance was defined as $P < 0.05$.

## Results
### Baseline patient characteristics

During the observation period from June 2015 to June 2016, 839 patients were admitted to the ICU. The details of study patient recruitment are shown in Additional file 4 [see Additional file 4]. A total of 232 patients were enrolled in this study. Table 1 shows the baseline characteristics of enrolled patients. The median age was 69.0 years (IQR 55.8–80.0 years) and 156/ 232 (67%) patients were male. Of 232 patients, 181 (78%) were admitted from the emergency department, 72 (31%) underwent mechanical ventilation and six (2.6%) received ECMO. The APACHE II and SOFA scores on admission were 16 (IQR 10–22) and 4 (IQR 2–7) and the average length of ICU stay and duration of mechanical ventilation were 1.8 and 2.1 days, respectively.

### Safety
#### Rehabilitation sessions and adverse events

A total of 587 rehabilitation sessions were conducted for 232 patients. The median number of rehabilitation sessions per patient was 1 (range 0–55 sessions). The relationship between rehabilitation sessions and adverse events is summarized in Table 2. During 587 rehabilitation sessions, 13 adverse events occurred. The primary outcome, the incidence rate of adverse events among all rehabilitation sessions was 2.2% (95% confidence interval [CI] 1.2–3.8%). The adverse events included seven episodes of patient intolerance, necessitating discontinuing the rehabilitation session, and six episodes of orthostatic hypotension with symptoms (Table 3). Thirteen adverse events occurred in 10 patients; 2 patients experienced adverse events several times. One patient had three adverse events as intolerance at same rehabilitation level (level 5), and the other patient had two adverse events as orthostatic hypotension with symptoms at different levels (level 2 and 3). There was no significant difference between the incidence rate in active rehabilitation, (levels 3 to 5, 387 sessions, 11 adverse events, 2.8%; 95% confidence interval [CI] 1.4– 5.0%) and the incidence rate for non-active rehabilitation, (levels 1 and 2, 200 sessions, 2 adverse events,

**Table 1** Baseline patient characteristics (n = 232)

| Variable | Values median [IQR] or number (%) |
|---|---|
| Age (years), median [IQR] | 69.0 [55.8–80.0] |
| Gender (male), n (%) | 156 (67%) |
| BMI (kg/m$^2$), median [IQR] | 21.1 [18.8–24.2] |
| Ambulatory prior to admission, n (%) | 208 (90%) |
| Admitted from | |
| Emergency room, n (%) | 181 (78%) |
| Hospital ward, n (%) | 51 (22%) |
| ICU admission diagnosis | |
| Sepsis, n (%) | 92 (40%) |
| Gastrointestinal, n (%) | 49 (21%) |
| Respiratory failure, n (%) | 29 (13%) |
| Trauma, n (%) | 28 (12%) |
| Drug abuse, n (%) | 12 (5%) |
| Others, n (%) | 22 (9%) |
| APACHE II score, median [IQR] | 16 [10–22] |
| SOFA on admission, median [IQR] | 4 [2–7] |
| Patients undergoing mechanical ventilation, n (%) | 72 (31%) |
| Patients receiving ECMO, n (%) | 6 (2.6%) |
| Patients receiving continuous analgesia (opiates), n (%) | 117 (50%) |
| Patients receiving continuous sedation, n (%) | 82 (35%) |
| Patients receiving vasopressors, n (%) | 87 (38%) |
| Patients receiving steroids, n (%) | 39 (17%) |
| Patients receiving neuromuscular blocking agents, n (%) | 2 (0.90%) |
| Patients receiving dialysis, n (%) | 34 (15%) |
| ICU length of stay (days), median [IQR] | 1.8 [1.2–3.7] |
| Mechanical ventilation period (days), median [IQR] | 2.1 [0.9–4.2] |
| Hospital length of stay (days), median [IQR] | 16.9 [9.3–36.1] |
| Ambulatory at discharge, n (%) | 184 (79%) |
| In-hospital mortality, n (%) | 11 (4.7%) |
| Discharged to | |
| Home, n (%) | 138 (60%) |
| Another hospital or rehabilitation center, n (%) | 72 (31%) |
| Nursing home, n (%) | 11 (4.7%) |

Data in table are presented as the median with the interquartile range or as a number with percentage in total patients

*BMI* body mass index, *IQR* interquartile range, *ICU* intensive care unit, *APACHE* Acute Physiology and Chronic Health Evaluation, *SOFA* Sequential Organ Failure Assessment, *ECMO* extracorporeal membrane oxygenation

**Table 2** Rehabilitation sessions and adverse events

| | Total number of sessions performed | Adverse events, n (%) | Total number of patients (n = 232)[a] |
|---|---|---|---|
| Rehabilitation level | | | |
| Level 1, n | 154 | 1 (0.60%) | 73 |
| Level 2 | | | |
| Total, n | 46 | 1 (2.2%) | 26 |
| Ergometer, n | 10 | 0 (0%) | 4 |
| Level 3, n | 169 | 7 (4.1%) | 74 |
| Level 4, n | 54 | 0 (0%) | 18 |
| Level 5 | | | |
| Total, n | 164 | 4 (2.4%) | 83 |
| Standing or marching at bedside, n | 103 | 4 (3.9%) | 42 |
| Ambulating in the ICU, n | 61 | 0 (0%) | 49 |
| Active rehabilitation, n | 387 | 11 (2.8%) | 143 |
| Total Rehabilitation sessions, n | 587 | 13 (2.2%) | |

Data are presented as number (%)

*ICU* intensive care unit

[a]This demonstrates the number of the patients who experienced the each rehabilitation levels

**Table 3** Type and frequency of adverse events

| | Adverse events (n = 13) | Event rate per 1000 rehabilitation sessions |
|---|---|---|
| Event | | |
| Patient intolerance[a] | 7 (54%) | 12 |
| Symptomatic orthostatic hypotension | 6 (46%) | 10 |
| Fall to knees or ground | 0 (0%) | 0 |
| Asynchrony with mechanical ventilation | 0 (0%) | 0 |
| Tachycardia or bradycardia | 0 (0%) | 0 |
| Arrhythmia | 0 (0%) | 0 |
| Myocardial infraction associated symptom | 0 (0%) | 0 |
| Tachypnea or bradypnea | 0 (0%) | 0 |
| Desaturation | 0 (0%) | 0 |
| Cardiopulmonary arrest | 0 (0%) | 0 |
| Bleeding | 0 (0%) | 0 |
| Inadvertent removal of medical devices | 0 (0%) | 0 |

Data are presented as number of occurrences with percentage

A total of 587 rehabilitation sessions were performed during the study period

[a]Patients' intolerance includes five episodes of extreme exhaustion and two episodes of exacerbation of abdominal pain in patients diagnosed with acute pancreatitis. There is no scale for exhaustion or pain

1.0%; 95% confidence interval [CI] 1.0–3.6%), (P = 0.15). There were no serious adverse events requiring additional treatment, such as cardiopulmonary resuscitation, an increase in vasopressor dose, the fraction of inspired oxygen, or the need for additional analgesia (Table 3).

## Relationship between medical devices and adverse events

Medical devices in place during the rehabilitation sessions are summarized in Table 4 Nearly all rehabilitation sessions were performed with peripheral venous catheters (99%), arterial lines (98%), and urinary bladder catheters (94%) in place. Other medical devices, such as chest or abdominal drains, or central venous catheters, were also in place during rehabilitation. Additional file 5 shows the details of rehabilitation sessions and adverse events related to mechanical ventilation and ECMO. Of 587

**Table 4** Relation between medical devices and adverse events.

| | Total number of sessions performed | Adverse events, n (%) |
|---|---|---|
| Medical devices in place during the session | | |
| Peripheral venous catheter, n | 582 | 13 (2.2%) |
| Arterial line | | |
| Total, n | 574 | 13 (2.3%) |
| Radial, n | 568 | 13 (2.3%) |
| Femoral, n | 6 | 0 (0%) |
| Central venous catheter | | |
| Total, n | 167 | 8 (4.8%) |
| Jugular, n | 112 | 5 (4.5%) |
| Subclavian, n | 18 | 0 (0%) |
| Femoral, n | 37 | 3 (8.1%) |
| Hemodialysis catheter | | |
| Total, n | 105 | 1 (1.0%) |
| Jugular, n | 96 | 1 (1.0%) |
| Femoral, n | 11 | 0 (0%) |
| Mechanical ventilator, n | 293 | 7 (2.4%) |
| Endotracheal tube, n | 183 | 5 (2.7%) |
| Tracheostomy tube, n | 127 | 3 (2.4%) |
| ECMO cannula, n | | |
| Total, n | 110 | 4 (3.6%) |
| Jugular, n | 110 | 4 (3.6%) |
| Femoral, n | 110 | 4 (3.6%) |
| Feeding tube, n | 419 | 10 (2.4%) |
| Urinary catheter, n | 550 | 12 (2.2%) |
| Chest tube, n | 83 | 3 (3.6%) |
| Abdominal drain, n | 112 | 2 (1.8%) |
| Total rehabilitation sessions | 587 | 13 (2.2%) |

Data are presented as number (%)
*ECMO* extracorporeal membrane oxygenation

rehabilitation sessions, 293 sessions (50%) were performed while the patient was undergoing mechanical ventilation and 110 sessions (19%) were performed with ECMO devices in place. The incidence rate of adverse events in patients undergoing mechanical ventilation was 2.4% and with ECMO was 3.6%. There were no adverse events directly related to medical devices, such as inadvertent removal.

## Compliance with the Maebashi EM protocol and participating staff at each level

Protocol compliance was reviewed, and there were no violations, such as rehabilitation sessions which were not conducted according to the Maebashi EM protocol. All rehabilitation sessions were conducted strictly according to the written protocol. ICU physicians attended 96% of active rehabilitation sessions, ICU nurses attended 99%, and physical therapists attended 71% (Fig. 3). During all sessions which ICU physicians did not attend, especially at levels 1 or 2, ICU physicians were present near the rehabilitation site in the ICU and monitored the hemodynamic and respiratory status of all patients.

## Rehabilitation outcomes

Rehabilitation outcomes during the study period are summarized in Table 5. The median number of days to the first protocolized rehabilitation session was 0.7 (IQR 0.0–0.9). A total of 62% of patients (n = 143) got out of bed during their ICU stay, and the median time to first getting out of bed was 1.2 (IQR 0.1–2.0) days.

## Subgroup analysis

There were 71 patients who stayed in the ICU for more than 72 h, including 41 (59%) who underwent mechanical ventilation, with mean APACHE II scores of 23 (IQR 18–28), and the length of ICU stay or mechanical ventilation were 5.2 days (IQR 3.8–7.8) or 3.9 days (IQR 2.1–6.8), respectively [see Additional file 6]. The rehabilitation outcomes in this subgroup are summarized in Table 5. The rehabilitation sessions began within 1 day (median 1.0 days; IQR 0.8–2.0 days), and 82% (58) of patients could get out of bed within 2 days (median 2.0 days; IQR 1.4–3.6 days).

## Discussion

This is the first study from Japan to demonstrate the safety of EM in the ICU. There are few studies focusing on the direct involvement of ICU physicians in EM. In this study, two important clinical outcomes were observed. First, EM conducted by ICU physicians according to a protocol, without a specialized EM team or an EM culture, results in a rate of adverse events similar to that reported in previous studies [12, 14, 16, 17, 25, 26, 28]. There were no adverse events related to in situ

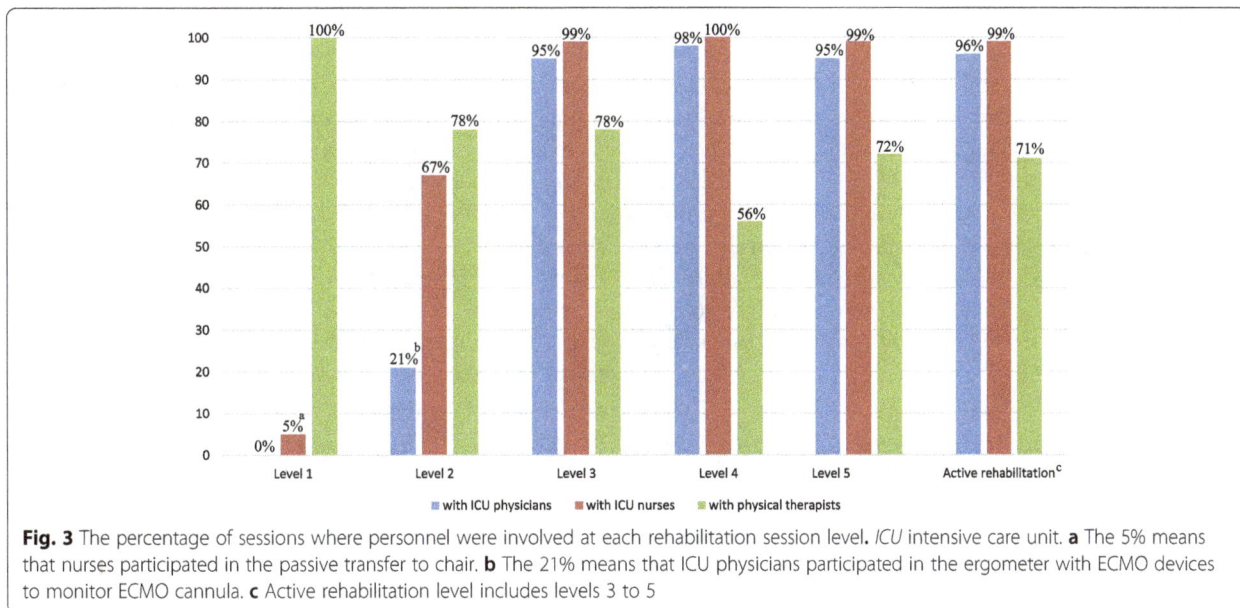

**Fig. 3** The percentage of sessions where personnel were involved at each rehabilitation session level. *ICU* intensive care unit. **a** The 5% means that nurses participated in the passive transfer to chair. **b** The 21% means that ICU physicians participated in the ergometer with ECMO devices to monitor ECMO cannula. **c** Active rehabilitation level includes levels 3 to 5

medical devices. Second, EM conducted by ICU physicians can be initiated in the acute phase of critical illness without serious adverse events requiring additional treatment or resuscitation. These results suggest that ICU physician-conducted EM is safely performed in an environment where EM was not routine practice, available resources are limited, and there is no specialized EM team, EM specialists, or an EM culture.

EM conducted by ICU physicians according to a protocol is performed at a safety level comparable to that reported in prior studies, in the absence of a specialized EM team, and in patients with a variety of medical devices in place. This study identified 13 adverse events (2.2%; 95% CI 1.2–3.8%), which did not require specific treatment and occurred at the incidence rate of adverse events similar to previous studies conducted in institutions with a specialized EM team [12, 14, 16, 17, 25, 30]. EM conducted in patients undergoing mechanical ventilation or ECMO, which have been considered

barriers to active rehabilitation or relatively high risk [25, 31], was also safely performed with a low incidence rate of adverse events (2.4 and 3.6%, respectively). In an ICU without a specialized team or an EM culture, the lack of specially trained personnel to manage safety during EM and provide leadership among multidisciplinary ICU staff [10, 32], limited numbers of personnel [18, 24], the presence of medical devices [25, 31] have all been considered major barriers to initiate EM in the ICU [19–21]. A questionnaire was given to members of the ICU staff to identify the barriers in the ICU, which revealed similar barriers for the initiation of EM [see Additional file 1]. ICU physicians are trained to lead and cooperate with other staff, to manage clinical problems and to deal with problems associated with medical devices [33]. The leadership, cooperation, and medical management skills of ICU physicians are essential to initiate EM in such an environment. This skill set matches some of the perceived difficulties of initiating EM in the

**Table 5** Outcomes of protocolized rehabilitation

| Variable | All study patients (n = 232)[a] Values median [IQR] or number (%) | Subgroup in the ICU ≧ 72 h (n = 71) Values median [IQR] or number (%) |
|---|---|---|
| Patients who could get out of bed, n (%) | 143 (62%) | 58 (82%) |
| Patients who could stand during ICU stay, n (%) | 82 (35%) | 31 (45%) |
| Patients who could ambulate during ICU stay, n (%) | 49 (21%) | 12 (17%) |
| Days to first rehabilitation session (days), median [IQR][a] | 0.7 [0.0–0.9] | 1.0 [0.8–2.0] |
| Days to first out of bed (days), median [IQR][a] | 1.2 [0.1–2.0] | 2.0 [1.4–3.6] |
| Days to first standing (days), median [IQR][a] | 1.2 [0.8–2.1] | 2.8 [1.7–4.9] |
| Days to first ambulating (days), median [IQR][a] | 1.0 [0.7–1.7] | 2.3 [1.2–2.9] |

Data in table are presented as the median with the interquartile range or as a number with percentage in total patients
*IQR* interquartile range, *ICU* intensive care unit
[a]Days counted from the time of ICU admission

ICU, making the ICU physician an ideal person to lead such an effort. The Maebashi EM protocol adopted a simple algorithm and simple rehabilitation content based on previous studies which were successively introduced in the ICU [see Additional file 2] and did not utilize specialized rehabilitation equipment such as electrical muscle stimulation. Due to the simplicity of the protocol, ICU physicians who are not specialized in rehabilitation can initiate and make clinical decisions regarding EM. In this study, ICU physicians were directly involved in over 95% of active rehabilitation sessions and safely provide protocolized EM.

EM, guided by an ICU physician conducted protocol, can be initiated in the acute phase of critical illness without serious adverse events requiring additional treatment. Prior studies showed that respiratory and hemodynamic instability, which are familiar problems in acute illness, are commonly perceived as barriers by some staff, such as nurses or physical therapists [19–21]. Another study pointed out that mobilization in the acute phase of critical illness may be difficult because of severity [34], though early initiation of rehabilitation is recommended to improve patient outcomes because of rapid muscle atrophy within 24 to 48 h after ICU admission [11, 35, 36].

Although the involvement of specialists or a specialized team have been recommended to promote EM in the acute phase of critical illness [37–40], many hospitals in Japan do not have a specialized team to conduct this therapy. In these situations, the ICU physician can play an important role. As part of their training, ICU physicians develop the requisite skills to manage respiratory and hemodynamic problems in acutely ill patients [33, 41]. Some studies suggest that the involvement of ICU physicians may reduce complications and potentially enhance the safety of ICU procedures [42–44]. If adverse events associated with critical illness occur, ICU physicians can cope with events immediately and appropriately. There were no serious adverse events requiring additional treatment or resuscitation in this study. ICU physicians play an important role as a safety net in the conduct of EM in the acute phase of critical illness.

In this study, the length of ICU stay (1.8 days) and the duration of mechanical ventilation (2.1 days) are shorter than previous studies [11, 15]. Patients who received mechanical ventilation represent 31% of enrolled patients. It may seem natural that many patients could get out of bed early in their ICU stay, since their critical illness was not so severe. Therefore, we conducted a subgroup analysis, focusing on patients who stayed in the ICU for more than 72 h (Table 5, [see Additional file 6]). The average length of ICU-stay (5.2 days) and duration of mechanical ventilation (3.9 days) were comparable to a prior study (5.9 and 3.4 days respectively) [11]. Patients in the sub-

group were more severely ill (median APACHE II score 23) and underwent mechanical ventilation more frequently (59%) compared to all enrolled patients. This subgroup analysis also confirmed the safety of the EM protocol (adverse events in 2.7%, and no serious adverse events) and showed positive rehabilitation outcomes (82% of the subgroup-patients could get out of bed within 2 days).

This study has several acknowledged limitations. First, patients with certain diseases were excluded. Due to relatively stringent patient selection criteria, severe critical ill patients were excluded and relatively mild severe patients were included, and the results of this study may not be generally applicable. Patients with diseases excluded from this study were immobilized for a long period and were thought not to be suitable for active rehabilitation strategies in the acute phase of critical illness, especially within 1 day. Other protocols or strategies might be necessary for patients with these excluded conditions. Patients with post-operative scheduled admission to the ICU were also excluded, because almost all of them stayed in the ICU for a very short period and were usually discharged early the next morning before receiving the rehabilitation sessions.

There may be unrecognized confounding factors associated with adverse events. For example, data regarding agitation, delirium, the rate of ICU-acquired weakness, or muscle atrophy were not collected in this study. Although the clinical workload of ICU physicians and nurses was increased due to this protocol, any relationship between an increase in daily work and adverse events was not examined.

Third, the statistical method to count adverse events and rehabilitation sessions was a repeated measurement which could influence the results. We used the method described in a previous study and a recent systematic review with a meta-analysis to enhance the comparability of safety among studies [10, 16, 25, 45]. It is important to take repeated measurement data into account when the sample size is calculated, which is a limitation of this study. The total number of patients was included to evaluate the rate of the adverse events per patient at each rehabilitation level, in addition to the rate of adverse events per session. This analysis allows consideration of the rate of adverse events without the influence of individual patient characteristics.

Fourth, this is a single-center observational study without a comparison group, which could introduce bias, limiting the ability to generalize these results to other hospitals. Further observation and verification, focusing on the other factors associated with the safety of EM or the short- and long-term effects of EM according to the protocol on clinical outcomes, is necessary to investigate the external validity and the utility of the Maebashi EM protocol.

## Conclusion

EM, performed according to the Maebashi EM protocol conducted by ICU physicians, without EM specialists, an EM specialized team or an EM culture, was performed with a safety level similar to that reported in previous studies which were conducted with a specialized team, even though patients had a variety of medical devices in place. Protocolized EM led by ICU physicians can be initiated in the acute phase of critical illness without serious adverse events requiring additional treatment.

## Additional files

**Additional file 1:** Barriers described by ICU physicians, ICU nurses, and physical therapists. (DOCX 15 kb)

**Additional file 2:** References for details of the Maebashi early mobilization protocol. (DOCX 17 kb)

**Additional file 3:** Example of each rehabilitation level. (DOCX 4361 kb)

**Additional file 4:** Details of exclusion criteria and a flow diagram of recruitment. *ICU* intensive care unit. There were no missing data. (PPTX 43 kb)

**Additional file 5:** Rehabilitation sessions and adverse events—mechanical ventilation and ECMO. (DOCX 15 kb)

**Additional file 6:** Characteristics of patients who stayed in the ICU more than 72 h. (DOCX 15 kb)

## Abbreviation

APACHE: Acute Physiology and Chronic Health Evaluation II; BMI: Body mass index; CI: Confidence interval; ECMO: Extracorporeal membrane oxygenation; EM: Early mobilization; ICU: Intensive care unit; IQR: Interquartile range; SOFA: Sequential Organ Failure Assessment

## Acknowledgements

The authors thank the early mobilization working group and the staff in the Japan Red Cross Hospital, including ICU physicians, nurses, and physical therapists for their collaboration to initiate early mobilization in ICU.

## Funding

This research did not receive any specific grant from funding agencies in the public, commercial, or not-for-profit sectors.

## Authors' contributions

KL and TO conducted the study design. KL, TO, HO, KJ, EA, and JO participate in creating the protocol and introducing the protocol in our ICU. MN helped in the data collection and the statistical analysis. TO, MN, DM, HS, and AL helped in the development of this manuscript and AL also checked the English grammar. KT advised the statistical methods. All authors read and approved the final manuscript.

## Competing interests

The authors declare that they have no competing interests in this section.

## Author details

[1]Advanced Medical Emergency Department and Critical Care Center, Japan Red Cross Maebashi Hospital, 3-21-36 Asahi-cho, Maebashi, Gunma 371-0014, Japan. [2]Department of Biostatistics, Nagoya University Graduate School of Medicine, Tsurumai-cho 64, Syowa-ku, Nagoya, Aichi 466-8560, Japan. [3]Department of Rehabilitation Medicine, Japan Red Cross Maebashi Hospital, 3-21-36 Asahi-cho, Maebashi, Gunma 371-0014, Japan. [4]Department of Nursing, Intensive Care Unit, Japan Red Cross Maebashi Hospital, 3-21-36 Asahi-cho, Maebashi, Gunma 371-0014, Japan. [5]Department of Surgery, Jichi Medical University, 3311-1 Yakushiji, Shimotsukeshi, Tochigi 329-0498, Japan. [6]Department of Emergency Medicine, Jichi Medical University, 3311-1 Yakushiji, Shimotsukeshi, Tochigi 329-0498, Japan.

## References

1. Harvey MA, Davidson JE. Postintensive care syndrome: right care, right now… and later. Crit Care Med. 2016;44:381–5.
2. Iwashyna TJ, Ely EW, Smith DM, Langa KM. Long-term cognitive impairment and functional disability among survivors of severe sepsis. JAMA. 2010;304:1787–94.
3. Griffith J, Hatch RA, Bishop J, Morgan K, Jenkinson C, Cuthbertson BH, et al. An exploration of social and economic outcome and associated health-related quality of life after critical illness in general intensive care unit survivors: a 12-month follow-up study. Crit Care. 2013;17:R100.
4. Hill AD, Fowler RA, Pinto R, Herridge MS, Cuthbertson BH, Long-term SDC. Outcomes and healthcare utilization following critical illness—a population-based study. Crit Care. 2016;20:76.
5. Oeyen SG, Vandijick DM, Benoit DD, Annemans L, Decruyenaere JM. Quality of life after intensive care: a systematic review of the literature. Crit Care Med. 2010;38:2386–400.
6. Needham DM, Davidson J, Cohen H, Hopkins RO, Weinert C, Wunsch H, et al. Improving long-term outcomes after discharge from intensive care unit: report from a stakeholders' conference. Crit Care Med. 2012;40:502–9.
7. Herridge MS, Cheung AM, Tansey CM, Matte-Martyn A, Diaz-Granados N, Al-Saidi F, et al. One-year outcomes in survivors of the acute respiratory distress syndrome. N Engl J Med. 2003;348:683–93.
8. Kamdar BB, Huang M, Dinglas VD, Colantuoni E, von Wachter TM, Hopkins RO, et al. Joblessness and lost earnings after ARDS in a 1-year national multicenter study. Am J Respir Crit Care Med. 2017;198:1012–20.
9. Hodgson CL, Stiller K, Needham DM, Tipping CJ, Harrold M, Baldwin CE, et al. Expert consensus and recommendations on safety criteria for active mobilization of mechanically ventilated critically ill adults. Crit Care. 2014;18:658.
10. Needham DM, Korupolu R, Zanni JM, Pradhan P, Colantuoni E, Palmer JB, et al. Early physical medicine and rehabilitation for patients with acute respiratory failure: a quality improvement project. Arch Phys Med Rehabil. 2010;91:536–42.
11. Schweickert WD, Pohlman MC, Pohlman AS, Nigos C, Pawlik AJ, Esbrook CL, et al. Early physical and occupational therapy in mechanically ventilated, critically ill patients: a randomized controlled trial. Lancet. 2009;373:1874–82.
12. Baily P, Thomsen GE, Spuhler VJ, Jewkes J, Bezdjian L, Veale K, et al. Early activity is feasible and safe in respiratory failure patients. Crit Care Med. 2007;35:139–45.
13. Klein K, Mulkey M, Bena JF, Albert NM. Clinical and psychological effects of early mobilization in patients treated in a neurological ICU: a comparative study. Crit Care Med. 2015;43:865–73.
14. Burtin C, Clerckx B, Robbeets C, Ferdinande P, Langer D, Troosters T, et al. Early exercise in critically ill patients enhances short-term functional recovery. Crit Care Med. 2009;37:2499–505.
15. Morris PE, Goad A, Thompson C, Taylor K, Harry B, Passmore L, et al. Early intensive care unit mobility therapy in the treatment of acute respiratory failure. Crit Care Med. 2008;36:2238–43.
16. Sricharoenchai T, Parker AM, Zanni JM, Nelliot A, Dinglas VD, Safety NDM. Of physical therapy interventions in critically ill patients: a single center prospective evaluation of 1110 intensive care unit admissions. J Crit Care. 2014;29:395–400.

17. Bourdin G, Barbier J, Burle JF, Durante G, Passant S, Vincent B, et al. The feasibility of early physical activity in intensive care unit patients: a prospective observational one-center study. Respir Care. 2010;55:400–7.

18. Zanni JM, Korupolu R, Fan E, Pradhan P, Janjua K, Palmer JB, et al. Rehabilitation therapy and outcomes in acute respiratory failure: an observational pilot project. J Crit Care. 2010;25:254–62.

19. Cameron S, Ball I, Cepinskas G, Choong K, Doherty TJ, Ellis CG, et al. Early mobilization in the critical care unit: a review of adult and pediatric literature. J Crit Care. 2015;30:664–72.

20. Dubb R, Nydahl P, Hermes C, Schwabbauer N, Toonstra A, Parker AM, et al. Barriers and strategies for early mobilization of patients in intensive care units. Ann Am Thorac Soc. 2016;13:724–30.

21. Parry SM, Knight LD, Connolly B, Baldwin C, Puthucheary Z, Morris P, et al. Factors influencing physical activity and rehabilitation in survivors of critical illness: a systematic review of quantitative and qualitative studies. Intensive Care Med. 2017;43:531–54.

22. Taito S, Sanui M, Yasuda H, Shime N, Lefor AK. Japanese SocietyOf education for physicians and trainees in intensive care (JSEPTIC) clinical trial group. Current rehabilitation practices in intensive care units: a preliminary survey by the Japanese Society of Education for Physicians and Trainees in Intensive Care (JSEPTIC) clinical trial group. J Intensive Care. 2016;4:66.

23. Parry SM, Remedios L, Denehy L, Knight LD, Beach L, Rollinson TC, et al. What factors affect implementation of early rehabilitation into intensive care unit practice? A qualitative study with clinicians. J Crit Care. 2017;38:137–43.

24. Jolley SE, Regan-Baggs J, Dickson RP, Hough CL. Medical intensive care unit clinician attitudes and perceived barriers towards early mobilization of critically ill patients: a cross-sectional survey study. BMC Anesthesiol. 2014;14:84.

25. Lee H, Ko YJ, Yang JH, Park CM, Jeon K, Park YH, et al. Safety profile and feasibility of early physical therapy and mobility for critically ill patients in the medical intensive care unit: beginning experiences in Korea. J Crit Care. 2015;30:573–7.

26. Pohlman MC, Schweickert WD, Pohlman AS, Nigos C, Pawlik AJ, Esbrook CL, et al. Feasibility of physical and occupational therapy beginning from initiation of mechanical ventilation. Crit Care Med. 2010;38:2089–94.

27. Vandenbroucke JP, von Elm E, Altman DG, Gotzsche PC, Mulrow CD, Pococke SJ, et al. Strengthening the reporting of observational studies in epidemiology (STROBE): explanation and elaboration. Epidemiology. 2007;18:805–35.

28. Taito S, Shime N, Ota K, Yasuda H. Early mobilization of mechanically ventilated patients in the intensive care unit. J Intensive Care. 2016;4:50.

29. Investigation KY. Of the freely available easy-to-use software 'EZR' for medical statistics. Bone Marrow Transplant. 2013;48:452–8.

30. Morris PE, Berry MJ, Files DC, Thompson JC, Hauser J, Flores L, et al. Standardized rehabilitation and hospital length of stay among patients with acute respiratory failure: a randomized clinical trial. JAMA. 2016;315:2694–702.

31. Jolley SE, Moss M, Needham DM, Caldwell E, Morris PE, Miller RR, et al. Point prevalence study of mobilization practices for acute respiratory failure patients in the United States. Crit Care Med. 2017;45:205–15.

32. Dammeyer J, Baldwin N, Packard D, Harrington S, Christopher J, Strachan CL, et al. Mobilizing outcomes: implementation of a nurse-led multidisciplinary mobility program. Crit Care Nurs Quart. 2013;36:109–19.

33. Guidelines committee. Society of Critical Care Medicine. Guidelines for the definition of an intensivist and the practice of critical care medicine. Crit Care Med. 1992;20:540–2.

34. Nordon-Craft A, MaloneD SM, Moss M. Reply: is an earlier and more intensive physical therapy program better? Am J Respir Crit Care Med. 2016;194:1032–3.

35. Hodgson CL, Berney S, Harrold M, Saxena M, Bellomo R. Clinical review: early patient mobilization in the ICU. Crit Care. 2013;17:207.

36. Pulthucheary ZA, Rawal J, McPhail M, Connolly B, Ratnayake G, Chan P, et al. Acute skeletal muscle wasting in critical illness. JAMA. 2013;310:1591–600.

37. Winkelman C, Peereboom K. Staff-perceived barriers and facilitators. Crit Care Nurse. 2010;30:S13–6.

38. Hanson CW 3rd, Deutschman CS, Anderson HL 3rd, Reilly PM, Behringer EC, Schwab CW, et al. Effects of an organized critical care service on outcomes and resource utilization: a cohort study. Crit Care Med. 1999;27:270–4.

39. Titsworth HL, HesterJ CT, Reed R, Guin P, Archibald L, et al. The effect of increased mobility on morbidity in the neurointensive care unit. J Neurosurg. 2012;116:1379–88.

40. Bassett RD, Vollman KM, Brandwene L, Murray T. Integrating a multidisciplinary mobility programme into intensive care practice (IMMPTP): amulticentre collaborative. Intensive Crit Care Nurs. 2012;28:88–97.

41. Gutche JT, Kohl BA. Who should care for intensivist care unit patietns? Crit Care Med. 2007;35:S18–23.

42. Pronovost PJ, Jenckes MW, Doman T, Garrett E, Breslow MJ, Rosenfeld BA, et al. Organizational characteristics of intensive care units related to outcomes of abdominal aortic surgery. JAMA. 1999;281:1310–7.

43. Pronovost PJ, Angus DC, Dorman T, Robinson KA, Dremsizov TT, Young TL. Physician staffing patterns and clinical outcomes in critically ill patients: a systematic review. JAMA. 2002;288:2151–62.

44. Young MP, Birkmeyer JD. Potential reduction in mortality rates using an intensivist model to manage intensive care units. Eff Clin Pract. 2000;6:284–9.

45. Nydahl P, Sricharoenchai T, Chandra S, Kundt FS, Huang M, Fischill M, et al. Safety of patient mobilization and rehabilitation in the intensive care unit. Systematic review with meta-analysis. Ann Am Thorac Soc. 2017;14:766–77.

# 23

# Predicting in-hospital mortality in pneumonia-associated septic shock patients using a classification and regression tree

Jaime L Speiser[1], Constantine J Karvellas[2,3]* iD, Geoffery Shumilak[4], Wendy I Sligl[4], Yazdan Mirzanejad[7], Dave Gurka[8], Aseem Kumar[9], Anand Kumar[5,6] and the Cooperative Antimicrobial Therapy of Septic Shock (CATSS) Database Research Group

## Abstract

**Background:** Pneumonia complicated by septic shock is associated with significant morbidity and mortality. Classification and regression tree methodology is an intuitive method for predicting clinical outcomes using binary splits. We aimed to improve the prediction of in-hospital mortality in patients with pneumonia and septic shock using decision tree analysis.

**Methods:** Classification and regression tree models were applied to all patients with pneumonia-associated septic shock in the international, multicenter Cooperative Antimicrobial Therapy of Septic Shock database between 1996 and 2015. The association between clinical factors (time to appropriate antimicrobial therapy, severity of illness) and in-hospital mortality was evaluated. Accuracy in predicting clinical outcomes, sensitivity, specificity, and area under receiver operating curve of the final model was evaluated in training ($n = 2111$) and testing datasets ($n = 2111$).

**Results:** The study cohort contained 4222 patients, and in-hospital mortality was 51%. The mean time from onset of shock to administration of appropriate antimicrobials was significantly higher for patients who died (17.2 h) compared to those who survived (5.0 h). In the training dataset ($n = 2111$), a tree model using Acute Physiology and Chronic Health Evaluation II Score, lactate, age, and time to appropriate antimicrobial therapy yielded accuracy of 73% and area under the receiver operating curve 0.75. The testing dataset ($n = 2111$) had accuracy of 69% and area under the receiver operating curve 0.72.

**Conclusions:** Overall mortality (51%) in patients with pneumonia complicated by septic shock is high. Increased time to administration of antimicrobial therapy, Acute Physiology and Chronic Health Evaluation II Score, serum lactate, and age were associated with increased in-hospital mortality. Classification and regression tree methodology offers a simple prognostic model with good performance in predicting in-hospital mortality.

**Keywords:** Pneumonia, Septic shock, Classification and regression tree, Antimicrobial therapy,

\* Correspondence: dean.karvellas@ualberta.ca
[2]Department of Critical Care Medicine, University of Alberta, 1-40 Zeidler-Ledcor Building, Edmonton, Alberta T6G-2X8, Canada
[3]Division of Gastroenterology and Hepatology, University of Alberta, Edmonton, Canada
Full list of author information is available at the end of the article

## Background

Pneumonia complicated by septic shock is associated with significant morbidity and mortality. It is a leading cause of hospitalization and death with an estimated 423,000 emergency department visits per year and 15.9 deaths per 100,000 individuals in the USA [1, 2]. Annual medical costs associated with pneumonia were in excess of $10 billion annually in 2011 [3]. Most existing literature in the prognostication of pneumonia is targeted at risk stratification of patients presenting to hospital to determine the optimal location of care by predicting risk of death. Little data exists on predicting in-hospital mortality in patients presenting with pneumonia complicated by septic shock.

The primary aim of this study was to use classification and regression tree (CART) methodology to predict in-hospital mortality of patients with pneumonia complicated by septic shock. CART methodology allows the development of predictive models using binary splits on variables which can be read like a flow chart [4, 5]. Gaining popularity in diverse medical fields [6–8], CART models offer an intuitive method for predicting outcomes by using processes familiar to clinicians (e.g., "high" versus "low" values of a predictor). We hypothesized that CART models predicting in-hospital mortality would have good overall performance in terms of predictive accuracy, sensitivity, specificity, and area under the receiver operating curve (AUROC). Specifically, the objectives for this study were to:

1. Assess overall demographic and clinical characteristics of patients with pneumonia-associated septic shock
2. Compare demographic and clinical characteristics of pneumonia-associated septic shock patients based on clinical outcomes
3. Develop a CART model containing variables suggested within current literature to predict in-hospital mortality for patients with pneumonia-associated septic shock
4. Assess performance of the CART model using predictive accuracy, sensitivity, specificity, and AUROC

## Methods

This was a nested cohort study within a retrospective database (the Cooperative Antimicrobial Therapy of Septic Shock (CATSS) Database) of patients with septic shock. Data was collected from 28 medical centers in Canada, the USA, and Saudi Arabia between 1996 and 2015. The details of the study design and data collection were described in a previous paper [9]. Approval was obtained from the Institutional Review Boards of all participating institutions. This study was written according

to the STROBE Guideline for reporting retrospective studies (see Additional file 1) [10].

### Study design: patients and setting

Clinical and microbiological data was extracted for all patients with pneumonia enrolled in the CATSS database. All patients in the CATSS database had septic shock, so that all patients included in our study had both pneumonia and septic shock. The diagnosis of pneumonia was made at the discretion of the physician and based on clinical, microbiological, and radiographic information. Only patients with a primary diagnosis of pneumonia were eligible for this study. Patient records and information were anonymized and de-identified prior to use in this analysis. Eligible patients with missing outcome data were excluded from the final analysis.

### Exposures and outcomes

Baseline patient characteristics including demographics and comorbid conditions were obtained at enrollment into the registry. Data collected within the first 24 h of septic shock diagnosis included serum bicarbonate level, serum lactate, bilirubin, creatinine, platelet count, international normalized ratio (INR), white blood cell (WBC) count, number of organ failures, and Acute Physiology And Chronic Health Evaluation II (APACHE II) score [11]. The primary outcome of interest was in-hospital mortality. Time to administration of appropriate antimicrobials was defined as the time of development of shock (hypotension with a mean arterial pressure < 65 mmHg and need for vasopressor support) to the time of receipt of antimicrobial therapy listed in the CATSS registry based on review of original patient records.

### Operational definitions

Septic shock was defined using the 1992 ACCP/SCCM guidelines [12]. Per that definition, patients were required to have documented or suspected infection, persistent hypotension requiring vasopressors, and at least two of the following four elements: (1) a heart rate of > 90 beats/min, (2) a respiratory rate > 20 breaths/min or arterial partial pressure of carbon dioxide ($PaCO_2$) of < 32 mmHg. (3) a core temperature of < 36 °C or > 38 °C, and (4) a WBC count < 4000/μL or > 12,000/μL or bands > 10%. Hypotension was considered to represent the initial onset of septic shock when it persisted despite adequate fluid resuscitation (2 l of crystalloid) [13]. Predetermined rules were used to define documented and suspected infections and to assign significance to clinical isolates as previously described [9]. Cases of septic shock caused by infections acquired > 48 h after hospital admission were classified as nosocomial cases.

Predetermined rules were used to assess the appropriateness and delays of initial empiric antimicrobial therapy [9, 13, 14]. For septic shock with positive cultures, initial antimicrobial therapy was considered appropriate if an antimicrobial with in vitro activity appropriate for the isolated pathogen or pathogens was the first new antimicrobial agent given after the onset of recurrent or persistent hypotension or was initiated within 6 h of the administration of the first new antimicrobial agent. Initial therapy not meeting these criteria was considered inappropriate [9]. For septic shock with negative cultures, initial antimicrobial therapy was considered appropriate when an antimicrobial agent consistent with broadly accepted norms for empiric management of the typical pathogens for the clinical syndrome was the new antimicrobial agent given after the onset of recurrent or persistent hypotension or was initiated within 6 h of administration of the first new antimicrobial agent [9]. The designation of appropriateness of empiric therapy of culture-negative infections was based on recommendations listed in the "Clinical Approach to Initial Choice of Antimicrobial Therapy" from the Sanford Guide to Antimicrobial Therapy (most recently available edition at the time of the case). Additionally, infectious disease physicians and microbiologists were consulted at the discretion of the clinical team to account for local practice patterns and regional bacterial resistance patterns during the study period. To evaluate the predictive performance of the models, specificity is defined as the proportion of correctly predicted outcomes of death and sensitivity is the proportion of correctly predicted outcomes of survival.

## CART analysis

CART is a type of decision tree algorithm which follows deterministic rules to develop prediction models for continuous or categorical outcomes. This is a popular method in clinical prediction modeling because CART offers models that are simple to use with no calculations or computer applications to obtain predictions [6–8]. Additionally, CART models offer clear interpretation by using high versus low values of clinical variables related to the outcome of interest based on optimal splitting criteria from an automated algorithm. Trees are read from top to bottom like a flow chart in order to obtain a prediction for a specified outcome (e.g., survived or died). Starting at the top of a tree, branches corresponding to observed clinical features are followed until a terminal node has been reached and the fraction of patients contained in each outcome group is displayed. These tables may be used to assess the probability that a patient falls within each outcome category.

CART models were developed using the following algorithm first introduced by Breiman [4].Trees were constructed firstly by selecting the variable that optimally separated outcome groups, and a binary split was made.

Then, from both of these subgroups, subsequent variables were selected with replacement (meaning that variables can be used more than once within a model) that optimally separated outcome groups, and second levels of binary splits were made. Variable splits were made recursively until stopping criteria were reached, in which case a terminal node occurred. At each terminal node was the outcome prediction for the specific subset of the data.

The features of CART described in the previous paragraph are advantageous compared to standard logistic regression for modeling binary outcomes. Potential deficiencies of logistic regression for clinical prediction modeling include cumbersome calculations (e.g., inserting numbers and exponentiation requires a calculator or application), unclear interpretation of results (e.g., log odds ratios are not intuitive, especially in the presence of interactions between predictor variables), and unsatisfied assumptions (e.g., linear relationship between predictors and outcome via the link function may be inappropriate). CART also includes a method for handling missing predictor data using surrogate splits while logistic regression requires missing data to be filled in using a separate imputation method for all observations prior to developing a prediction model. For these reasons, CART is a beneficial framework for developing clinical prediction models compared to logistic regression.

## Variables

The main outcome of interest was in-hospital mortality. Multiple variables were used in developing the prediction model. Clinical variables included age, sex, use of mechanical ventilation, location of infection acquisition (nosocomial or community), underlying immunosuppression, number of systems with end-organ dysfunction, time to appropriate antimicrobial therapy, body mass index, and APACHE II score. Biochemical variables included serum lactate, bilirubin, sodium, creatinine, INR, platelets, WBC count, and albumin. Microbiological variables included culture positivity, concomitant bacteremia/fungemia, isolated fungal and bacterial pathogens, and the presence of antimicrobial resistant organisms. All clinical predictors were collected at baseline unless otherwise noted.

## Statistical methods

Analyses were completed using RStudio software [15]. Patient characteristics were presented as mean (standard deviation (SD)) or $n$ (percent) and compared using $t$ tests and binomial tests using the R package *tableone* [16]. $P$ values of $< 0.05$ were considered statistically significant. CART models were constructed using a training dataset ($n = 2111$) and were assessed using a testing dataset ($n = 2111$). Training and test data were randomly split from the entire dataset. The R package *rpart* was used to develop the CART models [17]. Missing predictor data were handled using the method of surrogate splitting, which is a standard built-in feature of CART implementation using the *rpart* package. CART can sometimes produce models, which overfit data (i.e., they can model too many splits for a specific training dataset), which may not predict well for independent test data. One of the ways to reduce overfitting is by constraining the number of observations, which each terminal node of the tree must contain. We required that the minimum number of observations in terminal nodes of the CART was 100 (i.e., the tuning parameter for minimum bucket size was 100) to provide a sufficient amount of data relative to the total training sample for meaningful predictions within the final variable splits. Prediction models were assessed in terms of overall accuracy, sensitivity, and specificity using binomial estimates and confidence intervals. AUROC and its corresponding confidence intervals were determined using the R packages *ROCR* [18] and *cvAUC* [19].

## Results

### Overall demographic and clinical characteristics

In total, 4222 patients (61% male) with pneumonia and septic shock were included in the analysis (Table 1). The mean (SD) age of patients was 62 (17) years. Sixty-three percent ($n = 2652$) had positive cultures from clinical isolates, 21% ($n = 876$) had concomitant bacteremia, and 35% ($n = 1075$) had nosocomial infections. Of patients with positive cultures, the most common pathogens were *Staphylococcus aureus* ($n = 702$, 27%), *Streptococcus* spp. ($n = 658$, 25%), *Pseudomonas* spp. ($n = 267$, 10%), *Escherichia coli* ($n = 225$, 9%), *Klebsiella* spp. ($n = 183$, 7%), and *Haemophilus influenzae* ($n = 118$, 4.4%). Mean (SD) APACHE II score was 26 (8), and serum lactate was 4.1 (3.9) mmol/L at onset of septic shock. During ICU admission, 89% ($n = 3760$) required mechanical ventilation. Of 3048 patients who received appropriate antimicrobial therapy after the development of septic shock, the mean time to administration of antimicrobials was 10.9 h (SD = 18.6 h). Fifty-one percent ($n = 2141$) of patients died in hospital.

Of patients with pneumonia and septic shock, 2141 died in hospital and 2081 survived. Patients who died in hospital were significantly older (mean age of 65 versus 59) and had lower body mass index (28 versus 27) when compared to survivors (Table 2). The presence of concomitant bloodstream infection, empyema, positive microbiology, gram-negative pathogens, and fungal pathogens were associated with increased in-hospital mortality. Nosocomial pneumonia infections, higher APACHE II scores, and higher numbers of organ failures were also associated with worse outcomes (Table 2). Mechanical ventilation was more commonly used in patients who

died. Admission biochemistry revealed that patients who died had significantly lower platelets, higher lactate, higher INR, higher bilirubin, and lower albumin compared to patients who survived. There was no significant difference detected between the groups for white blood cell count, sodium, and creatinine. In-hospital mortality was significantly more common in patients who were immunocompromised. The mean time to administration of appropriate antimicrobial therapy was 5 h in patients who survived and 17 h in patients who died.

### CART model predicting in-hospital mortality

The overall dataset was randomly split into training data for model development and testing data for model validation. There were no significant differences detected between the training and test datasets. The CART model for predicting mortality in patients with pneumonia and septic shock is depicted in Fig. 1. Variables included within the model were the time to administration of appropriate antimicrobial therapy, APACHE II score, serum lactate, and age. The most important predictor of in-hospital mortality was the time to appropriate antimicrobial therapy.

The following features were associated with higher probability of death:

1. Time from onset of septic shock to administration of appropriate antimicrobial therapy > 6.6 h (node 1, probability of death = 0.76)
2. Time from onset of septic shock to administration of appropriate antimicrobial therapy < 6.6 h, APACHE > 28, and lactate > 6.3 mmol/L (node 5, probability of death = 0.817)
3. Time from onset of septic shock to administration of appropriate antimicrobial therapy < 6.6 h, APACHE > 28, lactate < 6.3 mmol/L, and age > 65 (node 7, probability of death = 0.670)

The following features were associated with higher probability of survival:

1. Time from onset of septic shock to administration of appropriate antimicrobial therapy < 6.6 h and APACHE < 28 (node 4, probability of survival = 0.744)
2. Time from onset of septic shock to administration of appropriate antimicrobial therapy < 6.6 h, APACHE > 28, lactate < 6.3 mmol/L, and age < 65 (node 8, probability of survival = 0.591)

There were 1174 patients who received appropriate antimicrobials before the onset of septic shock. In the training dataset used to develop the CART prediction model, these were treated as missing. The CART

**Table 1** Demographic and clinical characteristics of pneumonia-associated septic shock patients

| | Overall cohort (n = 4222) | |
|---|---|---|
| | N | Number (%) or mean (SD) |
| Demographics | | |
| Age | 4222 | 62 (17) |
| Sex (male) | 4222 | 2574 (61.0) |
| Body mass index | 2013 | 27 (8) |
| Microbiology characteristics | | |
| Concomitant bloodstream infection | 4222 | 876 (20.7) |
| Empyema | 4222 | 119 (2.8) |
| Culture positive | 4222 | 2652 (62.8) |
| Gram positive | 4222 | 1413 (33.5) |
| Gram negative | 4222 | 1073 (25.4) |
| Fungal | 4222 | 20 (0.8) |
| Hospital-acquired infection | 4222 | 1547 (36.6) |
| Community-acquired infection | 4222 | 2675 (63.4) |
| Organ failure/support | | |
| APACHE | 3995 | 26 (8) |
| Organ failure day 1 | 4222 | 3.8 (1.5) |
| Mechanical ventilation | 4222 | 3760 (89.1) |
| Biochemistry (admission) | | |
| WBC | 4031 | 16.3 (15.7) |
| Platelets | 4046 | 206 (136) |
| Sodium | 2488 | 137.2 (7.1) |
| Creatinine | 3829 | 189.9 (164.6) |
| Lactate | 2804 | 4.1 (3.9) |
| INR | 3695 | 1.7 (1.3) |
| Bilirubin | 3544 | 29.9 (64.6) |
| Albumin | 1506 | 22.7 (6.5) |
| Immunocompromised | 4222 | 561 (13.3) |
| Time delay from shock to appropriate antimicrobials (hours) | 3048 | 10.9 (18.6) |
| Primary outcome: in-hospital mortality | 4222 | 2141 (50.7) |

framework uses a method called surrogate splitting in order to handle any missing values, in which non-missing variables are used to make a "surrogate" split for any missing values. Thus, the patients who received appropriate antimicrobials before onset of septic shock were included in the CART model development. For use in practice for new observations of patients, one should follow the branch corresponding to time to appropriate antimicrobials < 6.6 within Fig. 1 (i.e., proceed to node 2).

### Predicting in-hospital mortality: an example

A patient with pneumonia and septic shock presented at the hospital with the following characteristics:

antimicrobials were administered 3 h after septic shock, APACHE II score of 30, lactate of 10.2 mmol/L, and age of 64. At the start, time to antibiotic administration is less than 6.6 h (true at node 1), so we follow the right branch to node 2. Next, the APACHE II score is > 28 is true, so we follow the left branch to node 3. Then, lactate is > 6.3 mmol/L, so we proceed to the left branch to node 5. Since there are no nodes under node 5, this is our final prediction for the model. The probability of death for the patient is 0.817, and the probability of survival is 0.183. Therefore, the patient is predicted to die in-hospital.

### Assessing performance

Performance measures and the associated confidence intervals for the CART model are presented in Table 3. In the training dataset, the CART prediction model for mortality yielded overall accuracy of 73%, specificity of 75%, and sensitivity of 71%. The model showed good overall performance, with training dataset AUROC of 0.75. In the testing dataset, the CART prediction model for mortality yielded accuracy of 69%, specificity of 72%, and sensitivity of 65%. The model had good overall performance, with testing dataset AUROC of 0.72.

### Discussion
#### Summary of key results

In this study, we evaluated a large multi-center cohort of patients with pneumonia complicated by septic shock. Overall mortality (51%) was high in this population. There were 3048 patients who received appropriate antimicrobial therapy after the development of septic shock with a mean time to appropriate antimicrobial therapy of 10.9 h. Patients who died in the hospital were significantly older and had significantly higher APACHE II scores, number of organ failures, and admission serum lactate. Time to administration of appropriate antimicrobial therapy remained the most important predictor of in-hospital mortality in this population. In the training set (n = 2111), a CART model using APACHE II score, lactate, age, and time to appropriate antimicrobial therapy yielded predictive accuracy of 73%, specificity 75%, sensitivity 71%, and AUROC 0.75. In the testing set (n = 2111), the CART model offered predictive accuracy of 69%, specificity 72%, sensitivity 65%, and AUROC 0.72.

The novelty of the study is the use of classification and regression tree (CART) methodology for the development of a simple, accurate prediction model for outcomes in pneumonia patients with septic shock. CART allows for development of prediction models using binary splits and offers an intuitive method for obtaining predictions of outcome using processes familiar to clinicians (e.g., "high" versus "low" values of a predictor). The nonparametric nature of CART offers results that are simple to use and does not require calculation of use

**Table 2** Demographic and clinical characteristics of pneumonia-associated septic shock patients by mortality

| | Died (n = 2141) | | Survived (n = 2081) | | P value |
|---|---|---|---|---|---|
| | N | Number (%) or mean (SD) | N | Number (%) or mean (SD) | |
| Demographics | | | | | |
| Age | 2141 | 64.6 (15.8) | 2081 | 58.8 (16.7) | < 0.001 |
| Sex (male) | 2141 | 1323 (61.8) | 2081 | 1251 (60.1) | 0.277 |
| Body mass index | 974 | 26.6 (7.8) | 1039 | 27.7 (7.7) | 0.001 |
| Microbiology characteristics | | | | | |
| Concomitant bloodstream infection | 2141 | 484 (22.6) | 2081 | 392 (18.8) | 0.003 |
| Empyema | 2141 | 45 (2.1) | 2081 | 74 (3.6) | 0.010 |
| Culture positive | 2141 | 1421 (66.4) | 2081 | 1231 (59.2) | < 0.001 |
| Gram positive | 2141 | 696 (32.5) | 2081 | 717 (34.5) | 0.191 |
| Gram negative | 2141 | 608 (28.4) | 2081 | 465 (22.3) | < 0.001 |
| Fungal | 2141 | 16 (0.7) | 2081 | 4 (0.2) | 0.009 |
| Hospital-acquired infection | 2141 | 957 (44.7) | 2081 | 590 (28.4) | < 0.001 |
| Organ failure/support | | | | | |
| APACHE | 2034 | 28.5 (8.0) | 1961 | 22.8 (6.7) | < 0.001 |
| Organ failure day 1 | 2141 | 4.2 (1.6) | 2081 | 3.4 (1.3) | < 0.001 |
| Mechanical ventilation | 2141 | 2005 (93.6) | 2081 | 1755 (84.3) | < 0.001 |
| Biochemistry (admission) | | | | | |
| WBC | 2052 | 16.3 (17.9) | 1979 | 16.4 (13.0) | 0.757 |
| Platelets | 2021 | 195 (143) | 2025 | 216 (128) | < 0.001 |
| Sodium | 1121 | 137.4 (7.2) | 1367 | 137.0 (7.0) | 0.192 |
| Creatinine | 1937 | 192.2 (164.6) | 1892 | 187.5 (164.6) | 0.377 |
| Lactate | 1447 | 5.1 (4.6) | 1357 | 3.1 (2.8) | < 0.001 |
| INR | 1848 | 1.9 (1.5) | 1847 | 1.6 (1.1) | < 0.001 |
| Bilirubin | 1768 | 39.7 (82.7) | 1776 | 20.1 (36.7) | < 0.001 |
| Albumin | 621 | 21.6 (6.3) | 885 | 23.5 (6.4) | < 0.001 |
| Immunocompromised | 2141 | 360 (16.8) | 2081 | 201 (9.7) | < 0.001 |
| Time delay from shock to appropriate antimicrobials (hours) | 1494 | 17.2 (23.6) | 1554 | 5.0 (5.6) | < 0.001 |

of an application. Models are easily read and interpreted using a flow chart diagram. These aspects of CART are advantageous compared to logistic regression, where calculations may be cumbersome (e.g., plugging in numbers and exponentiation requires a calculator or application), interpretation of results may be unclear (e.g., if there are interactions between two or more predictors), and assumptions may not be satisfied.

### Comparison with the literature
Patients with pneumonia complicated by septic shock are at substantial risk of poor outcomes. The 51% in-hospital mortality observed in this cohort is substantially higher than the reported mortality for population-level outcomes in patients with pneumonia and patients presenting with pneumonia and septic

shock [20, 21]. Despite these studies, a lack of data on predicting outcomes for patients with pneumonia and septic shock remained.

In this study, a mechanism for predicting the probability of in-hospital mortality was developed using CART methodology. Previous prediction models have focused on predicting patient outcomes for purposes of risk stratification at presentation to hospital with pneumonia [22–24]. Consistent with previous literature, our study highlights that the presence of septic shock and the severity of illness (APACHE II), age, lactate, and time to administration of appropriate antimicrobial therapy significantly impacts survival in patients with pneumonia. In our study, multivariable CART analysis demonstrated that the most important predictor of mortality was the increasing time from onset of septic shock to

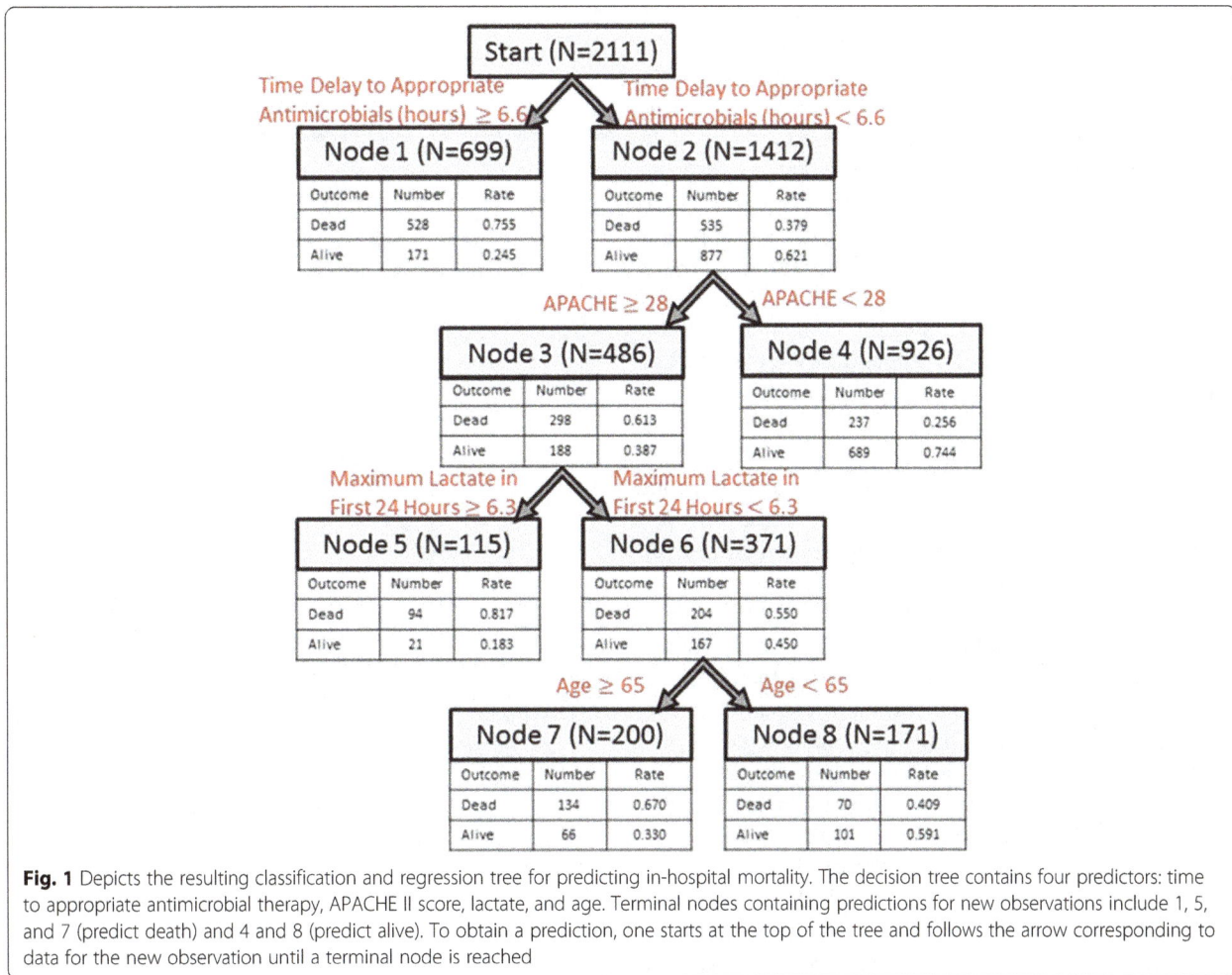

**Fig. 1** Depicts the resulting classification and regression tree for predicting in-hospital mortality. The decision tree contains four predictors: time to appropriate antimicrobial therapy, APACHE II score, lactate, and age. Terminal nodes containing predictions for new observations include 1, 5, and 7 (predict death) and 4 and 8 (predict alive). To obtain a prediction, one starts at the top of the tree and follows the arrow corresponding to data for the new observation until a terminal node is reached

administration of appropriate antimicrobial therapy. Additional predictors of in-hospital mortality included severity of illness (APACHE II score), high serum lactate, and older age. Our study complements previous research by highlighting the importance of early intervention and administration of appropriate antimicrobial therapy to optimize outcomes in patients with septic shock.

Though CART models have existed for several decades, there is a paucity of decision tree models available for predicting outcomes in critically ill patient populations. Wong et al. [25] use CART to analyze 355 children with septic shock to assess biomarkers and clinical variables. The resulting decision tree consisted of five

biomarker-based decision rules with ten variable splits. This work was primarily done to complement microarray work to explore potential gene products as targets in sepsis. Wong et al. subsequently applied the same five biomarkers along with lactate, age, and chronic disease status [26] in 672 adult patients with septic shock with and developed a clinical prediction model with an area under the receiver curve of 0.72 (validation set), similar to this study. Besides these two studies which primarily focused on gene products/potential novel biomarkers (both < 700 patients), the decision tree approach for prediction has not been previously used for a large population of adults with septic shock using readily available clinical information as in this study.

### Limitations

This study should be interpreted within the limitations of its design. This study is a retrospective analysis of prospectively collected data and only association, not causation, can be inferred. Given that this study was observational, we are unable to conclusively exclude sources of selection bias [27]. We implemented an

**Table 3** Performance measures (95% exact binomial confidence intervals) for the CART model prediction in-hospital mortality

| Model | Accuracy (95% CI) | Specificity (95% CI) | Sensitivity (95% CI) | AUROC (95% CI) |
|---|---|---|---|---|
| Training (n = 2111) | 0.73 (0.71, 0.75) | 0.75 (0.73, 0.78) | 0.71 (0.68, 0.74) | 0.75 (0.73, 0.78) |
| Testing (n = 2111) | 0.69 (0.67, 0.71) | 0.72 (0.70, 0.75) | 0.65 (0.62, 0.68) | 0.72 (0.69, 0.75) |

internal validation scheme that used randomly split training and testing datasets to build and evaluate the CART prediction model for mortality. External data should be used to further validate the CART model. Another limitation is that the average time to appropriate antimicrobial therapy was 6 h, which is greater than the current suggested 3-h completion of treatment. These guidelines changed over the course of the study period (from 1996 to 2016), so we included all data in order to have a larger sample size to develop a prediction model. Though current guidelines suggest completion of the sepsis bundle within 3 h [28], approximately one third of the patients in this study received appropriate antibiotic after 6 h. There are several reasons for the longer time to antibiotics: our study included appropriate use of antibiotics not just time to any usage of antibiotics, about half of the patients included in our study were ward patients which have higher time to appropriate antimicrobials compared to emergency room admissions, and the data range for our study is from 1996 to 2016 during which the time to antibiotics was substantially longer than the standard practice now. Despite these limitations, the strengths include inclusion of patients from 28 intensive care units across three geographic regions.

Limitations of CART modeling include the challenge of determining parameters for model building (e.g., deciding the minimum bucket size) and the possible variability of CART models, as discussed in statistical literature (e.g., [8, 29–32]) (Additional file 2). Inclusion of variables for age and APACHE II, which also used age for its calculation, highlights the importance of age for predicting outcomes of pneumonia-associated septic shock patients. Unlike traditional regression models, which can be negatively influenced by correlated variables, the CART model can adequately handle correlated variables due to the binary nature of splitting. However, these limitations are minimal compared to the beneficial simplicity and relatively high predictive accuracy of CART models.

## Conclusion
Overall mortality in patients with pneumonia and septic shock is high (51% in the CATSS dataset). Increasing time to appropriate antimicrobial therapy, APACHE II score, serum lactate, and age were significantly associated with in-hospital mortality. CART models offer simple prognostic models with good performance.

## Additional files

**Additional file 1:** STROBE guideline for reporting retrospective studies. (DOCX 38 kb)

**Additional file 2:** Benefits of CART, tree development, and limitations of CART models. (DOCX 17 kb)

### Abbreviations
APACHEII: Acute Physiology and Chronic Health Evaluation II score; AUROC: Area under the receiver operating curve; CART: Classification and regression tree; CATSS: Cooperative Antimicrobial Therapy of Septic Shock; CI: Confidence interval; ICU: Intensive care unit; INR: International normalized ratio; SD: Standard deviation; WBC: White blood cell

### The Cooperative Antimicrobial Therapy of Septic Shock (CATSS) Database Research Group
Yaseen Arabi, MD, King Saud Bin Abdulaziz University for Health Sciences, Riyadh, Saudi Arabia
Phillip Dellinger, MD, Cooper Hospital/University Medical Center, Camden NJ, USA
Sandra Dial, MD, McGill University, Montreal QC, Canada
Peter Dodek, MD, University of British Columbia, Vancouver BC, Canada
Paul Ellis, MD, University Health Network, Toronto, ON, Canada
Daniel Feinstein, MD, Moses H. Cone Memorial Hospital, Greensboro NC, USA
Dave Gurka, MD, Rush-Presbyterian-St. Luke's Medical Center, Chicago IL, USA
Jose Guzman, MD, Cleveland Clinic, Cleveland, OH, USA
Sean Keenan, MD, Royal Columbian Hospital, New Westminster BC, Canada
Andreas Kramer, MD, Foothills Hospital, Calgary AB, Canada
Aseem Kumar, PhD, Laurentian University, Sudbury, ON, Canada
Stephen Lapinsky, MD, Mount Sinai Hospital, Toronto ON, Canada
Denny Laporta, MD, Jewish General Hospital, Montreal QC, Canada
Bruce Light, MD, Winnipeg Regional Health Authority, Winnipeg MB, Canada
Dennis Maki, MD, University of Wisconsin Hospital and Clinics, Madison WI, USA
Greg Martinka, MD, Richmond General Hospital, Richmond BC, Canada
Yazdan Mirzanejad, MD, Surrey Memorial Hospital, Surrey, BC, Canada
Joseph E. Parrillo, MD, Hackensack University Medical Centre, Hackensack, NJ, USA
Gourang Patel, PharmD, Rush-Presbyterian-St. Luke's Medical Center, Chicago IL, USA
Brian Bookatz, MD, Brandon General Hospital, Brandon MD, Canada
Dan Roberts, MD, Winnipeg Regional Health Authority, Winnipeg MB, Canada
John Ronald, MD, Nanaimo Regional Hospital, Nanaimo BC, Canada
Dave Simon, MD, Rush-Presbyterian-St. Luke's Medical Center, Chicago IL, USA
Yoanna Skrobik, MD, Hôpital Maisonneuve Rosemont, Montreal QC, Canada
Gordon Wood, MD, Royal Jubilee Hospital/Victoria General Hospital, Victoria BC, Canada
Kenneth E. Wood, DO, University of Maryland Medical System, Baltimore MD, USA

### Associate Members of the CATSS Database Research Group
Muhammed Wali Ahsan, MD, Winnipeg MB, Canada
Mozdeh Bahrainian, MD, Madison WI
Rob Bohmeier, MD, University of Manitoba, Winnipeg MB, Canada
Lindsey Carter, MD, University of Manitoba, Winnipeg MB, Canada
Harris Chou, BSc, of British Columbia, Vancouver BC, Canada
Sofia Delgra, RN, King Saud Bin Abdulaziz University for Health Sciences, Riyadh, Saudi Arabia
Collins Egbujuo, MD, Winnipeg MB, Canada
Winnie Fu, MD, University of British Columbia, Vancouver BC, Canada
Catherine Gonzales, RN, King Saud Bin Abdulaziz University for Health Sciences, Riyadh, Saudi Arabia
Harleena Gulati, MD, University of Manitoba, Winnipeg MB, Canada
Oliver Gutierrez, MD, University of Manitoba, Winnipeg MB, Canada
Aparna Jindal, MD, University of Manitoba, Winnipeg MB, Canada
Erica Halmarson, MD, University of Manitoba, Winnipeg MB, Canada
Ziaul Haque, MD, Montreal QC, Canada
Johanne Harvey, RN, Hôpital Maisonneuve Rosemont, Montreal QC, Canada
Ehsan Koohpayehzadeh Esfahani, MD, University of Manitoba, Winnipeg MB, Canada
Farah Khan, MD, Toronto ON, Canada
Laura Kolesar, RN, St. Boniface Hospital, Winnipeg MB, Canada
Laura Kravetsky, MD, University of Manitoba, Winnipeg MB, Canada
Runjun Kumar, BSc, Washington University Medical School, St. Louis, MO, USA
Nasreen Merali, MD, Winnipeg MB, Canada
Sheri Muggaberg, MD, University of Manitoba, Winnipeg MB, Canada
Heidi Paulin, MD, University of Toronto, Toronto ON, Canada

Cheryl Peters, RN, MD, University of Manitoba, Winnipeg MB, Canada
Jody Richards, RN, Camosun College, Victoria BC, Canada
Honorata Serrano, RN, King Saud Bin Abdulaziz University for Health
Sciences, Riyadh, Saudi Arabia
Amrinder Singh, MD, Winnipeg MB Canada
Katherine Sullivan, MD, University of Manitoba, Winnipeg MB, Canada
Robert Suppes, MD, University of Manitoba, Winnipeg MB, Canada
Leo Taiberg, MD, Rush Medical College, Chicago IL, USA
Ronny Tchokonte, MD, Wayne State University Medical School, Detroit MI, USA
Omid Ahmadi Torshizi, MD, Montreal QC, Canada
Kym Wiebe, RN, St. Boniface Hospital, Winnipeg MB, Canada

## Authors' contributions

JLS performed the statistical and data analysis and drafted and extensively revised the final manuscript. CJK conceived the idea of the study and drafted and extensively revised the final manuscript. GS and WIS drafted and extensively revised the final manuscript. YM, DG, and AK collected the data and revised the final manuscript. AK is the principal investigator and responsible for CATSS database who developed the initial registry; provided content expertise, significant guidance on compilation of the database, and analysis and interpretation of data; and assisted extensively with the manuscript revision. All authors read and approved the final manuscript.

## Competing interests

The authors declare that they have no competing interests.

## Author details

Department of Biostatistical Sciences, Division of Public Health Sciences, Wake Forest School of Medicine, Winston-Salem, NC, USA. [2]Department of Critical Care Medicine, University of Alberta, 1-40 Zeidler-Ledcor Building, Edmonton, Alberta T6G-2X8, Canada. [3]Division of Gastroenterology and Hepatology, University of Alberta, Edmonton, Canada. [4]Division of Critical Care Medicine and Infectious Diseases, University of Alberta, Edmonton, Canada. [5]Section of Critical Care Medicine, University of Manitoba, Winnipeg, Canada. [6]Section of Infectious Diseases, University of Manitoba, Winnipeg, Canada. [7]Surrey Hospital, Surrey, BC, Canada. [8]Rush Medical College, Chicago, IL, USA. [9]Laurentian University, Sudbury, ON, Canada.

## References

1. Kochanek KD, Murphy SL, Xu J, Tejada-Vera B. Deaths: final data for 2014. National vital statistics reports: from the Centers for Disease Control and Prevention, National Center for Health Statistics. Natl Vital Stat Syst. 2016; 65(4):1–122.
2. Rui P, Kang K. National Hospital Ambulatory Medical Care Survey: 2014 emergency department summary tables. Centers for Disease Control and Prevention; 2014.
3. Pfuntner A, Wier LM, Steiner C. Costs for hospital stays in the United States, 2011: statistical brief# 168. 2006.
4. Breiman L, Friedman JH, Olshen RA, Stone CJ. Classification and regression trees. Monterrey, CA: Wadsworth and Brooks; 1984.
5. Loh WY. Fifty years of classification and regression trees. Int Stat Rev. 2014; 82(3):329–48.
6. Aguiar FS, Almeida LL, Ruffino-Netto A, Kritski AL, Mello FC, Werneck GL. Classification and regression tree (CART) model to predict pulmonary tuberculosis in hospitalized patients. BMC Pulm Med. 2012;12:40.
7. Garzotto M, Beer TM, Hudson RG, et al. Improved detection of prostate cancer using classification and regression tree analysis. J Clin Oncol. 2005; 23(19):4322–9.
8. Speiser JL, Lee WM, Karvellas CJ. Predicting outcome on admission and post-admission for acetaminophen-induced acute liver failure using classification and regression tree models. PLoS One. 2015;10(4):e0122929.
9. Kumar A, Ellis P, Arabi Y, et al. Initiation of inappropriate antimicrobial therapy results in a fivefold reduction of survival in human septic shock. Chest. 2009;136(5):1237–48.
10. von Elm E, Altman DG, Egger M, et al. Strengthening the Reporting of Observational Studies in Epidemiology (STROBE) statement: guidelines for reporting observational studies. BMJ. 2007;335(7624):806–8.
11. Knaus WA, Draper EA, Wagner DP, Zimmerman JE. APACHE II: a severity of disease classification system. Crit Care Med Oct. 1985;13(10):818–29.
12. Bone RC, Balk RA, Cerra FB, et al. Definitions for sepsis and organ failure and guidelines for the use of innovative therapies in sepsis. The ACCP/SCCM Consensus Conference Committee. American College of Chest Physicians/ Society of Critical Care Medicine. Chest. 1992;101(6):1644–55.
13. Kumar A, Roberts D, Wood KE, et al. Duration of hypotension before initiation of effective antimicrobial therapy is the critical determinant of survival in human septic shock. Crit Care Med Jun. 2006;34(6):1589–96.
14. Kumar A, Zarychanski R, Light B, et al. Early combination antibiotic therapy yields improved survival compared with monotherapy in septic shock: a propensity-matched analysis. Crit Care Med Sep. 2010;38(9): 1773–85.
15. RStudio Team. RStudio. Integrated development for R. RStudio, Inc. Boston, MA URL https://www.rstudio.com; 2015.
16. Yoshida K, Bohn J. tableone: Create "table 1" to describe baseline characteristics. R package version 2015 0. 7. 3; .
17. Therneau TM, Atkinson EJ. An introduction to recursive partitioning using the Rpart routines. Rochester: Mayo Foundation; 1997. MN
18. Sing T, Sander O, Beernwinkel N, Lengauer T. ROCR: visualizing classifier performance in R. Bioinformatics. 2005;21(20):3940–1.
19. LeDell E, Petersen M, van der Laan M, LeDell ME. Package 'cvAUC'. 2012.
20. Control CfD, Prevention. Compressed mortality file 1999–2013. CDC wonder on-line database, compiled from compressed mortality file 1999–2013 series 20 no. 2s, 2015. 2015.
21. Garcia-Vidal C, Ardanuy C, Tubau F, et al. Pneumococcal pneumonia presenting with septic shock: host-and pathogen-related factors and outcomes. Thorax. 2009;2009:123612 thx.
22. Fine MJ, Auble TE, Yealy DM, et al. A prediction rule to identify low-risk patients with community-acquired pneumonia. N Engl J Med. 1997;336(4): 243–50.
23. Lim W, Van der Eerden M, Laing R, et al. Defining community acquired pneumonia severity on presentation to hospital: an international derivation and validation study. Thorax. 2003;58(5):377–82.
24. Myint PK, Kamath AV, Vowler SL, Maisey DN, Harrison BD. Severity assessment criteria recommended by the British Thoracic Society (BTS) for community-acquired pneumonia (CAP) and older patients. Should SOAR (systolic blood pressure, oxygenation, age and respiratory rate) criteria be used in older people? A compilation study of two prospective cohorts. Age Ageing. 2006;35(3):286–91.
25. Wong HR, Salisbury S, Xiao Q, et al. The pediatric sepsis biomarker risk model. Crit Care. 2012;16(5):R174.
26. Wong HR, Lindsell CJ, Pettilä V, et al. A multibiomarker-based outcome risk stratification model for adult septic shock. Crit Care Med. 2014;42(4):781.
27. Connors AF Jr. Pitfalls in estimating the effect of interventions in the critically ill using observational study designs. Crit Care Med Jun. 2001;29(6): 1283–4.
28. Rhodes A, Evans LE, Alhazzani W, et al. Surviving sepsis campaign: international guidelines for management of sepsis and septic shock: 2016. Intensive Care Med. 2017;43(3):304–77.
29. Chun FKH, Karakiewicz PI, Briganti A, et al. A critical appraisal of logistic regression-based nomograms, artificial neural networks, classification and regression-tree models, look-up tables and risk-group stratification models for prostate cancer. BJU Int. 2007;99(4):794–800.
30. Hastie T, Tibshirani R, Friedman J, Hastie T, Friedman J, Tibshirani R. The elements of statistical learning. Vol 2. Paolo Alto: Springer; 2009.
31. Lemon SC, Roy J, Clark MA, Friedmann PD, Rakowski W. Classification and regression tree analysis in public health: methodological review and comparison with logistic regression. Ann Behav Med. 2003;26(3):172–81.
32. Province MA, Shannon W, Rao D. 19 classification methods for confronting heterogeneity. Adv Genet. 2001;42:273–86.

# 24

# Comparison of extracorporeal membrane oxygenation outcome for influenza-associated acute respiratory failure

Shinichiro Ohshimo[1], Nobuaki Shime[1*], Satoshi Nakagawa[2], Osamu Nishida[3], Shinhiro Takeda[4] and Committee of the Japan ECMO project

## Abstract

**Background:** Since the 2009 pandemic influenza, we have nationally established a committee of the extracorporeal membrane oxygenation (ECMO) project. This project involves adequate respiratory management for severe respiratory failure using ECMO. This study aimed to investigate the correlations between changes in respiratory management using ECMO in Japan and outcomes of patients with influenza-associated acute respiratory failure between 2009 and 2016.

**Methods:** We investigated the incidence, severity, characteristics, and prognosis of influenza-associated acute respiratory failure in 2016 by web-based surveillance. The correlations between clinical characteristics, ventilator settings, ECMO settings, and prognosis were evaluated.

**Results:** A total of 14 patients were managed with ECMO in 2016. There were no significant differences in age, sex, and the acute physiology and chronic health evaluation II score between 2009 and 2016. The maximum sequential organ failure assessment score and highest positive end-expiratory pressure were lower in 2016 than in 2009 ($p = 0.03$ and $p = 0.015$, respectively). Baseline and lowest partial pressure of arterial oxygen ($PaO_2$)/fraction of inspiratory oxygen ($F_IO_2$) ratios were higher in 2016 than in 2009 ($p = 0.009$ and $p = 0.002$, respectively). The types of consoles, circuits, oxygenators, centrifugal pumps, and cannulas were significantly changed between 2016 and 2009 ($p = 0.006$, $p = 0.003$, $p = 0.004$, $p < 0.001$, respectively). Duration of the use of each circuit was significantly longer in 2016 than in 2009 (8.5 vs. 4.0 days; $p = 0.0001$). Multivariate analysis showed that the use of ECMO in 2016 was an independent predictor of better overall survival in patients with influenza-associated acute respiratory failure (hazard ratio, 7.25; 95% confidence interval, 1.35–33.3; $p = 0.021$).

**Conclusions:** Respiratory management for influenza-associated acute respiratory failure using ECMO was significantly changed in 2016 compared with 2009 in Japan. The outcome of ECMO use had improved in 2016 compared with the outcome in 2009 in patients with influenza-associated acute respiratory failure.

**Keywords:** Acute respiratory distress syndrome, Mechanical ventilation, Prognosis, Survival, Complication

* Correspondence: nshime@hiroshima-u.ac.jp
[1]Department of Emergency and Critical Care Medicine, Graduate School of Biomedical and Health Sciences, Hiroshima University, 1-2-3 Kasumi, Minami-ku, Hiroshima 734-8551, Japan
Full list of author information is available at the end of the article

## Background

Influenza virus can occasionally induce severe respiratory failure, including acute respiratory distress syndrome. The Centers for Disease Control and Prevention reported that more than approximately 20,000 influenza-associated deaths annually occurred in the USA [1]. Extracorporeal membrane oxygenation (ECMO) can be a lifesaving method in patients with potentially reversible acute respiratory failure, including influenza-associated acute respiratory failure [2, 3]. However, Takeda et al. showed that the survival rate of influenza-associated acute respiratory failure managed with ECMO in Japan was inferior compared with that in other countries during the pandemic of H1N1 influenza in 2009 [4–6]. Inadequate use of ECMO equipment (cannula, pump, and oxygenator), insufficient understanding of the ECMO strategy by physicians and other medical staff, and insufficient centralization of ECMO treatment might have affected this poor survival rate in Japan [4].

Since the 2009 pandemic of H1N1 influenza, we have nationally established a committee of an ECMO project, which is expected to guide adequate respiratory management for severe respiratory failure using ECMO. Introduction and simulation education by the ECMO project includes the physiology of ECMO, cannulation techniques, repositioning of the cannula, monitoring skill, daily management, and troubleshooting.

This study aimed to investigate the incidence, severity, characteristics, and prognosis of pandemic of influenza-associated acute respiratory failure that occurred in Japan in 2016. We also aimed to evaluate the correlations between changes in respiratory management using ECMO and outcomes of patients with influenza-associated acute respiratory failure in 2009 and 2016.

## Methods

This study involved adult patients with acute respiratory failure that was associated with H1N1 influenza who were admitted to the institutes of the ECMO project from January to April in 2016. A database was created based on the information collected from the institutes that participated in this study. A total of 87 institutes participate in the ECMO project, and 463 patients with various kind of respiratory failure who underwent ECMO have been registered in the database. Among them, 14 patients in 2009 and 14 patients in 2016 who suffered from influenza-associated acute respiratory failure were analyzed in this study. Data extracted from a previous study [4] were simultaneously analyzed and compared with those in the ECMO 2016 group. Informed consent was obtained from each individual by document or the opt-out procedure. Collected data included baseline characteristics (age, sex, body weight, body temperature, acute physiology and chronic health

evaluation [APACHE] II score, and predicted death rate), sequential organ failure assessment (SOFA) score, administered drugs, ventilator settings, ECMO equipment and settings, and outcome. Maximum SOFA score was defined as the highest SOFA score before starting ECMO. Overall survival rate was defined as the survival rate during the follow-up. Inclusion criteria were as follows: (1) patients with influenza-associated acute respiratory failure who were treated in institutes that participated in the ECMO project and (2) age older than 20 years. Categorical differences between the survival and non-survival groups were compared using Fisher's exact test or the chi-square test. Numerical differences were compared using the Mann–Whitney $U$ test. Multivariate analysis was conducted after adjustment for the predicted death rate. All statistical analyses were performed using SPSS software (Abacus Concepts, Berkeley, CA, USA). All values are reported as median (interquartile), and all $p$ values less than 0.05 were considered statistically significant. This study was approved by the ethical committee in Hiroshima University with the approval number of E-390-1. Each institute obtained institutional ethics approval and consent to participate.

## Results

### Patients' characteristics

A total of 14 patients from 16 institutes participating in ECMO project were enrolled as the ECMO 2016 group in this study (Table 1). There were no significant differences in age, sex, weight, body mass index, and APACHE II score between the groups. Maximum SOFA scores in the ECMO 2016 group were significantly lower than those in the ECMO 2009 group. (ECMO 2009 group, 16 [12-19]; ECMO 2016 group, 11 [9-13]; $p = 0.030$). There were no significant differences in the underlying conditions, complications, and the use of rescue and adjunctive therapies (prone positioning, renal replacement therapy, non-invasive positive pressure ventilation) between the groups. The use of peramivir was significantly increased, and the use of oseltamivir was significantly decreased in 2016 compared with 2009. The baseline pressure of arterial oxygen/fraction of inspiratory oxygen ratio (80 vs 55; $p = 0.009$) and the lowest pressure of arterial oxygen/fraction of inspiratory oxygen ratio (70 vs 50; $p = 0.002$) were higher in 2016 compared with 2009. The highest positive end-expiratory pressure was lower in 2016 compared with 2009 (15 vs 24 cmH$_2$O; $p = 0.015$). The lowest compliance in 2016 was 31 (9–42) mL/cmH$_2$O.

### Changes in ECMO equipment

There were significant changes in the proportions of the console, circuit, oxygenator, and centrifugal pump between 2009 and 2016. The ECMO equipment models used in 2016 widely varied, whereas those in 2009 were almost

**Table 1** Baseline characteristics of the patients enrolled

| Year | 2009 | 2016 | p value |
|---|---|---|---|
| n | 14 | 14 | |
| Age | 54 (43–60) | 52 (43–63) | 0.70 |
| Sex (male/female) | 12/2 | 12/2 | > 0.99 |
| Weight (kg) | 70 (64–80) | 67 (59–78) | 0.50 |
| BMI | NA | 23 (22–27) | |
| Body temperature (°C) | | | |
|   On admission | 38.8 (37.1–39.1) | 37.5 (36.7–38.2) | 0.11 |
|   Maximum | 39.4 (38.7–39.8) | 38.2 (37.7–39.7) | 0.21 |
| APACHE II score | 17 (12–25) | 20 (5–37) | 0.30 |
| Predicted death rate (%) | 24.9 (14.6–54.1) | 38.0 (34.5–47.8) | 0.24 |
| Maximum SOFA score | 16 (12–19) | 11 (9–13) | 0.030 |
| Underlying condition | | | |
|   Immunosuppression | 0 (0) | 3 (21) | 0.22 |
|   Drug abuse | 1 (7) | 0 (0) | > 0.99 |
|   Pregnancy | 1 (7) | 0 (0) | > 0.99 |
|   COPD | 0 (0) | 2 (14) | 0.46 |
|   Chronic renal failure | 0 (0) | 2 (14) | 0.46 |
| Vaccination | 1 (7) | 1 (7) | > 0.99 |
| Influenza antigen/PCR (A/B) | 14 / 0 | 14 / 0 | > 0.99 |
| Complications | | | |
|   Acute renal failure | 7 (50) | 9 (64) | 0.70 |
|   Acute hepatic failure | 4 (29) | 1 (7) | 0.32 |
|   Culture-confirmed infection | 5 (36) | 10 (71) | 0.13 |
|   Shock | 4 (29) | 5 (36) | > 0.99 |
|   Cardiac failure | 0 (0) | 0 (0) | > 0.99 |
|   Respiratory failure | 1 (7) | 2 (14) | > 0.99 |
|   Neurological impairment | 0 (0) | 0 (0) | > 0.99 |
| Medical treatment | | | |
|   Peramivir | 5 (36) | 14 (100) | 0.001 |
|   Oseltamivir | 6 (43) | 0 (0) | 0.021 |
|   Zanamivir | 1 (7) | 1 (7) | > 0.99 |
|   Laninamivir | 0 (0) | 0 (0) | > 0.99 |
|   Antibiotics | 13 (93) | 13 (93) | > 0.99 |
|   gamma-globulin | 5 (36) | 3 (21) | 0.68 |
|   Corticosteroid | | | |
|    High-dose methylprednisolone | 9 (64) | 6 (43) | 0.45 |
|    Low dose | 7 (50) | 6 (43) | > 0.99 |
|   Sivelestat | 5 (36) | 1 (7) | 0.17 |
|   Vasoactive drugs | 13 (93) | 11 (79) | 0.24 |
| Rescue and adjunctive therapies | | | |
|   Prone | 3 (21) | 5 (36) | 0.68 |
|   Nitric oxide | 1 (7) | 2 (14) | > 0.99 |
|   CRRT | 7 (50) | 7 (50) | > 0.99 |

**Table 1** Baseline characteristics of the patients enrolled *(Continued)*

| Year | 2009 | 2016 | *p* value |
|---|---|---|---|
| HFOV | 0 (0) | 0 (0) | > 0.99 |
| APRV | 13 (93) | 5 (36) | 0.006 |
| NPPV | 3 (21) | 4 (29) | > 0.99 |
| Respiratory impairment before starting ECMO | | | |
| PaO$_2$/F$_I$O$_2$ before starting ventilation | 55 (46–65) | 80 (64–80) | 0.009 |
| PaO$_2$/F$_I$O$_2$ at starting ventilation | 78 (58–86) | 96 (72–150) | 0.09 |
| Lowest PaO$_2$/F$_I$O$_2$ during ventilation | 50 (41–52) | 70 (58–75) | 0.002 |
| PEEP at starting ventilation (cmH2O) | 10 (10–11) | 11 (8–14) | 0.48 |
| Highest PEEP during ventilation (cmH$_2$O) | 24 (17–30) | 15 (14–19) | 0.015 |
| PIP at starting ventilation (cmH$_2$O) | 25 (21–29) | 21 (18–27) | 0.17 |
| Highest PIP during ventilation (cmH$_2$O) | 30 (30–34) | 28 (25–30) | 0.10 |
| OI at starting ventilation | NA | 16 (3–21) | |
| Highest OI during ventilation | NA | 20 (8–27) | |

Data are expressed as median (interquartile) or number (%)

*BMI* body mass index, *APACHE* acute physiology and chronic health evaluation, *SOFA* sequential organ failure assessment, *COPD* chronic obstructive pulmonary disease, *PCR* polymerase chain reaction, *DIC* disseminated intravascular coagulation; *CRRT* continuous renal replacement therapy, *HFOV* high-frequency oscillatory ventilation, *APRV* airway pressure release ventilation, *NPPV* non-invasive positive pressure ventilation, *ECMO*, extracorporeal membrane oxygenation, *PaO$_2$/FIO$_2$* pressure of arterial oxygen/fraction of inspiratory oxygen ratio, *PEEP* positive end-expiratory pressure, *PIP* peak inspiratory pressure, *OI* oxygenation index, ICU intensive care unit, *NA* not available

homogeneous. The diameters of drainage and return cannulas were significantly larger in 2016 compared with 2009 (*p* = 0.0097, *p* = 0.022, respectively; Fig. 1). The durations of each circuit were 4.0 (3.3–4.9) days in 2009, and 8.5 (6.5–14.9) days in 2016, respectively (*p* = 0.0001).

### Approach sites and complications of ECMO

Table 2 shows the approach sites and complications of ECMO. A drainage cannula was inserted in the femoral vein in all of the patients, and a return cannula was inserted into the right jugular vein in 86% of patients in 2009. However, in 2016, the approach sites of drainage and return cannulas were markedly changed. Femoral and right jugular veins became used for either drainage or a

return cannula. There were no differences in the incidence of complications, such as oxygenator failure, blood clots, cannula-related problems, pump head complications, massive bleeding, hemolysis, and venous thrombosis. There were also no differences in the incidence of adverse events indirectly associated with the ECMO circuit, such as massive bleeding, hemolysis, disseminated intravascular coagulation, and venous thrombus.

### Outcomes of patients

Outcomes of the patients enrolled are shown in Table 3. Ventilator days before ECMO were shortened from 5.0 days (1.0–7.0 days) to 1.0 day (1.0–2.8 days), but this difference was not significant. Total ventilator days were

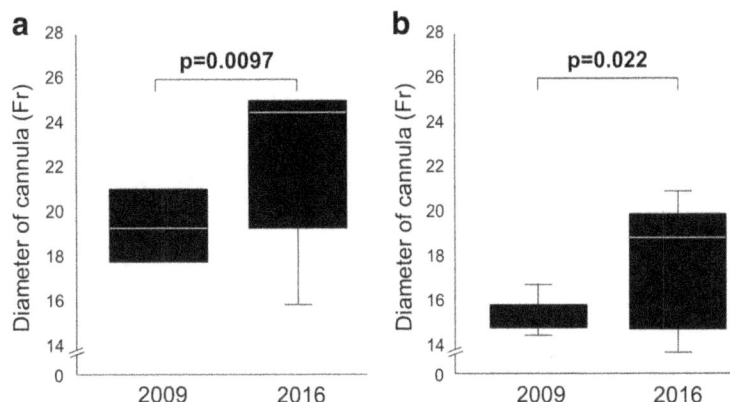

**Fig. 1** Diameters of the drainage and return cannulas. Box plot graph showing the diameters of **a** the drainage cannula and **b** return cannula used in 2009 and 2016. The diameters of both cannulas were significantly larger in 2016 compared with those in 2009

**Table 2** Approach sites and complications of ECMO

| Year | 2009 | 2016 | p value |
|---|---|---|---|
| Approach site of drainage cannula | | | 0.021 |
| Femoral vein | 14 (100) | 8 (57) | |
| Right jugular vein | 0 (0) | 6 (43) | |
| Approach site of return cannula | | | 0.0498 |
| Femoral vein | 2 (14) | 6 (43) | |
| Right jugular vein | 12 (86) | 6 (43) | |
| Femoral artery | 0 (0) | 2 (14) | |
| Adverse events directly related to the ECMO circuit | | | |
| Oxygenator failure | 7 (50) | 6 (43) | > 0.99 |
| Blood clots | | | |
| Oxygenator | 3 (21) | 8 (57) | 0.12 |
| Other circuit | 1 (7) | 2 (14) | > 0.99 |
| Cannula-related problems | 3 (21) | 3 (21) | > 0.99 |
| Pump head complications | 1 (7) | 1 (7) | > 0.99 |
| Adverse events indirectly related to the ECMO circuit | | | |
| Massive bleeding | | | |
| Surgical site | 4 (29) | 3 (21) | > 0.99 |
| Upper digestive tract | 4 (29) | 2 (14) | 0.65 |
| Cannulation site | 2 (14) | 2 (14) | > 0.99 |
| Pulmonary hemorrhage | 1 (7) | 0 (0) | > 0.99 |
| Hemolysis | 2 (14) | 1 (7) | > 0.99 |
| Disseminated intravascular coagulation | 10 (71) | 5 (36) | 0.13 |
| Venous thrombus | 2 (14) | 4 (21) | 0.50 |

*ECMO* extracorporeal membrane oxygenation

not significantly different between the ECMO 2016 group and the ECMO 2009 group. Duration of the use of each circuit was significantly longer in 2016 than in 2009 ($p = 0.0001$). There was no difference in the number of patients per institute in 2016 compared with 2009. The length of intensive care unit (ICU) stay was significantly longer in 2016 than in 2009 ($p = 0.038$). The overall survival rate tended to be better in 2016 compared with 2009 ($p = 0.054$).

**Overall survival**

Kaplan–Meier curves show the overall survival rates in each group (Fig. 2). There was a significant difference between the groups ($p = 0.007$, log-rank test). Univariate analysis demonstrated that the use of ECMO in 2016 (hazard ratio, 6.33; 95% confidence interval [CI], 1.35–33.3; $p = 0.019$) and the maximum SOFA score (hazard ratio, 0.86; 95% CI, 0.76–0.96; $p = 0.010$) were predictive factors of better overall survival. In multivariate analysis, the use of ECMO in 2016 (hazard ratio, 7.25; 95% CI, 1.35–33.3; $p = 0.021$) and the maximum SOFA score (hazard ratio, 0.81; 95% CI, 0.69–0.95; $p = 0.011$) were independent predictive factors of better overall survival (Table 4).

**Discussion**

In this study, we showed that the ECMO equipment used for acute respiratory failure in Japan was significantly changed in 2016 compared with 2009. Additionally, the overall survival rate had improved in patients with influenza-associated acute respiratory failure by 2016. Multivariate analysis showed that the use of

**Table 3** Outcomes of the patients enrolled

| Year | 2009 | 2016 | p value |
|---|---|---|---|
| Ventilator days before ECMO (days) | 5.0 (1.0–7.0) | 1.0 (1.0–2.8) | 0.11 |
| Total ventilator days (days) | 19 (9–25) | 27 (14–38) | 0.24 |
| Ventilator-free days (days) | 1.5 (0–10.5) | 7.5 (4–27) | 0.12 |
| Length of ECMO therapy (days) | 8.5 (4.5–10.0) | 10.0 (8.3–32.5) | 0.08 |
| Number of circuits used | 2.0 (1.3–3.0) | 1.0 (1.0–2.0) | 0.14 |
| Duration of each circuit (days) | 4.0 (3.3–4.9) | 8.5 (6.5–14.9) | 0.0001 |
| Number of patients (per institute) | 1.0 (1.0–1.0) | 1.0 (1.0–1.8) | 0.42 |
| Length of ICU stay (days) | 17 (9–26) | 29 (20–41) | 0.038 |
| Length of ICU stay in survived patients (days) | 24 (17–26) | 24 (20–38) | 0.57 |
| Length of hospital stay (days) | 25 (12–53) | 41 (27–65) | 0.14 |
| Length of hospital stay in survived patients (days) | 69 (40–77) | 42 (23–70) | 0.38 |
| Days alive (days) | 25 (14–46) | 43 (37–73) | 0.073 |
| Overall survival rate | 5 (36) | 11 (79) | 0.054 |
| In-hospital survival rate | 5 (36) | 11 (79) | 0.054 |
| 60-day survival rate | 5 (36) | 12 (86) | 0.018 |

Data are expressed as median (interquartile) or number (%)

*ECMO* extracorporeal membrane oxygenation, *ICU* intensive care unit, *NA* not available

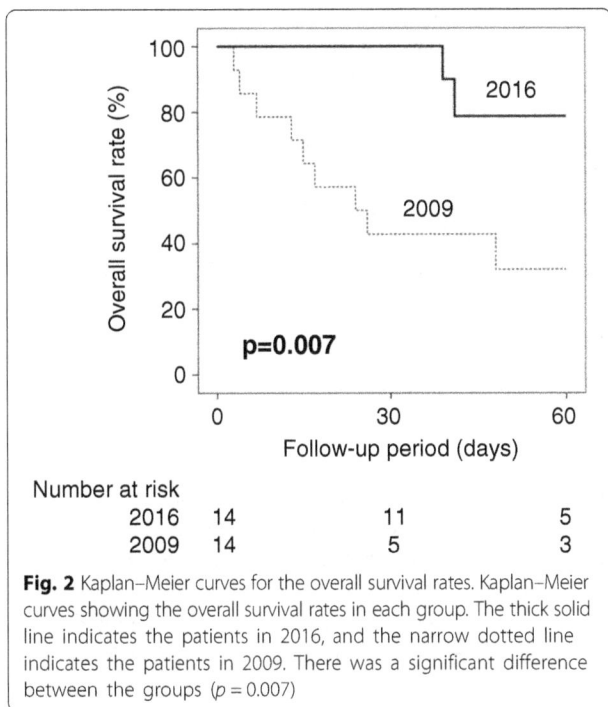

**Fig. 2** Kaplan–Meier curves for the overall survival rates. Kaplan–Meier curves showing the overall survival rates in each group. The thick solid line indicates the patients in 2016, and the narrow dotted line indicates the patients in 2009. There was a significant difference between the groups (p = 0.007)

ECMO in 2016 was an independent predictive factor for a favorable survival.

Takeda et al. showed that the survival rate of patients with 2009 H1N1 influenza-associated respiratory failure managed with ECMO was limited to 36% [4]. They also found that the majority of patients suffered from adverse events associated with the use of ECMO. Previous studies from Europe and Oceania showed the benefit of ECMO for influenza-associated acute respiratory failure [7]. The survival rates in patients with 2009 H1N1 influenza-associated

respiratory failure managed with ECMO were 92% in Sweden [6], 76% in the UK [5], 70% in Australia and New Zealand [8], 68% in Italy [9], and 56% in France [10]. Despite the variation in survival rate according to the country, the survival rates in these countries were always better than that in Japan. A recent meta-analysis regarding the benefit of ECMO for influenza-associated acute respiratory failure demonstrated the worst mortality in Japan of 65% compared with the other 12 countries included in this meta-analysis [11]. This finding might be partially explained by the insufficient knowledge and skill in Japan in 2009 regarding ECMO equipment and the relevant physiology.

Based on the insufficient survival rate in 2009, the ECMO project was established in Japan to improve the survival rate of influenza-associated respiratory failure. The educational activity by the ECMO project during these years included the lecture regarding physiology of ECMO, managements of bleeding, coagulation, infection and sedation, selection of pumps, oxygenators and cannulae, and the hands-on simulation for the replacement of oxygenators and total circuits, shift from venovenous to venoarterial ECMO, priming of circuits, and fixing mechanical problems. Activity and education by the committee of the ECMO project in Japan might have changed the strategy of ECMO use and promoted improvement of ECMO management, and consequently, the survival rate in patients with influenza-associated acute respiratory failure had improved in 2016. This was partly reflected by changes in oxygenators and pumps shifting to the long-term durability models, diameters of cannulas shifting to a larger size, and the duration of each circuit use becoming longer. In addition, the number of adverse events was similar in 2009 and 2016 despite the longer

**Table 4** Univariate and multivariate analyses for better in-hospital and out-of-hospital overall survival

| Variable | β | HR | (95%CI) | p value |
|---|---|---|---|---|
| Univariate analysis | | | | |
| Use of ECMO in 2016 | 1.85 | 6.33 | (1.35–33.3) | 0.019 |
| Baseline PaO2/FIO2Baseline PaO2/FIO2 | 0.05 | 1.05 | (0.98–1.11) | 0.15 |
| Lowest PaO2/FIO2Lowest PaO2/FIO2 | 0.03 | 1.03 | (0.98–1.08) | 0.27 |
| Highest PEEP (cmH2O) Highest PEEP (cmH2O) | − 0.07 | 0.93 | (0.85–1.02) | 0.12 |
| Maximum SOFA score | − 0.15 | 0.86 | (0.76–0.96) | 0.010 |
| Use of peramivir | 0.81 | 2.25 | (0.68–7.14) | 0.18 |
| Use of oseltamivir | − 0.85 | 0.43 | (0.12–1.47) | 0.18 |
| Use of APRV | − 0.36 | 0.70 | (0.18–2.63) | 0.60 |
| Size of drainage cannula | − 0.16 | 0.85 | (0.43–1.69) | 0.65 |
| Size of return cannula | 0.20 | 1.22 | (0.57–2.63) | 0.60 |
| Multivariate analysis | | | | |
| Use of ECMO in 2016 | 1.98 | 7.25 | (1.35–33.3) | 0.021 |
| Maximum SOFA score | − 0.21 | 0.81 | (0.69–0.95) | 0.011 |

HR hazard ratio, CI confidence interval, ECMO, extracorporeal membrane oxygenation, PaO2/FIO2 partial pressure of arterial oxygen/fraction of inspiratory oxygen ratios, PEEP positive end-expiratory pressure, SOFA sequential organ failure assessment, APRV airway pressure release ventilation

duration of each circuit, which might have associated with the improved management of ECMO.

Although the severity of an H1N1 influenza infection that occurred in Mexico and the USA in 2009 was similar to that of seasonal influenza, many patients developed severe respiratory failure that was not typical of conventional seasonal influenza [4]. Our study showed that the severity of influenza-associated acute respiratory failure in Japan in 2016 was similar to that of in 2009 according to the APACHE II score and predicted death rate. Despite the similar severity, we could have significantly improved the survival rate. Recent advances in technology (e.g., biocompatible artificial membranes, heparin-coated circuits, and smaller devices), and network organization with referral ECMO centers have contributed to the dramatic increase in the use of ECMO [12, 13]. However, despite these technological improvements, ECMO is still associated with many complications including bleeding, thrombosis, and nosocomial infection [14–16]. Additionally, in-hospital mortality still remains high (35%–45%), and long-term impairment in physical/psychological function is also significant [16, 17]. Considerable investment for high costs of resources, staffing, and training might be important for improving survival rate and reducing complications. Therefore, improvement in overall survival without any increase in complications observed in this study was impressive. Although this improvement in overall survival might have been associated with an application of ECMO in milder cases, multivariate analysis after adjustment for the SOFA score discounted this possibility.

Baseline and lowest $PaO_2/F_IO_2$ ratios were higher in 2016 than in 2009, suggesting better oxygenation and lower severity status of the enrolled patients in 2016. In addition, ECMO-associated equipment has been improved in 2016. However, the length of ICU stay was significantly longer in 2016, which was likely to be associated with the improved ability of longer management of ECMO with smaller number of complications.

Bleeding is a serious complication that is associated with ECMO and occurs in approximately 20% of patients [18, 19]. The main mechanisms of bleeding include excessive anticoagulation, thrombocytopenia, and consumption of coagulation factors. Use of ECMO circuits time-dependently activates plasma metalloproteinase-2, a pathway of platelet aggregation, with a subsequent increase in plasma soluble P-selectin concentrations [20]. The resultant platelet dysfunction persists after repeated transfusions of platelets to maintain sufficient platelet counts. Acquired von Willebrand syndrome could also be a complication associated with ECMO. This is characterized by loss of the high molecular weight of von Willebrand factor as a result of shear stress, which impairs binding of von Willebrand factor to platelets [21]. Therefore, adequate selection of ECMO equipment is essential to minimize the shear stress. A shift to the long-term durability models of oxygenators and pumps and to the larger size of diameter of cannulas could have contributed to the reduction in platelet dysfunction, resulting in the longer durability of each circuit in our study.

Previous studies have suggested that centralization of ECMO use to expert referral centers may contribute to improved survival [22, 23]. Propensity score matching analysis suggested that transfer to an ECMO center was associated with a 50% reduction in mortality [5]. Bryner et al. suggested that ECMO centers experiencing more than 30 cases/year were consistently associated with better survival [24]. However, concluding that use of ECMO itself improves survival is difficult because ECMO centers are usually centers of excellence, which can provide better overall intensive care [25]. No definite conclusion can be made because of the lack of randomized, controlled trials. However, adequate use of ECMO after the onset of acute respiratory failure can result in improved survival. Although centralization of ECMO use in Japan has been partially promoted, the number of patients per institute has not yet significantly increased.

Despite the similar severity according to the APACHE II score and predicted death rate, baseline $PaO_2/F_IO_2$ ratios before and during ventilation were significantly different in both groups. Higher $PaO_2/F_IO_2$ ratio in 2016 may have associated with less severity in lung injury or early initiation of ECMO. The indication criteria of ECMO are generally considered as patients with mortality risk of 50 to 80%, according to the Extracorporeal Life Support Organization Guidelines [26]. However, the use of ECMO can be associated with various severities of complications, and permissive hypoxemia is an emerging concept in which a lower level of arterial oxygenation can be accepted to avoid the harmful effects of high concentration of inspired oxygen and invasive mechanical ventilation [27]. Therefore, the indication criteria of ECMO might be reconsidered in the future studies.

Our study includes several potential limitations. First, this study was based on surveillance, which did not cover all patients who received ECMO. Second, several clinical items were not completely included because of the retrospective design. Further prospective studies are necessary for confirming the data observed in this study.

## Conclusions

In conclusion, the surveillance in Japan showed that the overall survival rate was significantly improved in patients with influenza-associated acute respiratory failure, who were managed with ECMO in 2016 compared with those in 2009. The procedures of respiratory management using ECMO have significantly changed in 2016. Adequate use of ECMO equipment and promoting better understanding of ECMO physiology in medical staff might have been associated with the improved survival rate in patients with influenza-associated acute respiratory failure in Japan.

## Abbreviations
APACHE: Acute physiology and chronic health evaluation; CI: Confidence interval; ECMO : Extracorporeal membrane oxygenation; $F_iO_2$: Fraction of inspiratory oxygen; $PaO_2$: Partial pressure of arterial oxygen; SOFA: Sequential organ failure assessment

## Acknowledgements
We thank the following institutes included in the ECMO registry (ecmo-kokyu-jsicm@jrcm.in.arena.ne.jp) for data collection of this study: Chiba University, Hiroshima General Hospital, Japanese Red Cross, Musashino Hospital, Jichi Medical University, Kobe University, Kurume University, Maebashi Red Cross Hospital, Nagasaki University, National Center for Global Health and Medicine, Niigata University, Nippon Medical School, Osaka City University, Osaka Women's and Children's Hospital, Tokyo Metropolitan Bokutoh Hospital, Tokyo Metropolitan Children's Medical Center, and Tsukuba University.
We thank Ellen Knapp, PhD, from Edanz Group (www.edanzediting.com/ac) for editing a draft of this manuscript.

## Funding
This work was supported by a Japan Society for the Promotion of Science (JSPS) KAKENHI Grant (Numbers JP 16K09541, 17K11573), Strategic Information and Communications R&D Promotion Programme (SCOPE), and the Japan Agency for Medical Research and Development (AMED).

## Authors' contributions
SO collected and analyzed the data and drafted the manuscript. NS supervised the study and revised the manuscript. SN, ON, and ST designed and organized the study, helped with data collection, and revised the manuscript. All authors read and approved the final manuscript.

## Competing interests
The authors declare that they have no competing interests.

## Author details
[1]Department of Emergency and Critical Care Medicine, Graduate School of Biomedical and Health Sciences, Hiroshima University, 1-2-3 Kasumi, Minami-ku, Hiroshima 734-8551, Japan. [2]Department of Critical Care and Anesthesia, National Center for Child Health and Development, Tokyo, Japan. [3]Department of Anaesthesiology and Critical Care Medicine, Fujita Health University School of Medicine, Aichi, Japan. [4]Kawaguchi Cardiovascular and Respiratory Hospital, Saitama, Japan.

## References
1. Centers for Disease Control and Prevention (CDC). Estimates of deaths associated with seasonal influenza — United States, 1976-2007. MMWR Morb Mortal Wkly Rep. 2010;59:1057–62.
2. Fan E, Pham T. Extracorporeal membrane oxygenation for severe acute respiratory failure: yes we can! (but should we?). Am J Respir Crit Care Med. 2014;189:1293–5.
3. Cooper DJ, Hodgson CL. Extracorporeal membrane oxygenation rescue for H1N1 acute respiratory distress syndrome: equipoise regained. Am J Respir Crit Care Med. 2013;187:224–6.
4. Takeda S, Kotani T, Nakagawa S, Ichiba S, Aokage T, Ochiai R, Taenaka N, Kawamae K, Nishimura M, Ujike Y, Tajimi K. Extracorporeal membrane oxygenation for 2009 influenza a (H1N1) severe respiratory failure in Japan. J Anesth. 2012;26:650–7.
5. Noah MA, Peek GJ, Finney SJ, Griffiths MJ, Harrison DA, Grieve R, Sadique MZ, Sekhon JS, McAuley DF, Firmin RK, Harvey C, Cordingley JJ, Price S, Vuylsteke A, Jenkins DP, Noble DW, Bloomfield R, Walsh TS, Perkins GD, Menon D, Taylor BL, Rowan KM. Referral to an extracorporeal membrane oxygenation center and mortality among patients with severe 2009 influenza a (H1N1). JAMA. 2011;306:1659–68.
6. Holzgraefe B, Broome M, Kalzen H, Konrad D, Palmer K, Frenckner B. Extracorporeal membrane oxygenation for pandemic H1N1 2009 respiratory failure. Minerva Anestesiol. 2010;76:1043–51.
7. Zangrillo A, Biondi-Zoccai G, Landoni G, Frati G, Patroniti N, Pesenti A, Pappalardo F. Extracorporeal membrane oxygenation (ECMO) in patients with H1N1 influenza infection: a systematic review and meta-analysis including 8 studies and 266 patients receiving ECMO. Crit Care. 2013;17:R30.
8. Davies A, Jones D, Bailey M, Beca J, Bellomo R, Blackwell N, Forrest P, Gattas D, Granger E, Herkes R, Jackson A, McGuinness S, Nair P, Pellegrino V, Pettila V, Plunkett B, Pye R, Torzillo P, Webb S, Wilson M, Ziegenfuss M. Extracorporeal membrane oxygenation for 2009 influenza a (H1N1) acute respiratory distress syndrome. JAMA. 2009;302:1888–95.
9. Patroniti N, Zangrillo A, Pappalardo F, Peris A, Cianchi G, Braschi A, Iotti GA, Arcadipane A, Panarello G, Ranieri VM, Terragni P, Antonelli M, Gattinoni L, Oleari F, Pesenti A. The Italian ECMO network experience during the 2009 influenza a (H1N1) pandemic: preparation for severe respiratory emergency outbreaks. Intensive Care Med. 2011;37:1447–57.
10. Roch A, Lepaul-Ercole R, Grisoli D, Bessereau J, Brissy O, Castanier M, Dizier S, Forel JM, Guervilly C, Gariboldi V, Collart F, Michelet P, Perrin G, Charrel R, Papazian L. Extracorporeal membrane oxygenation for severe influenza a (H1N1) acute respiratory distress syndrome: a prospective observational comparative study. Intensive Care Med. 2010;36:1899–905.
11. Sukhal S, Sethi J, Ganesh M, Villablanca PA, Malhotra AK, Ramakrishna H. Extracorporeal membrane oxygenation in severe influenza infection with respiratory failure: a systematic review and meta-analysis. Ann Card Anaesth. 2017;20:14–21.
12. MacLaren G, Combes A, Bartlett RH. Contemporary extracorporeal membrane oxygenation for adult respiratory failure: life support in the new era. Intensive Care Med. 2012;38:210–20.
13. Blum JM, Lynch WR, Coopersmith CM. Clinical and billing review of extracorporeal membrane oxygenation. Chest. 2015;147:1697–703.
14. Schmidt M, Zogheib E, Roze H, Repesse X, Lebreton G, Luyt CE, Trouillet JL, Brechot N, Nieszkowska A, Dupont H, Ouattara A, Leprince P, Chastre J, Combes A. The PRESERVE mortality risk score and analysis of long-term outcomes after extracorporeal membrane oxygenation for severe acute respiratory distress syndrome. Intensive Care Med. 2013;39:1704–13.
15. Cooper E, Burns J, Retter A, Salt G, Camporota L, Meadows CI, Langrish CC, Wyncoll D, Glover G, Ioannou N, Daly K, Barrett NA. Prevalence of venous thrombosis following Venovenous extracorporeal membrane oxygenation in patients with severe respiratory failure. Crit Care Med. 2015;43:e581–4.
16. Zangrillo A, Landoni G, Biondi-Zoccai G, Greco M, Greco T, Frati G, Patroniti N, Antonelli M, Pesenti A. Pappalardo F. A meta-analysis of complications and mortality of extracorporeal membrane oxygenation. Crit Care Resusc. 2013;15:172–8.
17. Rozencwajg S, Pilcher D, Combes A, Schmidt M. Outcomes and survival prediction models for severe adult acute respiratory distress syndrome treated with extracorporeal membrane oxygenation. Crit Care. 2016;20:392.
18. Munshi L, Telesnicki T, Walkey A, Fan E. Extracorporeal life support for acute respiratory failure. A systematic review and metaanalysis. Ann Am Thorac Soc. 2014;11:802–10.
19. Ried M, Bein T, Philipp A, Muller T, Graf B, Schmid C, Zonies D, Diez C,

Hofmann HS. Extracorporeal lung support in trauma patients with severe chest injury and acute lung failure: a 10-year institutional experience. Crit Care. 2013;17:R110.

20. Cheung PY, Sawicki G, Salas E, Etches PC, Schulz R, Radomski MW. The mechanisms of platelet dysfunction during extracorporeal membrane oxygenation in critically ill neonates. Crit Care Med. 2000;28:2584–90.

21. Heilmann C, Geisen U, Beyersdorf F, Nakamura L, Benk C, Trummer G, Berchtold-Herz M, Schlensak C, Zieger B. Acquired von Willebrand syndrome in patients with extracorporeal life support (ECLS). Intensive Care Med. 2012; 38:62–8.

22. Barbaro RP, Odetola FO, Kidwell KM, Paden ML, Bartlett RH, Davis MM, Annich GM. Association of hospital-level volume of extracorporeal membrane oxygenation cases and mortality. Analysis of the extracorporeal life support organization registry. Am J Respir Crit Care Med. 2015;191:894–901.

23. Peek GJ, Mugford M, Tiruvoipati R, Wilson A, Allen E, Thalanany MM, Hibbert CL, Truesdale A, Clemens F, Cooper N, Firmin RK, Elbourne D. Efficacy and economic assessment of conventional ventilatory support versus extracorporeal membrane oxygenation for severe adult respiratory failure (CESAR): a multicentre randomised controlled trial. Lancet. 2009;374:1351–63.

24. Bryner B, Cooley E, Copenhaver W, Brierley K, Teman N, Landis D, Rycus P, Hemmila M, Napolitano LM, Haft J, Park PK, Bartlett RH. Two decades' experience with interfacility transport on extracorporeal membrane oxygenation. Ann Thorac Surg. 2014;98:1363–70.

25. Wallace DJ, Milbrandt EB, Boujoukos A. Ave, CESAR, morituri te salutant! (hail, CESAR, those who are about to die salute you!). Crit Care. 2010;14:308.

26. Extracorporeal Life Support Organization (ELSO). General Guidelines for all ECLS Cases. https://www.elso.org/Portals/0/ ELSO%20Guidelines%20General%20All%20ECLS%20Version%201_4.pdf. Accessed 30 May 2018.

27. Gilbert-Kawai ET, Mitchell K, Martin D, Carlisle J, Grocott MP. Permissive hypoxaemia versus normoxaemia for mechanically ventilated critically ill patients. Cochrane Database Syst Rev. 2014;5:CD009931.

# 25

# Vasopressin versus norepinephrine in septic shock: a propensity score matched efficiency retrospective cohort study in the VASST coordinating center hospital

James A. Russell[1,2*], Hugh Wellman[3] and Keith R. Walley[1,2]

## Abstract

**Purpose:** It is not clear whether vasopressin versus norepinephrine changed mortality in clinical practice in the Vasopressin and Septic Shock Trial (VASST) coordinating center hospital after VASST was published. We tested the hypothesis that vasopressin changed mortality compared to norepinephrine using propensity matching of vasopressin to norepinephrine-treated patients in the VASST coordinating center hospital before (SPH1) and after (SPH2) VASST was published.

**Methods:** Vasopressin-treated patients were propensity score matched to norepinephrine-treated patients based on age, APACHE II, respiratory, renal, and hematologic dysfunction, mechanical ventilation status, medical/surgical status, infection site, and norepinephrine dose. The propensity score estimated the probability that a patient would have received vasopressin given baseline characteristics. For sensitivity analysis, we then excluded patients who had underlying severe congestive heart failure. The primary outcome was 28-day mortality.

**Results:** Vasopressin- and norepinephrine-treated patients were similar after matching in SPH1 (pre-VASST); vasopressin-treated patients ($n = 158$) had a significantly higher mortality than norepinephrine-treated patients ($n = 158$) (60.8 vs. 46.2%, $p = 0.009$). In SPH2 after matching, the 28-day mortality rates were not significantly different; 31.2% and 26.9% in the vasopressin ($n = 93$) and norepinephrine ($n = 93$) groups, respectively ($p = 0.518$). The day 1 vasopressin dose in SPH1 vs. SPH2 was 0.036 units/min (SD 0.009) vs. 0.032 units/min (SD 0.005), $p = 0.001$, significantly lower in SPH2 after VASST.

**Conclusions:** Before VASST, vasopressin use was associated with increased mortality compared to norepinephrine in the VASST coordinating center hospital. After VASST, there was no difference in mortality between vasopressin- and norepinephrine-treated patients. This may be the first retrospective propensity-matched cohort study of a sepsis treatment in a center that had previously coordinated a large pivotal randomized controlled trial of that treatment and could be a useful approach for other sepsis therapies.

**Keywords:** Septic shock, Vasopressin, Norepinephrine, Propensity match, Efficiency, Mortality, VASST

* Correspondence: Jim.Russell@hli.ubc.ca
[1]Centre for Heart Lung Innovation, St. Paul's Hospital, University of British Columbia, 1081 Burrard Street, Vancouver, BC V6Z 1Y6, Canada
[2]Division of Critical Care Medicine, St. Paul's Hospital, University of British Columbia, 1081 Burrard Street, Vancouver, BC V6Z 1Y6, Canada
Full list of author information is available at the end of the article

## Introduction

Vasopressin is deficient in septic shock [1, 2] and low-dose vasopressin infusion decreased norepinephrine dose requirements and organ dysfunction in early uncontrolled [3, 4] and controlled studies that were not powered for mortality [5]. The VASST trial (Vasopressin and Septic Shock Trial) [6] was a randomized blinded controlled trial of vasopressin vs. norepinephrine in septic shock powered for mortality. Although there was no overall statistically significant difference in mortality, some authors [7] and the Surviving Sepsis Campaign (SSC) [8] recommend the use of vasopressin in patients who are not responsive to norepinephrine. The Vasopressin vs. Norepinephrine as Initial Therapy in Septic Shock (VANISH) randomized controlled trial of vasopressin vs. norepinephrine used a higher dose and applied vasopressin earlier in septic shock but found no difference in acute kidney injury (the primary endpoint) or mortality [9] but did observe a reduction in the use of renal replacement therapy in vasopressin-treated patients. Efficacy trials such as VASST and VANISH should be followed by effectiveness studies to further assess whether publication of high-quality data alters practice and clinical outcomes.

Physicians have often been slow to adapt practice as new evidence is reported resulting in decreased compliance with guidelines and recommendations. It is possible that physicians would adapt practice more quickly and more widely in the centers that coordinated large pivotal trials that were incorporated into guidelines.

Studies of vasopressin use in clinical practice are limited. Physicians' indications for use of vasopressin vary widely, and there is potential overuse of vasopressin in a survey of American intensivists [10]. Vail et al. [11] found wide variability (5–20% use) in clinical use of vasopressin in septic shock across the USA, suggesting local institution policies and physician beliefs drive use of vasopressin [12]. Neither of these studies evaluated mortality. One observational study (not matched) found no difference in vasopressin- vs. norepinephrine-treated patients' mortality but did not address the period prior to or after VASST [13].

To date, there have been no efficiency studies comparing the mortality rates of vasopressin- vs. norepinephrine-treated septic shock patients in practice before and after the VASST results were known in the VASST coordinating center hospital. Thus, it is not clear whether vasopressin use changed and whether vasopressin alters mortality compared to norepinephrine in clinical practice. We took advantage of our being the VASST coordinating center hospital to test the hypothesis that vasopressin alters mortality compared to norepinephrine in septic shock using a propensity-matched cohort of patients treated clinically in a tertiary care center in the periods before and after the publication of VASST [6] in the VASST coordinating center hospital.

## Methods

### General

This study adheres to the STROBE Guidelines.

### Ethics

The retrospective observational and de-identified SPH cohort studies (SPH1 and SPH2) were approved by the St. Paul's Hospital ethics committee who agreed that no patient consent was necessary.

### Patient cohorts

#### Inclusion criteria

This was a single university-affiliated tertiary care center study of use of vasopressin in the center that was the coordinating center of VASST. Patients admitted to the intensive care unit (ICU) of St. Paul's Hospital in Vancouver, BC, Canada, who had two of four SIRS criteria who had suspected or proven infection and who were unresponsive to fluid resuscitation and received infusion of norepinephrine or vasopressin were included. Vasopressin and norepinephrine were given according to local clinical practice, i.e., choice of therapy was not randomized, controlled, or blinded. Less severe septic shock was defined as treatment with < 15 μg/min norepinephrine, and more severe septic shock was defined as treatment with ≥ 15 μg/min norepinephrine (the same definition as was used in VASST [6]).

Patients recruited prior to publication of VASST (2001–2007) were included in the SPH1 cohort, and patients recruited following the publication of VASST (2008–2012) were included in the SPH2 cohort.

Vasopressin may have different effects in patients who have underlying severe congestive heart failure (CHF) New York Heart Association IV (NYHA IV), so for sensitivity analysis, we excluded patients who had NYHA IV CHF in a separate analysis. We used the written section of the chart to determine whether patients had NYHA class IV heart failure. The diagnosis of heart failure was not confirmed by prior Echo, MUGA scan, or cardiac catheterization results. The self-reporting of symptoms at rest was based on histories obtained from the patients and their families.

### Matching vasopressin-treated to norepinephrine-treated patients

Vasopressin was likely given according to individual patient preference and likely varied widely [14]. Therefore, a well-matched control group is fundamental to the validity of this non-randomized study. Accordingly, the current study incorporated a robust, well-accepted matching strategy. After meeting the eligibility criteria, norepinephrine-treated patients were matched with vasopressin-treated patients using a computerized optimal matching algorithm incorporating baseline demographic and disease characteristics that had been identified a priori as likely influencing, first, the decision to prescribe vasopressin or, second, the probability of death. The number of matched control patients for each vasopressin-treated patient varied from one to three to increase the precision in the estimation of the differences between groups [15, 16].

Matching variables were baseline age, gender, APACHE II score, organ dysfunction (respiratory, renal, and coagulation), use of mechanical ventilation, underlying medical vs. surgical diagnosis, norepinephrine dose, and propensity score.

The matching strategy combined minimum-distance matching using "calipers" that force the matches for selected variables to fall within specified tolerances. A propensity score of the estimated probability that a patient would have received vasopressin given their key baseline characteristics was calculated, and patients were selected as matches had to be within a prespecified tolerance on this score. Combining the use of propensity scores with covariate matching is superior to the use of either strategy alone [17]. Individual variables were used to compute a multivariate distance (Mahalanobis distance). The Mahalanobis distance is a statistical measure of the distance between a point P and a distribution D and so measures how many standard deviations a point P is from the mean of the distribution D [18]. The Mahalanobis distance measures the number of standard deviations from P to the mean of D.

A propensity score of the estimated probability that a patient would have received vasopressin given their key baseline characteristics was calculated because combining both the propensity score and covariate matching is superior to the use of either strategy alone [19]. The intended clinical variables for the calculation of the Mahalanobis distance and the reasons these variables are shown in Additional file 1: Table S1.

The propensity score was estimated using a logistic regression model for the treatment group using the matching variables included in the calculation of Mahalanobis distances. Calipers were applied to selected key variables to ensure close matches. For age, a maximum 5-year difference was chosen. The propensity score caliper was set at 0.6 standard deviations (of the average propensity score) because this often decreases bias [20–22].

## Outcomes
The primary outcome variable was 28-day mortality.

## Statistical analyses
Baseline characteristics of vasopressin- and norepinephrine-treated patients were compared using parametric procedures (independent $t$ test), non-parametric procedures (Wilcoxon rank sum test), or the Fisher exact test as appropriate. The primary analysis comparing 28-day mortality between the two treatment groups was performed using an unadjusted chi-square test according to treatment received. Conditional logistic regression was done to adjust for any baseline characteristics that remained significantly different ($p < 0.05$) between vasopressin- and norepinephrine-treated patients. Results are presented as absolute and relative risks and 95% confidence intervals. Kaplan-Meier curves describing the estimated probability of survival in the two treatment arms as a function of time from admission into the study were compared using the log-rank test statistic. Statistical significance was noted for $p < 0.05$.

## Results
### Overall SPH1 (pre-VASST)
In SPH1, there were 165 vasopressin-treated and 558 norepinephrine-treated patients before matching; at baseline, the vasopressin-treated patients were significantly younger, had higher APACHE II, and had more frequent renal, coagulation, and hepatic dysfunction, more often had underlying chronic disease and had a lower dose of norepinephrine (Table 1). After matching, vasopressin-treated ($n = 158$) and norepinephrine-treated ($n = 158$) patients were well matched (Table 1).

There was a significantly higher mortality rate in the vasopressin- (60.8%) vs. norepinephrine-treated patients (46.2%), $p = 0.009$ (Table 1) in SPH1. This difference in mortality represents an absolute risk reduction of 14.6% and a number needed to treat to save one life of 6.8.

### Sensitivity analysis—exclusion of patients who had NYHA IV CHF in SPH1 (pre-VASST)
We excluded patients who had underlying NYHA IV CHF in SPH1. There were 145 vasopressin-treated patients and 525 norepinephrine-treated before matching (Table 2). Before matching, vasopressin-treated patients were significantly younger, had higher APACHE II scores, were more frequently male, had more frequent renal, coagulation, hepatic, and CNS dysfunction, and were receiving a higher dose of norepinephrine at baseline (Table 2). After matching, there were 140 vasopressin-treated and 140 norepinephrine-treated patients (Table 2). The matching strategy and technique was quite successful; after matching, vasopressin- and norepinephrine-treated patients were well matched (Table 2).

After excluding patients who had NYHA IV CHF and then matching, the vasopressin-treated mortality remained significantly higher (62.9%) than that of the

**Table 1** Baseline characteristics and mortality before and after matching in SPH1

| Variable | Norepinephrine | Vasopressin | p |
|---|---|---|---|
| Baseline characteristics before matching of norepinephrine- vs. vasopressin-treated patients in SPH1 | | | |
| Age (years), $X \pm$ SD | $60.7 \pm 16.2$ | $56.1 \pm 15.7$ | < 0.001 |
| APACHE II, $X \pm$ SD | $25.6 \pm 8.0$ | $28.8 \pm 8.9$ | < 0.001 |
| Gender (% male) | 61.8 | 73.3 | 0.007 |
| Surgical (%) | 39.2 | 35.2 | 0.146 |
| Respiratory (%) | 88.3 | 92.1 | 0.17 |
| Renal (%) | 68.1 | 81.2 | < 0.001 |
| Coagulation (%) | 23.3 | 36.4 | < 0.001 |
| Hepatic (%) | 14.3 | 22.4 | 0.013 |
| Neurological (%) | 64.7 | 79.4 | < 0.001 |
| Ventilated (%) | 92.7 | 89.1 | 0.142 |
| Any chronic disease (%) | 44.8 | 55.8 | 0.013 |
| Norepinephrine dose (ug/min) | $13.2 \pm 14.8$ | $21.4 \pm 21.7$ | < 0.001 |
| Baseline characteristics after matching of norepinephrine- vs. vasopressin-treated patients in SPH1 | | | |
| Age (years), $X \pm$ SD | $57.1 \pm 15.1$ | $56.4 \pm 15.4$ | 0.65 |
| APACHE II, $X \pm$ SD | $28.1 \pm 8.3$ | $28.4 \pm 8.4$ | 0.782 |
| Gender (% male) | 67.1 | 72.8 | 0.27 |
| Surgical (%) | 34.8 | 34.8 | 1 |
| Respiratory (%) | 93.0 | 91.8 | 0.671 |
| Renal (%) | 74.7 | 81.0 | 0.176 |
| Coagulation (%) | 28.5 | 36.1 | 0.149 |
| Hepatic (%) | 18.4 | 22.2 | 0.401 |
| Neurological (%) | 69.0 | 78.5 | 0.055 |
| Ventilated (%) | 94.3 | 89.2 | 0.101 |
| Any chronic disease (%) | 51.9 | 54.4 | 0.652 |
| Norepinephrine dose (ug/min) | $15.9 \pm 16.7$ | $19.8 \pm 18.9$ | 0.139 |
| Mortality of norepinephrine- vs. vasopressin-treated patients in SPH1 | | | |
| 28-day mortality (%) | 46.2 | 60.8 | 0.009 |

**Table 2** Baseline characteristics and mortality of norepinephrine- vs. vasopressin-treated patients in SPH1 before and after matching. Sensitivity analysis after exclusion of patients who had underlying NYHA IV CHF

| Variable | Norepinephrine | Vasopressin | p |
|---|---|---|---|
| Baseline characteristics norepinephrine- vs. vasopressin-treated patients in SPH1 before matching | | | |
| Age (years), $X \pm$ SD | $60.2 \pm 16.3$ | $55.5 \pm 15.5$ | < 0.001 |
| APACHE II, $X \pm$ SD | $25.5 \pm 8.0$ | $29.0 \pm 8.7$ | < 0.001 |
| Gender (% male) | 61.3 | 73.1 | 0.009 |
| Surgical (%) | 28.2 | 31.0 | 0.503 |
| Respiratory (%) | 88.6 | 92.4 | 0.183 |
| Renal (%) | 68.4 | 82.8 | < 0.001 |
| Coagulation (%) | 23.4 | 38.0 | < 0.001 |
| Hepatic (%) | 13.9 | 22.8 | 0.01 |
| Neurological (%) | 64.8 | 80.0 | < 0.001 |
| Ventilated (%) | 92.4 | 89.0 | 0.188 |
| Any chronic disease (%) | 41.3 | 49.7 | 0.073 |
| Norepinephrine dose (ug/min) | $13.6 \pm 15.0$ | $21.8 \pm 22.0$ | < 0.001 |
| Baseline characteristics norepinephrine- vs. vasopressin-treated patients in SPH1 after matching | | | |
| Age (years), $X \pm$ SD | $56.8 \pm 14.9$ | $56.1 \pm 15.3$ | 0.644 |
| APACHE II, $X \pm$ SD | $28.5 \pm 8.2$ | $28.8 \pm 8.4$ | 0.831 |
| Gender (% male) | 66.4 | 72.9 | 0.242 |
| Surgical (%) | 31.4 | 31.4 | 1 |
| Respiratory (%) | 92.9 | 92.1 | 0.821 |
| Renal (%) | 77.1 | 82.1 | 0.299 |
| Coagulation (%) | 28.6 | 37.9 | 0.099 |
| Hepatic (%) | 18.6 | 23.6 | 0.305 |
| Neurological (%) | 71.4 | 79.3 | 0.127 |
| Ventilated (%) | 93.6 | 89.3 | 0.2 |
| Any chronic disease (%) | 47.9 | 48.6 | 0.905 |
| Mortality of norepinephrine- vs. vasopressin-treated patients in SPH1 after matching | | | |
| 28-day mortality (%) | 46.4 | 62.9 | 0.006 |

norepinephrine-treated patients (46.4%) ($p = 0.006$ unadjusted; $p = 0.02$ adjusted) (Table 2).

### Overall SPH 2 (post-VASST)

In SPH2, there were 525 vasopressin-treated and 145 norepinephrine-treated patients before matching; at baseline, the vasopressin-treated patients had higher APACHE II and norepinephrine dose (Table 3). After matching, there was no difference in any baseline characteristic between vasopressin-treated ($n$ = 93) and norepinephrine-treated ($n$ = 93) patients (Table 3).

In SPH2, the 28-day mortality rates were much lower than in SPH1 and not significantly different between vasopressin-treated and norepinephrine-treated patients,

26.9% and 31.2% in the norepinephrine and vasopressin groups, respectively ($p = 0.518$) (Table 3).

We compared the vasopressin doses of SPH1 vs. SPH2 and found that day 1 vasopressin dose in SPH 1 vs. SPH2 was 0.036 units/min (SD 0.009) vs. 0.032 units/min (SD 0.005), $p = 0.001$, significantly lower in SPH2 (Additional file 1: Figure S1).

### Sensitivity analysis—exclusion of patients who had NYHA IV CHF in SPH2 (post-VASST)

We excluded patients who had underlying NYHA IV CHF in SPH2. There were 93 vasopressin-treated patients and 214 norepinephrine-treated before matching (Table 4). Before matching, vasopressin-treated patients

**Table 3** Baseline characteristics and mortality of patients who had septic shock according to norepinephrine- vs. vasopressin-treated infusion prior to and after matching in SPH2

| Variable | Norepinephrine | Vasopressin | p |
|---|---|---|---|
| Baseline characteristics norepinephrine- vs. vasopressin-treated patients prior to matching in SPH2 | | | |
| Age (years), $X \pm SD$ | 61.4 ± 16.8 | 60.9 ± 13.9 | 0.574 |
| APACHE II, $X \pm SD$ | 21.1 ± 7.2 | 23.9 ± 6.4 | < 0.001 |
| Gender (% male) | 66.4 | 62.4 | 0.617 |
| Surgical (%) | 21 | 22.6 | 0.761 |
| Renal (%) | 18.2 | 22.6 | 0.376 |
| Hepatic (%) | 10.2 | 15.1 | 0.232 |
| Neurological (%) | 36.5 | 32.3 | 0.48 |
| Ventilated (%) | 82.7 | 82.8 | 0.985 |
| Any chronic disease (%) | 45.3 | 50.5 | 0.401 |
| Norepinephrine dose (ug/min) | 14.2 ± 13.6 | 19.2 ± 5.9 | < 0.001 |
| Baseline characteristics norepinephrine- vs. vasopressin-treated patients after matching in SPH2 | | | |
| Age (years), $X \pm SD$ | 61.4 ± 14.5 | 60.9 ± 13.9 | 0.812 |
| APACHE II, $X \pm SD$ | 23.8 ± 6.5 | 23.9 ± 6.4 | 0.939 |
| Gender (% male) | 30.1 | 37.6 | 0.278 |
| Surgical (%) | 19.3 | 22.6 | 0.589 |
| Renal (%) | 20.4 | 22.6 | 0.721 |
| Hepatic (%) | 15.1 | 15.1 | 1 |
| Neurological (%) | 40.3 | 32.3 | 0.13 |
| Ventilated (%) | 88.2 | 82.8 | 0.298 |
| Any chronic disease (%) | 50.5 | 50.5 | 1 |
| Norepinephrine dose (ug/min) | 16.9 ± 14.6 | 19.2 ± 15.9 | 0.242 |
| Mortality of norepinephrine- vs. vasopressin-treated patients after matching in SPH2 | | | |
| 28-day mortality (%) | 26.9 | 31.2 | 0.518 |

**Table 4** Baseline characteristics and mortality of norepinephrine- vs. vasopressin-treated patients before and after matching in SPH2. Sensitivity analysis after exclusion of patients who had underlying NYHA IV CHF

| Variable | Norepinephrine | Vasopressin | p |
|---|---|---|---|
| Baseline characteristics norepinephrine- vs. vasopressin-treated patients before matching in SPH2 | | | |
| Age (years), $X \pm SD$ | 61.4 ± 16.8 | 60.9 ± 13.9 | 0.574 |
| APACHE II, $X \pm SD$ | 21.1 ± 7.2 | 23.9 ± 6.4 | < 0.001 |
| Gender (% male) | 66.4 | 62.4 | 0.617 |
| Surgical (%) | 21.0 | 22.6 | 0.761 |
| Renal (%) | 18.2 | 22.6 | 0.376 |
| Hepatic (%) | 10.3 | 15.1 | 0.232 |
| Neurological (%) | 36.5 | 32.3 | 0.48 |
| Ventilated (%) | 82.7 | 82.8 | 0.985 |
| Any chronic disease (%) | 45.3 | 50.5 | 0.401 |
| Norepinephrine dose (ug/min) | 14.2 ± 13.6 | 19.2 ± 15.9 | < 0.001 |
| Baseline characteristics norepinephrine- vs. vasopressin-treated patients after matching in SPH2 | | | |
| Age (years), $X \pm SD$ | 61.4 ± 14.5 | 60.9 ± 13.9 | 0.812 |
| APACHE II, $X \pm SD$ | 23.8 ± 6.5 | 23.9 ± 6.4 | 0.939 |
| Gender (% male) | 69.9 | 62.4 | 0.278 |
| Surgical (%) | 19.3 | 22.6 | 0.589 |
| Renal (%) | 20.4 | 22.6 | 0.721 |
| Hepatic (%) | 15.1 | 15.1 | 1 |
| Neurological (%) | 43 | 32.3 | 0.13 |
| Ventilated (%) | 88.2 | 82.8 | |
| Any chronic disease (%) | 50.5 | 50.5 | 1 |
| Norepinephrine dose (ug/min) | 16.9 ± 14.6 | 19.2 ± 15.9 | 0.242 |
| Mortality of norepinephrine- vs. vasopressin-treated patients after matching in SPH2 | | | |
| 28-day mortality (%) | 26.9 | 31.2 | 0.518 |

had significantly higher APACHE II scores and were receiving a higher dose of norepinephrine at baseline (Table 4). After matching, there were 93 vasopressin-treated and 93 norepinephrine-treated patients (Table 4). After matching, there were no significant differences in baseline characteristics between the vasopressin- vs. norepinephrine-treated patients (Table 4). After excluding patients who had NYHA IV CHF and then propensity matching, the mortality rates were lower in SPH1 and there was no significant difference in 28-day mortality rates of the vasopressin-treated (31.2%) vs. the norepinephrine-treated (26.9%) patients ($p$ = 0.52 unadjusted; $p$ = 0.49 adjusted) (Table 4).

## Discussion

In this single center—VASST coordinating center hospital—propensity-matched retrospective cohort study of patients who had septic shock, patients treated with

vasopressin had significantly higher mortality than norepinephrine-treated patients in the period before VASST [6] was published. After the publication of VASST, there was no difference in mortality between vasopressin- and norepinephrine-treated patients. This suggests—but does not prove—there may have been a change in vasopressin prescribing and a change in vasopressin- vs. norepinephrine treatment-related outcomes. To our knowledge, this is the first propensity-matched retrospective cohort study of a sepsis treatment in a center that had previously coordinated a large pivotal randomized controlled trial of that treatment.

We used propensity matching on several key variables to mitigate bias based on selection of patients who received vasopressin. The logical basis for matching was first to simulate in a non-randomized population a vasopressin-treated and non-vasopressin-treated (control) group that is as comparable as possible at baseline and so that differences in outcomes can be better attributed to the vasopressin treatment or not. The logic of the specific matching variables was to match for variables that are associated with use of vasopressin: age, gender, APACHEII score, organ dysfunction (respiratory, renal, and coagulation), use of mechanical ventilation, underlying medical vs. surgical diagnosis, and norepinephrine dose.

Heart failure patients were excluded because severe heart failure (NYHA class IV) is a contraindication to use of vasopressin because vasopressin can decrease cardiac output. In a clinical observational cohort study, some patients with heart failure could have received vasopressin and could have been worsened by vasopressin-induced decrease in cardiac output. Thus, the exclusion of heart failure patients addresses potential bias (overestimation of mortality in vasopressin-treated patients) and adds robustness to the study. The use of inotropic agents was not the reason to exclude heart failure patients.

After excluding patients who had NYHA IV CHF and then propensity matching, there was a difference in the 28-day mortality between the norepinephrine-treated patients of SPH1 (46.4%) and those of SPH2 (26.9%) (Tables 2 and 4) that may be due to the difference in severity of illness. In SPH1, APACHE II score was $28.5 \pm 8.2$ in the norepinephrine group and $28.8 \pm 8.4$ in the vasopressin group, whereas in SPH2, APACHE II score was $23.8 \pm 6.5$ in the norepinephrine group and $23.9 \pm 6.4$ in the vasopressin group (Tables 2 and 4).

We do not know the cause of mortality difference between SPH1 and SPH2, and there may be factors related to mortality other than the dose of vasopressin. We speculate that changes in availability of ICU beds or referrals from the emergency, and other sites may have resulted in a change in severity of illness and mortality of SPH 2 compared with SPH1.

We clarify that the sepsis 2.0 definition was used in the original VASST trial inclusion and exclusion criteria [23]. Thus, we also used this definition in our current retrospective cohort study so that we could compare the results of VASST to the results of our retrospective cohort study.

Since Landry and colleagues' [1, 2] discovery of a vasopressin deficiency in septic shock, subsequent small uncontrolled [3, 4] or controlled trials [5] were the available evidence, and the use of vasopressin was uncertain in septic shock. The VASST randomized controlled trial showed that there was no overall difference in mortality between vasopressin- and norepinephrine-treated patients [6]. However, in the stratum of patients who had less severe shock (norepinephrine infusion less than 15 μg/min at time of randomization), there was a very strong trend to decreased mortality in the vasopressin compared to the norepinephrine-treated group ($p = 0.05$).

So, skeptics interpreted that there was no benefit of vasopressin, some authors [7, 24, 25] and the Surviving Sepsis Campaign [8, 26] recommended vasopressin for patients not responding to norepinephrine, and others likely used vasopressin in patients who had less severe shock (based on the VASST stratum results). The authors have been on record as recommending 0.01–0.04 units/min vasopressin in patients with more severe shock and that we recommend starting vasopressin earlier when patients have less severe shock because this is the subgroup that appeared to have benefit in the original VASST analysis and in the retrospective analyses that used the sepsis 3.0 definition [15, 23]. One meta-analysis suggested efficacy of vasopressin vs. norepinephrine in septic shock [16].

The VANISH randomized controlled trial used a higher dose of vasopressin and applied vasopressin earlier than did VASST, but also found no difference in acute kidney injury (the primary endpoint of VANISH) or mortality of vasopressin- vs. norepinephrine-treated patients [9].

Randomized controlled trials (such as VASST and VANISH) assess efficacy of a drug in a highly selected group of patients carefully selected to test whether the drug can decrease the primary endpoint under trial conditions. Efficacy trials should be followed by effectiveness trials to better assess benefits and risks of drugs such as vasopressin in the broader range of patients in clinical practice. Indeed, despite inherent methodological limitations (lack of randomization and blinding), comparative effectiveness research is ramping up in the USA [19, 27, 28] and has shown effectiveness of drugs and devices (e.g., drug-eluting stents [29]) used in practice.

Physicians may not widely adapt new evidence into clinical practice when new evidence is reported so outcomes do not improve as soon or as well as expected. We speculated that physicians would alter vasopressin use quickly and widely in the VASST coordinating center hospital after the VASST results were known. Furthermore, there had been no propensity-matched cohort studies of use of vasopressin vs. norepinephrine in septic shock before and after the publication of VASST [6]. In our current study, before VASST was published, vasopressin was associated with increased mortality compared to norepinephrine and our study suggests—but does not prove—that after publication of VASST, physicians were more selective in prescribing vasopressin such that the difference in mortality between vasopressin- and norepinephrine-treated patients disappeared after VASST. This interpretation is supported by the significantly lower vasopressin dose used after VASST (SPH2) than before VASST (SPH1). Finally, if we assume that randomized controlled trial results align most closely with the true effects of vasopressin in septic shock, then it is satisfying to see that our propensity-matched efficiency study post-VASST aligned well with the overall negative results of the two large randomized controlled trials of vasopressin in septic shock, VASST [23] and VANISH [9]. These randomized controlled trials found no difference in mortality between vasopressin and norepinephrine.

But one could ask how the current study could change physicians' practice. The current study is important because it validates the results of VASST in clinical practice, albeit in the VASST coordinating center hospital. It is an important first step in moving from the VASST efficacy trial to an efficiency trial in the VASST coordinating center, which could be followed by a broader multi-center efficiency trial to compare vasopressin versus norepinephrine in clinical practice of septic shock. We speculate that our current study results could apply to other hospitals that also use vasopressin vs. norepinephrine in septic shock.

How did the clinical equipoise regarding vasopressin in septic shock translate into practice in other studies? There is indirect evidence of possible overuse of vasopressin in practice based on a survey of US intensivists' vasopressor preferences [14]. There is also very wide inter-institutional variation in the use of vasopressin for septic shock in the USA; mean hospital use of vasopressin was 12%, with a range of 0 to 70% [11]. Lower age and respiratory dysfunction were clinical features associated with use of vasopressin as was hospital of admission [11].

Although the reasons for changes in mortality rates of vasopressin vs. norepinephrine are not known, one possible explanation was the use of higher doses of vasopressin in the VASST coordinating center hospital before VASST than after VASST was known. The day 1 vasopressin dose in SPH 1 vs. SPH2 was 0.036 units/min (SD 0.009) vs. 0.032 units/min (SD 0.005), $p = 0.001$, significantly lower in SPH2. In VASST, the blinded vasopressin infusion was started at 0.01 units/min and titrated to a maximum of 0.03 units/min [23] while in VANISH, the vasopressin dose was up to 0.06 units/min [9]. Higher dose vasopressin is associated with increased risk of adverse events [25, 30, 31] such as vital organ and digital ischemia, which may have contributed to increased mortality in our propensity-matched efficiency study. We were concerned about the difference in mortality between SPH1 and SPH2 because our study showed significantly lower vasopressin dose used after VASST than before VASST may have resulted in lower 28-day mortality. However, this interpretation is limited because of the severity and mortality differences between SPH1 and SPH2.

The differences in mortality between vasopressin -treated vs. non-vasopressin-treated patients in SPH1 vs. SPH2 could be related to the differences in vasopressin

benefits (lowering norepinephrine dose, decreasing organ dysfunction) vs. side effects (cardiac, gut, digital and renal ischemia [23, 30], and arrhythmias) related to mechanisms such as effects of vasopressin on vascular tone, immune effects (such as cytokines) [32, 33], vascular permeability, renal blood flow and function [9, 34], and von Willebrand factor release. We did not assess these possible mechanisms in this clinical study.

The strengths of our study are efficiency evaluation of vasopressin vs. norepinephrine in the hospital that coordinated VASST, the quality of the matching that removed differences in baseline characteristics between vasopressin- and norepinephrine-treated patients, and sensitivity analysis by excluding patients who had New York Heart Association class IV congestive heart failure in a separate analysis.

The limitations of the study are the lack of control by randomization and blinding (so there could be remaining confounding by indication), the single-center design (the single-center design of our study limits generalizability), the use of the sepsis 2.0 (vs. the sepsis 3.0) definition in VASST, and the lack of control of secular changes in management of septic shock before and after VASST (but these would have had to favor vasopressin outcomes in some unknown way). We do not know how many patients were self-reported NYHA class IV heart failure but did not have confirmation such as by echocardiography or cardiac catheterization. The sample size was a convenience sample size of the available patients in the SPH and SPH2 cohorts. We only included patients who had all of the data required for the current study, and so there was no missing data. The difference in day 1 vasopressin dose between SPH1 vs. SPH2 (0.036 vs. 0.032 units/min) was statistically different ($p = 0.001$), but it is not entirely certain how much of a clinical impact this difference would have made on mortality. Another limitation is that we do not have other clinical variables including use of corticosteroids, need for positive pressure ventilation, time to first appropriate antibiotic, other concomitant vasopressor use, fluid volume during resuscitation, and transfusion(s).

## Conclusions

Before VASST was published, vasopressin may have increased mortality compared to norepinephrine in the VASST coordinating center hospital. After the VASST results were known, there was no difference in mortality between vasopressin- and norepinephrine-treated patients. This is the first propensity-matched cohort study of a sepsis treatment in a center that had previously coordinated a large pivotal randomized controlled trial of that treatment—this approach may be useful for other sepsis therapies.

## Additional file

**Additional file 1: Table S1.** Rationale for Mahalanobis distance variable selection in the propensity matching of vasopressin to norepinephrine-treated patients with septic shock. Figure S1. Doses of vasopressin in SPH1 and SPH2. The dose of vasopressin (mean ± SD) in SPH2 was significantly lower than that in SPH1 ($p = 0.001$). (DOCX 26 kb)

## Abbreviations
APACHE II: Acute Physiology and Chronic Health Evaluation II; CHF: Congestive heart failure; ICU: Intensive care unit; NYHA IV: New York Heart Association IV; SD: Standard deviation; SPH: St. Paul's Hospital; SSC: Surviving Sepsis Campaign; USA: United States of America; VANISH: Vasopressin vs. Norepinephrine as Initial Therapy in Septic Shock; VASST: Vasopressin and Septic Shock Trial

## Acknowledgements
We thank the patients and families who were cared for in SPH ICU because this has increased our understanding of the treatment of septic shock. We also thank the many dedicated clinicians (doctors, nurses, therapists, and others) who cared for these critically ill patients and comforted their families. Support for VASST is from the Canadian Institutes of Health Research, Grant number: MCT 44152.

## Funding
Not applicable.

## Authors' contributions
JAR, HW, and KW are responsible for the conception and design, and analysis and interpretation. JAR and KW drafted the manuscript for important intellectual content. All authors read and approved the final manuscript.

## Authors' information
Not applicable

## Competing interests
Dr. Russell reports patents owned by the University of British Columbia (UBC) that are related to PCSK9 inhibitor(s) and sepsis and related to the use of vasopressin in septic shock. Dr. Russell is an inventor on these patents. Dr. Russell is a founder, Director and shareholder in Cyon Therapeutics Inc. (developing a sepsis therapy (PCSK9 inhibitor)). Dr. Russell has share options in Leading Biosciences Inc. Dr. Russell is a shareholder in Molecular You Corp. Dr. Russell reports receiving consulting fees in the last 3 years from the following:

1. Asahi Kesai Pharmaceuticals of America (AKPA) (developing recombinant thrombomodulin in sepsis).
2. La Jolla Pharmaceuticals (developing angiotensin II; Dr. Russell chaired the DSMB of a trial of angiotensin II from 2015 to 2017)—no longer actively consulting.
3. Ferring Pharmaceuticals (manufactures vasopressin and was developing selepressin)—no longer actively consulting.
4. Cubist Pharmaceuticals (now owned by Merck; formerly was Trius Pharmaceuticals; developing antibiotics)—no longer actively consulting.
5. Leading Biosciences (was developing a sepsis therapeutic that is no longer in development)—no longer actively consulting.
6. Grifols (sells albumin)—no longer actively consulting.
7. CytoVale Inc. (developing a sepsis diagnostic)—no longer actively consulting.

Dr. Russell reports having received an investigator-initiated grant from Grifols (entitled "Is HBP a mechanism of albumin's efficacy in human septic shock?") that is provided to and administered by UBC.

## Author details
[1]Centre for Heart Lung Innovation, St. Paul's Hospital, University of British Columbia, 1081 Burrard Street, Vancouver, BC V6Z 1Y6, Canada. [2]Division of Critical Care Medicine, St. Paul's Hospital, University of British Columbia, 1081 Burrard Street, Vancouver, BC V6Z 1Y6, Canada. [3]GenomeDx Biosciences Inc., 1038 Homer Street, Vancouver, BC V6B 2W9, Canada.

## References
1. Landry DW, Levin HR, Gallant EM, Ashton RC Jr, Seo S, D'Alessandro D, et al. Vasopressin deficiency contributes to the vasodilation of septic shock. Circulation. 1997;95(5):1122–5.
2. Landry DW, Levin HR, Gallant EM, Seo S, D'Alessandro D, Oz MC, et al. Vasopressin pressor hypersensitivity in vasodilatory septic shock. Crit Care Med. 1997;25(8):1279–82.
3. Holmes CL, Walley KR, Chittock DR, Lehman T, Russell JA. The effects of vasopressin on hemodynamics and renal function in severe septic shock: a case series. Intensive Care Med. 2001;27(8):1416–21.
4. Malay MB, Ashton RC Jr, Landry DW, Townsend RN. Low-dose vasopressin in the treatment of vasodilatory septic shock. J Trauma. 1999;47(4):699–703 Discussion -5.
5. Patel BM, Chittock DR, Russell JA, Walley KR. Beneficial effects of short-term vasopressin infusion during severe septic shock. Anesthesiology. 2002;96(3): 576–82.
6. Russell JA, Walley KR, Singer J, Gordon AC, Hebert PC, Cooper DJ, et al. Vasopressin versus norepinephrine infusion in patients with septic shock. N Engl J Med. 2008;358(9):877–87.
7. Parrillo JE. Septic shock—vasopressin, norepinephrine, and urgency. N Engl J Med. 2008;358(9):954–6.
8. Dellinger RP, Levy MM, Rhodes A, Annane D, Gerlach H, Opal SM, et al. Surviving Sepsis Campaign: international guidelines for management of severe sepsis and septic shock, 2012. Intensive Care Med. 2013;39(2): 165–228.
9. Gordon AC, Mason AJ, Thirunavukkarasu N, Perkins GD, Cecconi M, Cepkova M, et al. Effect of early vasopressin vs norepinephrine on kidney failure in patients with septic shock: the VANISH randomized clinical trial. JAMA. 2016; 316(5):509–18.
10. Hsu JL, Liu V, Patterson AJ, Martin GS, Nicolls MR, Russell JA. Potential for overuse of corticosteroids and vasopressin in septic shock. Crit Care. 2012; 16(5):447.
11. Vail EA, Gershengorn HB, Hua M, Walkey AJ, Wunsch H. Epidemiology of vasopressin use for adults with septic shock. Ann Am Thorac Soc. 2016; 13(10):1760–7.
12. Russell JA. Physician culture and vasopressin use in septic shock. Ann Am Thorac Soc. 2016;13(10):1677–9.
13. Nguyen HB, Lu S, Possagnoli I, Stokes P. Comparative effectiveness of second vasoactive agents in septic shock refractory to norepinephrine. J Intensive Care Med. 2017;32(7):451–9.
14. Hammond DA, Cullen J, Painter JT, McCain K, Clem OA, Brotherton AL, et al. Efficacy and Safety of the Early Addition of Vasopressin to Norepinephrine in Septic Shock. J Intensive Care Med. 2017;885066617725255.
15. Russell JA, Lee T, Singer J, Boyd JH, Walley KR, Vasopressin, et al. The Septic Shock 3.0 definition and trials: a vasopressin and septic shock trial experience. Crit Care Med. 2017;45(6):940–8.
16. Serpa Neto A, Nassar AP, Cardoso SO, Manetta JA, Pereira VG, Esposito DC, et al. Vasopressin and terlipressin in adult vasodilatory shock: a systematic review and meta-analysis of nine randomized controlled trials. Crit Care. 2012;16(4):R154.
17. Rosenbaum PR, Rubin DB. The bias due to incomplete matching. Biometrics. 1985;41(1):103–16.

Vasopressin versus norepinephrine in septic shock: a propensity score matched efficiency...

207

18. De Sanctis R, Vigano A, Giuliani A, Gronchi A, De Paoli A, Navarria P, et al. Unsupervised versus supervised identification of prognostic factors in patients with localized retroperitoneal sarcoma: a data clustering and Mahalanobis distance approach. Biomed Res Int. 2018;2018:2786163.

19. Feudtner C, Schreiner M, Lantos JD. Risks (and benefits) in comparative effectiveness research trials. N Engl J Med. 2013;369(10):892–4.

20. Miettinen OS. The matched pairs design in the case of all-or-none responses. Biometrics. 1968;24(2):339–52.

21. Miettinen OS. Individual matching with multiple controls in the case of all-or-none responses. Biometrics. 1969;25(2):339–55.

22. Ming K, Rosenbaum PR. Substantial gains in bias reduction from matching with a variable number of controls. Biometrics. 2000;56(1):118–24.

23. Russell JA, Walley KR, Singer J, Gordon AC, Hébert PC, Cooper DJ, Holmes CL, Mehta S, Granton JT, Storms MM, Cook DJ, Presneill JJ, Ayers D for the VASST investigators. Interaction of vasopressin infusion, corticosteroid treatment and mortality of septic shock. Crit Care Med. 2009;37(3):811–18.

24. Angus DC, van der Poll T. Severe sepsis and septic shock. N Engl J Med. 2013;369(9):840–51.

25. Wu JY, Stollings JL, Wheeler AP, Semler MW, Rice TW. Efficacy and outcomes after vasopressin guideline implementation in septic shock. Ann Pharmacother. 2017;51(1):13–20.

26. Dellinger RP, Levy MM, Carlet JM, Bion J, Parker MM, Jaeschke R, et al. Surviving Sepsis Campaign: international guidelines for management of severe sepsis and septic shock: 2008. Crit Care Med. 2008;36(1):296–327.

27. VanLare JM, Conway PH, Sox HC. Five next steps for a new national program for comparative-effectiveness research. N Engl J Med. 2010;362(11):970–3.

28. Selby JV, Lipstein SH. PCORI at 3 years—progress, lessons, and plans. N Engl J Med. 2014;370(7):592–5.

29. Tu JV, Bowen J, Chiu M, Ko DT, Austin PC, He Y, et al. Effectiveness and safety of drug-eluting stents in Ontario. N Engl J Med. 2007;357(14):1393–402.

30. Anantasit N, Boyd JH, Walley KR, Russell JA. Serious adverse events associated with vasopressin and norepinephrine infusion in septic shock. Crit Care Med. 2014;42(8):1812–20.

31. Russell JA. Bench-to-bedside review: vasopressin in the management of septic shock. Crit Care. 2011;15(4):226.

32. Russell JA, Fjell C, Hsu JL, Lee T, Boyd J, Thair S, et al. Vasopressin compared with norepinephrine augments the decline of plasma cytokine levels in septic shock. Am J Respir Crit Care Med. 2013;188(3):356–64.

33. Russell JA, Walley KR. Vasopressin and its immune effects in septic shock. J Innate Immun. 2010;2(5):446–60.

34. Gordon AC, Russell JA, Walley KR, Singer J, Ayers D, Storms MM, et al. The effects of vasopressin on acute kidney injury in septic shock. Intensive Care Med. 2010;36(1):83–91.

# 26

# Predictors associated with unplanned hospital readmission of medical and surgical intensive care unit survivors within 30 days of discharge

Tetsu Ohnuma[1,2], Daisuke Shinjo[1,3], Alan M. Brookhart[2] and Kiyohide Fushimi[1*] (iD)

## Abstract

**Background:** Reducing the 30-day unplanned hospital readmission rate is a goal for physicians and policymakers in order to improve quality of care. However, data on the readmission rate of critically ill patients in Japan and knowledge of the predictors associated with readmission are lacking. We investigated predictors associated with 30-day rehospitalization for medical and surgical adult patients separately.

**Methods:** Patient data from 502 acute care hospitals with intensive care unit (ICU) facilities in Japan were retrospectively extracted from the Japanese Diagnosis Procedure Combination (DPC) database between April 2012 and February 2014. Factors associated with unplanned hospital readmission within 30 days of hospital discharge among medical and surgical ICU survivors were identified using multivariable logistic regression analysis.

**Results:** Of 486,651 ICU survivors, we identified 5583 unplanned hospital readmissions within 30 days of discharge following 147,423 medical hospitalizations (3.8% readmitted) and 11,142 unplanned readmissions after 339,228 surgical hospitalizations (3.3% readmitted). The majority of unplanned hospital readmissions, 60.9% of medical and 63.1% of surgical case readmissions, occurred within 15 days of discharge. For both medical and surgical patients, the Charlson comorbidity index score; category of primary diagnosis during the index admission (respiratory, gastrointestinal, and metabolic and renal); hospital length of stay; discharge to skilled nursing facilities; and having received a packed red blood cell transfusion, low-dose steroids, or renal replacement therapy were significantly associated with higher unplanned hospital readmission rates.

**Conclusions:** From patient data extracted from a large Japanese national database, the 30-day unplanned hospital readmission rate after ICU stay was 3.4%. Further studies are required to improve readmission prediction models and to develop targeted interventions for high-risk patients.

**Keywords:** Hospital readmission, Rehospitalizations, Intensive care unit, Critical illness, Predictors, Outcomes research

* Correspondence: kfushimi.hci@tmd.ac.jp
[1]Department of Health Policy and Informatics, Tokyo Medical and Dental University Graduate School, 1-5-45 Yushima, Bunkyo-ku, Tokyo 1138519, Japan
Full list of author information is available at the end of the article

## Background

Hospital readmission adversely affects patients and healthcare systems. The rate of hospital readmission is an important problem faced by the Japanese health care system. Readmission may occur because of unresolved acute illness, ongoing chronic illness, the development of new medical complications, or from gaps in outpatient care [1, 2]. In the post-intensive care setting, early hospital readmission is an indicator of poor-quality care of these vulnerable patients. Indeed, patients admitted to intensive care units (ICUs) who survive to hospital discharge have a higher 6-month mortality rate post-discharge than patients hospitalized without critical illness. In addition, they experience significant morbidity subsequent to their ICU stay [3, 4].

Unplanned hospital readmission is a more informative marker of clinical deterioration than all-cause hospital readmission since planned readmissions do not indicate poor-quality care [5, 6]. Only one study assessed predictors associated with readmission of critically ill patients using claims data [2]. In that study, admissions scheduled at least 24 h in advance were considered operationally planned admissions and were not included in the definition of re-hospitalization; hence, this definition might have underestimated the true prevalence of readmission.

Identifying predictors associated with unplanned hospital readmission may inform policymakers and facilitate identification of high-risk patients to be targeted for future interventions. However, such data are currently lacking in Japan. Therefore, the aim of this study was to determine the predictors associated with unplanned hospital readmission of ICU survivors within 30 days of hospital discharge by using routine admissions data from the Japanese Diagnosis Procedure Combination (DPC) database. In addition, because we hypothesized that medical and surgical patients would have different predictors for readmission, we analyzed medical and surgical patients separately.

## Methods

### Data source

The Tokyo Medical and Dental University ethics committee approved this study and waived the requirement for informed consent. The DPC database is a Japanese case-mix classification system linked to a payment system. Details of the DPC have been described elsewhere [7, 8]. In short, by 2011, data from more than 1400 acute care hospitals were included in the DPC database, covering approximately 50% of patients discharged from all Japanese hospitals. The database includes data on baseline patient information; diagnosis, according to the International Classification of Diseases and Injuries, 10th revision (ICD-10); medical procedures; medications; materials; discharge destination; and information regarding hospital readmission.

### Study population

Data of all patients admitted to ICU between April 2012 and February 2014 who survived to hospital discharge were retrospectively extracted from the DPC database using ICU bed utilization billing codes. Patients who required only step-down unit care (high care unit care) were not included. Exclusion criteria were as follows: missing data on admission, admission dates, or discharge dates; age less than 18 years; and hospital length of stay (LOS) > 365 days. Data of patients who were readmitted to other hospitals were unavailable because patient registration numbers differ at each hospital.

### Data collection and classification

We divided the hospital readmission cohort into medical and surgical cases. Patients who underwent any surgery were considered surgical cases. All other patients were considered medical cases. The cause, type (planned or unplanned), and outcome of hospital readmission were obtained from the DPC database. Planned hospital readmissions were not counted as re-hospitalization events in this analysis because we were interested in investigating hospital readmissions that are potentially preventable. Subsequent hospital readmissions were counted if they met the inclusion criteria.

We used the Charlson comorbidity index (CCI) to quantify the burden of comorbid illness [9]. Level of consciousness was assessed at admission using the Japan Coma Scale score: 0 (alert), 1–3 (delirious), 10–30 (somnolent), and 100–300 (comatose) [10]. The category of primary diagnosis of each patient was defined using ICD-10 coding, as presented in Additional file 1: Table S1. The categories considered were cardiac, respiratory, neurologic, gastrointestinal, malignancy, metabolic and renal, and other. Hospital-level characteristics, academic status (teaching or non-teaching), and size (< 399, 400–799, and > 800 beds) were captured. Hospital LOS was categorized into four groups: 1–15, 16–30, 31–45, and > 46 days.

Data on the use of a vasopressor, stress ulcer prophylaxis, blood products (packed red blood cells [pRBC], fresh frozen plasma [FFP], and platelets), low-dose steroids, total parental nutrition (TPN), any antibiotic, renal replacement therapy (RRT), and ventilation were extracted from the DPC database.

### Outcomes

The primary outcome was unplanned hospital readmission within 30 days of discharge following the index hospitalization. Unplanned readmission rates for the medical and surgical cohorts were calculated by dividing the number of survivors readmitted by the total number of survivors in each cohort. Diagnosis on hospital readmission was categorized using primary ICD-10 diagnosis categories.

## Statistical analysis

Data were presented as means ± standard deviation, medians and interquartile ranges (IQR), or percentages, as appropriate. Length of ICU stay was calculated based on the number of days billed. We used multivariable logistic regression to identify predictors associated with 30-day unplanned hospital readmission. The results were presented as odds ratios and 95% confidence intervals. We examined the following co-variables: teaching hospital; hospital size; age; sex; CCI score; category of primary diagnosis; coma on admission; hospital LOS; discharge destination; and requirement for vasopressors, stress ulcer prophylaxis, blood product (pRBC, FFP, platelet) transfusion, steroids, anticoagulant therapy, TPN, antibiotics, RRT, ventilation, and tracheostomy. Multicollinearity between covariates was assessed using variance inflation factor and tolerance values. To assess the model performance, we calculated the area under the receiver operating characteristic curve. The curves measured the model's ability to distinguish between readmission and no readmission by evaluating the C-statistic. A C-statistic equals to one indicates perfect discrimination, whereas a C-statistic of 0.5 indicate that the ability of the model to discriminate is due to chance. All analyses were performed using R statistical software, version 3.3.0 (R Foundation for Statistical Computing, Vienna, Austria).

## Results

### Characteristics of survivors

We enrolled 559,240 patients from 502 hospitals who were admitted to ICU for at least 1 day between April 2012 and February 2014. Overall hospital mortality was 9.1% (medical, 18.1% and surgical, 6.5%). After excluding patients for the reasons outlined in Fig. 1, the final cohort included 486,651 ICU patients who survived to hospital discharge. The 30-day unplanned hospital readmission rates following medical and surgical admissions were 3.8% (5583 of 147,423) and 3.3% (11,142 of 339,228), respectively. In the medical group, 5102 (3.6%) of all unique patients admitted were readmitted once, 383 (0.3%) were readmitted twice, and 77 (0.1%) were readmitted three times or more. In the surgical group, 10,573 (3.2%) of all unique patients admitted were readmitted once, 520 (0.2%) were readmitted twice, 45 (0.01%) were readmitted three times or more.

The characteristics of the cohorts of medical and surgical survivors are shown in Tables 1 and 2. The mean age of patients was 69.7 ± 14.4 years for the medical cohort and 68.2 ± 14.3 years for the surgical cohort. The median ICU stay was 2 (IQR, 1–4) days for medical and 1 (IQR, 1–3) day for surgical cases, and the median length of hospital stay was 17 (IQR, 10–32) days for medical and 22 (IQR, 15–37) days for surgical cases. Medical patients were discharged home (76.3%), transferred to another hospital (20.6%), or discharged to a skilled nursing facility (2.2%). On the other hand, 84.5% of surgical patients were discharged home,

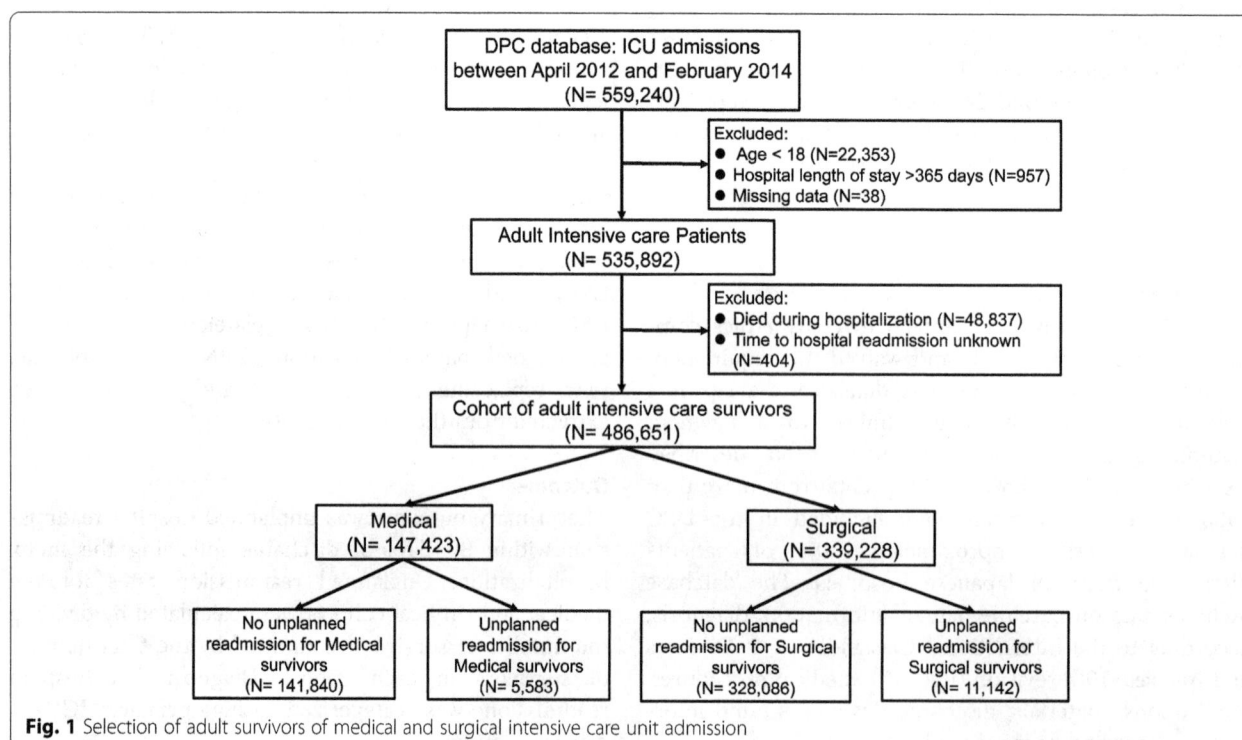

**Fig. 1** Selection of adult survivors of medical and surgical intensive care unit admission

**Table 1** Baseline characteristics of survivors in medical and surgical intensive care units

| Characteristic | Medical | | Surgical | |
| --- | --- | --- | --- | --- |
| | No unplanned readmission | Unplanned readmission | No unplanned readmission | Unplanned readmission |
| | (n = 141,840) | (n = 5583) | (n = 328,086) | (n = 11,142) |
| Hospital characteristics | | | | |
| Teaching, n (%) | 23,329 (17.2) | 794 (14.9) | 100,516 (31.9) | 2840 (26.6) |
| Size, n (%) | | | | |
| < 399 beds | 49,826 (36.7) | 2012 (37.7) | 74,587 (23.7) | 2654 (24.9) |
| 400–799 beds | 62,135 (45.8) | 2568 (48.1) | 154,905 (49.2) | 5575 (52.2) |
| > 800 beds | 23,715 (17.5) | 759 (14.2) | 85,576 (27.2) | 2451 (22.9) |
| Age, mean (SD), year | 69.7 (14.4) | 70.1 (14.2) | 68.2 (14.3) | 68.7 (14.2) |
| Men, n (%) | 89,565 (63.1) | 3450 (61.8) | 193,766 (59.1) | 7109 (63.8) |
| BMI, mean (SD) | 22.9 (4.4) | 22.2 (4.2) | 22.7 (4.3) | 22.4 (4.0) |
| CCI, median (IQR) | 1 (0–2) | 1 (0–2) | 1 (0–2) | 1 (0–2) |
| 0, n (%) | 52,063 (36.7) | 1686 (30.2) | 137,257 (41.8) | 3836 (34.4) |
| 1, n (%) | 45,830 (32.3) | 1683 (30.1) | 87,625 (26.7) | 3040 (27.3) |
| 2, n (%) | 26,809 (18.9) | 1251 (22.4) | 56,597 (17.3) | 2146 (19.3) |
| ≥ 3, n (%) | 17,138 (12.1) | 963 (17.2) | 46,607 (14.2) | 2120 (19.0) |
| Primary category of diagnosis on admission n (%) | | | | |
| Cardiac | 69,882 (49.3) | 2792 (50.0) | 49,981 (15.2) | 1807 (16.2) |
| Respiratory | 8626 (6.1) | 549 (9.8) | 5853 (1.8) | 257 (2.3) |
| Neurologic | 31,903 (22.5) | 799 (14.3) | 61,290 (18.7) | 1822 (16.4) |
| Gastrointestinal | 4336 (3.1) | 252 (4.5) | 25,473 (7.8) | 1180 (10.6) |
| Malignancy | 7158 (5.0) | 330 (5.9) | 138,309 (42.2) | 4645 (41.7) |
| Metabolic and renal | 5055 (3.6) | 297 (5.3) | 6507 (2.0) | 329 (3.0) |
| Other | 14,880 (10.5) | 564 (10.1) | 40,673 (12.4) | 1102 (9.9) |
| Coma on admission, n (%) | 8697 (6.1) | 285 (5.1) | 6157 (1.9) | 198 (1.8) |
| ICU stay, median (IQR), days | 2 (1–4) | 2 (1–5) | 1 (1–3) | 1 (1–3) |
| Hospital stay, median (IQR), days | 18 (10–32) | 21 (12–37) | 22 (15–37) | 26 (17–44) |
| 1–15 days, n (%) | 62,371 (44.0) | 1936 (34.7) | 93,430 (28.5) | 2364 (21.2) |
| 16–30 days, n (%) | 41,160 (29.0) | 1823 (32.7) | 125,972 (38.4) | 4125 (37.0) |
| 31–45 days, n (%) | 16,266 (11.5) | 783 (14.0) | 49,191 (15.0) | 1994 (17.9) |
| > 45 days, n (%) | 22,043 (15.5) | 1041 (18.6) | 59,493 (18.1) | 2659 (23.9) |
| Discharge destination | | | | |
| Home, n (%) | 107,590 (75.9) | 4572 (81.9) | 276,386 (84.2) | 9821 (88.1) |
| Other hospital, n (%) | 29,937 (21.1) | 698 (12.5) | 46,441 (14.2) | 1072 (9.6) |
| Skilled nursing facility, n (%) | 3099 (2.2) | 230 (4.1) | 2458 (0.7) | 154 (1.4) |
| Other, n (%) | 1214 (0.9) | 83 (1.5) | 2800 (0.9) | 95 (0.9) |

*SD* standard deviation, *BMI* body mass index, *CCI* Charlson comorbidity index, *IQR* interquartile range, *ICU* intensive care unit

13.9% were transferred to another hospital, and 0.8% were discharged to a skilled nursing facility.

During the index hospitalization, the proportions of medical and surgical cases, respectively, requiring various treatments were as follows: vasopressors, 27 vs 43%; stress ulcer prophylaxis, 76 vs 78%; pRBCs, 11 vs 33%; low-dose steroids, 4 vs 7%. Ventilation was required for a median of 4 (2–9)

days for medical and 2 (1–6) days for surgical patients, and 7% of medical and 6% of surgical patients received RRT.

### Timing of and reasons for unplanned hospital readmission

The majority of 30-day unplanned hospital readmissions occurred within 15 days of initial hospital

**Table 2** Treatments received in medical and surgical intensive care units during hospitalization

| Characteristic | Medical | | Surgical | |
|---|---|---|---|---|
| | No unplanned readmission | Unplanned readmission | No unplanned readmission | Unplanned readmission |
| | ($n = 141,840$) | ($n = 5583$) | ($n = 328,086$) | ($n = 11,142$) |
| Vasopressor, n (%) | 26,513 (18.7) | 1136 (20.3) | 93,209 (28.4) | 3319 (29.8) |
| Stress ulcer prophylaxis, n (%) | 107,214 (75.6) | 4266 (76.4) | 256,934 (78.3) | 9277 (83.3) |
| Blood product usage | | | | |
| pRBC, n (%) | 15,930 (11.2) | 891 (16.0) | 109,216 (33.3) | 4937 (44.3) |
| FFP, n (%) | 2563 (1.8) | 147 (2.6) | 23,040 (7.0) | 1006 (9.0) |
| Platelets, n (%) | 4050 (2.9) | 224 (4.0) | 33,954 (10.3) | 1468 (13.2) |
| Steroid use, n (%) | 5812 (4.1) | 303 (5.4) | 20,556 (6.3) | 838 (7.5) |
| Anticoagulant therapy, n (%) | 86,280 (60.8) | 3296 (59.0) | 232,864 (71.0) | 8163 (73.3) |
| TPN, n (%) | 36,037 (25.4) | 1574 (28.2) | 130,747 (39.9) | 4998 (44.9) |
| Antibiotic usage, n (%) | 64,532 (45.5) | 2972 (53.2) | 269,500 (82.1) | 9399 (84.4) |
| RRT | | | | |
| Number, n (%) | 9722 (6.9) | 609 (10.9) | 19,073 (5.8) | 998 (9.0) |
| Duration, days, median (IQR) | 3 (2–6) | 3 (2–5) | 4 (2–6) | 3 (2–6) |
| Ventilation | | | | |
| Number, n (%) | 27,731 (19.6) | 1459 (26.1) | 82,005 (25.0) | 3395 (30.5) |
| Duration, days, median (IQR) | 4 (2–9) | 4 (2–8) | 2 (1–6) | 2 (1–6) |
| Tracheostomy n (%) | 2626 (1.9) | 91 (1.6) | 8978 (2.7) | 295 (2.6) |

*pRBC* packed red blood cells, *FFP* fresh frozen plasma, *TPN* total parental nutrition, *RRT* renal replacement therapy, *IQR* interquartile range

discharge; 60.9% of the medical and 63.1% of the surgical readmissions occurred within 15 days, while 32% of readmissions in each cohort occurred within the first 7 days of discharge (Additional file 2: Figure S1). The most common categories of diagnosis assigned to ICU survivors at the time of unplanned hospital readmission were cardiac (31.5%) for medical cases and malignancy (19.6%) for surgical cases (Table 3). The

in-hospital mortality rate was 10.5% for medical and 7.5% for surgical ICU survivors who were rehospitalized.

### Predictors associated with 30-day unplanned hospital readmission

In the multivariable logistic regression analysis, the factors associated with increased 30-day unplanned hospital

**Table 3** Reasons for and outcomes of 30-day unplanned hospital readmissions of ICU survivors

| Category of primary diagnosis, n (%) | Medical | | Surgical | |
|---|---|---|---|---|
| | At readmission | At initial index admission | At admission | At initial index admission |
| | ($n = 5583$) | ($n = 147,423$) | ($n = 11,142$) | ($n = 339,228$) |
| Cardiac | 1758 (31.5) | 72,674 (49.3) | 1298 (11.6) | 51,788 (15.3) |
| Malignancy | 345 (6.2) | 7488 (5.1) | 2184 (19.6) | 14,2954 (42.1) |
| Respiratory | 738 (13.2) | 9175 (6.2) | 1138 (10.2) | 6110 (1.8) |
| Neurologic | 636 (11.4) | 32,702 (22.2) | 1022 (9.2) | 63,112 (18.6) |
| Gastrointestinal | 640 (11.5) | 4588 (3.1) | 1298 (11.6) | 26,653 (7.9) |
| Metabolic and renal | 575 (10.3) | 5352 (3.6) | 991 (8.9) | 6836 (2.0) |
| Other | 891 (16.0) | 15,444 (10.5) | 2457 (22.1) | 41,775 (12.3) |
| Outcomes | | | | |
| Hospital length of stay, median (IQR) | 15 (8–28) | | 14 (8–26) | |
| Hospital mortality, % | 585 (10.5) | | 836 (7.5) | |

*ICU* intensive care unit, *IQR* interquartile range

readmission rate were similar for medical and surgical patients (Table 4 and Additional file 1: Table S2). The area under the receiver operating characteristic curve was 0.64 (0.63–0.65) for the medical patients and 0.62 (0.61–0.63) for the surgical patients (Additional file 3: Figure S2).

**Table 4** Predictors associated with 30-day unplanned hospital readmission of ICU survivors

| Variable | Medical (n = 147,840) OR (95% CI) | Surgical (n = 339,228) OR (95% CI) |
|---|---|---|
| Teaching hospital | – | 0.79 (0.75–0.84) |
| Hospital size | | |
| < 399 beds | Reference | Reference |
| 400–799 beds | 0.98 (0.93–1.05) | 0.99 (0.94–1.04) |
| > 800 beds | 0.77 (0.69–0.87) | 0.90 (0.84–0.97) |
| CCI | 1.10 (1.08–1.12) | 1.05 (1.04–1.06) |
| Category of primary admission diagnosis | | |
| Cardiac | Reference | Reference |
| Respiratory | 1.30 (1.17–1.45) | 1.51 (1.31–1.75) |
| Neurologic | 0.64 (0.58–0.70) | 1.02 (0.95–1.09) |
| Gastrointestinal | 1.18 (1.02–1.36) | 1.59 (1.46–1.73) |
| Malignancy | 0.85 (0.75–0.97) | 1.18 (1.10–1.26) |
| Metabolic and renal | 1.25 (1.10–1.43) | 1.58 (1.38–1.79) |
| Other | 0.93 (0.84–1.03) | 0.99 (0.91–1.08) |
| Coma on admission | 0.87 (0.76–0.99) | |
| Hospital length of stay | | |
| 1–15 days | Reference | Reference |
| 16–30 days | 1.44 (1.34–1.54) | 1.21 (1.14–1.27) |
| 31–45 days | 1.62 (1.47–1.78) | 1.43 (1.34–1.53) |
| > 45 days | 1.58 (1.43–1.75) | 1.56 (1.46–1.68) |
| Discharge destination | | |
| Home | Reference | Reference |
| Other hospital | 0.48 (1.47–1.78) | 0.53 (0.50–0.57) |
| Skilled nursing facility | 1.46 (1.26–1.69) | 1.46 (1.23–1.73) |
| Others | 1.38 (1.02–1.65) | 0.88 (0.70–1.08) |
| Stress ulcer prophylaxis | – | 1.22 (1.15–1.29) |
| pRBC infusion | 1.16 (1.05–1.28) | 1.43 (1.37–1.51) |
| Low-dose steroid | 1.14 (1.01–1.29) | 1.08 (1.00–1.16) |
| Anticoagulation | 0.81 (0.76–0.87) | – |
| TPN | – | 1.05 (1.00–1.09) |
| Antibiotics | 1.09 (1.02–1.17) | – |
| RRT | 1.28 (1.15–1.41) | 1.24 (1.15–1.34) |
| Ventilation | 1.18 (1.09–1.27) | – |
| Tracheostomy | – | 0.83 (0.74–0.95) |

*ICU* intensive care unit, *OR* odds ratio, *CI* confidence interval, *CCI* Charlson comorbidity index, *pRBC* packed red blood cells, *FFP* fresh frozen plasma, *TPN* total parental nutrition, *RRT* renal replacement therapy

## Discussion

In a large database of acute care hospitals in Japan, the key findings show that the overall cumulative 30-day unplanned hospital readmission rate following ICU admission was 3.4% (medical cases, 3.8%; surgical cases, 3.3%). For both medical and surgical patients, CCI; category of primary diagnosis (respiratory, gastrointestinal, and metabolic and renal); hospital LOS; discharge destination (skilled nursing facility); and receipt of pRBC transfusion, low-dose steroids, or RRT were associated with higher rates of unplanned hospital readmission.

Hospital readmission has become a major concern, especially in the realm of critical care medicine, as hospital readmissions affect patient quality of life, morbidity, and mortality [2, 4, 11, 12]. In addition, Krumholz and others [1, 13] proposed the idea of a post-hospital syndrome, namely, that patients become vulnerable to new health impairments for a transient period following hospitalization as a result of physical and cognitive disability, nutritional impairment, sleep deprivation, and continued delirium that increases their susceptibility to further illness post-discharge. While the spectrum of readmission diagnoses is largely diverse, respiratory infection, heart failure, digestive disorders, and renal disorders are common reasons for readmission [1, 14]. In fact, our findings showed that the proportions of respiratory, gastrointestinal, and metabolic and renal reasons for ICU admission were higher for readmission than for initial admission. Critically ill survivors of recent hospitalization are more vulnerable [15] and have a higher risk of unplanned hospital readmission [2]. Therefore, appropriate methods to identify patients at higher risk of readmission are essential to improve quality of care after discharge.

We found that the cumulative prevalence proportion of 30-day unplanned hospital readmission (3.6%) was similar to the reported proportion of heart failure in the DPC database [16]. On the other hand, a recent study using an administrative database in New York State revealed that the cumulative incidence of early unplanned rehospitalization within 30 days of discharge for survivors of critical illness was 16.2% [2]. Among all acute care, nonfederal hospitals in California, the all-cause 30-day readmission rates were 20.4, 23.6, and 17.7% for sepsis, congestive heart failure, and acute myocardial infarction, respectively [17]. Our results suggest that there is a discrepancy between re-hospitalization rates in Japan and the USA. Several possible factors, such as the Japanese social context, the universal health care system, and the demographics of the cohort, may explain why critically ill survivors in Japan showed lower rehospitalization rates than those in the USA. Notably, hospital LOS would be an important reason. Patients in Japan are generally hospitalized for longer periods than patients in the USA [18]; the LOS in Japan was twice as long as in the

USA in one report [19]. In Japan, general wards are often used to provide rehabilitation and nursing care in addition to acute medical care for prolonged periods [16]. This practice might mitigate post-hospital syndrome and reduce gaps in outpatient care. Furthermore, we included patients under 60 years old; this group has the lowest rate of hospital readmission [2]. These factors contributed to the lower unplanned hospital readmission rates observed in Japan in the present study.

To examine the difference between medical and surgical cases, we divided ICU survivors into two groups; the rate of hospital readmission for surgical cases was lower than for medical cases. On the other hand, Hua et al. showed that non-surgical and surgical ICU survivors had the same cumulative rehospitalization rate (16.5% for non-surgical vs 15.9% for surgical; $P = .87$) [2]. Unlike hospital readmission of medical patients, readmission of surgical patients often results from delayed recognition of surgical procedure complications [20, 21]. Thus, the shorter the hospital LOS in general, the greater the possibility that complications will be identified after discharge. However, early medical follow-up of patients who are discharged after a surgical procedure is often performed in Japan [22], leading to lower rates of unplanned hospital readmission [5].

We identified several predictors associated with increased 30-day unplanned hospital readmission. Longer hospital LOS and discharge to skilled nursing facilities were identified as predictors in other studies assessing early rehospitalization [2, 5, 23–25]. Longer hospital LOS during the initial hospitalization is indicative of a more critically ill patient or the development of postoperative complications that might lead to rehospitalization [2, 5, 24, 26]. Additionally, past research has suggested that hospital readmission of patients discharged to skilled nursing facilities is higher than that of patients discharged to other destinations [23, 27]. A significant variation exists in the quality of care across skilled nursing facilities in Japan [28] and there is a paucity of reported data about care metrics. Better inpatient care, more complete predischarge resolution of certain problems, more effective care transitions to the home/community setting, and closer follow-up after discharge are important ways to reduce hospital readmissions.

Measures to prevent re-hospitalization remain elusive, as Walraven et al. in a recent systematic review reported that only 27% of hospital readmissions were preventable [29]. While most of predictors for hospital readmission in the present study can be considered as markers of severity of illness, RBC transfusion, which is possibly associated with increased risk of nosocomial infection, acute lung injury and acute kidney injury, [30] will be a potential target for intervention to reduce readmission rate. Future studies will be required to confirm this hypothesis.

## Strengths and limitations

There are several strengths to our study. First, we were able to investigate 30-day unplanned hospital readmissions in a large nationwide cohort of ICU survivors in Japan. As planned hospital readmissions do not reflect poor-quality care [5, 31, 32], we analyzed only unplanned hospital readmission as the primary outcome in this study. Second, adult patients of all ages were available in the DPC database, which accounted for whole adult ICU population. Third, the outcomes of and reasons for patients being readmitted to hospital were evaluated. This allowed us to identify the timing of hospital readmission and to evaluate the mortality associated with these hospital readmissions in the 30 days after discharge following the index hospitalization.

The present study also has several limitations. First, as our data source was an administrative database, we do not have information regarding patients who were readmitted to other hospitals, or information regarding out-of-hospital deaths. Also, we were not able to link data among patients transferred to another hospital. Hence, the true readmission rate may have been underestimated. However, death within 30 days post-discharge is a rare event [31]. Second, because our data were from Japan, our findings may not be generalizable to other countries with different healthcare systems, although some predictors such as longer index hospitalization, and discharge to a skilled nursing in the present study were also identified in other studies in other countries [2, 33, 34]. Third, data on some of the potential predictors, such as laboratory data, functional status, degree of social support, and adherence to medical treatment, were unavailable. Furthermore, our risk adjustment may have been limited due to the lack of general severity scoring models (Acute Physiology and Chronic Health Evaluation, Simplified Acute Physiology Score, or Sequential Organ Failure Assessment score), although we used treatments and procedures during the ICU stay as the surrogate measure. Fourth, information of end-of-life decisions to limit life-sustaining therapies was not available in our data, which could affect clinicians' decisions not to readmit those patients. Fifth, information with regards to ICU and hospital discharge policy (senior decision or not, criteria, contribution of social workers, or relation with the family members) was unavailable. Finally, data on quality of care by medical professionals in the ICU that contributed to the care of each patient were lacking.

## Conclusion

In a large national database in Japan, the prevalence proportion of unplanned rehospitalization within 30 days of hospital discharge following ICU admission was 3.4%. We also found that critically ill patients with a higher CCI score; whose initial category of primary diagnosis was respiratory, gastrointestinal, or metabolic and renal;

who had a longer hospital LOS; who were discharged to a skilled nursing facility; or who required pRBC infusion, low-dose steroids, or RRT during the index admission had a higher risk of 30-day unplanned hospital readmission. Further studies are required to improve readmission prediction modeling and targeted interventions for high-risk patients.

## Additional files

**Additional file 1: Table S1.** International classification the codes used to categorize the primary diagnosis. **Table S2.** Risk factors associated with 30–day unplanned hospital readmission of intensive care unit surgical patients for planned initial admission and urgent initial admission. (DOCX 25 kb)

**Additional file 2: Figure S1.** Distribution of the timing of 30-day readmission of medical or surgical intensive care unit survivors. The denominator was 5583 for medical intensive care unit survivors and 11,142 for surgical intensive care unit survivors. (PPTX 40 kb)

**Additional file 3: Figure S2.** Receiver operating characteristic curves for medical and surgical patients. (PPTX 48 kb)

## Abbreviations
CCI: Charlson comorbidity index; DPC: Diagnosis procedure combination; FFP: Fresh frozen plasma; ICD-10: International Classification of Diseases and Injuries 10th revision; ICU: Intensive care unit; IQR: Interquartile ranges; LOS: Length of stay; pRBC: Packed red blood cell; RRT: Renal replacement therapy; TPN: Total parental nutrition

## Acknowledgements
The authors have no additional acknowledgements.

## Funding
Dr. Fushimi is supported in part by Grants-in-Aid for Research on Policy Planning and Evaluation (Ministry of Health, Labour and Welfare, Japan, H25-SEISAKU-SITEI-010 and H26-SEISAKU-SITEI-011), and by JSPS KAKENHI (grant number 24590604). Dr. Shinjo has received Grant-in-Aid for Young Scientists (B) from the Japan Society for the Promotion of Science, Japan (JSPS KAKENHI, Grant Number 16K19284). Dr. Ohnuma has received the 19th Grant of the Institute for Health Economics and Policy. Dr. Brookhart has received investigator-initiated research funding from the National Institutes of Health and through contracts with the Agency for Healthcare Research and Quality's DEcIDE program and the Patient Centered Outcomes Research Institute. Within the past three years, he has received research support from Amgen and AstraZeneca and has served as a scientific advisor for Amgen, Merck, GSK, and UCB (honoraria/payment received by the institution). Merck, GSK, and UCB provide financial support the UNC Center for Pharmacoepidemiology, which has supported some of Dr. Brookhart's students. He has received consulting fees from RxAnte, Inc. and World Health Information Consultants. The funding organizations had no role in the design and conduct of the study; in the collection, analysis, and interpretation of the data; or in the preparation, review, or approval of the manuscript.

## Authors' contributions
KF had full access to all of the data in the study and takes responsibility for the integrity of the data and the accuracy of the data analysis. TO participated in the study design, drafting of the article, analysis and interpretation of data, and revision of the article for intellectual content. DS participated in the study design and revision of the article for intellectual content. AB participated in critical revision for intellectual content. Fushimi participated in the study design, interpretation of data, and revision of the

article for intellectual content. All authors read and approved the final manuscript.

## Competing interests
The authors declare that they have no competing interests.

## Author details
[1]Department of Health Policy and Informatics, Tokyo Medical and Dental University Graduate School, 1-5-45 Yushima, Bunkyo-ku, Tokyo 1138519, Japan. [2]Department of Epidemiology, Gillings School of Global Public Health, University of North Carolina, Chapel Hill, USA. [3]The Database Center of the National University Hospital, The University of Tokyo Hospital, Tokyo, Japan.

## References
1. Dharmarajan K, Hsieh AF, Lin Z, et al. Diagnoses and timing of 30-day readmissions after hospitalization for heart failure, acute myocardial infarction, or pneumonia. JAMA. 2013;309:355–63.
2. Hua M, Gong MN, Brady J, et al. Early and late unplanned rehospitalizations for survivors of critical illness*. Crit Care Med. 2015;43:430–8.
3. Hofhuis JG, Spronk PE, van Stel HF, et al. The impact of critical illness on perceived health-related quality of life during ICU treatment, hospital stay, and after hospital discharge: a long-term follow-up study. Chest. 2008;133:377–85.
4. Wunsch H, Guerra C, Barnato AE, et al. Three-year outcomes for Medicare beneficiaries who survive intensive care. JAMA. 2010;303:849–56.
5. Jencks SF, Williams MV, Coleman EA. Rehospitalizations among patients in the Medicare fee-for-service program. N Engl J Med. 2009;360:1418–28.
6. Sacks GD, Dawes AJ, Russell MM, et al. Evaluation of hospital readmissions in surgical patients: do administrative data tell the real story? JAMA Surg. 2014;149:759–64.
7. Umegaki T, Nishimura M, Tajimi K, et al. An in-hospital mortality equation for mechanically ventilated patients in intensive care units. J Anesth. 2013;27:541–9.
8. Ohnuma T, Shinjo D, Fushimi K. Hospital mortality of patients aged 80 and older after surgical repair for type a acute aortic dissection in Japan. Medicine (Baltimore). 2016;95:e4408.
9. Sundararajan V, Quan H, Halfon P, et al. Cross-national comparative performance of three versions of the ICD-10 Charlson index. Med Care. 2007;45:1210–5.
10. Shigematsu K, Nakano H, Watanabe Y. The eye response test alone is sufficient to predict stroke outcome—reintroduction of Japan coma scale: a cohort study. BMJ Open. 2013;3
11. Lilly CM, Zuckerman IH, Badawi O, et al. Benchmark data from more than 240,000 adults that reflect the current practice of critical care in the United States. Chest. 2011;140:1232–42.
12. Garland A, Olafson K, Ramsey CD, et al. Epidemiology of critically ill patients in intensive care units: a population-based observational study. Crit Care. 2013;17:R212.
13. Krumholz HM. Post-hospital syndrome—an acquired, transient condition of generalized risk. N Engl J Med. 2013;368:100–2.
14. Vashi AA, Fox JP, Carr BG, et al. Use of hospital-based acute care among patients recently discharged from the hospital. JAMA. 2013;309:364–71.
15. Harvey MA. The truth about consequences—post-intensive care syndrome in intensive care unit survivors and their families. Crit Care Med. 2012;40:2506–7.
16. Aizawa H, Imai S, Fushimi K. Factors associated with 30-day readmission of patients with heart failure from a Japanese administrative database. BMC Cardiovasc Disord. 2015;15:134.
17. Chang DW, Tseng CH, Shapiro MF. Rehospitalizations following sepsis: common and costly. Crit Care Med. 2015;43:2085–93.
18. Murthy S, Wunsch H. Clinical review: international comparisons in critical care—essons learned. Crit Care. 2012;16:218.
19. Sirio CA, Tajimi K, Taenaka N, et al. A cross-cultural comparison of critical care delivery: Japan and the United States. Chest. 2002;121:539–48.
20. Graboyes EM, Liou TN, Kallogjeri D, et al. Risk factors for unplanned hospital readmission in otolaryngology patients. Otolaryngol Head Neck Surg. 2013;149:562–71.
21. Shahian DM, He X, O'Brien SM, et al. Development of a clinical registry-based 30-day readmission measure for coronary artery bypass grafting surgery. Circulation. 2014;130:399–409.

22. Honda M, Hiki N, Nunobe S, et al. Unplanned admission after gastrectomy as a consequence of fast-track surgery: a comparative risk analysis. Gastric Cancer. 2015;

23. Mor V, Intrator O, Feng Z, et al. The revolving door of rehospitalization from skilled nursing facilities. Health Aff (Millwood). 2010;29:57–64.

24. Kansagara D, Englander H, Salanitro A, et al. Risk prediction models for hospital readmission: a systematic review. JAMA. 2011;306:1688–98.

25. Sun A, Netzer G, Small DS, et al. Association between index hospitalization and hospital readmission in sepsis survivors. Crit Care Med. 2016;44:478–87.

26. Donze J, Aujesky D, Williams D, et al. Potentially avoidable 30-day hospital readmissions in medical patients: derivation and validation of a prediction model. JAMA Intern Med. 2013;173:632–8.

27. Neuman MD, Wirtalla C, Werner RM. Association between skilled nursing facility quality indicators and hospital readmissions. JAMA. 2014;312:1542–51.

28. Nakanishi M, Hattori K, Nakashima T, et al. Health care and personal care needs among residents in nursing homes, group homes, and congregate housing in Japan: why does transition occur, and where can the frail elderly establish a permanent residence? J Am Med Dir Assoc. 2014;15(76):e1–6.

29. van Walraven C, Bennett C, Jennings A, et al. Proportion of hospital readmissions deemed avoidable: a systematic review. CMAJ. 2011;183:E391–402.

30. Dupuis C, Sonneville R, Adrie C, et al. Impact of transfusion on patients with sepsis admitted in intensive care unit: a systematic review and meta-analysis. Ann Intensive Care. 2017;7:5.

31. van Walraven C, Dhalla IA, Bell C, et al. Derivation and validation of an index to predict early death or unplanned readmission after discharge from hospital to the community. CMAJ. 2010;182:551–7.

32. van Walraven C, Jennings A, Taljaard M, et al. Incidence of potentially avoidable urgent readmissions and their relation to all-cause urgent readmissions. CMAJ. 2011;183:E1067–72.

33. Goodwin AJ, Rice DA, Simpson KN, et al. Frequency, cost, and risk factors of readmissions among severe sepsis survivors. Crit Care Med. 2015;43:738–46.

34. Liu V, Lei X, Prescott HC, et al. Hospital readmission and healthcare utilization following sepsis in community settings. J Hosp Med. 2014;9:502–7.

# 27

# Effect of norepinephrine dosage on mortality in patients with septic shock

Hitoshi Yamamura[1]* , Yu Kawazoe[2], Kyohei Miyamoto[3], Tomonori Yamamoto[4], Yoshinori Ohta[5] and Takeshi Morimoto[6]

## Abstract

**Background:** Use of high-dose norepinephrine is thought to have an immunosuppressive action that increases mortality. This study aimed to evaluate the correlation between norepinephrine dosage and prognosis of patients with septic shock.

**Methods:** This study was a nested cohort of the DExmedetomidine for Sepsis in Intensive Care Unit Randomized Evaluation (DESIRE) trial. We evaluated 112 patients with septic shock and an initial Sequential Organ Failure Assessment Cardiovascular (SOFA-C) category score > 2 and initial lactate level > 2 mmol/L. We divided the patients into two groups according to the norepinephrine dosage administered over the initial 7 days: high dose ($\geq$ 416 µg/kg/week) (H group, $n = 56$) and low dose (< 416 µg/kg/week) (L group, $n = 56$). The primary outcome of interest was 28-day mortality. Secondary outcomes were ventilator-free days, initial 24-h infusion volume, initial 24- to 48-h infusion volume, and the need for renal replacement therapy. For comparisons between the H group and L group, we used the chi-square test or Fisher's exact test for categorical variables and the $t$ test or Wilcoxon rank sum test for continuous variables. For time-to-event outcomes, Cox proportional hazards models were used. Kaplan-Meier survival curves were created for graphical representation.

**Results:** Patient characteristics appeared to be similar between the two groups except for the SOFA-C score and fibrinogen degradation product level. The cumulative incidence of death at 28 days was 29.9% (16 patients) in the L group and 29.7% (15 patients) in the H group ($p = 0.99$). The median number of 28-day ventilator-free days was 20 (0, 25) in the L group and 16 (0, 22) in the H group ($p < 0.05$). Initial infusion volume at 0–24 h in the H group was significantly higher than that in the L group ($p = 0.004$). Infusion volume at 24–48 h in the H group was also significantly higher than that in the L group ($p = 0.03$).

**Conclusions:** No statistically significant difference was observed in 28-day mortality between patients with septic shock treated with high-dose norepinephrine compared with those treated with low-dose norepinephrine. However, the number of ventilator-free days in the L group was higher than that in the H group.

**Keywords:** Norepinephrine, Septic shock, Ventilator-free days

* Correspondence: yamamura@hirosaki-u.ac.jp
[1]Department of Disaster and Critical Care Medicine, Hirosaki University School of Medicine, 5 Zaifuchou, Hirosaki, Aomori 036-8562, Japan
Full list of author information is available at the end of the article

## Background

Norepinephrine is the vasopressor of first choice for patients with septic shock [1]. Norepinephrine recruits unstressed volume through alpha adrenergic effects on venous and arterial vessels and might recruit volume to the macrovasculature. However, norepinephrine is also thought to have an immunosuppressive action that causes a poor prognosis [2, 3]. Previous reports showed that norepinephrine dosage was associated with intensive care unit (ICU) mortality, with an especially high mortality rate at doses above 1 μg/kg per min [2]. From this previous study, the high-dose usage of norepinephrine was thought to cause high mortality in patients with sepsis. As another problem, in the treatment strategy of septic shock, it is important to include early recognition, fluid resuscitation, and maintenance of the blood pressure. However, if massive fluid resuscitation is required, this can cause pulmonary edema and prolonged the number of ventilator days. In this study, we aimed to evaluate the correlation between norepinephrine dosage and prognosis and the number of ventilator-free days (VFD) of patients with septic shock.

## Methods

### Patient selection

The DExmedetomidine for Sepsis in Intensive Care Unit Randomized Evaluation (DESIRE) trial was conducted from February 2013 to January 2016 [4]. This trial was a multicenter, randomized, controlled trial that enrolled 201 adult patients with sepsis undergoing ventilation. It was designed to assess the effects of a sedation strategy with dexmedetomidine compared with that without dexmedetomidine. The results of this trial in the 201 patients showed that treatment with dexmedetomidine vs that without dexmedetomidine did not significantly reduce the number of VFD (20 vs 18 days) or 28-day

mortality (23 vs 31%, hazard ratio 0.69). This sub-analysis of the 201 randomized patients included those with septic shock. Septic shock was defined as a Sequential Organ Failure Assessment (SOFA) score > 2 for the cardiovascular category and a lactate level > 2 mmol/L at randomization. We enrolled 112 patients and divided the patients into two groups according to the total dosage of norepinephrine administered over the initial 7 days: low dose (< 416 μg/kg/week) (L group, $n = 56$) and high dose (≥ 416 μg/kg/week) (H group, $n = 56$) (Fig. 1).

### Treatment protocol

The treatment protocol for sepsis was based on the Guidelines for the Management of Sepsis [1]. In the resuscitation from septic shock-induced hypoperfusion, we initially administered an adequate amount of crystalloid on admission to maintain a mean arterial pressure of 65 mmHg, central venous pressure of 8–12 mmHg, and urinary output of > 0.5 mL/kg/h. Following fluid resuscitation, if the blood pressure could not be maintained, we used norepinephrine or vasopressin as the vasopressor.

### Measurements

We collected data on the initial serum lactate level, SOFA score, and Acute Physiology and Chronic Health Evaluation II (APACHE II) score at randomization. White blood cell (WBC) count, levels of fibrinogen, D-dimer, fibrinogen degradation products (FDP), C-reactive protein (CRP), and procalcitonin (PCT) and norepinephrine dosage were assessed. Infusion volume was assessed on the first and second days, and the dosages of other vasopressors were assessed on the first 7 days after randomization.

The primary outcome of interest was 28-day mortality. For other outcomes, patients were followed in the hospital

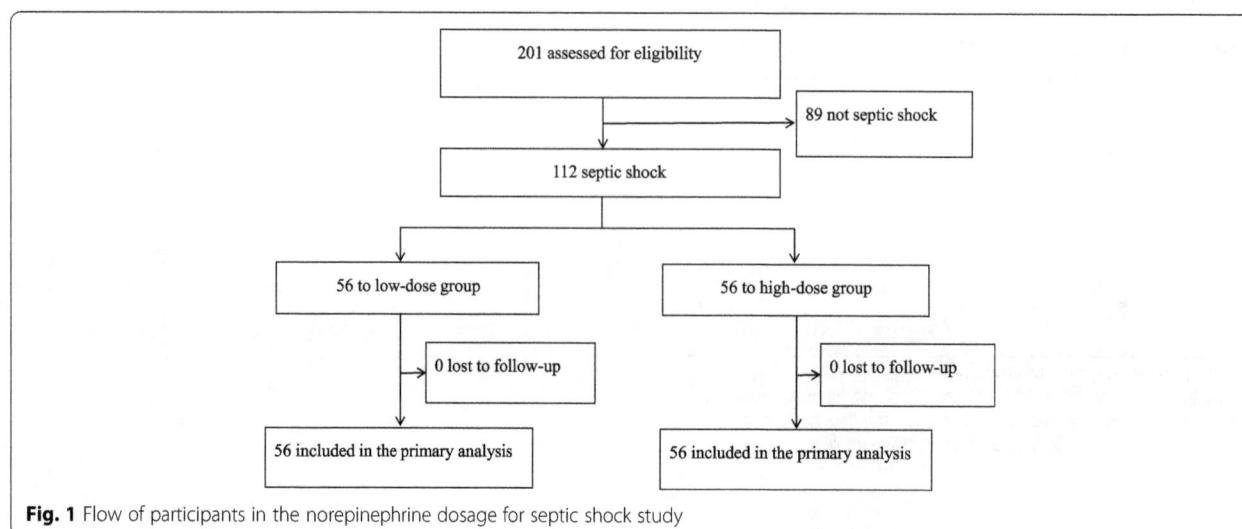

**Fig. 1** Flow of participants in the norepinephrine dosage for septic shock study

from enrollment for 28 days or until discharge or death if earlier. Secondary outcomes included the number of VFD, defined as the number of days without use of a ventilator during the 28-day study period, initial 24-h infusion volume, initial 24- to 48-h infusion volume, and the need for renal replacement therapy including continuous renal replacement therapy and hemodialysis.

### Statistical analysis

Continuous variables are presented as the mean ± standard deviation (SD) or the median and interquartile range (IQR). Categorical variables are presented as numbers and percentages (%). For comparisons between the H group and L group, we used the chi-square test or Fisher's exact test for categorical variables and the $t$ test or Wilcoxon rank sum test for continuous variables.

For time-to-event outcomes (time to ICU discharged death), Cox proportional hazards models were used. Kaplan-Meier survival curves were created for graphical representation of these time-to-event outcomes. When examining 28-day mortality, patients were censored at the time of last contact while alive or at 28 days from enrollment, whichever came first. Censoring for hospital discharge analyses occurred at the time of death or, rarely, at study withdrawal. To account for any effect of site and for baseline imbalances, a Cox proportional hazards regression model was used with patients nested within site, and site treated as a random effect with the following covariates included in the model: APACHE II score > 23, age > 65, emergency operation, infection site is lung, and treated with dexmedetomidine. A two-sided $p$ value of < 0.05 was considered statistically significant, and all analyses were performed using JMP Pro software (version 12.2; SAS Institute Inc., Cary, NC, USA).

### Results

Patient characteristics appeared to be similar between the two groups except for the Sequential Organ Failure Assessment Cardiovascular (SOFA-C) score and FDP level (Table 1). In the H group, use of another vasopressor, such as dobutamine, and total vasopressin dosage within 7 days were significantly higher than those in the L group. Causes of sepsis were lung ($n = 29$), abdomen ($n = 52$), and others ($n = 31$).

As the primary outcome, the cumulative incidence of death at 28 days was not significantly different between the two groups: 29.9% (16 patients) in the L group and 29.7% (15 patients) in the H group ($p = 0.99$) (Fig. 2). The analysis adjusted for infusion volume over the first 24 h also did not show a significant difference ($p = 0.38$). The median 28-day VFD in the L group was significantly higher than that in the H group (20 [0, 25] vs 16 [0, 20] days: $p < 0.05$) (Fig. 3). Using the Cox proportional hazards model to adjust for all five of the covariates,

VFD was incorporated into the model, with similar results compared with the primary analysis. The dose of norepinephrine used was significantly different between the two groups on each of the first 7 days. Especially, the highest dose of norepinephrine administered was in the H group on day 2 at 345.1 (170.9) µg/kg (Fig. 4).

Initial infusion volume at 0–24 h in the H group was significantly higher than that in the L group (7829 [5689, 10,676] vs 5544 [3985, 8000] mL, $p = 0.004$). Infusion volume at 24–48 h in the H group was also significantly higher than that in the L group (3530 [2382, 4612] vs 2689 [1962, 3916] mL, $p = 0.03$). Within the first 3 days after admission, 7 patients died in the H group and 9 patients died in the L group. The cumulative incidences of death at 28 days except for the patients with death within 3 days were not significantly different between the two groups: 32.8% in the L group and 28.4% in the H group ($p = 0.39$). Renal replacement therapy was performed in 32 patients in the H group and in 18 patients in the L group.

### Discussion

Septic shock is defined as a subset of sepsis in which underlying abnormalities of circulatory and cellular metabolism are profound enough to substantially increase mortality [5]. Norepinephrine is the vasoactive agent of first choice for patients with septic shock after adequate volume resuscitation [1]. Our results showed that the dosage of norepinephrine did not affect the mortality of patients with septic shock, but the number of VFD was lower in the H group. The reason for the difference in the number of VFD between the two groups was that the infusion volume in the H group was significantly higher than that in the L group. Massive infusion volumes can bring about pulmonary dysfunction and cardiovascular failure. Generally, such conditions require ventilator support. Thus, we thought that the factors contributing to the lower number of VFD in the H group were the unstable circulatory status and massive infusion volume administered. A previous report showed that a norepinephrine dosage of 1 µg/kg per minute was associated with an ICU death rate of 90% and suggested that a dosage of norepinephrine greater than 1 µg/kg per minute is an independent factor associated with mortality in patients with septic shock [2]. However, the study by Martin and colleagues had a few problems related to fluid treatment for septic shock. The non-survivors group did not receive the same resuscitation infusion volume as the survivors group. Crystalloid was 1.0 L (0.0–2.5) in the 168 survivors vs 1.0 L (0.0–2.0) in the 156 non-survivors, and cumulative fluid administration was 1.5 L (0.9–3.0) in the 168 survivors vs 1.0 L (0.5–2.0) in the 156 non-survivors [2]. These results indicate that the non-survivors were not infused

**Table 1** Patient characteristics

| | L group (n = 56) | H group (n = 56) | p value |
|---|---|---|---|
| Age, years | 70.8 ± 13.4 | 70.5 ± 14.4 | 0.92 |
| Male sex, n (%) | 33 (58) | 36 (64) | 0.56 |
| Body weight, kg | 53.9 ± 11.2 | 54.7 ± 11.9 | 0.72 |
| COPD (%) | 4 (7.1) | 3 (5.3) | 0.70 |
| Soft tissue infection (%) | 4 (7.1) | 4 (7.1) | 1.00 |
| Emergency surgery (%) | 28 (50.1) | 23 (41.1) | 0.34 |
| Site of infection (%) | | | |
|   Lung | 16 (29) | 13 (23) | |
|   Abdomen | 29 (52) | 23 (41) | |
|   Urinary tract | 4 (7) | 8 (14) | |
|   Skin and soft tissue | 1 (2) | 6 (11) | |
|   Others | 6 (11) | 6 (11) | |
| APACHE II score | 25 (19, 33) | 25 (20, 30) | 0.89 |
| SOFA score | 10 (8, 12) | 10 (8, 12) | 0.63 |
| SOFA-R score | 2 (1, 3) | 2 (1, 3) | 0.65 |
| SOFA-P score | 0.5 (0, 2) | 1 (0, 2) | 0.23 |
| SOFA-L score | 0 (0, 1) | 0 (0, 1) | 0.65 |
| SOFA-C score | 3 (3, 4) | 4 (3, 4) | 0.007 |
| SOFA-N score | 0 (0, 3) | 1 (0, 2) | 0.63 |
| SOFA-K score | 1.5 (0, 3) | 1 (0, 2) | 0.34 |
| Systolic BP, mmHg | 109 (26) | 105 (28) | 0.31 |
| Mean BP, mmHg | 73 (16) | 72 (18) | 0.75 |
| Lactate level, mmol/L | 4.5 (3.0, 7.8) | 4.4 (3.6, 6.6) | 0.94 |
| Urine output, mL/day | 1240 (298, 2302) | 1279 (378, 2566) | 0.84 |
| WBC, mm$^3$ | 8500 (4500, 14,109) | 5000 (2250, 13,930) | 0.18 |
| FDP, μg/dL | 15.8 (7.5, 28.0) | 23.6 (10.5, 52) | 0.02 |
| Fibrinogen, mg/dL | 337 (243, 532) | 403 (271, 583) | 0.26 |
| CRP, mg/dL | 11.9 (5.2, 24.4) | 16.1 (5.4, 27.3) | 0.76 |
| PCT, ng/mL | 29.3 (3.2, 81.5) | 40.0 (12.9, 100) | 0.11 |
| Catecholamine | | | |
|   Total dopamine dosage (μg/kg) | 15,727 (6180, 36,150) | 28,532 (12,321, 43,407) | 0.15 |
|   Total dobutamine dosage (μg/kg) | 6191 (3652, 14,796) | 23,051 (13,931, 35,760) | 0.003 |
| Total vasopressin dosage (IU) | 9.8 (5.1, 15.4) | 30.2 (12, 54.2) | 0.05 |
| Hospital length of stays, days | 29 (31) | 33 (29) | 0.12 |
| Renal replacement therapy (%) | 18 (32) | 32 (57) | 0.008 |

Data are shown as mean ± SD, number of subjects (%), or median (IQR), as appropriate

*SD* standard deviation, *COPD* chronic obstructive pulmonary disease, *IQR* interquartile range, *APACHE II* Acute Physiology and Chronic Health Evaluation II, *SOFA* Sequential Organ Failure Assessment, *SOFA-R* Sequential Organ Failure Assessment Respiration score, *SOFA-P* Sequential Organ Failure Assessment Coagulation score, *SOFA-L* Sequential Organ Failure Assessment Liver score, *SOFA-C* Sequential Organ Failure Assessment Cardiovascular score, *SOFA-N* Sequential Organ Failure Assessment Central nervous system score, *SOFA-K* Sequential Organ Failure Assessment Renal score, *BP* blood pressure, *WBC* white blood cell, *FDP* fibrinogen degradation products, *CRP* C-reactive protein, *PCT* procalcitonin

with an adequate amount of resuscitation volume in the initial period.

In our study, the H group received an adequate amount of resuscitation fluid compared with the L group over the initial 24 h and at 48 h. The most important treatment strategy for patients with septic shock is initial fluid resuscitation and maintenance of the blood pressure. If patients with septic shock receive adequate infusion of fluid volume, the dose of norepinephrine may not be related to patient prognosis.

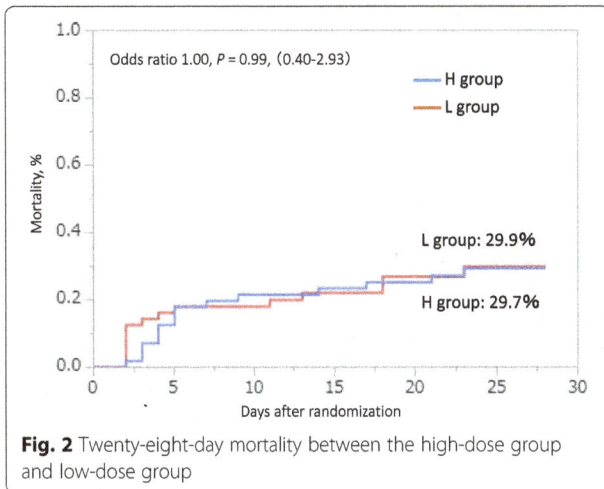

**Fig. 2** Twenty-eight-day mortality between the high-dose group and low-dose group

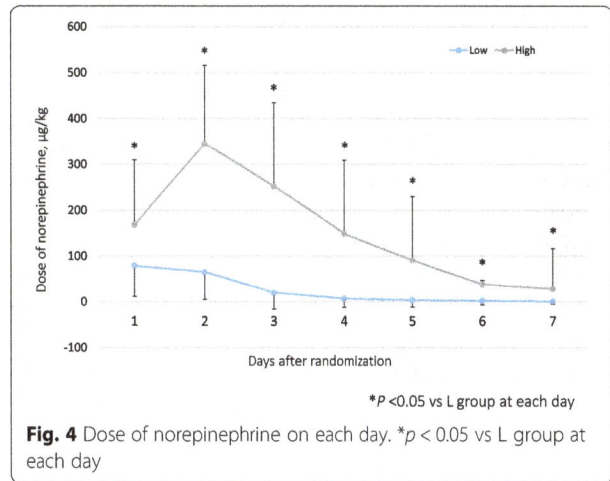

**Fig. 4** Dose of norepinephrine on each day. *$p < 0.05$ vs L group at each day

In previous in vitro and animal studies, norepinephrine was shown to exert multiple anti-inflammatory actions [6, 7]. Exogenous norepinephrine infused into the portal vein of rats resulted in elevation of serum levels of IL-10 and IL-1 beta [8, 9]. Another study showed neutrophils incubated with norepinephrine displayed an immunosuppressive phenotype [10–12]. These studies indicate that epinephrine may have anti-inflammatory effects. In contrast, clinical studies have not investigated norepinephrine in relation to immunosuppressive reactions. Some studies investigating the correlation of the dosage of norepinephrine with mortality indicated that a high norepinephrine level is associated with high mortality in patients with septic shock [13]. However, no study found any correlation between the dosage of norepinephrine and immunological parameters. The blocking action of endogenous catecholamine with β-blockers has improved the prognosis in patients with sepsis [14, 15] and reduced secondary infection in

pediatric burn patients [16]. These clinical studies suggested that a high catecholamine level may have led to immunoparalysis [17, 18].

In our study, some alternative vasopressors were also used to treat the patients with septic shock. More dobutamine, vasopressin, and renal replacement therapy were used in the H group than in the L group. However, mortality was not significantly different between the two groups. Our results indicated that renal replacement therapy and total dobutamine dosage also did not affect mortality. We surmise that because of the greater inflammatory action in the H group, the patients did not respond to the epinephrine effect and required the use of vasopressin and another vasopressor to maintain their blood pressure. The patients in a severe condition died earlier, and as a result, the doses of norepinephrine or another vasopressor in these patients might be smaller. We also assessed the incidence of death at 28 days after excluding the patients who died within 3 days. However, there was no significant difference between the two groups, and thus we thought that the early death of some patients had no influence on mortality.

Several adverse effects of catecholamines were reported previously, such as pulmonary edema, bowel ischemia, immunomodulation, increase cellular energy expenditure, and hyperglycemia [19–21]. Generally, we believed that a high concentration of catecholamine would increase mortality and worsen patient prognosis. However, our results were contrary to those of previous reports and did not indicate that high norepinephrine usage worsened mortality or caused organ dysfunction such as bowel ischemia and pulmonary edema although we did not measure the actual catecholamine concentration in serum. We think that high-dose norepinephrine may be used safely with no associated complications.

This study has several limitations. First, it was a nested cohort of a randomized control study, and use of a vasopressor other than norepinephrine was not allowed by

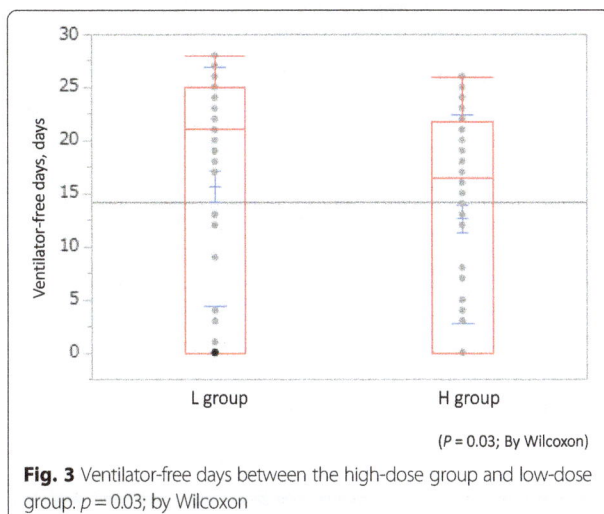

**Fig. 3** Ventilator-free days between the high-dose group and low-dose group. $p = 0.03$; by Wilcoxon

the treatment protocol. Our study concentrated on the use of noradrenaline as the initial vasopressor, and use of another vasopressor was uneven. Second, use of an alternate vasopressor other than norepinephrine was left to each physician's judgment. Third, we cannot determine to what extent the mechanism of norepinephrine contributed to the change in mortality. Also, the duration of shock was similar because there was no significant difference in initial lactate levels and APACHE II scores between the two groups. However, the initial SOFA-C score was different. We attribute this difference in SOFA-C score to the catecholamine dosage in the two groups because the initial blood pressure was not different between the groups. The early recognition and treatment of septic shock in our patients may be one factor influencing our results. However, the greater inflammatory action occurring in the H group required a high-dose vasopressor.

## Conclusions

There was no statistically significant difference in 28-day mortality between the patients with septic shock treated with high-dose norepinephrine vs those treated with low-dose norepinephrine. However, the number of VFD was significantly higher in the group treated with low-dose norepinephrine than in the group treated with high-dose norepinephrine.

### Abbreviations

APACHE II: Acute Physiology and Chronic Health Evaluation II; CRP: C-reactive protein; FDP: Fibrinogen degradation products; ICU: Intensive care unit; IQR: Interquartile range; PCT: Procalcitonin; SD: Standard deviation; SOFA: Sequential Organ Failure Assessment; SOFA-C: Sequential Organ Failure Assessment Cardiovascular; VFD: Ventilator-free days; WBC: White blood cell

### Acknowledgements

We would like to thank the DESIRE Trial Investigators: Akihiro Fuke, MD (Osaka City General Hospital, Osaka, Japan); Atsunori Hashimoto, MD (Hyogo College of Medicine, Nishinomiya, Japan); Hiroyuki Koami, MD (Saga University Hospital, Saga, Japan); Satoru Beppu, MD (National Hospital Organization Kyoto Medical Center, Kyoto, Japan); Yoichi Katayama, MD (Sapporo Medical University, Sapporo, Japan); and Makoto Itoh, MD (Yamaguchi Grand Medical Center, Yamaguchi, Japan).

### Funding

The original study was supported in part by a noncontractual research grant to Wakayama Medical University provided by Hospira Japan.

### Authors' contributions

HY made substantial contributions in data acquisition and writing of the manuscript. HY, YO, and TM contributed to the study design, statistical analysis, interpretation of data, and final approval of the manuscript. YK, TY, and KM made equally substantial contributions in data acquisition and reviewing the manuscript. HY critically revised the manuscript for important intellectual content. TM supervised the study. All authors read and approved the final manuscript.

### Competing interests

Dr. Yamamura reports receipt of lecture fees from Hospira Japan, Nipro, and Asahi Kasei and educational consulting fees from Toray Industries, CSL Behring, Teijin Pharma, and Nihon Pharmaceutical. Dr. Kawazoe reports receipt of lecture fees from Hospira Japan and Pfizer Japan and a scholarship from Hospira Japan. Dr. Miyamoto reports receipt of lecture fees from Becton Dickinson and Pfizer Japan. Dr. Morimoto reports receipt of lecture fees from AbbVie, AstraZeneca, Daiichi-Sankyo, Kowa, Kyorin, Mitsubishi-Tanabe, and Pfizer Japan and consulting fees from Asahi Kasei and Boston Scientific. Dr. Tomonori Yamamoto and Dr.Yoshinori Ohta, have no competing interests. The other authors declare no competing interests.

### Author details

[1]Department of Disaster and Critical Care Medicine, Hirosaki University School of Medicine, 5 Zaifuchou, Hirosaki, Aomori 036-8562, Japan. [2]Division of Emergency and Critical Care Medicine, Tohoku University, Sendai, Japan. [3]Department of Emergency and Critical Care Medicine, Wakayama Medical University, Wakayama, Japan. [4]Department of Trauma and Critical Care Medicine, Osaka City University, Osaka, Japan. [5]Division of General Medicine, Hyogo College of Medicine, Nishinomiya, Japan. [6]Department of Clinical Epidemiology, Hyogo College of Medicine, Nishinomiya, Japan.

### References

1. Rhodes A, Evans LE, Alhazzani W, Levy MM, Antonelli M, Ferrer R, et al. Surviving sepsis campaign: international guidelines for management of sepsis and septic shock: 2016. Intensive Care Med. 2017;43:304–77.
2. Martin C, Medam S, Antonini F, Alingrin J, Haddam M, Hammad E, et al. Norepinephrine: not too much, too long. Shock. 2015;44:305–9.
3. Stolk RF, van der Poll T, Angus DC, van der Hoeven JG, Pickkers P, Kox M. Potentially inadvertent immunomodulation: norepinephrine use in sepsis. Am J Respir Crit Care Med. 2016;194:550–8.
4. Kawazoe Y, Miyamoto K, Morimoto T, Yamamoto T, Fuke A, Hashimoto A, et al. Effect of dexmedetomidine on mortality and ventilator-free days in patients requiring mechanical ventilation with sepsis: a randomized clinical trial. JAMA. 2017;317:1321–8.
5. Singer M, Deutschman CS, Seymour CW, Shankar-Hari M, Annane D, Bauer M, et al. The third international consensus definitions for sepsis and septic shock (sepsis-3). JAMA. 2016;315:801–10.
6. Lyte M, Freestone PP, Neal CP, Olson BA, Haigh RD, Bayston R, et al. Stimulation of Staphylococcus epidermidis growth and biofilm formation by catecholamine inotropes. Lancet. 2003;361:130–5.
7. Lyte M, Bailey MT. Neuroendocrine-bacterial interactions in a neurotoxin-induced model of trauma. J Surg Res. 1997;70:195–201.
8. Zhou M, Das P, Simms HH, Wang P. Gut-derived norepinephrine plays an important role in up-regulating IL-1beta and IL-10. Biochim Biophys Acta. 2005;1740:446–52.
9. Woiciechowsky C, Asadullah K, Nestler D, Eberhardt B, Platzer C, Schoning B, et al. Sympathetic activation triggers systemic interleukin-10 release in immunodepression induced by brain injury. Nat Med. 1998;4:808–13.
10. Tsuda Y, Kobayashi M, Herndon DN, Suzuki F. Impairment of the host's antibacterial resistance by norepinephrine activated neutrophils. Burns. 2008;34:460–6.
11. Dunser MW, Ruokonen E, Pettila V, Ulmer H, Torgersen C, Schmittinger CA, et al. Association of arterial blood pressure and vasopressor load with septic shock mortality: a post hoc analysis of a multicenter trial. Crit Care. 2009;13:R181.
12. Povoa PR, Carneiro AH, Ribeiro OS, Pereira AC. Influence of vasopressor agent in septic shock mortality. Results from the Portuguese Community-Acquired Sepsis Study (SACiUCI study). Crit Care Med. 2009;37:410–6.
13. Yoshigi M, Hu N, Keller BB. Dorsal aortic impedance in stage 24 chick embryo following acute changes in circulating blood volume. Am J Phys. 1996;270(5 Pt 2):H1597–606.
14. Morelli A, Ertmer C, Westphal M, Rehberg S, Kampmeier T, Ligges S, et al. Effect of heart rate control with esmolol on hemodynamic and clinical outcomes in patients with septic shock: a randomized clinical trial. JAMA. 2013;310:1683–91.
15. Macchia A, Romero M, Comignani PD, Mariani J, D'Ettorre A, Prini N, et al. Previous prescription of beta-blockers is associated with reduced mortality among patients hospitalized in intensive care units for sepsis. Crit Care Med. 2012;40:2768–72.

16. Jeschke MG, Norbury WB, Finnerty CC, Branski LK, Herndon DN. Propranolol does not increase inflammation, sepsis, or infectious episodes in severely burned children. J Trauma. 2007;62:676–81.

17. Boomer JS, To K, Chang KC, Takasu O, Osborne DF, Walton AH, Bricker TL, et al. Immunosuppression in patients who die of sepsis and multiple organ failure. JAMA. 2011;306:2594–605.

18. Leentjens J, Kox M, van der Hoeven JG, Netea MG, Pickkers P. Immunotherapy for the adjunctive treatment of sepsis: from immunosuppression to immunostimulation. Time for a paradigm change? Am J Respir Crit Care Med. 2013;187:1287–93.

19. Dunser MW, Hasibeder WR. Sympathetic overstimulation during critical illness: adverse effects of adrenergic stress. J Intensive Care Med. 2009;24: 293–316.

20. Schmittinger CA, Torgersen C, Luckner G, Schroder DC, Lorenz I, Dunser MW. Adverse cardiac events during catecholamine vasopressor therapy: a prospective observational study. Intensive Care Med. 2012;38:950–8.

21. de Montmollin E, Aboab J, Mansart A, Annane D. Bench-to-bedside review: beta-adrenergic modulation in sepsis. Crit Care. 2009;13:230.

# Permissions

All chapters in this book were first published in JIC, by BioMed Central; hereby published with permission under the Creative Commons Attribution License or equivalent. Every chapter published in this book has been scrutinized by our experts. Their significance has been extensively debated. The topics covered herein carry significant findings which will fuel the growth of the discipline. They may even be implemented as practical applications or may be referred to as a beginning point for another development.

The contributors of this book come from diverse backgrounds, making this book a truly international effort. This book will bring forth new frontiers with its revolutionizing research information and detailed analysis of the nascent developments around the world.

We would like to thank all the contributing authors for lending their expertise to make the book truly unique. They have played a crucial role in the development of this book. Without their invaluable contributions this book wouldn't have been possible. They have made vital efforts to compile up to date information on the varied aspects of this subject to make this book a valuable addition to the collection of many professionals and students.

This book was conceptualized with the vision of imparting up-to-date information and advanced data in this field. To ensure the same, a matchless editorial board was set up. Every individual on the board went through rigorous rounds of assessment to prove their worth. After which they invested a large part of their time researching and compiling the most relevant data for our readers.

The editorial board has been involved in producing this book since its inception. They have spent rigorous hours researching and exploring the diverse topics which have resulted in the successful publishing of this book. They have passed on their knowledge of decades through this book. To expedite this challenging task, the publisher supported the team at every step. A small team of assistant editors was also appointed to further simplify the editing procedure and attain best results for the readers.

Apart from the editorial board, the designing team has also invested a significant amount of their time in understanding the subject and creating the most relevant covers. They scrutinized every image to scout for the most suitable representation of the subject and create an appropriate cover for the book.

The publishing team has been an ardent support to the editorial, designing and production team. Their endless efforts to recruit the best for this project, has resulted in the accomplishment of this book. They are a veteran in the field of academics and their pool of knowledge is as vast as their experience in printing. Their expertise and guidance has proved useful at every step. Their uncompromising quality standards have made this book an exceptional effort. Their encouragement from time to time has been an inspiration for everyone.

The publisher and the editorial board hope that this book will prove to be a valuable piece of knowledge for researchers, students, practitioners and scholars across the globe.

# List of Contributors

**Akira Ushiyama**
Department of Environmental Health, National Institute of Public Health, Saitama, Japans

**Hanae Kataoka and Takehiko Iijima**
Department of Perioperative Medicine, Division of Anesthesiology, Showa University, School of Dentistry, Tokyo, Japan

**Takahiro Hirayama**
Department of Clinical Engineering, Okayama University Hospital, 2-5-1 Shikata-cho, Kita-ku, Okayama city 700-8558, Japan

**Takahiro Hirayama, Toyomu Ugawa and Atsunori Nakao**
Department of Emergency and Critical Care Medicine, Okayama University Graduate School
of Medicine, Dentistry and Pharmaceutical Sciences, Okayama University Hospital, 2-5-1 Shikata-cho, Kita-ku, Okayama city 700-8558, Japan

**Nobuyuki Nosaka**
Department of Pediatrics, Okayama University Hospital, 2-5-1 Shikata-cho, Kita-ku, Okayama city 700-8558, Japan

**Yasumasa Okawa, Soichiro Ushio, Yoshihisa Kitamura and Toshiaki Sendo**
Department of Pharmacy, Okayama University Hospital, 2-5-1 Shikata-cho, Kita-ku, Okayama city 700-8558, Japan

**Nobuyuki Nosaka**
Department of Pediatrics, Division of Infectious Diseases and Immunology, Cedars-Sinai Medical Center, 8700 Beverly Blvd., Los Angeles, CA 90048, USA

**Tushna Vandevala, Louisa Pavey and Nai-Feng Chang**
1School of Social and Behavioural Sciences, Criminology and Sociology, Faculty of Arts and Social Sciences, Kingston University, Penrhyn Road, Kingston, Surrey KT1 2EE, UK

**Olga Chelidoni and Anna Cox**
School of Health Sciences, Faculty of Health and Medical Sciences, University of Surrey, Guildford, Surrey GU2 7XH, UK

**Ben Creagh-Brown**
Intensive Care Unit, Royal Surrey County Hospital, Egerton Road, Guildford, Surrey GU2 7XX, UK

Surrey Perioperative Anaesthesia Critical Care Collaborative Research Group (SPACeR), Department of Clinical and Experimental Medicine, Faculty of Health and Medical Sciences, University of Surrey, Guildford GU2 7XH, UK

**Naoki Ehara, Akinori Wakai, Tetsuro Nishimura and Daikai Sadamitsu**
Traumatology and Critical Care Medical Center, National Hospital Organization Osaka National Hospital, 2-1-14 Hoenzaka Chuo-ku, Osaka, Osaka 540-0006, Japan

**Tomoya Hirose, Tadahiko Shiozaki, Nobuto Mori, Mitsuo Ohnishi and and Takeshi Shimazu**
Department of Traumatology and Acute Critical Medicine, Osaka University Graduate School of Medicine, 2-15 Yamadaoka, Suita, Osaka 565-0871, Japan

**Mira John, Dorothee Halfkann, Julika Schoen, Beate Sedemund-Adib, Sebastian Stehr and Michael Hueppe**
Clinic for Anaesthesiology and Intensive-Care Medicine, UKSH Campus Luebeck, Ratzeburger Allee 160, 23538 Luebeck, Germany

**E. Wesley Ely**
Pulmonary and Critical Care Medicine, Vanderbilt University, Nashville, Tennessee, USA
Geriatric Research Education Clinical Center (GRECC) of the Tennessee Valley Veterans Administration, Nashville, Tennessee, USA

**Stefan Klotz**
Department of Cardiac and Thoracic Vascular Surgery, UKSH Campus Luebeck, Luebeck, Germany

**Finn Radtke**
Clinic for Anaesthesiology and Operative Intensive-Care Medicine, Charité University Hospital Berlin, Berlin, Germany

**Hiroyuki Yamada, Tatsuo Tsukamoto and Motoko Yanagita**
Department of Nephrology, Graduate School of Medicine, Kyoto University, 54 Shogoin-Kawahara-cho, Sakyo-ku, Kyoto 606-8507, Japan

**Hiroyuki Yamada, Hiromichi Narumiya and Masako Deguchi**
Department of Metabolism, Nephrology and Rheumatology, Japanese Red Cross Kyoto Daini

Hospital, 355-5 Haruobi, Kamigyo-ku, Kyoto 602-8026, Japan

**Hiromichi Narumiya, Kazumasa Oda, Satoshi Higaki and Ryoji Iizuka**
Department of Emergency, Japanese Red Cross Kyoto Daini Hospital, 355-5 Haruobi,
Kamigyo-ku, Kyoto 602-8026, Japan

**Midori Uozumi and Kazuyuki Ono**
Emergency and Critical Care Medicine, Dokkyo Medical University, Mibumachi, Shimotsuga-gun, Tochigi, Japan

**Masamitsu Sanui, Tetsuya Komuro, Yusuke Iizuka, Tadashi Kamio, Hiroshi Koyama, Hideyuki Mouri and Tomoyuki Masuyama**
Department of Anesthesiology and Critical Care Medicine, Division of Critical Care Medicine, Jichi Medical University Saitama Medical Center, 1-847 Amanumacho, Omiya-ku, Saitama-shi, Saitama 330-8503, Japan

**Alan Kawarai Lefor**
Department of Surgery, Jichi Medical University, 3311-1 Yakushiji, Shimotsuke-shi, Tochigi 329-0498, Japan

**Alexander Fletcher Sandersjöö, Jiri Bartek Jr., Adrian Elmi-Terander and Bo-Michael Bellander**
Department of Neurosurgery, Karolinska University Hospital, Stockholm, Sweden

**Alexander Fletcher Sandersjöö, Jiri Bartek Jr., Eric Peter Thelin and Bo-Michael Bellander**
Department of Clinical Neuroscience, Karolinska Institutet, Stockholm, Sweden

**Jiri Bartek Jr**
Department of Neurosurgery, Copenhagen University Hospital Rigshospitalet, Copenhagen, Denmark

**Eric Peter Thelin**
Division of Neurosurgery, Department of Clinical Neurosciences, Cambridge Biomedical Campus, University of Cambridge, Cambridge, UK

**Anders Eriksson and, Mikael Broman**
ECMO Center Karolinska, Department of Pediatric Perioperative Medicine and Intensive Care, Karolinska University Hospital, Stockholm, Sweden

**Mikael Broman**
Department of Physiology and Pharmacology, Karolinska Institutet, Stockholm, Sweden

**Laure Calvet, Alexandre Lautrette and Bertrand Souweine**
Service de Réanimation Médicale, Hôpital Gabriel Montpied, CHU de Clermont-Ferrand, BP 69, 63003 Clermont-Ferrand, Cedex 1, France

**Bruno Pereira**
Département de biostatistique, CHU de Clermont-Ferrand, Clermont-Ferrand, France

**Anne-Françoise Sapin and Gabrielle Mareynat**
Laboratoire d'hématologie, CHU de Clermont-Ferrand, Clermont-Ferrand, France

**Alexandre Lautrette and Bertrand Souweine**
Université Clermont Auvergne, CNRS, LMGE, F-63000 Clermont-Ferrand, France

**Zhongheng Zhang**
Department of Emergency Medicine, Sir Run-Run Shaw Hospital, Zhejiang University School of Medicine, No 3, East Qingchun Road, Hangzhou 310016, Zhejiang Province, China

**Melanie Kowalsk and Michael J. Dooley**
Pharmacy Department, Alfred Health, 55 Commercial Road, Melbourne, VIC 3004, Australia

**Melanie Kowalski**
Intensive Care Unit, Alfred Health, Melbourne, Australia

**Hayden J. McRobbie**
Wolfson Institute of Preventive Medicine, London, UK
Queen Mary University of London, London, UK

**Melanie Kowalski, Andrew A. Udy and Michael J. Dooley**
Monash University, Melbourne, Australia

**Vu Dinh Phu, Dao Tuyet Trinh, Dong Phu Khiem, Tran Ngoc Quang, Nguyen Hong Ha and Nguyen Van Kinh,**
National Hospital for Tropical Diseases, Hanoi, Vietnam

**Vu Dinh Phu, Behzad Nadjm, Nguyen Thi Hoang Mai, James Campbell, Quynh-Dao Dinh, Duong Bich Thuy, Huong Nguyen Phu Lan, Quynh-Dao Dinh, Duong Bich Thuy, Huong Nguyen Phu Lan, Lam Minh Yen, Guy E. Thwaites, H. Rogier van Doorn and C. Louise Thwaites**
Oxford University Clinical Research Unit, Hanoi, Vietnam

Behzad Nadjm, James Campbell, Hoang Nguyen Van Minh, Guy E. Thwaites, H. Rogier van Doorn and C. Louise Thwaites
Centre for Tropical Medicine and Global Health, University of Oxford, Oxford, UK

Nguyen Hoang Anh Duy, Huynh Thi Loan, Huong Nguyen Phu Lan, Nguyen Van Hao and Nguyen Van Vinh Chau
Hospital for Tropical Diseases, Ho Chi Minh City, Vietnam

Dao Xuan Co, Ha Son Binh, Hoang Minh Hoan, Đang Quoc Tuan and Nguyen Gia Binh
Bach Mai Hospital, Hanoi, Vietnam

Mattias Larsson
Karolinska Institutet, Stockholm, Sweden

Hakan Hanberger
Linköping University, Linköping, Sweden

Nguyen Van Hao
University of Medicine and Pharmacy, Ho Chi Minh City, Vietnam

Heiman F. Wertheim
Department of Medical Microbiology and Radboud Center for Infectious Diseases, Radboudumc, Nijmegen, Netherlands

Nguyen Thi Hoang Mai, James Campbell, Duong Bich Thuy, Huong Nguyen Phu Lan, Lam Minh Yen, Guy E. Thwaites and C. Louise Thwaites
Oxford University Clinical Research Unit, Ho Chi Minh City, Vietnam

Ayahiro Yamashita, Masaki Yamasaki, Hiroki Matsuyama and Fumimasa Amaya
Department of Anesthesiology, Kyoto Prefectural University of Medicine, Kajiicho 465, Kamigyo-Ku, Kyoto 602-8566, Japan

Hiroki Matsuyama
Department of Anesthesia, Japanese Red Cross Kyoto Daiichi Hospital, Kyoto, Japan

Yasumasa Kawano, Shinichi Morimoto, Yoshito Izutani, Kentaro Muranishi, Hironari Kaneyama, Kota Hoshino, Takeshi Nishida and Hiroyasu Ishikura
Department of Emergency and Critical Care Medicine, Fukuoka University Hospital, Faculty of Medicine, 7-45-1 Nanakuma, Jonan-ku, Fukuoka 8140180, Japan

Emilio Rodrigo, Lara Belmar and Angel Luis Martín de Francisco
Nephrology Service, IDIVAL-Hospital Marqués de Valdecilla, University of Cantabria, Santander, Spain

Borja Suberviola, Álvaro Castellanos and Juan Carlos Rodríguez-Borregán
Intensive Care Unit, IDIVAL-Hospital Marqués de Valdecilla, University of Cantabria, Santander, Spain

Miguel Santibáñez
School of Nursing, IDIVAL-Hospital Marqués de Valdecilla, University of Cantabria, Santander, Spain

Claudio Ronco
Department of Nephrology Dialysis and Transplantation, International Renal Research Institute of Vicenza (IRRIV), San Bortolo Hospital, Vicenza, Italy

Masahiro Ojima, Ryosuke Takegawa, Tomoya Hirose, Mitsuo Ohnishi, Tadahiko Shiozaki and Takeshi Shimazu
Department of Traumatology and Acute Critical Medicine, Osaka University Graduate School of Medicine, Suita, Osaka, Japan

Khie Chen Lie
Department of Internal Medicine, Cipto Mangunkusumo Hospital, Jakarta, Indonesia

Chuen-Yen Lau
Collaborative Clinical Research Branch, Division of Clinical Research, National Institute of Allergy and Infectious Diseases, National Institutes of Health, Bethesda, USA

Nguyen Van Vinh Chau
Department of Internal Medicine, Hospital for Tropical Diseases, Ho Chi Minh City, Vietnam Department of Internal Medicine, Oxford University Clinical Research Unit, Ho Chi Minh City, Vietnam

T. Eoin West
Division of Pulmonary and Critical Care Medicine, Department of Medicine, University of Washington, Seattle, WA, USA
Department of Global Health, University of Washington, Seattle, WA, USA

Direk Limmathurotsakul
Centre for Tropical Medicine and Global Health, Nuffield Department of Medicine, University of Oxford, Oxford, UK

Mahidol-Oxford Tropical Medicine Research Unit, Faculty of Tropical Medicine, Mahidol University, Bangkok, Thailand
Department of Tropical Hygiene, Faculty of Tropical Medicine, Mahidol University, 420/6 Rajvithi Road, Bangkok 10400, Thailand

**Richard J. Nies, Roman Pfister, Felix S. Nettersheim and and Guido Michels**
Department III of Internal Medicine, Heart Center, University Hospital of Cologne, Kerpener Str. 62, 50937 Cologne, Germany

**Carsten Müller and Nicole Nosseir**
Center of Pharmacology, Department of Therapeutic Drug Monitoring, University Hospital of Cologne, Gleueler Str. 24, 50931 Cologne, Germany

**Philipp S. Binder**
St. Katharinen-Hospital GmbH, Kapellenstrasse 1-5, 50226 Frechen, Germany

**Kathrin Kuhr**
Institute of Medical Statistics and Computational Biology, University of Cologne, Kerpener Str. 62, 50937 Cologne, Germany

**Matthias Kochanek**
Department I of Internal Medicine, University Hospital of Cologne, Kerpener Str. 62, 50937 Cologne, Germany

**Richard J. Nies**
Department of Cardiology, University Hospital of Cologne, Kerpener Str. 62, 50937 Cologne, Germany

**Olga Rubio, Anna Arnau and Sílvia Cano**
Hospital Sant Joan De Déu, Fundació Althaia Xarxa Universitaria de Manresa, C/ Dr. Joan Soler s. n., 08243 Manresa, Spain

**Pablo Monedero**
Clínica Universitaria de Navarra, Pamplona, Spain

**Elisabeth Zabala**
Hospital Clínico Universitario de Barcelona, Barcelona, Spain

**Cristina Murcia**
Hospital Josep Trueta, Girona, Spain

**Jordi Mancebo**
Hospital de la Santa Creu I Sant Pau, Barcelona, Spain

**Charles Sprung**
Hadassh Hebrew University Medical Center, Jerusalem, Israel

**Rafael Fernández**
Hospital Sant Joan de Deu, Fundació Althaia Xarxa Universitaria de Manresa, Manresa, Spain

**Sulagna Bhattacharjee and Souvik Maitra**
Department of Anaesthesiology, Pain Medicine and Critical Care, All India Institute of Medical Sciences, Room No. 5011, 5th Floor Teaching block, Ansari Nagar New Delhi 110029, India

**Kapil D. Soni**
Department of Trauma Critical Care, Jai Prakash Narayan Apex Trauma Centre, All India Institute Medical Sciences, New Delhi, India

**Tomoya Hirose, Hiroshi Ogura, Hiroki Takahashi, Masahiro Ojima, Kang Jinkoo, Youhei Nakamura, Takashi Kojima and Takeshi Shimazu**
Department of Traumatology and Acute Critical Medicine, Osaka University Graduate School of Medicine, 2-15 Yamadaoka, Suita, Osaka 565-0871, Japan

**Keibun Liu, Takayuki Ogura, Kenji Fujiduka, Dai Miyazaki, Hiroyuki Suzuki and Mitsuaki Nishikimi**
Advanced Medical Emergency Department and Critical Care Center, Japan Red Cross Maebashi Hospital, 3-21-36 Asahi-cho, Maebashi, Gunma 371-0014, Japan

**Kunihiko Takahashi and Mitsunobu Nakamura**
Department of Biostatistics, Nagoya University Graduate School of Medicine, Tsurumai-cho 64, Syowa-ku, Nagoya, Aichi 466-8560, Japan

**Hiroaki Ohtake and Hitoshi Oosaki**
Department of Rehabilitation Medicine, Japan Red Cross Maebashi Hospital, 3-21-36 Asahi-cho, Maebashi, Gunma 371-0014, Japan

**Emi Abe**
Department of Nursing, Intensive Care Unit, Japan Red Cross Maebashi Hospital, 3-21-36 Asahi-cho, Maebashi, Gunma 371-0014, Japan

**Alan Kawarai Lefor**
Department of Surgery, Jichi Medical University, 3311-1 Yakushiji, Shimotsukeshi, Tochigi 329-0498, Japan

**Takashi Mato**
Department of Emergency Medicine, Jichi Medical University, 3311-1 Yakushiji, Shimotsukeshi, Tochigi 329-0498, Japan

**Jaime L Speiser**
Department of Biostatistical Sciences, Division of Public Health Sciences, Wake Forest School of Medicine, Winston-Salem, NC, USA

**Constantine J Karvellas**
Department of Critical Care Medicine, University of Alberta, 1-40 Zeidler-Ledcor Building, Edmonton, Alberta T6G-2X8, Canada

Division of Gastroenterology and Hepatology, University of Alberta, Edmonton, Canada

**Geoffery Shumilak and Wendy I Sligl**
Division of Critical Care Medicine and Infectious Diseases, University of Alberta, Edmonton, Canada

**Anand Kumar**
Section of Critical Care Medicine, University of Manitoba, Winnipeg, Canada
Section of Infectious Diseases, University of Manitoba, Winnipeg, Canada

**Yazdan Mirzanejad**
Surrey Hospital, Surrey, BC, Canada

**Dave Gurka**
Rush Medical College, Chicago, IL, USA

**Aseem Kumar**
Laurentian University, Sudbury, ON, Canada

**Shinichiro Ohshimo and Nobuaki Shime**
Department of Emergency and Critical Care Medicine, Graduate School of Biomedical and Health Sciences, Hiroshima University, 1-2-3 Kasumi, Minami-ku, Hiroshima 734-8551, Japan

**Satoshi Nakagawa**
Department of Critical Care and Anesthesia, National Center for Child Health and Development, Tokyo, Japan

**Osamu Nishida**
Department of Anaesthesiology and Critical Care Medicine, Fujita Health University School of Medicine, Aichi, Japan

**Shinhiro Takeda**
Kawaguchi Cardiovascular and Respiratory Hospital, Saitama, Japan

**James A. Russell, and Keith R. Walley James A. Russell and Keith R. Walley**
Centre for Heart Lung Innovation, St. Paul's Hospital, University of British Columbia, 1081 Burrard Street, Vancouver, BC V6Z 1Y6, Canada

Division of Critical Care Medicine, St. Paul's Hospital, University of British Columbia, 1081 Burrard Street, Vancouver, BC V6Z 1Y6, Canada

**Hugh Wellman**
GenomeDx Biosciences Inc., 1038 Homer Street, Vancouver, BC V6B 2W9, Canada

**Tetsu Ohnuma, Daisuke Shinjo and Kiyohide Fushimi**
Department of Health Policy and Informatics, Tokyo Medical and Dental University Graduate School, 1-5-45 Yushima, Bunkyo-ku, Tokyo 1138519, Japan

**Tetsu Ohnuma and Alan M. Brookhart**
Department of Epidemiology, Gillings School of Global Public Health, University of North Carolina, Chapel Hill, USA

**Daisuke Shinjo**
The Database Center of the National University Hospital, The University of Tokyo Hospital, Tokyo, Japan

**Hitoshi Yamamura**
Department of Disaster and Critical Care Medicine, Hirosaki University School of Medicine, 5 Zaifuchou, Hirosaki, Aomori 036-8562, Japan

**Yu Kawazoe**
Division of Emergency and Critical Care Medicine, Tohoku University, Sendai, Japan

**Kyohei Miyamoto**
Department of Emergency and Critical Care Medicine, Wakayama Medical University, Wakayama, Japan

**Tomonori Yamamoto**
Department of Trauma and Critical Care Medicine, Osaka City University, Osaka, Japan.

**Yoshinori Ohta**
Division of General Medicine, Hyogo College of Medicine, Nishinomiya, Japan

**Takeshi Morimoto**
Department of Clinical Epidemiology, Hyogo College of Medicine, Nishinomiya, Japan

# Index